GENERAL
MEDICAL
CONDITIONS
in the Athlete

The Latest *Evolution* in Learning.

Evolve provides online access to free learning resources and activities designed specifically for the textbook you are using in your class. The resources will provide you with information that enhances the material covered in the book and much more.

Visit the Web address listed below to start your learning evolution today!

Think outside the book...*evolve.*

GENERAL

MEDICAL CONDITIONS
in the Athlete

Micki Cuppett, EdD, ATC
Coordinator, Athletic Training
University of South Florida
Tampa, Florida

Katie M. Walsh, EdD, ATC
Director of Sports Medicine and Athletic Training
East Carolina University
Greenville, North Carolina

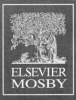

ELSEVIER
MOSBY

ELSEVIER
MOSBY

11830 Westline Industrial Drive
St. Louis, Missouri 63146

GENERAL MEDICAL CONDITIONS IN THE ATHLETE
Copyright © 2005, Mosby Inc.

NOTICE

Knowledge and best practice in this field are constantly changing. As new research and experience broaden our knowledge, changes in practice, treatment and drug therapy may become necessary or appropriate. Readers are advised to check the most current information provided (i) on procedures featured or (ii) by the manufacturer of each product to be administered, to verify the recommended dose or formula, the method and duration of administration, and contraindications. It is the responsibility of the practitioner, relying on their own experience and knowledge of the patient, to make diagnoses, to determine dosages and the best treatment for each individual patient, and to take all appropriate safety precautions. To the fullest extent of the law, neither the Publisher nor the Authors assume, any liability for any injury and/or damage to persons or property arising out or related to any use of the material contained in this book.

ISBN-13: 978-0-323-02623-9
ISBN-10: 0-323-02623-0

Printed in the United States of America

Last digit is the print number: 9 8 7 6 5 4

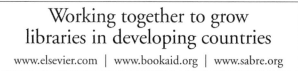

Working together to grow
libraries in developing countries

www.elsevier.com | www.bookaid.org | www.sabre.org

ELSEVIER   BOOK AID International   Sabre Foundation

To my sons, Derek and Kyle, who literally grew up in the athletic training room and have been an inspiration for me to contribute to the growth of the athletic training profession, if only in this small way. And to Rick, whose never-ending encouragement and belief in me has inspired me to pursue things I never thought possible. I look forward to finally being together.

Micki Cuppett

This book is dedicated to the memory of my father, Kevin Brendan Walsh, who instilled in his eight children a lifelong love of learning; to my mother, Phyllis Fletcher Walsh Kelly, who is a timeless tribute to beauty, grace, and determination; and to my wonderful bonus dad, Gerald Kelly, who has allowed me the great fortune of having three terrific parents in one lifetime!

Katie M. Walsh

CONTRIBUTORS

Dorraine Reynolds, PharmD
Assistant Professor and Director of the Outpatient
  Pharmacy
Creighton University Medical Center
Omaha, Nebraska
  Chapter 3: Basic Principles of Pharmacology

Arnold Ramirez, MD
Director of Sports Medicine Fellowship Program
Bayfront Medical Center
St. Petersburg, Florida
Assistant Professor
University of South Florida College of Medicine
Tampa, Florida
  Chapter 4: Respiratory Disorders

Bryan W. Smith, MD, PhD
Medical Consultant
Atlantic Coast Conference
Greensboro, North Carolina
  Chapter 5: Cardiovascular Disorders

Daniel J. Van Durme, MD
Professor and Chair
Department of Family Medicine and Rural Health
Florida State University College of Medicine
Tallahassee, Florida
  Chapter 6: Gastrointestinal Disorders

Joseph M. Garry, MD
Associate Professor of Family Medicine and
  Exercise and Sport Science
Brody School of Medicine
East Carolina University
Greenville, North Carolina
  Chapter 7: Genitourinary and Gynecological Disorders

M. Craig Whaley, MD
Eastern Carolina Internal Medicine Group
New Bern, North Carolina
  Chapter 7: Genitourinary and Gynecological Disorders

Rose Snyder, MS, ATC, CSCS, OPA-C
William Clay Ford Center for Athletic
  Medicine
Detroit, Michigan
  Chapter 8: Neurological Disorders

Sara McDade, MD
William Clay Ford Center for Athletic Medicine
Detroit, Michigan
  Chapter 8: Neurological Disorders

David Eichenbaum, MD
Chief Resident
Department of Ophthalmology
University of South Florida College of Medicine
Tampa, Florida
  Chapter 9: Disorders of the Eye

Charles B. Slonim, MD, FACS
Affiliate Professor of Ophthalmology
University of South Florida College of Medicine
Tampa, Florida
  Chapter 9: Disorders of the Eye

Richard Figler, MD
Family Practice Center
East Carolina University
Greenville, North Carolina
  Chapter 11: Systemic Disorders

Patrick Sexton, EdD, ATC, CSCS
Director of Athletic Training Education
Minnesota State University, Mankato
Mankato, Minnesota
Chapter 13: Dermatological Conditions

Todd Kanzenbach, MD
University Health Services
Minnesota State University, Mankato
Mankato, Minnesota
Chapter 13: Dermatological Conditions

Larry Collins, PA, ATC
Florida Orthopedic Institute
Temple Terrace, Florida
Chapter 14: Musculoskeletal Disorders

Layne Prest, PhD, LMFT
Associate Professor and Director of Behavior
Medicine
Department of Family Medicine
University of Nebraska Medical Center
Omaha, Nebraska
Chapter 15: Mental Health Issues in Athletes

Monique Butcher-Mokha, PhD, ATC
Associate Professor of Athletic Training
Department of Sport and Exercise Sciences
Barry University
Miami Shores, Florida
Chapter 16: Special Populations

REVIEWERS

Linda Gazzillo Diaz, EdD, ATC
William Paterson University
Wayne, New Jersey

Nicole Dinn, MSc(c), B Kin, PFLC, CSCS, NLKA, CFC
Memorial University of Newfoundland
St. John's, Newfoundland, Canada

James M. Lynch, MD
Florida Southern College
Lakeland, Florida

Stacey L. Ocander, EdD, ATC
Associate Dean
Nebraska Wesleyan University
Lincoln, Nebraska

PREFACE

The role of the athletic trainer (AT) in caring for physically active individuals continues to expand to more diverse populations. Today, ATs provide medical coverage to youngsters, teens, young and mature adults, and special needs athletes. In all of these groups, underlying or preexisting medical conditions may be a concern. The AT is often the first person to learn about a medical problem and, therefore, the one in a position to determine if the athlete has a minor illness or a potentially serious condition. Therefore it is imperative that the AT be able to recognize and appreciate potentially serious medical conditions and understand when to seek additional medical consultation and care.

Although ATs have traditionally received excellent preparation and have therefore become very adept at orthopedic examination, general medical conditions have often been relegated to a few chapters in athletic-training texts. In 1999, however, the National Athletic Trainers' Association adopted educational competencies and proficiencies specific to medical conditions, which challenged ATs to learn and perform general medical skills.

Unfortunately, the resources designed, written, and produced for athletic training programs to cover general medical conditions have been limited. Many practitioners have adapted resources aimed at other professions to teach the concepts of general medical conditions as well as nontraumatic conditions that ATs regularly see. Our goal in writing *General Medical Conditions in the Athlete* is to fill this gap in the athletic training literature and provide a comprehensive text on general medical conditions in the athlete.

The text begins with an overview of the basic information presented in subsequent chapters, including a discussion of the role of the AT as an initial health care provider and physician extender and the importance of the preparticipation examination. This introductory chapter also explains communication tools, policies, rules, legal concerns, and regulations associated with medical care and stresses prevention of disease transmission along with the process of reporting communicable diseases to health networks.

The second chapter, Medical Evaluation Techniques and Equipment, discusses the basic evaluation tools that will assist the reader throughout the remainder of the book. A thorough explanation of health history, observation and inspection, palpation, and pertinent tests used for the diagnosis of medical conditions is presented. Photographs and carefully detailed procedures instruct the reader in the use of special equipment and techniques for the general medical examination.

The remaining text follows a systematic approach to discuss common conditions and diseases by body system. Most chapters follow a similar template, beginning with an overview of the relevant anatomy and physiology as it relates to the body system; then identifying specific conditions; explaining signs and symptoms, referral and diagnostic tests, differential diagnoses, and treatment; and, finally, discussing prognosis and implications for participation. If a specific condition has related age or gender-specific considerations, those issues are also discussed. Implications for the pediatric athlete as well as the mature athlete, if relevant, are also included.

Features

Content is expanded and reinforced by special features that include Key Point and Red Flag boxes and Web Resource listings in each chapter. Over 400 illustrations aid the reader's comprehension of the anatomy, physiology, and pathophysiology. Two inserts in full color repeat photographs essential to accurate assessment of eye, ear, nose, throat and mouth disorders, and dermatological conditions. Pharmacological tables provide easy access to a full range of drug categories that include generic and trade names, therapeutic uses, adult dosage information, and possible adverse effects. Important terminology is highlighted throughout the chapters, and an expanded glossary appears at the end of the text. Appendixes containing pertinent information to health care assessment are located with the glossary.

Supplements

This educational package includes a DVD-ROM, that has been carefully constructed to reinforce health assessment and physical examination techniques. The DVD provides video instruction of many examination techniques, audio and video interactive exercises, memory matches, and study tools. Video demonstrations, as well as the audio and video interactive exercises, are identified and cross-referenced in the text by a DVD icon that appears in the appropriate margin. A fully indexed, interactive directory is also available on the DVD to help the user find specific information, including illustrations, video segments, and animations. In addition, this text is supported by an Elsevier Evolve website, which offers educational adoptees access to similar study and comprehension resources online at *http://evolve.elsevier.com/cuppett/athlete*.

A Textbook and Reference Source

We are athletic training educators and practitioners who have pooled our experience and worked with our colleagues in athletic training and medicine to design this textbook and the DVD interactive resource. We present it to you as an informative and easy to use instructional tool for beginning and advanced students, as well as an indispensable reference guide for practitioners in the field. We look forward to your feedback and suggestions for future editions.

Micki Cuppett and Katie M. Walsh
c/o Health Professions II
Elsevier Inc.
1600 John F. Kennedy Blvd., Suite 1800
Philadelphia, PA 19103-2899

ACKNOWLEDGMENTS

We wish to thank the many people who made this project possible. First of all, we thank the chapter contributors for providing their knowledge of the subject matter and expertise in their fields. They made our job so much easier and ensured a strong and accurate product. We appreciate their spectacular responses to a tight timeline and their ongoing support of the project.

We also thank the Elsevier team, which has made publication of this first edition an enjoyable process. We are fortunate that Executive Editor Marion Waldman convinced us to start this project in the first place. Her vision for a new line of athletic training textbooks and her efforts in bringing resources together for this book provided the backbone for this venture and will not be forgotten. Marion is always the calming force who makes sure projects proceed on schedule.

Our special thanks go to Sue Bredensteiner, our developmental editor, for her organizational and editorial skills. Her continuous communications kept us on task, and her editorial experience provided tremendous guidance. Her ongoing efforts will always be appreciated. We are also thankful to Marjory Fraser, senior development editor in Health Professions II, for her guidance and supervision.

We are grateful to the production team as well: Melissa Lastarria, publishing services manager; Gail Michaels, project manager; and Paula Ruckenbrod, designer, for her outstanding cover and interior book designs.

We also recognize the tremendous marketing efforts of Derril Trakalo, marketing manager, and Allison Wyffels, marketing coordinator, who are aggressively promoting this book to make it a centerpiece in the athletic training field.

The accompanying DVD started off as a small ancillary project but soon grew into a major production, largely fueled by the creative thinking of Rachelle Brunton, project manager of the Media Innovation Team at the University of South Florida, and Paul Coker, executive producer at Elsevier. Christine Brown of the Media Innovation Team put all the pieces together for a dynamic DVD designed to enhance the reader's experience with this multimedia package. The media team's creativity and ability to think "big" is greatly appreciated. Special thanks also go to Claudia Jarimillo, executive producer of the Media Innovation Team, and her production crew for the countless hours of shooting and editing video components produced especially for this DVD.

We also thank the Athletic Training Faculty and Staff at East Carolina University and the University of South Florida for their help, advice, and understanding while we were working on this project. Many of our colleagues kindly allowed us to use their photographs in the text and the DVD. A particular note of thanks goes to Chuck Baldwin, photographer for the College of Health and Human Performance at East Carolina University, for taking many of the photos in the book, and to Kip Sloan of Performance Computer and Photo Services for contributing a number of action shots, including the photo of the basketball player and athletic trainer on the cover. And special thanks go to Chuck Slonim, MD, for providing most of the photos of eye disorders and trauma.

We also want to recognize the efforts of the undergraduate and graduate athletic training students at East Carolina University and the University of South Florida for their input and assistance. Thanks to our students who volunteered to be in the photographs and DVD filming. Special thanks also to Valerie Rich, Marci Wulf, and Travis Irwin for help with the acquisition of illustrations and development of the glossary.

Additional thanks go to Ann Marie Santos and her colleagues at Sports 'n Spokes magazine, published by the Paralyzed Veterans of America, for sharing photographs of wheelchair athletes.

Finally, we recognize and appreciate the tenacity of our friendship, which began at a professional meeting and evolved into "Hey, we can do this project!" It has stood strong throughout our vision of improving the educational experience in the field of medicine for the athletic trainer. We have learned that with vision, drive, and determination, anything is possible if good friends keep pulling and pushing each other in the same direction with a common goal.

ABOUT THE AUTHORS

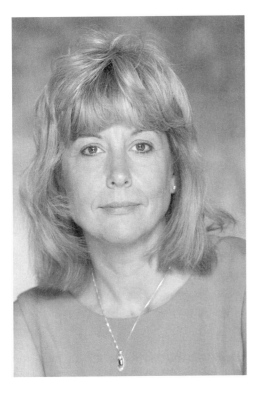

Marchell (Micki) Cuppett is the athletic training program coordinator and an assistant professor at the University of South Florida. A graduate of the University of North Dakota and the University of Northern Iowa, Dr. Cuppett has twenty years of experience as an educator. She has taught and developed curriculum in physical assessment, prevention of physical injuries, therapeutic modalities, clinical instruction in athletic training, general medical conditions in the athlete, and

topics in sports medicine at the University of Northern Iowa, the United States Military Academy, and the University of Nebraska at Omaha. In her current role she is responsible for all aspects of the athletic training education program and program accreditation.

Her published research includes physical fitness and performance variables, documentation of clinical skills using personal digital assistants, prevalence of migraines in basketball players, exertional compartment syndrome related to runners with type I diabetes, anatomy and pathology of the sacroiliac joint, and standardized protocol for the initial evaluation and documentation of mild brain injury. She has conducted regional and national presentations on athletic training education and digital equipment. She is a reviewer for academic publications and a national consultant for athletic training education programs.

Dr. Cuppett serves the University of South Florida as chair of the Committee on Athletic Fees, she is chair-elect of the College of Education Technology Committee, and she serves on numerous other committees in the School of Physical Education, Wellness, and Sport Studies.

Dr. Cuppettt works with the National Athletic Trainers' Association Board of Certification on the Role Delineation Committee, Continuing Education Committee, and as an examiner training facilitator and test site administrator. In addition, she is the District 9 representative to the NATA Educational Multimedia Committee.

Dr. Cuppett has been an athletic trainer in clinical settings, high schools, colleges, and military settings before becoming an academic program director.

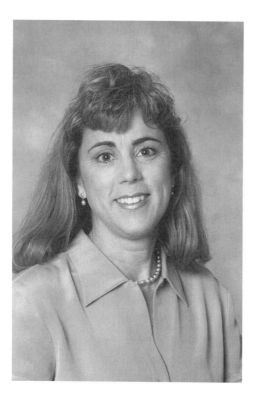

Katie M. Walsh is director of Sports Medicine and Athletic Training at East Carolina University. A graduate of Oregon State University, Illinois State University, and the University of Southern California in Los Angeles, Dr. Walsh has worked as an educator and athletic trainer for over twenty-five years. She has taught and developed curricula in all aspects of athletic training, sports medicine practicum, therapeutic rehabilitation in sports medicine, therapeutic exercise, and advanced care and prevention of athletic injuries. In her current role she is responsible for the undergraduate and graduate athletic training programs in the College of Health and Human Performance.

Her published research includes infection and disease transmission in the athletic training setting, preevaluation exams, proactive emergency action planning, rehabilitation of postsurgical hand and finger injuries in the athlete, the NATA position on lightning safety for athletics, and the efficacy of the rapid-form cervical vacuum immobilizer in cervical spine immobilization of the equipped football player. She has conducted national and international presentations on treatment, athletic trainer education programs, lightning and liability, and the development of emergency action plans. She is associate editor for *Athletic Therapy Today,* a reviewer for the *Journal of Athletic Training* and other academic publications, and a national consultant for athletic training education programs.

Dr. Walsh serves on the East Carolina University Personnel Committee. She works with the National Athletic Trainers' Association Joint Review Committee on Athletic Training and chairs the site review team, is chair of the Mid-Atlantic Athletic Trainers' Association Program Committee, and is vice president for the North Carolina Athletic Trainers' Association. In 2000, she received the North Carolina Athletic Trainers' Association College and University Athletic Trainer of the Year Award.

Dr. Walsh has been the head athletic trainer for the Chicago Power Men's Professional Soccer Team and the Illinois Sportsmedicine and Orthopaedic Centers in Chicago. In addition, she has been the athletic trainer for women and men's teams representing the United States during various international tours and for the U.S. Soccer Federation for national and international tours. She has been a volunteer athletic trainer for the Olympic Training Center in Colorado Springs, Colorado and the Centennial Olympic Games in Atlantic, Georgia.

TABLE OF CONTENTS

Introduction to General Medical Conditions

Katie M. Walsh

OBJECTIVES

At the conclusion of this chapter, the reader should be able to do the following:

1. Discuss the basic differences between orthopedic and general medical assessment.
2. Understand the importance of a preparticipation examination in relation to medical history.
3. Appreciate proper communication as a valuable tool in the general medical assessment of the physically active person.
4. Apply principles of disease transmission prevention.
5. Implement and use the regulations and laws that govern care and privacy of patients.
6. Understand the levels of and need for the reporting system of infectious diseases.

INTRODUCTION

Most textbooks used in athletic training programs concentrate on the knowledge and skills used for orthopedic assessment and provide a systematic overview of athletic injuries. Emphasis is on the student's learning how to follow the history, inspection/observation, palpation, special tests (HIPS/HOPS) plan in taking a history and determining what decisions to make regarding return to play. In these orthopedic situations, an injury is usually obvious because it has been witnessed by the athletic trainer, and a thorough history may shed light on the type of damage sustained.

Unlike the typical athletic injury, medical conditions are not always immediately apparent in an assessment. This book is a comprehensive resource for health care

students and providers that includes general medical conditions by body system, their mechanism of acquisition, signs, symptoms, referral, treatment, and return-to-participation criteria. Its purpose is not only to provide information but also to help the reader develop a framework for decision making. We assume that the reader is versed in basic human anatomy and physiology and can build on that knowledge. The text also includes associated chapters on pharmacology and special populations.

This chapter provides an overview of the basic information necessary for understanding subsequent chapters. It reviews the preparticipation examination (PPE), communication tools, the prevention of disease transmission, legal concerns, and the importance of reporting communicable infectious diseases to health networks.

THE ROLE OF THE ATHLETIC TRAINER IN GENERAL MEDICAL CONCERNS

The certified athletic trainer is often the person who has the first opportunity to identify a medical issue for an athlete. An athlete who is feeling ill commonly turns to the athletic trainer because the athletic trainer is the most accessible health care provider. The athletic trainer working with a team has established a rapport with athletes and is familiar with their previous medical history and normal performance. This may allow the athletic trainer to detect a condition that otherwise might go unnoticed. The athletic trainer working with college or professional teams is also responsible for the health care of the entire team while on the road. Although many medical problems are orthopedic, the conditions an athletic trainer encounters also can include infections, colds, and other maladies, which need to be identified and properly treated in order for the athlete to continue to participate in sports at optimal levels.

In 1999 the National Athletic Trainers' Association (NATA) published a new series of educational competencies that focused on several areas not previously part of the athletic trainers' educational process[1]: pathology of injury and illness, pharmacology, and general medical conditions and disabilities. These competencies have become part of athletic training educational curricula throughout the country.

Recently, the Board of Certification for Athletic Trainers released a new *Role Delineation Study*[2] that included several major changes in the role of the athletic trainer, particularly the change of Domain II, previously known as Recognition, Evaluation and Assessment. The recent role delineation changed the domain name to Clinical Evaluation and Diagnosis.[2] Previously, certified athletic trainers (ATCs) were limited by the Board of Certification role delineation to having a clinical impression rather than diagnosing a particular medical condition. The new Domain II represents the athletic training profession's

recognition that the athletic trainer does indeed use the diagnostic decision-making process common to physicians and other health practitioners.

The certified athletic trainer has also taken on a greater role in the general health care of the physically active, thereby requiring greater emphasis on the clinical evaluation and diagnosis of general medical problems. This is a result, in part, of advances in medical science that enable athletes with medical conditions who would formerly have been excluded from participation to participate at the highest levels. It also is the result of expanding employment opportunities for athletic trainers. Certified athletic trainers are now employed in industries, inpatient hospitals, outpatient clinics, and other nontraditional workplaces as well as the traditional realms of interscholastic, intercollegiate, and professional sports.[3,4] Athletic trainers also serve as physician extenders in many states and see a more diverse population, including the pediatric athlete (Figure 1-1) and physically active mature and older adults.[5]

Learning more about medical conditions and their assessment is therefore a part of the comprehensive

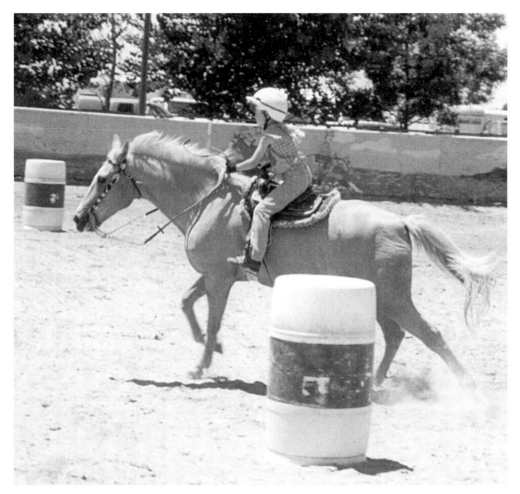

Figure 1-1 Physically active people who are involved in a variety of activities may require the support, knowledge, and skills of a certified athletic trainer. (Courtesy Tam Stainbrook.)

educational process of the athletic trainer. A recent study on the continuing educational needs of athletic trainers revealed that staying abreast of the latest techniques and continuing the learning process throughout their careers were some of the most important reasons cited for completing continuing education.[6] The athletic trainers included in this study expressed a desire to obtain information on general medical conditions more frequently than other orthopedic conditions because those conditions had been well covered previously in the athletic training curricula.[6]

Preparticipation Examination

Generally, the PPE is the first interaction a health care provider has with an athlete. This exam is not a true physical but a screening procedure that sheds light on potential problems associated with activity. The American Academy of Family Physicians (AAFP) recommends that all athletes have a PPE for the primary purpose of identifying any medical problems or conditions that could affect participation in sports.[7] Without these exams, an athlete with systemic illnesses or a family history of cardiovascular disease may not be discovered or treated appropriately. The AAFP along with other medical societies requires the PPE to be signed by either a medical doctor (MD) or doctor of osteopathy (DO). Some states or school districts allow a health care provider other than a DO or MD to administer a PPE, but it is important to be aware of the different education credentials that each provider

has achieved. Table 1-1 lists an overview of various health care providers with their educational backgrounds, including the number of postbaccalaureate years required to obtain the particular degree, and their ability to prescribe medications.

Student athletes are required to have a comprehensive PPE on entry into middle or high school or transfer to a new school. The AAFP recommends these comprehensive evaluations at 2- to 3-year intervals for older students, with annual updates on a comprehensive health history, problem-focused areas, and vital signs.[7] Although some in the medical community still contend that PPEs are not thorough enough, especially in the realm of conditions related to sudden death, these evaluations have come a long way from the mass gymnasium physicals of 20 years ago.[8,9]

According to the National Collegiate Athletics Association (NCAA), PPEs are also required for a student's entrance into the intercollegiate athletics program (Figure 1-2), and an updated annual health history should follow.[10] Although many institutions use this exam largely as a medical history that focuses on orthopedic issues, it is also a venue to address medical problems.[11,12] According to the NCAA, the college athlete's PPE should answer questions relating to current immunizations, allergies, and illnesses, in addition to containing cardiovascular, neurological, and musculoskeletal system assessments.[10] Medical history questions extrapolated from the suggested sports PPE are found in Appendix A. (Note the types of history questions asked in Appendix A, which relate to the different body systems and include mental health.)

Table 1-1	Health Care Providers					
Degree	Title	BS/BA	MS/MA	PhD	Postgraduate education	Prescribing authority
MD	Medical doctor	X			+7 years	X
DO	Doctor of osteopathy	X			+7 years	X
DC	Doctor of chiropractics	X				
ATC	Certified athletic trainer	X	X	X		
DPM	Doctor of podiatry	X			+4 years	X
PT	Physical therapist	X	X	X		
OT	Occupational therapist	X	X	X		
RD	Registered dietitian	X	X			
PTA	Physical therapy assistant (associate's degree)	X				
PA	Physician's assistant (intensive 26-month program)	X	X	X		X
NP	Nurse practitioner	X	X			X
RN	Registered nurse (diploma, associate's or baccalaureate degree)	X	X	X		
LPN PhD	Licensed practical nurse (1-year technical degree) Psychologist	X	X	X		
EMT	Emergency medical technician (initial 6-week course)					
EMT-P	Paramedic (various levels, including CPR, intubation, or IV administration)	X				

CPR, Cardiopulmonary resuscitation; *IV,* intravenous.

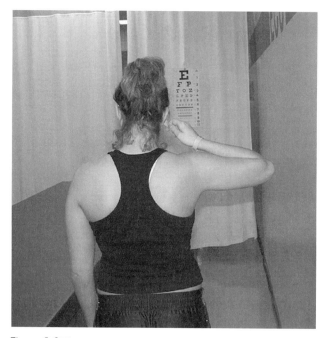

Figure 1-2 The preparticipation exam includes a thorough medical history and physical assessment. The Snellen chart for visual acuity is often used as a part of this exam.

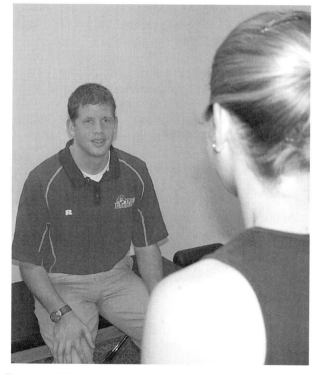

Figure 1-3 Athletic trainers use an open posture to facilitate discussion when talking with athletes. Note that the athletic trainer is sitting down rather than standing above the athlete and is leaning forward in a posture that encourages discussion and questions.

Proper administration of the PPE requires good communication skills, which are also critical to assessment of medical conditions. The health care provider must be aware of tone, body positioning, and language when having dialogue with athletes.

Communication

Because the PPE is largely concerned with symptoms, the nature of questions asked when acquiring a health or illness history from an athlete is just as critical as the information gained from them. One way to improve this dialogue between the practitioner and the athlete is to ask open-ended questions, such as "Why have you come into the athletic training clinic today?"

The athletic trainer can also facilitate and encourage communication by slightly leaning toward the athlete, maintaining eye contact, having an open posture, repeating key words the athlete uses, and using simple phrases for encouragement, such as "go on" or "mm-hmmm."[13] Being empathetic—e.g., "that sounds difficult"—and allowing pauses that give the athlete time to add to comments reassures the athlete that the athletic trainer is listening carefully (Figure 1-3). Asking about the athlete's feelings associated with symptoms is also appropriate in medical assessment. Last, a good practitioner can summarize and interpret the athlete's comments by saying, "I hear you say ..." rather than empathetically injecting words or opinions into the conversation during the subjective review of symptoms.[13]

Along with verbal communication skills, the athletic trainer must be sensitive to cultural, ethnic, and gender issues when working with an athlete. In certain cultures, touching is impermissible because it violates a personal space. Knowing the athletes or asking them if they are comfortable is a good beginning. An athlete will more freely give medical history if the health care provider uses a quiet and private place to communicate.

The athletic trainer must always be aware of the surroundings when communicating with an athlete about a medical issue. When a practitioner assesses an athlete of a different gender, a person of the athlete's gender should be present in the room as well. Using proper draping and maintaining privacy during physical examinations or discussion of private topics are critical.

Communication with Health Professionals

Federal regulations allow health care providers to exchange information in the medical care of a given patient. This discussion can occur after the patient signs permission under the Health Information Portability and Accountability Act (HIPAA). Certain medical terms common to the allied health profession are not often used in athletic training because they are medical rather than orthopedic in nature. However, athletic trainers should be familiar with these terms so that they can discuss medical conditions on the same intellectual

Table 1-2	Common Medical Terminology
Term	**Definition**
Adventitious	Coming from an external source; occurring spontaneously
Afebrile	Without a fever; also apyretic
Biopsy	Removal and examination of tissue
Comorbid	Two or more possibly unrelated medical conditions existing at the same time
Constitutional	Relating to the body as a whole
Erythema	Redness of the skin brought about by capillary dilation
Febrile	Having a fever
Malaise	A general feeling of discomfort or uneasiness; often the first symptom of an illness or infection
Morbidity	Consequences of a given illness
Mortality	Death from a particular illness or disease
Palliative or supportive treatment	Reducing the severity of an illness or disease without curing it
Prodromal	Preillness symptoms
Purulent	Pus filled
Sequela, sequelae	A condition occurring as a consequence of a given illness or disease
Suppurative	Pus forming

level as other health care providers. Because some of these communications may be in written notes, athletic trainers need to understand standard abbreviations as well. Appendix B lists many common abbreviations that relate to medical care. Table 1-2 lists terminology used to describe medical conditions and situations that are used throughout this text.

Medical History

A medical health history taken to ascertain the extent of a medical condition or illness is vastly different from an orthopedic history. In an athletic injury, the condition is typically contained within one joint, muscle, or bone and usually involves only the musculoskeletal system. Conversely, a medical condition may involve many body systems, may be difficult to describe, and may not be at all obvious. An athletic trainer needs to appreciate the different types of questions asked in a health history about a medical condition compared with a history for an orthopedic injury. Typical orthopedic questions include the mechanism of injury; sounds associated with the onset (e.g., snap, crunch, pop); and immediate disability associated with the injury, such as swelling, inability to bear weight, deformity, and radiculopathy. Questions in a medical health history review the entire body and include respiratory, gastrointestinal, and neurological symptoms. Questions relating to symptoms are critical because symptoms

Box 1-1	Sample Questions for a Medical Health History

- Describe your symptoms.
- How long have you had these symptoms?
- Do your symptoms interfere with activities of daily living?
- Are you currently taking any medications, vitamins, or supplements?
- Do your symptoms tend to occur at a specific time (after eating, when exercising, after exposure to an allergen, at night, etc.)?
- Do your symptoms come and go, or are they constant?
- Are you sleeping well and according to your normal habits?
- Do you feel more fatigued than usual?
- Have you recently changed your diet, medication, activity level, or personal habits?
- Are you under more stress than typical?
- Are you having normal bowel and bladder function (ask if gastrointestinal in nature)?
- Is there anything else going on that you would like to discuss?

cannot be measured objectively yet may give clues about the athlete's condition. Box 1-1 gives examples of questions to consider and seek answers to for a medical condition.

Other aspects of a medical history include duration of signs and symptoms, onset (e.g., rapid, insidious, gradual), and disability from symptoms (Key Points—Signs and Symptoms). Some medical situations may be life threatening and require complex information to make a correct but timely decision. The end result for the athletic trainer is a decision about how to treat the athlete and when or to whom to refer. A basic upper respiratory infection or cold may be treated by over-the-counter medications whereas a long-term infection of the respiratory tract or asthma requires physician intervention and medication.

KEY POINTS
Signs and Symptoms

Although generally used together when assessing a medical condition, signs and symptoms are not synonymous.
- **Signs** refer to something that the athletic trainer sees or feels, such as a temperature, respiration, heart beat, blood pressure.
- **Symptoms** refer to something the athlete feels, such as a headache, nausea, dizziness, or pain.

Prevention of Disease Transmission

Everyone who works in the health care field appreciates the need to prevent disease transmission. Protection from infection and maintaining a sanitary environment are two critical elements in caring for patients with illnesses. Another prevention technique is immunization from specific diseases by vaccine. Chapter 12 discusses vaccination as well as established standards for preventing the spread of disease and illnesses.

Occupational Safety and Health Administration

The Occupational Safety and Health Administration (OSHA) is an organization that sets standards to protect health care workers and their patients. OSHA standards apply only to established relationships between employers and employees and do not extend federal protections to students.[14] However, students who could potentially be exposed to hazardous waste in facilities where they practice or observe should follow the safety standards set forth by OSHA, receive training, and have ready access to precautionary materials, such as barriers and proper disposal containers.

OSHA has a right to inspect any facility under its auspices without prior notification, and it has the power to suspend or shut down a facility, as well as impose hefty fines for noncompliance with standards.[15,16] The most familiar OSHA requirement affecting athletic medical care concerns the bloodborne pathogen (BBP) standard. Athletic trainers must be intimately familiar with this standard because many athletes are at risk of open wounds in the course of their activities and subsequently have potential for the transmission of infection.

OSHA Standards for Bloodborne Pathogens

The BBP standard is intended to safeguard health care workers against hazards resulting from exposure to infectious body fluids and covers anyone who could reasonably anticipate having occupational exposure to infectious waste (e.g., blood). Included in this standard is a description of how to formulate an individualized institutional or setting exposure control plan. A written document outlines steps to take and specific people to call in the event of an exposure to infectious waste. An exposure may range from a needle stick to having blood spilled onto intact skin. All health care workers must have an operating knowledge of their employer's plan, access to personal protective equipment, BBP training, and knowledge about who to contact should an exposure occur.[17]

The BBP standard uses the phrase **universal precautions** to emphasize that all human waste should be treated as if it is infectious and that health care workers and patients must be protected in every situation in which they might be exposed to body fluid, including contact with mucous membranes in the eyes, mouth, or nose; genital secretions; or blood. Any sharp object that may be contaminated with infectious waste, such as needles, scalpels, or broken glass, is also considered potentially hazardous material.[17] Box 1-2 has suggestions for handling infectious waste.

Box 1-2   Handling Infectious Waste

- All infectious waste must be placed in closeable, leakproof approved container for storage, transporting, or shipping.
- An OSHA-approved plan for proper disposal of infectious-waste bags and sharps units must be on hand and followed.
- Gloves must be worn when personnel handle infectious laundry.
- Laundry contaminated with infectious waste must be separated from other materials to be cleaned.
- Personal protective equipment (gowns, masks, gloves) shall be properly disposed of before leaving the treatment room or upon contamination.
- While wearing gloves, personnel may clean blood stains on material (uniforms, towels) with hydrogen peroxide in cold water and immediately rinse.
- Only red hazardous-waste bags should be used to dispose of infectious materials.
- In the absence of antibacterial soap and running water, personnel should use antibacterial wipes or gels to sanitize hands often.
- Personnel should avoid putting hands to face (eyes, nose, mouth) when around ill patients or working with infectious waste.

Data from Klossner D, editor: *2004-2005 NCAA sports medicine handbook,* Indianapolis, 2004-2005, National Collegiate Athletics Association; U.S. Department of Labor Occupational Safety & Health Administration: Bloodborne pathogens—1910.1030. U.S. Department of Labor. Available at http://www.osha.gov/pls/oshaweb/owadisp.show_document?p_table=STANDARDS&p_id=10051. Accessed September 2004; Howe W: Preventing infectious disease in sports, *Physician Sportsmedicine* 31(2):23-29, 2003.

Barriers to Bloodborne Pathogens

Barriers are devices worn to protect both the health care worker and patient against the spread of disease. The traditionally accepted barrier is latex gloves, but OSHA also requires access to face and eye protection, gowns, and mouthpieces for resuscitation.[10,17] Health care workers with allergies to latex must be provided with an alternate material suitable as a barrier against transmission of BBPs.

All health care workers must have ready access to barriers that fit properly in order to retard infection from hazardous materials. Ideally, soap and water are the best methods to clean hands before and following glove use (Box 1-3). If soap and water are not readily available, commercial disinfectant single-use wipes can sanitize hands (Figure 1-4).

Workers should remove and properly dispose of soiled barriers before leaving the treatment area. Brightly labeled red infectious waste bags are the most common means of storing such waste until it can be disposed of per OSHA protocol. These bags must be contained in a sturdy, leakproof container with a lid and located in an easily accessible area for all to use.

Sharps containers are specially built units that have one-way valves (Figure 1-5) and are used to accommodate sharp instruments such as needles and scalpels that may have infectious materials on them. These containers should never be opened or over-stuffed. Intercollegiate sports medicine guidelines

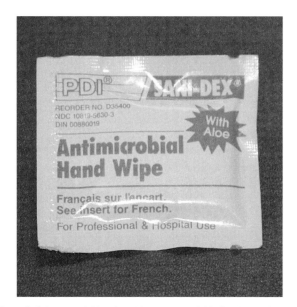

Figure 1-4 Commercial hand sanitizers are available for times when soap and water are not available.

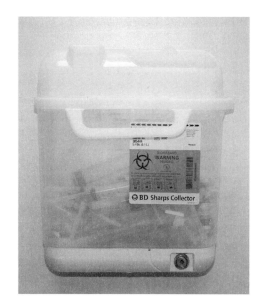

Figure 1-5 A Sharps container is a self-contained, one-way locking box or device that holds used sharp instruments including needles and scalpels. Note that this particular container is locked to the wall so that only an OSHA-approved provider is able to remove the container for proper disposal.

Box 1-3   Correct Glove Use

1. Thoroughly wash all aspects of both hands and fingers with liberal use of an antibacterial soap and plenty of water.

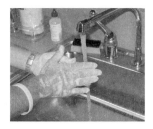

2. Dry hands with a disposable single-use hand towel.
3. Apply gloves without touching the external surfaces of the gloves.

When the procedure requiring gloves is complete:
4. Use the gloved index finger and thumb of one hand; gently pinch the glove at the wrist and pull toward finger tips.
5. Invert the glove, and remove all but index finger and thumb.
6. Repeat the procedure with the second hand, inverting the glove as it is removed.

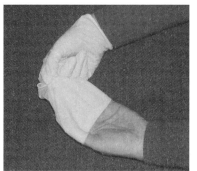

7. Fold gloves inside out and dispose of them in a red (OSHA-approved) bag.
8. Thoroughly wash and dry hands as described above.

---

require that all necessary materials, such as barriers, bleach, waste receptacles, and wound coverings, comply with universal precautions and be available to all health care providers.[10]

The NCAA has specific regulations that address bleeding athletes or those with blood on their uniforms.[10,18] These regulations specifically mandate a bleeding athlete be removed from activity until the bleeding has been stopped and the wound covered with a dressing sturdy enough to withstand the demands of activity.[10] Again, this guideline and the requirements of storing and disposing of infectious waste are intended to protect both the athlete and athletic trainer from transmitting diseases.

Disinfection

Another component of prevention in the spread of infections is disinfection of surfaces used for examination and treatment (Figure 1-6) and of soiled materials, including uniforms and clothing. Disinfection is a critical aspect of every athletic training facility because of its potential to stop the spread of disease. The simple acts of sterilizing treatment tables following use and washing hands frequently can diminish disease transmission considerably. Many infections, such as hepatitis B, are quite hardy and can live outside the body if not obliterated properly (see Chapter 12).

Products claiming to have disinfectant properties must be reviewed and registered by the Environmental Protection Agency (EPA) before being sold. Registered disinfectants include data that all the microorganisms listed on the product label are indeed eradicated by

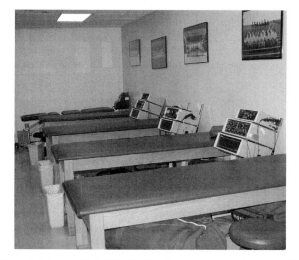

Figure 1-6 An athletic training facility should always be clean and disinfected to prevent the transmission of disease.

Box 1-4 OSHA Disinfectant Agents Mandates

- Contaminated surfaces must be sprayed to saturation with the disinfectant.
- HIV-1 disinfection requires 30 seconds of saturation.
- Hepatitis B virus disinfection requires 10 minutes of saturation.

From the U.S. Department of Labor Occupational Safety and Health Administration: What does OSHA currently accept as "appropriate" disinfectants to prevent the spread of HIV and HBV? U.S. Department of Labor. Available at http://www.osha-slc.gov/html/faq-bbp.html. Accessed September 2004.

---

correct use of the product. The difference between a disinfectant and a disinfectant-cleaner is that a disinfectant merely kills microorganisms, whereas a combination cleaner removes soils and disinfects in one step. Regulations governing how these cleaners and disinfectants are dispersed include the following: If the material is removed from its original container, it must have all the product information transferred to the second receptacle including a notation that the cleaner was moved from a gallon container to a spray bottle.

When sanitizing surfaces soiled with possible BBPs, OSHA recommends the proper use of barriers, cleaning all blood from the surface and properly disposing of the waste, and then disinfecting the area. OSHA mandates that disinfectant agents approved by the EPA for contaminated surfaces be used to wet down the surface for 30 seconds for human immunodeficiency virus (HIV-1) and 10 minutes for hepatitis B virus disinfection (Box 1-4).[19] The *2004-2005 NCAA Sports Medicine Handbook* suggests using a 1:10 ratio of freshly prepared bleach to water solution for disinfecting surfaces but cites references before 1995.[10] More current research calls for a 1:9 ratio of bleach to water solution to have an effective disinfectant.[20]

Household chlorine bleach contains 5.25% active sodium hypochlorite and 94.75% water. Although it is extremely effective against staphylococcus and streptococcus bacteria, salmonella, *Escherichia coli*, certain fungi, and influenza A and B, it is not a cleaner. The EPA and U.S. Department of Agriculture have deemed chlorine bleach safe for use in food preparation and as a disinfectant. It is registered with the EPA for appropriate use as a hospital disinfectant and the Centers for Disease Control and Prevention have written guidelines for its use in health care facilities.[21]

A popular disinfectant-cleaner is quaternary ammonium chlorides (quats), which are formulated with the active ingredient benzalkonium chloride. Quats are effective in destroying a broad spectrum of harmful microorganisms, staphylococcus and streptococcus bacteria, herpes simplex, HIV, fungi, and antibiotic-resistant bacteria such as methicillin-resistant *Staphylococcus aureus*.[22]

Legal Considerations

As with everything else, legal ramifications must be considered when caring for athletes. Certified athletic trainers hired for the purpose of providing evaluation and prevention of illnesses and injuries have a duty to their employer, and subsequently their athlete patients, to render appropriate medical care (Figure 1-7). The word *duty* in this situation is a legal term, one of the four components necessary to prove negligence. Breaching a duty and thereby causing harm is negligence. Athletic trainers also have other types of duty to their athlete patients. Among them are maintaining skills and knowledge, providing a reasonable standard of care, medical referral, and upholding patients' right to privacy.

Standard of Care

Negligence is conduct falling below an established and expected standard of care validated by law for the protection of others, which results in physical or mental harm or damage to another. Typically, case law assists in interpreting what a given standard of care should be in a specific situation. In the case of *Kleinknecht v. Gettysburg College*, the court held that the college had a duty to protect against medical crisis, specifically to adopt a policy that might avoid life-threatening emergencies.[23] In another case, the presence of a qualified medical person at certain practices but not others was not deemed in itself to be a violation of the standard of care owed an athlete.[24] In this situation, the athletic trainer was always present at higher-risk sports events. A serious wrist injury occurred at a different venue but was not caused nor worsened by the failure of the athletic trainer to habitually attend football practice but not gymnastics.

The privilege of being a certified and often state-licensed or registered athletic trainer does carry with it certain obligations. Athletic trainers are held to a higher standard than are physical education teachers

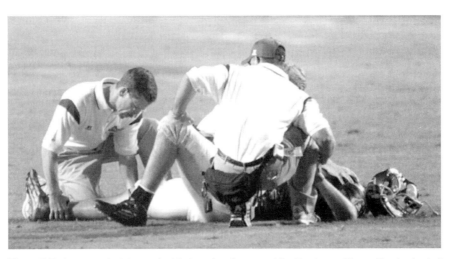

Figure 1-7 The team physician and athletic trainer have an obligation to provide quality standard of care for athletes. (Courtesy Kip Sloan.)

or personal trainers because of their training, experience, and national certification examination. The NATA Code of Ethics has several references in its principles regarding the expected level of care to patients by its members.[25,26] Athletic trainers would be wise to review their job description to clearly delineate their roles and responsibilities and to appreciate the understood standard of expected care.

Because most athletic trainers do not see as great a volume of medical conditions as they do orthopedic problems, athletic trainers must also work within established guidelines, such as under the direction of a team physician, especially when working with medical disorders. Appreciating the need for referral for medical attention beyond the scope of practice of the athletic trainer is critical, especially in medical situations.

Medical Referral

All people working with injured or ill patients know that delay in medical attention may result in lasting damage or, in medical conditions, death. Case law has been consistent in siding with the plaintiff in situations where an athletic trainer delayed or denied an injured athlete opportunity to be referred to a physician in a timely fashion.[26] The NATA Code of Ethics has a mandate to refer injured athletes for further medical attention.[25] Because many team physicians may hold only an orthopedic specialty, athletic trainers should have a family practice–trained MD or DO available for medical condition referrals for their athletes.

Right to Privacy

The right of the athlete to have personal medical information protected against dissemination to outside parties is of utmost importance. These outside agents may be the media, coaches, or even parents if the athlete is over 18 years of age and can function as an adult. Although citing an orthopedic reason for the inability of a given athlete to participate is a common practice, most athletes do not give permission to reveal medical conditions preventing full activity. Even when athletes sign a form allowing medical information to be shared with certain parties, such as coaches, insurance secretaries, professional scouts, and the media, this form usually allows revealing injuries that are typically orthopedic in nature and does not cover medical issues such as sexually transmitted diseases (STDs) or other infections.

Case law has routinely protected the athlete from violations of patient privacy, citing reasons ranging from discrimination against the patient with HIV to the American Disability Act protecting the athlete with autoimmune deficiency syndrome (AIDS).[27] Disclosure of medical information without expressed permission is illegal and falls under two federal acts.

Federal Regulations

Two acts, HIPAA and the Family Education Rights and Privacy Act (FERPA), govern personal health information (PHI), depending on the age of the athlete.

HIPAA

HIPAA, also known as Public Law 104-191, was enacted in August 1996 and implemented on April 14, 2003. It is the first federally mandated act to protect patient privacy, oversee medical records, and allow patients more control over how and to whom their personal health information is disclosed.[28] Specifically, the law allows patients to access their medical records and request corrections if factual errors are discovered. It provides limits to use and sharing of PHI outside of health care agencies, e.g., a life insurance company. The act dictates how PHI may be disseminated in given situations: verbally or electronically. The U.S. Department of Health and Human Services Office for Civil Rights provides oversight and enforcement of HIPAA.[28]

FERPA

FERPA, also known as the Buckley Amendment, was created in 1974 to protect the privacy of student education records and applies to any school receiving funds from the U.S. Department of Education.[29,30] It functions similarly to HIPAA in that it allows a person access to and limits disclosure of his educational records. Parents have a right to inspect a child's educational records until the student is 18 years old. After the student becomes an adult, the rights transfer from the parent to the student.[29]

The act allows only certain parties access to educational records without prior permission in given situations. An example is "appropriate officials in cases of health and safety emergencies."[29] An educational record may contain biographical information, grade point averages, records of student conduct, and test scores. Disclosing without prior consent that a particular athlete is not a rocket scientist, weighs a certain amount, is an orphan, took remedial reading classes, or plagiarized is a violation of this act. The consequences of disclosure range from loss of certain federal funds to prosecution of a criminal offense.[30]

Medical Records

Adequate records on the health care of athletes must be kept, and everyone who has access to these records must appreciate and abide by confidentiality and the athletes' right to privacy.[10] These records must be maintained and stored with limited access in accordance with institutional and state regulatory acts and must also be safeguarded against improper disclosure at all times. Limited access includes monitoring daily injury reports, athletes' status, results of diagnostic tests, and accessibility to medical files. Even daily treatment logs, e-mails with identifiable information, and fax transmissions need to be considered private information. Unsecured files, open storage areas, or unprotected computers without password encryption are examples of inappropriate medical record storage.

Abbreviations used among health care workers are considered appropriate and legal methods of keeping notations on medical records. The athletic trainer and other health care providers must be familiar with these abbreviations because they save time and space when writing notes into charts. A list of the abbreviations associated with common medical conditions is listed in Appendix B.

Reporting Communicable Diseases

A physician has a legal obligation to report certain medical conditions to public health authorities, such as some STDs or tuberculosis. Subsequent chapters identify which medical conditions are reportable and to whom. The rationale behind reporting these conditions is to protect the public from an outbreak of the disease; the courts have ruled that certain medical conditions' risks of exposure outweigh the patient's right to privacy.

A five-class reporting system for communicable diseases is used in the United States. When a physician has confirmed a certain infectious disease, the disease but not the person is reported to the correct state or federal agency.[20] On rare occasions, such as with an STD, the infectious individual is reported, and any partners who may have been infected are contacted.

The purpose of reporting communicable diseases is two-fold: to isolate a given disease and retard its spread and to generate data regarding current disease trends so they may be prevented in the future. An overview of the reporting system is confined here to the local level. Basic reporting is collected on two levels: report of cases and report of epidemics.

Reporting Individual Cases

Local health officials in conjunction with state and federal agencies decide which individual cases are to be routinely reported and develop policy for the responsible person to follow in the reporting, information to be collected and documented, and method of report transmission. Physicians and health care workers who have knowledge of a reportable illness are required by law to report it. Hospitals generally have a specific officer who handles such reports, but smaller units often have similar protocols, policies, and procedures regarding reporting communicable diseases. Minimal data for these reports include the patient's name, address, diagnosis, age, gender, and date of report. The right of privacy is paramount to an individual but so is the right of the greater community to prevent the spread of a communicable disease and protect unsuspecting individuals. Collective reports can simply list the number of cases for a given disease in a very specific timeframe.

Reporting Epidemics

Reporting outbreaks of epidemics of specific diseases is also important. Epidemics must be identified and contained as expeditiously as possible, and the physician or health care provider is crucial in the management of reports of these outbreaks.

There are five identified classes for reporting these diseases:

- Class 1: Case report universally required by International Health Regulations or as a disease under surveillance by the World Health Organization (WHO). These comprise the internationally quarantinable diseases such as plague, cholera, or yellow fever. The specific diseases in this category were first identified in 1969 and updated as recently as 2002 before distribution to the World Health Assembly.

Diseases listed in Class 1 are to be immediately reported to WHO because they are considered of urgent international public health importance. A subcategory of Class 1 includes louse-borne typhus fever, paralytic poliomyelitis, malaria, and influenza. These diseases must be reported as urgent to state or federal agencies by fax, e-mail, or telephone with a subsequent daily or weekly update as dictated by law.

- Class 2: Case report regularly required wherever the disease occurs. The first subcategory includes diseases such as typhoid fever, diphtheria, and agents used by bioterrorists, including anthrax, botulism, and smallpox. The second subcategory comprises diseases that require a less urgent notification, within 1 week as opposed to a same-day report. An example of a disease in this category is leprosy.
- Class 3: Diseases selectively reportable in recognized endemic areas. These include three subcategories to specific regions, counties, or states that may have a particular proclivity for an infectious disease. Many states have no diseases in Class 3.
- Class 4: Obligatory report of epidemics but no case report required. Class 4 diseases are to be reported immediately and include staphylococcal foodborne intoxication.
- Class 5: Official report not ordinarily required for sporadic and uncommon infectious diseases, as well as those having no practical measures for containment, such as the common cold and sinusitis.

WEB RESOURCES

HIPAA
http://www.hhs.gov/ocr/hipaa/
Information on the health information privacy act

FERPA
http://www.ed.gov/policy/gen/guid/fpco/ferpa/index.html
Educational privacy

OSHA
http://www.osha.gov/
General OSHA information

BBP
http://www.osha.gov/SLTC/bloodbornepathogens/index.html
Bloodborne pathogen information

PPEs
http://www.amssm.org/
Information on preparticipation exams recommended for athletes

NATA
http://www.nata.org
The NATA Code of Ethics, as well as the scope of practice for certified athletic trainers

OSHA and ATCs
http://www.osha.gov/pls/oshaweb/owadisp.show_document?p_table=INTERPRETATIONS&p_id=23466
Bloodborne pathogen information for certified athletic trainers by OSHA

SUMMARY

The athletic trainer is in a unique position to detect medical conditions in the athlete and to determine the appropriate course of action. It is imperative that the athletic trainer be familiar with the techniques for evaluating these conditions and the signs and symptoms that may indicate a medical condition. Assessment of medical conditions in athletes requires a slightly different approach from orthopedic assessment. The chief complaint may be largely symptomatic and requires good communication skills on the part of the athletic trainer to elicit full disclosure of pertinent information. The PPE may represent the first disclosure of a medical problem so the form should be carefully crafted and reviewed to ensure that it covers a broad medical spectrum.

Because ill athletes may be a source of infection for others in the program and community, it is important for the athletic trainer to follow OSHA protocols. Knowledge and application of recognized disease transmission prevention standards are critical in both caring for the ill athlete and maintaining a sanitary workplace.

Athletes may be cared for in a school or university setting, but the mandates for a medical facility still need to be followed, including the maintenance of accurate and private records. Federal law requires that records be safely secured and that the contents remain undisclosed to protect the best interest of the athlete. In addition, the recognized system of reporting infectious disease is a vital component of public health. It is up to the treating physician to report a given disease to the proper public health agency and protect the public from additional disease transmission.

REFERENCES

1. National Athletic Trainers' Association (NATA): *Athletic training educational competencies*, ed 3, Dallas, 1999, NATA.
2. Board of Certification: *Role delineation study*, ed 5, Omaha, 2004, Board of Certification, Inc.
3. Trampf D, Oliphant J: Licensed athletic trainers: a traditional, unique, and proactive approach in Wisconsin sports medicine, *Wisconsin Medical Journal* 103(1):33-34, 2004.
4. Cormier J, York A, Domholdt E, Kegerreis S: Athletic trainer utilization in sports medicine clinics, *Journal of Orthopedic Sports Physical Therapy* 17(1):36-43, 1993.
5. Holm L: A new twist. Using certified athletic trainers as physician extenders, *Medical Group Management Association Coonex* 4(4):27-28, 2004.
6. Cuppett M: Self-perceived continuing education needs of certified athletic trainers, *Journal of Athletic Training* 36(4):388-395, 2001.
7. American Academy of Family Physicians: Periodic health examinations. July 2004 (rev 4.4). Available at http://www.aafp.org/x7661.xml. Accessed September 2004.
8. Koester M, Amundson C: Preparticipation screening of high school athletes, *The Physician and Sportsmedicine* 31(8):35-38, 2003.

9. Joy E, Paisley T, Price RJ, et al: Optimizing the collegiate preparticipation physical evaluation, *Clinics of Sports Medicine* 14(3):183-187, 2004.

10. Klossner D, editor: *2004-2005 NCAA sports medicine handbook*, ed 17, Indianapolis, 2004-2005, National Collegiate Athletics Association.

11. Carek P, Mainous AI: A thorough yet efficient exam identifies most problems in school athletes—applied evidence: research findings that are changing clinical practice, *Journal of Family Practice*, pp 1-3, February 2003.

12. American Medical Society for Sports Medicine: Preparticipation exam, Available at http://www.amssm.org/. Accessed September 2004.

13. Bickley L: *Bates' guide to physical examination and history taking*, ed 8, New York, 2003, Lippincott Williams & Wilkins.

14. United States Department of Labor Occupational Safety & Health Administration: Applicability of bloodborne pathogens standard to athletic trainers; handling of contaminated laundry. Available at http://www.osha.gov/pls/oshaweb/owadisp.show_document?p_table=INTERPRETATIONS&p_id=23466. Accessed September 2004.

15. United States Department of Defense: OSHA fines Batavia, NY commercial laundry $140,850 for not protecting workers against bloodborne hazards, US Department of Defense. Available at http://www.osha.gov/pls/oshaweb/owadisp.show_document?p_table=NEWS_RELEASES&p_id=11015. Accessed September 2004.

16. Kern S: OSHA knocking on doctors' doors, *Nevada Journal of Medicine* 89(6):467-468, 1992.

17. United States Department of Labor Occupational Safety & Health Administration: Bloodborne pathogens—1910.1030, United States Department of Labor. Available at http://www.osha.gov/pls/oshaweb/owadisp.show_document?p_table=STANDARDS&p_id=10051. Accessed September 2004.

18. Halpin T, editor: *NCAA 2003 wrestling rules and interpretations*, Indianapolis, 2003, National Collegiate Athletic Association.

19. United States Department of Labor Occupational Safety & Health Administration: What does OSHA currently accept as "appropriate" disinfectants to prevent the spread of HIV and HBV? US Department of Labor. Available at http://www.osha-slc.gov/html/faq-bbp.html. Accessed September 2004.

20. Chin J: *Control of infectious diseases manual*, ed 17, Washington, DC, 2000, American Public Health Association.

21. Birnbach N, Burgess N, Doswell W, et al: The disinfecting power of an old standby: chlorine bleach. Available at http://nsweb.nursingspectrum.com/cfforms/GuestLecture/Bleach.cfm. Accessed September 2004.

22. McFadden R: Cleaning and disinfecting the indoor environment: chlorine bleach, quats and phenolics, Coastwide Laboratories. Available at http://www.coastwidelabs.com/Technical%20Articles/quatbleach.htm. Accessed September 2004.

23. *Kleinknecht v Gettysburg College*, 786 F. Supp. 449 (M.D. Pa. 1992).

24. *Kennedy v Syracuse University*, No. 94-CV-269, 1995 U.S. Dist. LEXIS 13539 (N.D.N.Y. September 12, 1995).

25. National Athletic Trainers' Association: Code of ethics, NATA. Available at http://www.nata.org/about/codeofethics.htm. Accessed September 2004.

26. West S, Ciccolella M: Issues in the standard of care for certified athletic trainers. *Journal of Legal Aspects of Sport* 14(1):63-74, 2004.

27. Wong G, Apostolopoulou A: Infection detection: HIV testing policies ought to be put in place before problems arise, *Athletic Business* 12:24-26, 1999.

28. United States Department of Health & Human Services: Medical privacy—national standards to protect the privacy of personal health information. Available at http://www.hhs.gov/ocr/hipaa/. Accessed September 2004.

29. United States Department of Education: Family educational rights and privacy act (FERPA), US Department of Education. Available at http://www.ed.gov/policy/gen/guid/fpco/ferpa/index.html. Accessed September 2004.

30. Ness R: Family educational rights and privacy act and athletics, *Journal of Legal Aspects of Sport* 5(1):45-51, 1995.

CHAPTER 2

Medical Evaluation Techniques and Equipment

Micki Cuppett and
Katie M. Walsh

OBJECTIVES

At the completion of this chapter, the reader should be able to do the following:

1. Describe a basic general medical examination including a comprehensive history and physical examination.
2. Describe and demonstrate the proper use of evaluation tools and techniques for assessment of general health.
3. Appreciate the value of knowing normal ranges for urine and blood laboratory studies.
4. Understand the basics of palpation, percussion, and auscultation in a general medical examination.

INTRODUCTION

This chapter focuses on the evaluation techniques and equipment used in a general medical examination. It introduces the use of the otoscope and ophthalmoscope as well as the stethoscope; presents basic techniques in palpation, percussion, and auscultation; and discusses general information about normal vital signs and laboratory results. The chapters that follow present a more detailed explanation of both normal and abnormal results of the examination techniques specific to each body system. Subsequent chapters also assume that the reader has reviewed and understood this chapter and is familiar with the equipment and techniques used in a general medical examination.

EXAMINATION OF THE ATHLETE WITH A GENERAL MEDICAL CONDITION

The examination of an athlete with a nonorthopedic condition may present the athletic trainer with a challenge. Often, there is no specific onset and there may be few signs that anything is wrong. Each evaluation of a medical problem begins with taking a thorough history and is followed by an overall systemic review and, finally, an examination specific to the condition. The athletic trainer must rely heavily on the athlete's history to guide the examination. Evaluating a general medical condition requires a systematic approach, much like the history, inspection/observation, palpation, and special tests (HIPS/HOPS) of the typical orthopedic evaluation.

Comprehensive Medical History

The most common approach to taking a comprehensive medical history begins by identifying and recording an athlete's age and gender. If ethnicity, marital status, occupation, and religion are important to the diagnosis or treatment, they may be documented as well. Next, the athlete's chief complaint is identified, (Key Points—Athlete's Chief Complaint) including the present illness, onset, and setting when symptoms were first apparent. Descriptions of the chief complaint that assist the examiner include the following: location of discomfort, quality or quantity of symptoms, frequency, onset, duration, and any associated factors that aggravate or alleviate symptoms. Athletes should be asked if they are currently using medications, supplements, vitamins, home remedies, or **poultices.** Also, the examiner needs to know whether the athlete has shared or borrowed teammates' or roommates' prescription medications.

The next sections of a comprehensive history for an athlete with a medical condition include past medical history, current health status, and family history. Past history incorporates childhood and adult illnesses as well as accidents and injuries. Keep in mind that adult illnesses also may include psychiatric, obstetrical, or gynecological conditions and surgery. Typically, the patient's current health status covers alcohol, drug, and tobacco use; exercise; diet; and immunizations. The examiner asks questions about any history of allergies and specific reactions to the antigens and ensures that the athlete is up-to-date with routine screening tests, such as Pap smears and breast and testicular self-exams. It may also be appropriate to explore the reported environmental safety of the home and workplace.

A look into the patient's family history may provide critical information that can be quite useful in pointing out a susceptibility for a given illness or disease and prove helpful in the examination and care of the athlete (Key Points—Family Health History). Diabetes, heart disease, hypertension, kidney disease, cardiovascular disorders (e.g., deep vein thrombosis [DVT], stroke), allergies, asthma, mental illness, and addictions are all examples of diseases with a genetic tendency. The age, current health, or cause and age of death of immedi-

ate family members are also critical factors in family health history. Some physicians add a category—personal and social history—to assist them in understanding their patients better. This category covers a patient's education, occupation, significant others, home life, daily activities, hobbies, and important beliefs. Although these areas are not necessarily crucial to a specific diagnosis of a given condition, some physicians believe they profoundly affect the overall health and attitude toward wellness in their patients.[1]

Review of Body Systems

The review of body systems is the athletic trainer's primary focus in the evaluation of medical conditions. Indeed, most health care professionals use the comprehensive medical history and review of body systems in assessing orthopedic injuries as well as medical issues. Traditionally, all systems are reviewed, unlike in an orthopedic assessment where only the anatomical area or system believed to be affected is considered. A medical review differs from an orthopedic evaluation, in which the examiner may stop after determining that there is crepitus rather than continuing to look for ligamentous injury. For example, in an orthopedic injury, if the athlete has a clearly displaced fractured femur, the examiner does not continue the initial evaluation to determine if the anterior cruciate ligament (ACL) is intact.

The goal of the review of body systems during an examination for a general medical condition is to enable the athletic trainer to gather enough information to make an intelligent decision about patient referral and, if necessary, referral to a specific type of practitioner.

The review of systems always begins with a general assessment of an athlete's condition: weight and associated changes, fatigue, fever, and any reported sleep disturbances. Then the review continues system by system, starting with the skin and descending from head to toe. When assessing the skin, the examiner looks for obvious rashes, sores, dryness, color change, lumps, or swelling and asks the athlete about itching or skin dryness.

A good mnemonic to help remember the order of the first part of the review of systems is HEENT, which stands for head, eyes, ears, nose, and throat. Beginning with signs and symptoms associated with the head, the examiner inquires about the following: headaches, seizures, **syncope,** tremors, paralysis, or history of a head injury. Essential questions to ask about the eyes concern visual acuity, the need to wear corrective lenses (i.e., glasses, contacts), surgical history that may include procedures that correct vision, date and results of last eye examination, and any history of redness, tearing, **diplopia,** floaters, pain, dryness, or disease of the eye.

Questions linked to the ears relate to symptoms of **tinnitus,** vertigo, earaches, and signs of ear dysfunction, such as discharge. Patients with nasal problems or conditions of the accompanying sinuses can present with discharge, sinus pain, itching, sneezing, or stuffiness, whereas mouth and throat problems are manifested by hoarseness, sores, caries, halitosis, or bleeding gums. Pain or stiffness in the neck can indicate an infectious disease, and enlarged glands are palpable signs of a response to changes in the body. Questions about breast discomfort, lumps, or nipple discharge may be relevant if the examiner is given information that points to pathology of the breast tissue. These questions may be pertinent to both genders.

The review of systems continues with the respiratory, cardiovascular, and gastrointestinal systems and follows the same cephalocaudal order. Signs associated with respiratory problems include the presence of excessive sputum, altered respiratory sounds, or **hemoptysis.** The cardiovascular system encompasses the heart and blood vessels including blood pressure. Symptoms of cardiovascular anomalies encompass murmurs, **dyspnea,** chest pain, vasovagal responses, hypertension, or syncope. Gastrointestinal problems may manifest with symptoms such as heartburn, nausea, constipation, or food intolerance. Signs include vomiting; change in frequency, consistency, or color of stools; rectal bleeding; diarrhea; gas; or jaundice.[2]

Next in this descending order of specific systems come the urinary and gynecological systems. Any change in frequency, incontinence, pain, or discolored urine may indicate genitourinary system pathology. A male patient who complains of penile sores, discharge, or hesitancy in voiding should be referred to a physician.

Gynecological disorders include delayed onset of menses, **oligomenorrhea, dysmenorrhea, polymenorrhea,** severe cramping, late menstrual period, abnormal pain, discharge, or vaginal sores. The examiner questions the patient about these symptoms if gynecological issues are raised when discussing her current health history.

After the cephalocaudal systems review, the evaluation goes on to other prevalent body systems: peripheral vascular, musculoskeletal, neurological, hematological, endocrine, and psychiatric. Important areas to explore include complaints of loss of sensation in the extremities, pitting edema, soreness and swelling in multiple joints, and abnormal fatigue.[3] Specific questions pertaining to these systems are discussed later in the appropriate chapters. After the review of all systems, the athletic trainer begins a physical examination of the patient.

PHYSICAL EXAMINATION

Again, the athletic trainer follows the universally accepted cephalocaudal sequence for the physical examination (Box 2-1). The general survey includes observation of the athlete's apparent state of health, level of consciousness, signs of distress, height and weight, skin color, obvious lesions, and hygiene. These are noted as the athlete enters the examination area. The practitioner continues the physical assessment in the same order as the previously described review of systems, beginning with the vital signs and skin and advancing from the head down the body. The proper evaluation tools should be ready to expedite the examination.

Box 2-1 Sequence of Symptom Review and Physical Examination			
General • Fatigue and energy • Desired weight • Fever **Diet** • Appetite • Supplements • Restrictions **Skin, Hair, Nails** • Appearance • Color **Head and Neck** • Supple neck • Headache • LOC • Dizziness **Eyes** • Visual acuity • Corrective lenses • Visual disturbances	**Ears** • Vertigo • Tinnitus • Hearing acuity • Discharge **Nose** • Functional • Congestions • History of bleeding **Throat and Mouth** • Hoarseness • Sore throat • Dental issues • Chewing tobacco **Gastrointestinal** • Heartburn • Vomiting • Diarrhea • Constipation **Lymphatic System** • Swelling	• Pitting edema • Tender **Endocrine** • Heat or cold tolerance • Weight or energy change **Female** • FMP/LMP • Regularity • Symptoms **Male** • Testicular pain or swelling **Breasts** • Swelling • Lumps • Pain **Chest and Lungs** • SOB • Dyspnea • Night sweats • Cough • Sputum	**Cardiovascular** • Chest pain • Exercise history • Exertional SOB • Chest pain **Hematology** • Bruising history **Genitourinary** • Urine frequency, volume, color • Dysuria **Musculoskeletal** • Joint or muscle pain or swelling • Neurological symptoms **Mental Status** • Eating, sleeping, social habits • Mood • Concentration

LOC, Level of consciousness; *FMP,* first menstrual period; *LMP,* last menstrual period; *SOB,* shortness of breath.

Vital Signs

Assessment of all vital signs includes height and weight, blood pressure, heart and respiratory rate and rhythm, and body temperature.

Height and Weight

Recording an athlete's height and weight is essential because it provides a baseline for future reference. Height is often critical to athletes but is typically of only mild interest to the health care practitioner. Weight is more critical because a drastic change in weight, whether gain or loss, can indicate a health problem and needs to be followed up in a timely fashion.

Height is typically measured using a stadiometer or, particularly with extremely tall athletes, a tape measure fastened to the wall. The athlete removes shoes and stands with the back to the stadiometer or wall, placing all weight on the heels. When using a stadiometer, the athletic trainer stands at the side of the athlete and raises the stadiometer to the athlete's height. The horizontal arm rests at the crown of the athlete's head. The height measurement is read on the instrument's vertical scale (Figure 2-1, *A*). If not using a stadiometer,

the athletic trainer must accurately mark increments on the wall or fasten a tape measure to the wall. The athletic trainer stands to the side of the athlete (on a stool if necessary) and uses a flat surface on a sagittal plane along the crown of the athlete's head to evenly mark the height measurement on the wall (Figure 2-1, *B*). Height may be recorded in either centimeters or inches and should be indicated as such on the medical record (see Appendix C for a conversion chart).

Normal body weight is measured without shoes or excessive clothing. Weight is a confidential measurement, so the health care practitioner needs to ensure privacy for the athlete during weighing when possible. Weight is typically recorded in medical records in kilograms but may also be recorded in pounds (see Appendix D for a conversion chart showing pounds to kilograms). During preseason or excessively warm days, take weight measurements several times each day (preexercise and postexercise) to monitor proper hydration levels and prevent heat illnesses.[4,5] Standardization of measurements can be improved by following the same procedures each time height and weight are measured, for example, measuring both height and weight in the morning and having athletes wear a standard attire of gym shorts and T-shirt. More accurate

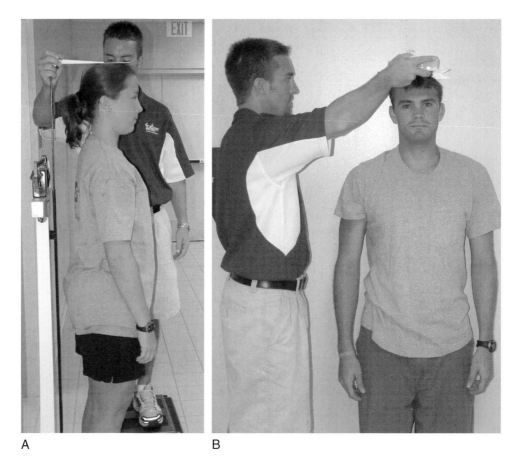

A   B

Figure 2-1 A, An athletic trainer measures the athlete's height with a stadiometer. B, The athletic trainer stands to the side of the athlete when measuring his height with a clipboard against the wall.

assessments of body composition exclusive of height and weight charts include hydrostatic weighing, skin-fold calipers, bioimpedance, and body mass index (BMI) (see Appendix E for a BMI chart).

Blood Pressure

A stethoscope and sphygmomanometer of the correct size will measure blood pressure properly (Key Points—Use of Blood Pressure Cuff). This is especially important for the athletic trainer, who often must evaluate extremely muscular or large athletes for whom a regular size blood pressure cuff is too small. Using a cuff that is too small results in a reading that is incorrect and abnormally too high. Normal resting blood pressure is measured after the athlete has been resting quietly for a period of time; it is never measured immediately following any exertion, such as practice or hurrying to an appointment.[6,7]

KEY POINTS
Use of Blood Pressure Cuff

- A blood pressure cuff that is too small should not be used.
- A cuff that is too small gives an abnormally high blood pressure reading.

The athlete is positioned in a quiet area with the selected arm free of clothing and positioned so that the brachial artery is roughly at heart level, which can be done by having the athlete rest the arm on a table next to the chair. The sphygmomanometer is placed around the upper arm with the lower end of the cuff about 2.5 cm above the antecubital crease (Figure 2-2). The cuff is snugly secured around the arm with the Velcro fasteners; and the aneroid dial is positioned toward the examiner. The diaphragm of the stethoscope is placed lightly over the brachial artery, touching the skin.

The cuff is inflated first to greater than 200 mm Hg and then gradually deflated at a rate of 2 to 3 mm Hg/sec. While deflating the cuff, the examiner listens for two consecutive beats, which will indicate the systolic pressure, and notes the numerical value when this occurs on the aneroid dial. The examiner continues deflating the blood pressure cuff slowly until the sound becomes muffled and finally disappears. The level at which the sound disappears is the diastolic pressure; this is often referred to as the fifth **Korotkoff sound** (the last of a series of sounds produced by distention of an artery by the cuff). Systolic pressure is related to the ventricles of the heart contracting, whereas diastolic pressure represents the relaxation phase of the ventricles. The effect of the cuff on arterial blood flow is related to the auscultatory findings (Box 2-2). Chapter 5 gives more details on cardiac output and blood pressure, and Table 2-1 shows normal and abnormal blood pressure readings for adults.

Pulse Rate and Rhythm

The examiner takes the heart rate by feeling the radial pulse with the pads of the index and middle fingers (Figure 2-3). Once the pulse is found, one counts the number of beats in 15 seconds and multiplies by 4 to estimate a normal regular heart beat (60 to 72 beats/min). The pulse is described by its rate, rhythm, and force (Box 2-3). The examiner notes any irregular rhythms and further evaluates by auscultating with the stethoscope at the cardiac apex,[3] keeping in mind that it is normal for athletes to have **bradycardia**, a pulse rate of 60 beats/min or less. The pulse is also easily palpable at the carotid artery, the posterior tibial artery, and other pulse points (Figure 2-4). Table 2-2 lists the location of palpable pulses. Pulse characteristics at the distal extremities give the examiner information about the status of blood flow to those extremities.

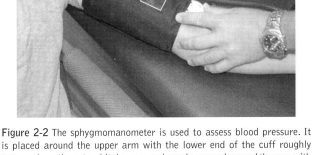

Figure 2-2 The sphygmomanometer is used to assess blood pressure. It is placed around the upper arm with the lower end of the cuff roughly 2.5 cm above the antecubital crease and snugly secured around the arm with the Velcro fasteners; the aneroid dial is positioned toward the examiner.

Table 2-1	American Heart Association Recommended Blood Pressure Levels*	
Blood Pressure	**Systolic (mm Hg)**	**Diastolic (mm Hg)**
Normal	<120	<80
Prehypertension	120-139	80-89
High Blood Pressure (Hypertension)		
Stage 1 (mild)	140-159	90-99
Stage 2 (moderate)	≥160	≥100
Severe	>180	>110

Modified from American Heart Association: What is high blood pressure? Available at www.americanheart.org/presenter.jhtml?identifier=2112. Accessed October 2004.
*A physician should evaluate low or high readings.

Box 2-2 Understanding Korotkoff Sounds When Assessing Blood Pressure

PHASE	QUALITY	DESCRIPTION	RATIONALE
Cuff correctly inflated	No sound		Cuff inflation compresses brachial artery. Cuff pressure exceeds heart's systolic pressure, occluding brachial artery blood flow.
I	Tapping	Soft, clear tapping, increasing in intensity	The SYSTOLIC pressure. As the cuff pressure lowers to reach intraluminal systolic pressure, the artery opens, and blood first spurts into the brachial artery. Blood is at very high velocity because of small opening of artery and large pressure difference across opening. This creates turbulent flow, which is audible.
Auscultatory gap*	No sound	Silence for 30–40 mm Hg	Sounds temporarily disappear during end of phase I, then reappear in phase II. Common with hypertension. If undetected, results in falsely low systolic or falsely high diastolic reading.
II	Swooshing	Softer murmur follows tapping	Turbulent blood flow through still partially occluded artery.
III	Knocking	Crisp, high-pitched sounds	Longer duration of blood flow through artery. Artery closes just briefly during late diastole.
IV	Abrupt muffling	Sound mutes to a low-pitched, cushioned murmur; blowing quality	Artery no longer closes in any part of cardiac cycle. Change in quality, not intensity.
V	Silence		Decreased velocity of blood flow, Streamlined blood flow is silent. The last audible sound (marking the disappearance of sounds) is DIASTOLIC pressure. The fifth Korotkoff sound is now used to define diastolic pressure in all age groups.

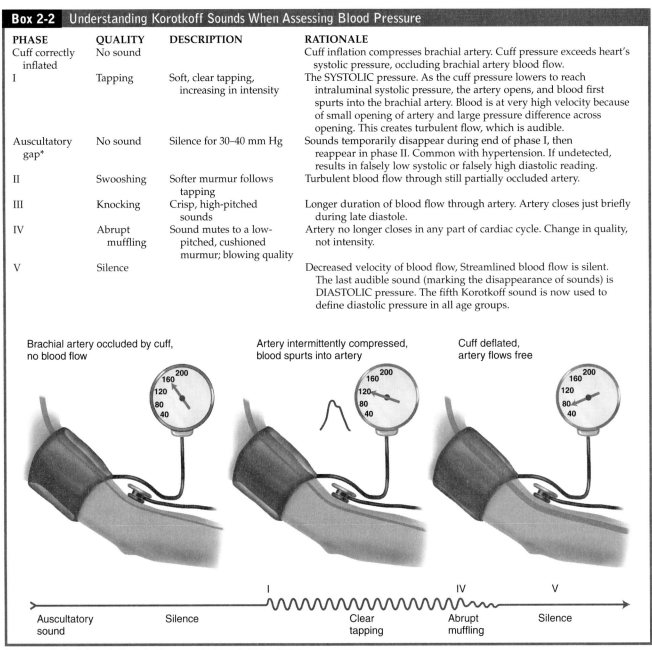

From Jarvis C: *Physical examination & health assessment*, ed 4, Philadelphia, 2004, Saunders, p 186.
*This is an abnormal finding.

Box 2-3 Pulse Rate, Rhythm, and Force

Rate
Bradycardia: <60 beats/min
Tachycardia: >100 beats/min

Rhythm
Sinus arrhythmia: heart rate speeds up at peak of inspiration and slows to normal with expiration

Force
4+:	Bounding
3+:	Increased
2+:	Normal
1+:	Weak, thready
0:	Absent

Respiratory Rate and Rhythm

Evaluation of respiration includes the rate, effort, and depth of inspiration as well as the ratio of inspirations to expirations. The rate is quantified by counting the number of respirations in 1 minute. Normal respiration rate for an adult is 12 to 20 breaths/min.[3] When assessing the rate, the examiner evaluates the athlete's effort by watching for symmetry and the use of accessory muscles (sternocleidomastoid, trapezius, intercostals) to assist in breathing.

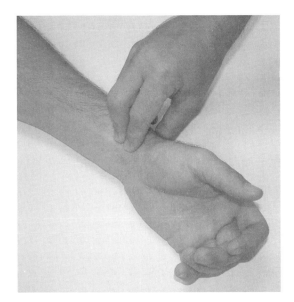

Figure 2-3 A pulse can be taken at the radial artery in the wrist.

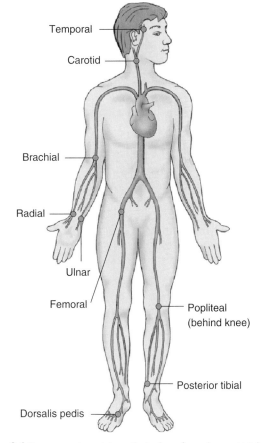

Figure 2-4 Common pulse points on the body surface where arterial pulses can be assessed. (From Monahan FD, Neighbors M: *Medical-surgical nursing: foundations in clinical practice,* ed 2, Philadelphia, 1998, WB Saunders.)

Temperature

Assessment of temperature can be omitted if there is no reason to suspect fever or heat-related illness. It may be wise, however, to record the temperature of any athlete presenting with a nonorthopedic complaint because temperature sometimes provides a defining clue to the severity of the condition. Normal temperature fluctuates considerably from the commonly reported oral temperature of 37° C (98.6° F); it may be as low as 35.8° C (96.4° F) in the early morning hours and as high as 37.3° C (99.1° F) in the evening (see Appendix F for Celsius to Fahrenheit conversion).[8] Rectal temperatures are higher than oral temperatures by 0.4° to 0.5° C, but this difference is also quite variable. In addition, athletes who have just finished a workout, recently experienced a heat modality (e.g., warm whirlpool or Hydrocollator), or drunk a hot beverage can present with a slightly elevated temperature.

It is important to maintain thermometer sanitation. Glass thermometers, although used less frequently today because of environmental concerns about mercury,[3] must be sanitized with either alcohol swabs or another approved cleaning medium. Electronic thermometers must be covered by single-use plastic covers to ensure sanitation, and tympanic thermometers likewise must have single-use protective covers.

Oral temperature can be measured by either a glass or electronic thermometer. Care must be taken with the glass thermometer to shake down the mercury to 35° C (96° F) or below before inserting it under the tongue; it needs to be left in place for 3 to 5 minutes for accurate measurement.

A plastic probe cover is always used on electronic thermometers. The examiner turns the unit on and places it under the patient's tongue; it generally takes

Table 2-2	Location of Palpable Pulses
Pulse	**Location**
Radial	Palpated with gentle pressure on the radial and ventral side of the wrist
Brachial	Palpated medial to the biceps tendon
Carotid	Palpated in the neck, medial and below the angle of the jaw
Popliteal	Palpated with a firm pressure in the popliteal fossa (posterior knee)
Posterior tibial	Palpated just posterior and inferior to the medial malleolus
Dorsalis pedis	Palpated on the medial side of the dorsum of the foot

Modified from Seidel HM, Ball JW, Dains JE, Benedict GWL: *Mosby's guide to physical examination,* ed 5, St Louis, 2003, Mosby, p 471.

only 10 seconds before beeping that an accurate reading is available (Figure 2-5).

The examiner measures rectal temperature if the patient is unconscious or suspected of having a heat-related illness to provide a better indicator of core temperature. The athlete is placed on the side with the hip flexed. A probe cover is used with an electronic

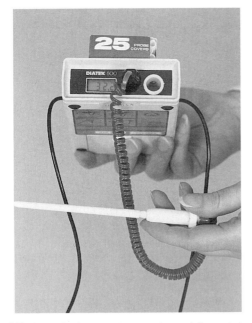

Figure 2-5 Electronic thermometers can be used for rectal, oral, or axillary temperature measurement; a probe cover is always used to ensure sanitation. (From Seidel HM, Ball JW, Dains JE, Benedict GW: *Mosby's guide to physical examination,* ed 5, St Louis, 2003, Mosby, p 59.)

rectal thermometer. The examiner lubricates the tip of the thermometer with petroleum jelly or KY jelly before inserting into the anal canal. Glass thermometers must remain in place for 3 minutes; electronic thermometers beep when ready, generally within 10 to 15 seconds.

Tympanic thermometers are increasingly common, are safe, and measure temperature very quickly. However, their reliability has been questioned especially in the athletic setting or in the assessment of heat-related illness. In suspected heat-related conditions, rectal temperature is the only current method shown to reliably measure core temperature (Key Points—Core Temperature).[5]

KEY POINTS
Core Temperature

- When assessing conditions of suspected heat illness, one should use a rectal thermometer.
- A rectal temperature is the only temperature measurement that has proven a reliable measure of core body temperature.

To use the tympanic thermometer, the examiner places the covered probe of the tympanic thermometer so that the beam has a direct route to the tympanic membrane (Figure 2-6). The auditory canal needs to be free from excessive cerumen. Within 2 to 3 seconds the tympanic temperature will register on the thermometer. Temperatures taken with the tympanic thermometer are generally 0.8° C (1.4° F) higher than normal oral temperatures.[3,7]

Another method sometimes used to measure temperature is the axillary method, in which a thermometer is placed in the axilla for 10 minutes. This method is not

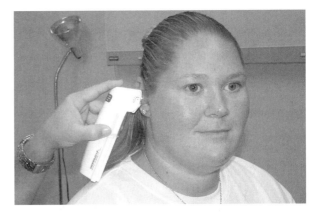

Figure 2-6 Tympanic thermometers are increasingly common, are safe, and measure temperature very quickly but may not be as reliable as electronic models for heat-related illnesses.

as accurate as either oral or rectal temperatures and is often as much as 1° F (or .5° C) lower than an oral temperature taken simultaneously.[9]

Evaluation Tools

Stethoscope

A good-quality acoustic stethoscope is sufficient for the athletic trainer to perform most examinations. More sophisticated stethoscopes (magnetic, electronic, stereophonic, or Doppler) are used by other medical specialists to auscultate less obvious sounds. An acoustic stethoscope contains a diaphragm and bell that are heavy enough to lay firmly on the body surface and thick, heavy tubing to conduct the sound.[7,10] Earpieces fit snugly and comfortably (Figure 2-7).

To correctly use the stethoscope, the examiner holds the end piece between the fingers, pressing the diaphragm (used for high-pitched sounds) firmly against the bare skin. When using the bell (for low-pitched sounds), the examiner holds it lightly on the skin to ensure that the entire bell is in contact with the skin. The tubing should not rub against itself or any other surface because extraneous noises will occur. Similarly, the environment must be quiet and free of noises. The examiner listens not only for the presence or absence of sound but also to its intensity, pitch, duration, and quality.[7]

Ophthalmoscope

The ophthalmoscope is an instrument used to view the internal structures of the eye (Figure 2-8). The head of the instrument contains a light source, which allows the examiner to visualize the inner eye through a series of lenses and apertures to allow for near or far focusing (Figure 2-9). The most commonly used aperture projects a large, round beam. Other apertures include the small aperture, the slit lamp aperture to examine

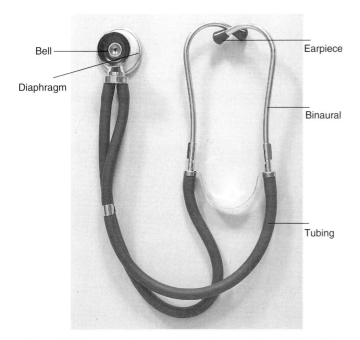

Figure 2-7 The parts of an acoustic stethoscope. (From Seidel HM, Ball JW, Dains JE, Benedict GW: *Mosby's guide to physical examination,* ed 5, St Louis, 2003, Mosby, p 66.)

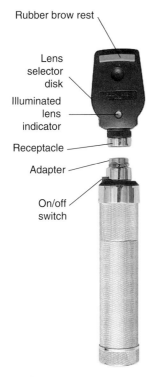

Figure 2-8 The parts of an ophthalmoscope. (From Seidel HM, Ball JW, Dains JE, Benedict GW: *Mosby's guide to physical examination,* ed 5, St Louis, 2003, Mosby, p 69.)

the anterior eye, the red-free filter aperture that shines a green beam to check the optic disc, and the grid aperture used to estimate size of fundal lesions.[7]

The diopter (magnification power of the lens) of the ophthalmoscope may be changed by turning the lens

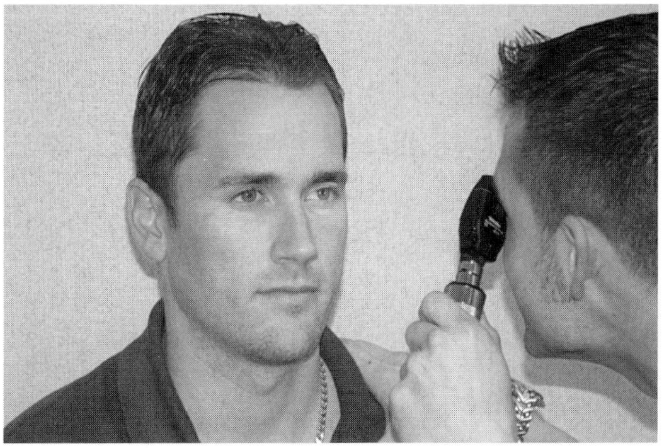

Figure 2-9 Athletic training students are encouraged to practice as much as possible with the ophthalmoscope because it takes considerable experience to be able to visualize the internal structures of the eye.

selector disk to the corresponding magnification.[3,7,8,11] The black numbers indicate positive magnification power, and the red numbers show the negative. Turning the wheel clockwise selects positive lenses, and rotating it counterclockwise selects negative lenses. Lens numbers range from +/−20 to +/−140 magnification power. The range of plus and minus lenses can compensate for myopia or hyperopia in both the examiner and the patient.[7] It is interesting to note that the abbreviations seen on a prescription for corrective lenses refer to the right and left eyes: oculus dexter (OD) to the right eye and oculus sinister (OS) to the left eye.

The heads of both the ophthalmoscope and the otoscope (used to view the ear and nose) typically share a common handle containing a rechargeable battery. The heads are interchangeable and can easily be converted from one instrument to the other. To change from an otoscope head to an ophthalmoscope head, the examiner pushes down on the head that is currently on the handle while turning to unlock the attachment, inserts the other head, and fastens it to the handle in the same manner.

Both instruments are turned on the same way, namely, by pushing the on/off switch while turning the black rheostat clockwise to the desired intensity of light.

Otoscope

The examiner visualizes the external auditory canal and tympanic membrane using an otoscope (Figure 2-10). As described previously, the otoscope usually shares the base and handle with the ophthalmoscope. The otoscope consists of a lamp to direct the light for illumination and disposable speculums, which protect it from contamination. The disposable speculums come in different sizes, and each is attached to the otoscope by placing it and then twisting clockwise approximately one-half turn to secure it on the instrument.

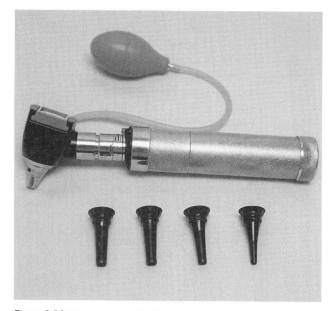

Figure 2-10 The otoscope, with different sizes of specula and a pneumatic attachment. The rechargeable base is often interchangeable with the ophthalmoscope. (From Seidel HM, Ball JW, Dains JE, Benedict GW: *Mosby's guide to physical examination,* ed 5, St Louis, 2003, Mosby, p 73.)

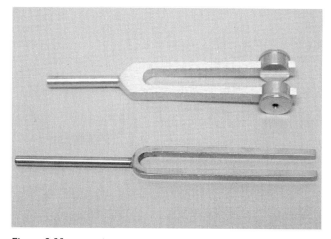

Figure 2-11 Tuning forks are used for assessment of vibratory sensations and screening for auditory perception. (From Seidel HM, Ball JW, Dains JE, Benedict GW: *Mosby's guide to physical examination,* ed 5, St Louis, 2003, Mosby, p 75.)

The instrument also has a viewing window that magnifies the area being visualized. Some otoscopes also contain a pneumatic attachment used to test the integrity of the tympanic membrane. In addition, the instrument can be used as a nasal speculum.

Tuning Fork

A tuning fork is used as a diagnostic tool for many different conditions. The most common uses are to check vibratory sensation or auditory sensitivity. A tuning fork with a frequency of 500 to 1000 Hz mimics the range of normal speech and is used for auditory evaluation.[12] The examiner squeezes the fork or taps the prongs against the opposite hand to activate it while holding the tuning fork at its base (Figure 2-11).

Snellen Chart

The Snellen chart is a quick and easy-to-use screening tool for far vision and is used most frequently during preparticipation exams to screen an athlete's vision. The chart contains graduated sizes of letters with standardized acuity numbers at the end of each line (Figure 2-12). The athlete is asked to read the lines of the chart while standing 20 feet away and covering one eye. The number corresponding to the row of smallest letters the athlete can read measures visual acuity. Although the athlete is allowed to err in calling out a particular number or letter, two wrong answers on a line indicate inability to correctly read at that distance. Visual acuity is recorded as a fraction with

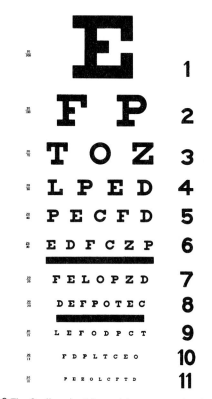

Figure 2-12 The Snellen chart is used to measure visual acuity. (From Palay DA, Krachmer JH: *Ophthalmology for the primary care practitioner,* St Louis, 1998, Mosby.)

the numerator of 20 indicating the distance away from the chart and the denominator being the distance from which a person with normal vision could read the lettering.[13] A measurement of 20/20 is considered normal vision, with denominators larger than 20 indicating poorer vision. A person with a measurement of 20/200 is considered legally blind. One must remember that this is a screening tool for far visual acuity only and does not measure near vision or dynamic visual acuity. Referring an athlete to an optometrist or ophthalmologist for a complete visual assessment may be warranted. An athlete who normally wears corrective lenses is screened without those corrective lenses and the results of the exam are noted as being without corrective lenses. Near vision is assessed using the Rosenbaum or Jaeger charts or a newspaper.[8]

Diagnostic Tests

Many common diagnostic tests are used to confirm specific conditions. An athletic trainer needs to be familiar with these tests, what they are used for, and what the results indicate. Common imaging techniques are described in Table 2-3. Two of the most traditional laboratory exams, urinalysis (UA) and complete blood count (CBC), are discussed below.

Urinalysis

Athletic trainers rarely perform laboratory tests with the possible exception of Chemstrips, but they do need to appreciate the normal values of these examinations. Throughout this text, the abnormal values of common tests and what they indicate in a specific condition or disease are discussed. Here, emphasis is on the common normal values found in urinalysis and CBC.

A UA is performed if the practitioner has reason to suspect a malady in the kidneys and urinary system. In the athletic environment, this may be a simple dipstick in a container of urine if **hematuria** is suspected. These dipsticks or Chemstrips are flexible coated paper with multiple test components on each stick; they are dipped into collected urine and subsequently held to a chart on the bottle's label to see if the color reaction matches a given component of urine. Common assessments check pH, red blood cells (a sign of injury), white blood cells (a sign of infection), glucose, specific gravity, and protein values. The bottle containing the sticks is dark in color to prevent light from penetrating and altering the sticks' reliability; it must be tightly sealed to preserve the reactive chemicals on each stick. The side of the bottle is labeled with a chart for each value (i.e., blood or pH) with associated color squares that indicate the amount or level of the value (Figure 2-13). Each value has a specific time frame for correct reaction response, typically from immediately to 2 minutes, and it is important to read the stick within the allotted time frame to obtain accurate results.

A physician may order an UA for various reasons. The presence of blood in the urine (e.g., hematuria) can indicate a kidney injury or occur benignly after an intense workout. The color of urine can reveal dehydration or may be the by-product of certain medications. Normally glucose is not present in the urine unless high levels exist in the body,[14] which might indicate diabetes. The presence of ketones also can reveal diabetes or a fasting athlete. The pH refers to the acidity or alkaline levels of the urine[8]; a higher acid reading can be found with diabetes or dehydration, whereas an alkaline reading indicates infections in the kidney or urinary tract.[15,16]

Specific gravity in urine indicates its concentration and attests to the athlete's hydration levels as well as the kidney's ability to process fluids.[15] Urine tests can also indicate drug use, electrolyte levels, and the presence

Table 2-3	Common Imaging Techniques	
Test	**Description**	**Type of Tissue**
Magnetic resonance imaging (MRI)	Uses radio frequency to view structures; considered superior to CT for central nervous system (CNS) tissues	CNS, organs, soft tissue, cartilage
Computed tomography (CT)	Provides cross sections of tissues 100× more sensitive than radiographs	Soft tissues, stress fractures, tumors, bleeding
Myelogram	Radiograph taken of a given area following a radiopaque injection that allows for illumination of specific structures	Spinal cord, meninges, specific cells in bone marrow
Radiograph	Picture using high-speed electrons that can penetrate most objects	Bony structure integrity, certain masses and tumors
Electrocardiogram (ECG)	A record of the heart's electrical activity	Heart
Bone scan	CT performed of a given area following a radiopaque injection that allows for illumination of specific structures	Stress fractures, osteoarthritis, bone activity levels
Mammogram	A radiograph of the soft tissues of the breast	Breast tissue, certain masses
Colonoscopy	Visualization into the colon	Colon
Endoscopy	Visualization into a specific body cavity	Bronchoscope (upper respiratory) Laparoscope (abdomen) Gastroscope (upper gastrointestinal)
Venogram, phlebogram	A radiograph of a vein is taken following injection of a radiopaque injection into the vein	Veins

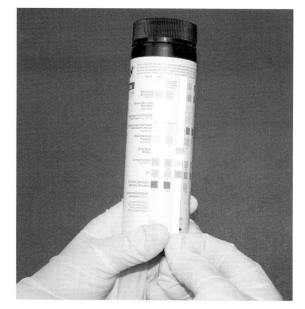

Figure 2-13 The label on the Chemstrip bottle can be used to assess strips for results of urinalysis.

Table 2-4	Normal Values for Urine
Color	Light yellow to amber
pH	Acidic
Specific gravity	1.003-1.030
Red blood cells	<5/HPF
White blood cells	<5/HPF
Protein	Negative
Glucose	Negative
Ketones	Negative
Nitrites	Negative
Casts	None
Crystals	None

From Copstead LEC, Banasik JL: *Pathophysiology: biological and behavioral perspectives,* ed 2, Philadelphia, 2000, WB Saunders, p 644.
HPF, High-powered field.

of infection. Collected urine should be refrigerated if it will not be assessed within 1 hour. Normal values for urine are found in Table 2-4.

Complete Blood Count

Human blood is composed of 52% to 62% plasma and 38% to 48% cells.[17] A typical adult has about 5 L of blood, which is typed A, B, or O, and Rh positive or negative.

Blood plasma is largely water; the three chief cell components are erythrocytes (red blood cells [RBCs]), leukocytes (white blood cells [WBCs]), and thrombocytes (platelets). Leukocytes are further divided into five types of cells: neutrophils, basophils, lymphocytes, monocytes, and eosinophils.[17] The function of RBCs is to carry oxygen to working tissues, whereas the WBCs

Table 2-5	Complete Blood Count (CBC) Normal Values
Component	**Normal Range**
WBC count	$3.8\text{-}10.8 \times 10^3/\mu l$
WBC differential: absolute neutrophils	1500-7800 cells /µl
WBC differential: absolute eosinophils	50-550 cells/µl
WBC differential: absolute basophils	0-200 cells/µl
WBC differential: absolute lymphocytes	850-4100 cells/µl
WBC differential: absolute monocytes	200-1100 cells/µl
RBC count	Males: $4.4\text{-}5.8 \times 10^6/\mu l$ Females: $3.9\text{-}5.2 \times 10^6/\mu l$
RBC MCV	78-102 fl
RBC mean corpuscular Hb	27-33 pg
RBC mean corpuscular Hb concentration	32-36 g/dl
RBC distribution width	≤15%
Hb	Males: 13.8-17.2 g/dl Females: 12.0-15.6 g/dl
Hct	Males: 41%-50% Females: 35%-46%

Data from Noble J: *Textbook of primary care medicine,* ed 3, St Louis, 2001, Mosby; Bickley LS, Szilagyi PG: *Bate's guide to physical examination and history taking,* ed 8, Philadelphia, 2003, Lippincott Williams & Wilkins; *Mosby's medical, nursing & allied health dictionary,* ed 3, St Louis, 2002, Mosby.
WBC, White blood cell; *RBC,* red blood cell; *MCV,* mean corpuscular volume; *Hb,* hemoglobin; *Hct,* hematocrit.

primarily fight invasion of unrecognized or foreign elements in the body.

A CBC is a laboratory work-up on a blood sample. It looks for specific components in designated units (per microliter [µl]) of whole blood.[14] It can indicate the overall health of a person and provide information regarding the ratios of cells per microliter of blood. A CBC does not typically furnish information on cell shape or blood type (i.e., ABO). Table 2-5 shows normal CBC values for adults.

In addition to a simple count of blood cells, the CBC also provides information about hemoglobin (i.e., iron) and hematocrit (volume of cells to plasma). Abnormal blood values indicate a variety of conditions described in subsequent chapters. Common disorders such as anemia can be present when hemoglobin or hematocrit levels are low. High WBC counts can indicate infections ranging from a skin infection to mononucleosis to leukemia; low RBCs and platelets can be caused by internal bleeding.

Evaluation Techniques

Neurological Testing

Neurological tests provide information about sensory, motor, and deep tendon reflexes, which may indicate pathology associated with the central nervous system

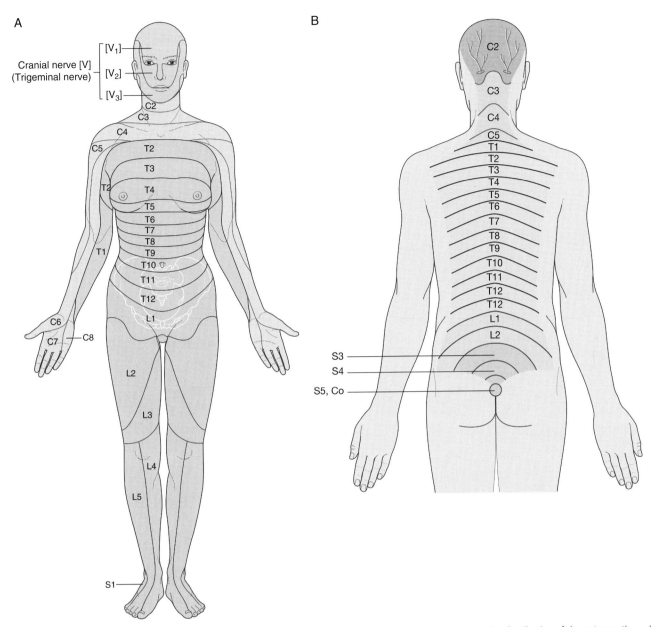

Figure 2-14 Dermatomes are the areas of the skin supplied by a single nerve or nerve root. The illustration shows the distribution of dermatomes through the body. **A,** Anterior view. **B,** Posterior view. (From Drake RL, Vogl W, Mitchell AW: Gray's anatomy for students, Philadelphia, 2005, Churchill Livingstone, pp 22, 25.)

or peripheral nerve trauma. The examiner performs neurological testing whenever an athlete complains of paresthesia, heightened sensations, or muscular weakness.

A dermatome is a specific area of skin innervated by a dorsal or sensory nerve root. These areas tend to make a circular pattern over the body and are associated with very specific nerve roots (Figure 2-14). Myotomes are a single muscle or group of muscles innervated by a single ventral or motor nerve.[3] A detailed description of dermatome and myotome evaluation is found in Chapter 8.

A deep tendon reflex (DTR) is an involuntary motor reaction to a stimulus. This reflex depends on several conditions, beginning with the hammer stimulus.

The dorsal fibers of sensory nerves transmit impulses from the hammer tap on the stretched tendon to sensory receptors in the muscle and along to the spinal cord. In the gray matter of the spinal cord, a reflex action can occur if the dorsal fibers synapse with the ventral or motor fibers, which in turn travel back to stimulate the muscle to contract (Figure 2-15). This reflex will not occur if the athlete's synapses are not functioning correctly, there is damage or disease to either dorsal or ventral nerve fibers, or there is an incongruent muscle. The instruments used to test these pathological conditions are called the reflex or neurological hammer. When doing a neurological assessment of an individual, it is important to test bilaterally to note any response differences.

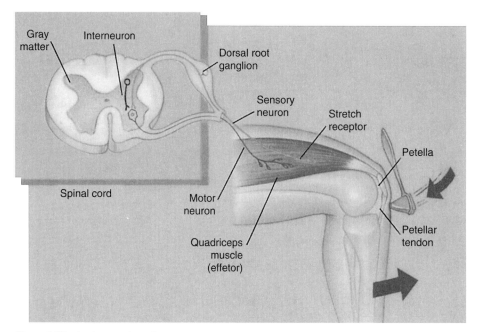

Figure 2-15 The deep tendon reflex arc. (From Thibodeau GA, Patton KT: *Anatomy and physiology,* ed 5, St Louis, 2003, Mosby.)

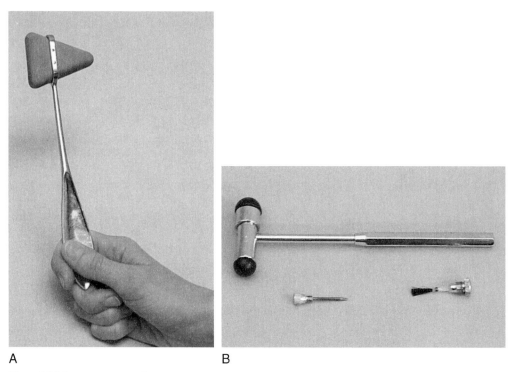

A   B

Figure 2-16 A, Reflex hammer. **B,** Neurological hammer. (From Seidel HM, Ball JW, Dains JE, Benedict GW: *Mosby's guide to physical examination,* ed 5, St Louis, 2003, Mosby, pp 76-77.)

Reflex and Neurological Hammers

The reflex hammer is commonly used to test DTRs. The examiner holds it loosely between the thumb and index finger (Figure 2-16, *A*). The wrist is snapped rapidly downward when striking the tendon to elicit the best reflex response. Common locations for DTRs are the insertion of the biceps brachii, distal triceps tendon, distal brachioradialis tendon, patella tendon, and Achilles tendon. The ulnar aspect of the hand or the fingertips can provide the same effect and be used in place of the hammer when necessary. DTRs have a common rating scale for responses (Table 2-6). When using the reflex hammer, the examiner places the athlete in a relaxed position (sitting is best) and provides slight tension on the tendon to be tested. The tendon should be palpated first to make certain to strike it correctly rather than the muscle.

A neurological hammer is a reflex hammer that also includes a brush and a sharp implement to use when eliciting the sensations a patient can feel, thereby assessing the integrity of dermatomes (Figure 2-16, *B*). Athletes close their eyes during the test. This ensures a non-discriminatory assessment because the athletes cannot witness the application of the tool. The pointed end of the tool is used to lightly depress the skin over a given dermatome, and the athletes are asked if they perceive any sensation; the same dermatome on the contralateral side is then tested. Care must be taken when using the sharp implement to prevent puncturing the skin. Likewise, the brush is used to lightly brush a specific area and then test with the same sensation to the opposite limb. Other instruments that can provide a sharp, dull, and brushing effect can be used to conduct these sensory tests.

When assessing myotomes, the examiner asks the athlete to move and then resist a given muscle group. The examiner then compares bilaterally. Tests of dermatomes and myotomes are common in orthopedic assessment and are used in many neurological assessments as well.

Cranial Nerve Assessment

Cranial nerve assessment is another area of testing valuable to the athletic trainer. When an athlete has a suspected head injury, evaluation of these nerves is critical. Familiarity with their source and function is also important to numerous neurological conditions. Table 2-7 provides an overview of these critical nerves, and Chapter 8 covers the neurological system in depth.

Palpation

Palpation involves the use of the hands and fingers to gain information about a patient's condition through the sense of touch. The athletic trainer typically is proficient in palpation of orthopedic conditions and can gain valuable information about general medical conditions through the use of systematic palpation. The athletic trainer uses the fingertips for palpation during the general medical exam to feel for texture and quality of the skin as well as temperature, underlying masses, rigidity, fluid, or crepitus. The ulnar surface to the hand should be used to palpate vibrations during inspiration or expiration because it is more sensitive (Figure 2-17) whereas the dorsal surface of the hand is best for estimating temperature.

Palpation may be done with one hand or bimanually with both hands. The examiner uses palpation with or after visual inspection, except when assessing the abdomen where palpation is completed after auscultation. Light palpation is performed at a depth of approximately 1 cm and is useful for feeling skin and underlying tissue. Light palpation always is done before deep palpation. It helps the examiner to gain

Table 2-6 Deep Tendon Reflex Grades

Grade	Response
0	No reflex
1	Sluggish muscle
2	Active or expected response
3	Slightly hyperactive
4	Brisk, hyperactive with intermittent or transient clonus

From Seidel HM, Ball JW, Dains JE, Benedict GW: *Mosby's guide to physical examination*, ed 5, St Louis, 2003, Mosby, p 798.

Table 2-7 Cranial Nerve Function

Source	Nerve	Sense	System
CN I	Olfactory nerve	Smell	Sensory
CN II	Optic nerve	Vision	Sensory
CN III	Oculomotor	Extraocular muscle movement Pupillary light reflex	Motor
CN IV	Trochlear nerve	Extraocular (upward) muscle movement	Motor
CN V	Trigeminal nerve	Muscles of mastication	Sensory/motor
CN VI	Abducens nerve	Extraocular (lateral) muscle movement	Motor
CN VII	Facial nerve	Muscles of facial expression Taste Tears and saliva	Sensory/motor
CN VIII	Vestibulocochlear nerve	Balance Hearing	Sensory
CN IX	Glossopharyngeal nerve	Taste Sensation of the mouth	Sensory/motor
CN X	Vagus nerve	Swallowing Gag reflex	Motor Sensory
CN XI	Spinal accessory nerve	Sternocleidomastoid, trapezius movement	Motor
CN XII	Hypoglossal nerve	Tongue movement	Motor

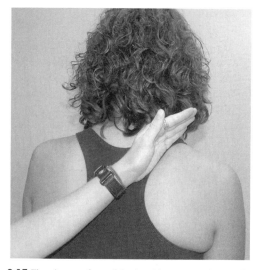

Figure 2-17 The ulnar surface of the hand is most sensitive in feeling the vibrations during inspiration and expiration.

the patient's trust, identify areas of tenderness, and establish a systematic method of palpation from superficial to deep tissues. Deep palpation may approach 4 cm and must be done carefully because it may elicit tenderness or disrupt underlying tissue (Figure 2-18). It is important that the patient be relaxed during palpation because muscle guarding, especially of the abdominal region, will prevent the clinician from obtaining significant information from the examination. The patient is draped with consideration given to privacy and modesty, and only the area being palpated is exposed.

Percussion

Percussion is the process of assessing sounds transmitted through the organs and cavities of the body and is generated by tapping. It involves striking one object (fingers or hand) against another to produce vibrations and subsequent sound waves. The techniques of percussion are the same regardless of the structure being percussed and include either direct or indirect percussion.

Direct percussion involves lightly striking the chest or abdominal wall with the ulnar aspect of the fist. Indirect percussion involves the finger of one hand acting as the hammer, striking the finger of the other hand that is resting on the body part being percussed (Figure 2-19). The striking action creates a vibration or resonance that with training and practice can be identified and quantified.

Practice is necessary to become proficient with percussion technique. The downward snap of the striking finger originates from the wrist and not the forearm or shoulder. The tap is sharp and rapid with the tip of the finger not the pad. The ulnar surface of the fist may also be used for percussion and is generally used to elicit tenderness over solid organs, such as the liver or kidneys.

Percussion-generated sounds may be recognized by different characteristics, including intensity, pitch, and location. The general percussion tone over air is loud, over fluid it is less loud, and over solid areas it is soft.[7] Common sounds produced by percussion are listed in Table 2-8. It is often difficult to quantify percussion tones, especially for the novice examiner. The examiner should practice identifying tones from various parts of the body to learn how to quantify them, specifically noting the change from one tone to another when moving from percussing a known air-filled body part, such as the lungs, to the abdomen or a muscle.

Auscultation

Auscultation is the skilled listening by a trained ear for sounds produced by the body. Most body sounds,

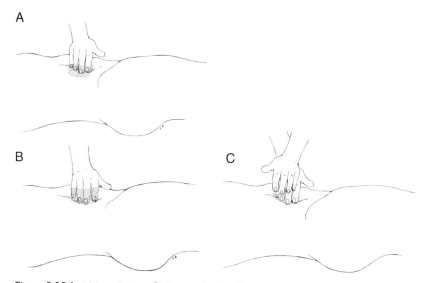

Figure 2-18 A, Light palpation. **B,** Deep palpation. **C,** Bimanual palpation. (From Potter PA, Weilitz PB: *Pocket guide to health assessment,* St Louis, 2003, Mosby, p 40.)

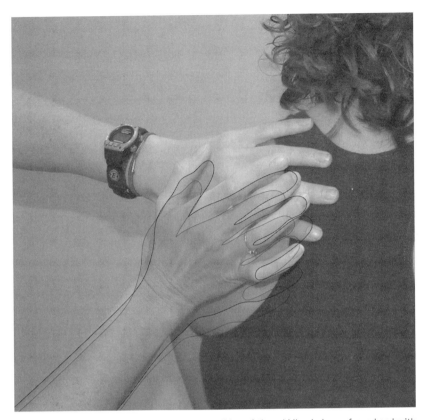

Figure 2-19 Indirect percussion involves the striking of the middle phalanx of one hand with the tip of the index or middle fingers of the opposite hand to elicit sounds over various structures of the chest and abdomen. The illustration shows the repetitive movement of the fingertip of the middle finger of the right hand against the middle finger of the left hand.

Table 2-8	Sounds Produced by Percussion				
Sound	Intensity	Pitch	Duration	Quality	Common Location
Tympany	Loud	High	Moderate	Drumlike	Enclosed, air-containing space
Resonance	Moderate to loud	Low	Long	Hollow	Normal lung
Hyperresonance	Very loud	Very low	Longer than resonance	Booming	Emphysematous lung
Dullness	Soft to moderate	High	Moderate	Thudlike	Liver
Flatness	Soft	High	Short	Flat	Muscle

From Potter PA, Weilitz PB: *Pocket guide to health assessment*, St Louis, 2003, Mosby, p 43.

including the heart, lung, and bowel, are not audible without the use of a stethoscope. Auscultation takes practice so that the sounds can be identified and isolated from each other.

Certain basic principles apply to auscultation regardless of the system being examined:

- Perform auscultation after history, observation, and palpation in order to gather as much information as possible from other sources first.
- Perform auscultation in a quiet environment.
- Listen for the presence or absence of sounds as well as their frequency, loudness, quality, and duration.
- Make sure the earpieces of the stethoscope fit comfortably following the angles of the ear canal.

- Point the earpieces of the stethoscope toward the face.

As mentioned previously, auscultation of the abdomen is done before palpation.

The examiner uses the part of the stethoscope that best relays the pitch of the sound sought. The diaphragm is used for high-pitched sounds, such as bowel, lung, and normal heart sounds, whereas the bell is used for low-pitched sounds (Key Points—Using a Stethoscope).[3]

KEY POINTS
Using a Stethoscope

- The bell is used to hear low-pitched sounds.
- The diaphragm is used to hear high-pitched sounds.

Abnormal heart and vascular sounds have a lower pitch and may be heard better by the bell.[10] Table 2-9 describes common characteristics of sounds heard during auscultation. Specific placement of the stethoscope for auscultation of lung, heart, and bowel sounds is discussed in chapters covering respiratory, cardiac, and gastrointestinal disorders.

Table 2-9	Characteristics of Sound
Characteristic	**Description**
Frequency	Number of sound wave cycles generated per second by a vibrating object. The higher the frequency, the higher the pitch of a sound and vice versa.
Loudness	Amplitude of a sound wave. Auscultated sounds are described as *loud* or *soft*.
Quality	Sounds of similar frequency and loudness from different sources. Terms such as *blowing* or *gurgling* describe quality of sound.
Duration	Length of time sound vibrations last. Duration of sound is *short*, *medium*, or *long*.

From Potter PA, Weilitz PB: *Pocket guide to health assessment*, St Louis, 2003, Mosby, p 46.

WEB RESOURCES

Medem Medical Library—part of the Medem network
http://www.medem.com/MedLB/articleslb.cfm?sub_cat=554
An online source of comprehensive, peer-reviewed health care information for practitioners as well as easy-to-understand patient handouts

Virtual Hospital sponsored by the University of Iowa
http://www.vh.org/
The user can search for a topic in this indexed digital database; information on many medical disorders

Medline Plus
http://www.nlm.nih.gov/medlineplus/medlineplus.html
A gateway to refereed articles through Medline as well as pictures, medical encyclopedias, and dictionaries; useful for all medical conditions

A Practical Guide to Clinical Medicine—University of California San Diego School of Medicine
http://medicine.ucsd.edu/clinicalmed/links.html
A comprehensive physical examination and clinical education site for medical students and other health care professionals; offers medical examination information for the major systems of the body; has many links to pictures and videos

Merck Medicus
http://www.merckmedicus.com/pp/us/hcp/hcp_home.jsp
Links to medical sources on the Internet; links to medical libraries, presentations, *The Merck Manual*, drug references, and patient handouts

WebMD and Medscape from WebMD
http://www.webmd.com/
http://www.medscape.com/px/urlinfo
General information aimed at the patient on numerous medical conditions; Medscape gives more specific information

SUMMARY

An athletic trainer must be comfortable with general examination techniques in order to differentiate among the many disorders discussed in this text and to provide the best possible care for athletes. The athletic trainer is often the first person the athlete approaches with a medical complaint. The examination begins with a thorough history of the chief complaint followed by pertinent history of other conditions, personal health history, and family health history. The athletic trainer then observes or inspects the problem area for changes in color, deformity, and swelling. Palpation follows to determine delicate differences in temperature, texture, and pliability of the skin.

Many techniques discussed in this chapter, such as palpation, percussion, and auscultation, are important skills for the athletic trainer to master but take considerable practice. Although athletic trainers do not actually perform diagnostic laboratory tests nor order them, it also is important that they understand what each test does and are familiar with normative values for each test.

REFERENCES

1. Noble J: *Textbook of primary care medicine*, ed 3, St Louis, 2001, Mosby.
2. Rakel RE: *Saunders manual of medical practice*, ed 2, Philadelphia, 2000, WB Saunders.
3. Jarvis C: *Physical examination & health assessment*, ed 4, Philadelphia, 2004, WB Saunders.
4. Binkley H, Beckett J, Casa D, et al: National Athletic Trainers' Association position statement: exertional heat illnesses, *Journal of Athletic Training* 37(3):329-343, 2002.
5. National Athletic Trainers' Association (NATA): *Heat illness task force*, Dallas, 2003, NATA.
6. Anderson MK, Hall SJ, Martin M: *Foundations of athletic training: prevention, assessment, and management*, ed 3, Philadelphia, 2004, Lippincott Williams & Wilkins.
7. Seidel HM, Ball JW, Dains JE, Benedict GW: *Mosby's guide to physical examination*, ed 5, St Louis, 2003, Mosby.
8. Bickley LS, Szilagyi PG: *Bate's guide to physical examination and history taking*, ed 8, Philadelphia, 2003, Lippincott Williams & Wilkins.
9. Dinarello C, Gelfand JA: Fever and hyperthermia. In Braunwald E, Fauci AS, Isselbacher KJ, et al, editors: *Harrison's manual of medicine*, ed 15, Boston, 2003, McGraw-Hill.
10. Potter PA, Weilitz PB: *Pocket guide to health assessment*, ed 5, St Louis, 2003, Mosby.
11. Bradford CA: *Basic ophthalmology for medical students and primary care residents*, San Francisco, 1999, American Academy of Ophthalmology.
12. Epstein O, Perkin GD, Cookson J, de Bono DP: *Clinical examination*, ed 3, St Louis, 2003, Mosby.
13. Dorman K, Mishriki Y: Primary care of the eye. In Noble J, editor: *Textbook of primary care medicine*, ed 3, St Louis, 2001, Mosby, pp 1629-1663.

14. Beers M, Berkow R, editors: *The Merck manual of diagnosis and therapy*, ed 17, Whitehouse Station, NJ, 1999, Merck Research Laboratories.
15. Prentice W: *Arnheim's principles of athletic training*, ed 11, Boston, 2003, McGraw-Hill.
16. Delmez J, Windus D: Generalist's guide to diagnostic tests. In Noble J, editor: *Textbook of primary care medicine*, ed 3, Philadelphia, 2001, Mosby, pp 1343-1352.
17. Thomas C, editor: *Taber's cyclopedic medical dictionary*, Philadelphia, 1997, FA Davis.

CHAPTER 3

Basic Principles of Pharmacology

Dorraine Reynolds and
Micki Cuppett

OBJECTIVES

At the completion of this chapter, the reader should be able to do the following:
1. Describe the basics of pharmaceutics and pharmacokinetics including dosage forms, routes of administration, and drug storage.
2. Access various drug information resources to obtain more information about a drug.
3. List the basic drug classifications, their indications, their contraindications, and their typical use.

INTRODUCTION

This chapter introduces the reader to the regulatory, pharmacological, and pharmaceutical information that athletic trainers must be familiar with and understand. Important regulatory agencies discussed in relation to athletic trainers include the Food and Drug Administration (FDA), the Drug Enforcement Administration (DEA), and the National Collegiate Athletic Association (NCAA). The basic principles of pharmacology cover pharmacokinetics, routes of administration, drug storage and resources, pharmacodynamics, indications and contraindications, and special considerations for athletes. Content about pharmaceuticals is organized by drug categories and identifies available drug forms and dosages, routes of administration, correct methods for storage of specific drugs, and side effects. Drug information resources also are reviewed and include web-based and personal digital assistant (PDA) options. This chapter is designed as an overview and lists additional sources for continued reading and expanded content.

REGULATION OF PHARMACEUTICALS

It is important for athletic trainers to understand the legal regulations that apply to the use of medications. Two entities of the U.S. federal government are charged to control the use of pharmaceutical products: the Food and Drug Administration (FDA) and the Drug Enforcement Administration (DEA). The equivalent agency in Canada to the FDA is the Canadian Health Products Food Branch (HPFB). The HPFB is responsible for regulating food and health products, including pharmaceuticals, biological agents, and genetic therapies.[1] The HPFB is one of six branches of Health Canada, which all report to the deputy and associate deputy ministers of health.

Drug Enforcement Administration

The DEA lies within the Department of Justice. Its function is to ensure compliance with the Controlled Substances Act of 1970 and implement the regulations found in Title 21, Code of Federal Regulations, Part 1300 to the end. The DEA registers health care practitioners who will be prescribing or dispensing those drugs that are considered controlled substances and advises them on how to comply with controlled substance regulations.

Controlled substances are drugs that have a high potential for abuse (e.g., morphine, codeine). The DEA has established five categories or "schedules" of controlled substances (I-V). Table 3-1 lists drugs that are classified as controlled substances and are placed into one of these five categories on the basis of their likelihood for abuse.

Table 3-1	Drug Enforcement Administration Schedules of Controlled Substances	
Schedule	**Description**	**Examples of Drugs***
I	Drugs with no accepted medical use in the United States High abuse potential	Opium Hallucinogens (heroin, LSD, mescaline) Marijuana
II	Drugs with a high abuse potential Severe psychic or physical dependence liability Tightly controlled prescribing requirements including written prescription (NO verbal orders) from physician No refills without additional prescription from physician	Morphine Cocaine Oxycodone Oxycodone combination products (Percocet) Methamphetamine
III	Drugs with less abuse potential than those in schedule I or II Contain limited quantities of narcotic or nonnarcotic ingredients	Benzphetamine Stimulants Depressants Clortermine Narcotic drugs Anabolic steroids
IV	Drugs with less abuse potential than those in schedule III	Barbital Phenobarbital Oxazepam
V	Drugs with less abuse potential than those in schedule IV Class consists of preparations containing limited quantities of certain narcotic ingredients generally for antitussive and antidiarrheal purposes	<200 mg of codeine or opium per 100 g

LSD, Lysergic acid diethylamide.
*Examples of drugs in each schedule are not an all-inclusive list.

Food and Drug Administration

The FDA is an agency of the Department of Health and Human Services. Its mission is to "promote and protect the public health by helping safe and effective products reach the market in a timely way and to monitor products for continued safety after they a re in use."[2]

The FDA is responsible for approving manufacturers who may produce medications for consumption, the approval of new chemical formulations for marketing and sale as either prescription or nonprescription such as over-the-counter products, and the approval of generic drug products that must exhibit the bioequivalence to a brand-name product (Key Points—Bioequivalence).

KEY POINTS
Bioequivalence

Bioequivalence is the quality of having the same drug strength and providing an equivalent amount of drug to the target tissue in the same dosage form as another sample of a given drug substance. For example, for two drugs to be considered bioequivalent, they must meet the following criteria:
• Have the same dosage form (e.g., tablet, suspension)
• Have the same drug strength
• Provide equivalent blood levels or tissue levels of the drug

The FDA is also charged with determining how drugs may be marketed and sold in the United States, including the drug's indications, information contained in the product's package insert, and how the drug is manufactured. Pharmaceutical product manufacturers must meet very stringent manufacturing guidelines and pass FDA inspections. The drug products that they produce must consistently pass dissolution and bioequivalence tests. It is important to remember that the FDA does not oversee the marketing or sale of food supplements and herbal products, many of which are used by athletes, and neither does any other government agency.

Administration Versus Dispensing

Most states regulate both administering and dispensing drugs. It is important that the athletic trainer understand the differences between these two actions. Dispensing is the act of delivering a medication to an ultimate user pursuant to a medical order issued by a practitioner authorized to prescribe. This includes the packaging, labeling, or compounding necessary to prepare the medication for such delivery. A facility that dispenses prescription medication must have a separate DEA certification.[3] Administration is the act of applying a medication by injection, inhalation, ingestion, or any other means to the body of a patient in a single dose (Key Points—Administration Versus Dispensing).[4]

Both dispensing and administration require a written prescription from a physician. Dispensing medications is beyond the scope of the athletic training profession. It is important, however, that the athletic training facility comply with both state and federal regulations governing prescription medications. Most states require that an athletic training facility has a DEA certificate and a signed agreement with a physician in cases in which medical staff serve as an "agency" in the care of the physician's patients. In these situations, the athletic trainer is acting as an agent assigned by the DEA and is not acting under the scope of the state practice acts for athletic trainers; at no time does the agent make any discretionary decisions about the administration or dosage of a medication. Companies such as SportPharm, Inc. are used by several major colleges and universities as well as by professional athletic teams to help ensure compliance with these regulations.[3] The 50 states have different legislation about administration and dispensing of medications. The athletic trainer, team physician, and team pharmacist must work together to ensure that state and federal regulations are being met.

PHARMACOLOGY

Pharmacology is the science of drugs and includes pharmacokinetics and pharmacodynamics. **Pharmacodynamics** is the study of the actions of the drug on the body, including mechanism of action and medicinal effect (i.e., the biochemical and physiological effects of the drug). This may involve a stimulatory or inhibitory reaction at the receptor type. **Pharmacokinetics,** on the other hand, is the study of how the body acts on the drug. Pharmacokinetics includes the absorption, distribution, metabolism, and elimination of the drug in the body.

To better understand how drugs work within the body, it is important to know the process by which a drug gets into the body, is distributed, is metabolized, and finally is eliminated from the body. The methods of absorption, distribution, metabolism, and elimination (Key Points—Pharmacokinetics) are discussed here.

Absorption is the process of getting the drug into the body. Drugs may be absorbed through various routes including rectal, intestinal, and dermal tissue. Which route is used depends on many different patient-related and drug-related factors. The age, level of consciousness, and disease being treated are patient-related considerations; drug-related factors include solubility and stability. The desired route of absorption will

determine the formulation used; a rectal absorption will generally indicate using a suppository, but tablets, capsules, liquids, and suspensions may also be absorbed rectally.

Absorption is a major influence on the bioavailability of a drug. The bioavailability of a drug describes how much of the drug is available to the tissues after its administration. Bioavailability is an important concept in drug development, especially as it pertains to generic drugs. In order for any generic drug to be considered equivalent to a brand-name preparation, it must be demonstrated to have bioavailability that is equal to the brand-name product.

Distribution refers to the process of moving the drug throughout the body. Most drugs are distributed throughout most or all of the body's tissues, but this distribution is not necessarily even. For example, many drugs do not cross the blood-brain barrier to enter the central nervous system (CNS). Factors such as the drug's pH, **hydrophilicity** (i.e., water solubility), and **lipophilicity** (i.e., fat solubility) will affect its distribution throughout the body. The concept of volume of distribution is used to describe the effective space in the body available to contain a drug. It is the ratio of the total amount of drug in the body to the plasma concentration of drug. Drugs with a high volume of distribution have lower plasma concentrations and are more greatly distributed into extravascular spaces. Drugs with a lower volume of distribution have higher plasma concentration and less distribution into extravascular tissues.

Metabolism is the complex process by which a drug is changed into one or more chemical entities that differ from the parent drug. These entities may be active metabolites that have a pharmacological effect or inactive metabolites with no pharmacological effect. Drug metabolism occurs primarily in the liver through the action of various hepatic enzymes, although some metabolism does occur in a few other tissues in the body (e.g., lung).

Elimination is the process of getting the drug out of the body. A drug and its metabolites are eliminated through some combination of renal or fecal excretion.

Although some drugs are completely eliminated either through renal or fecal excretion, most drugs and their metabolites undergo elimination through a combination of these two mechanisms. In individuals with renal or hepatic impairment, the rate of drug elimination will be slowed to a degree dependent on the level of impairment. This means that the dose of a drug or the frequency of taking the drug will often need to be adjusted in individuals with renal or hepatic dysfunction.

Two concepts used to describe the elimination of a drug from the body are clearance and half-life. Clearance is the measure of the body's ability to eliminate a drug. It describes the volume of blood that is cleared of a drug over a given period of time, usually expressed in milliliters per minute. Drugs with a higher clearance rate will be removed from the body more quickly. Creatinine clearance is the rate of removal of creatinine from the serum into the urine. It is used as a measure of renal function. The normal creatinine clearance for men is 100 ml/min; for women it is 80 ml/min. In individuals with impaired renal function, it is important to know the creatinine clearance. In pharmaceutical reference books, dosage adjustments for renal impairment are given on the basis of creatinine clearance.

Half-life is the length of time that it takes for blood levels or tissue levels of a drug to decrease by one half. The clearance rate of a drug and the drug's volume of distribution will determine the half-life of the drug. The half-life is directly proportional to the volume of distribution and inversely proportional to the clearance (Key Points—Half-Life). This means that a drug

KEY POINTS
Half-Life

The length of time it takes for levels of a drug to decrease by one half; determined by distribution and clearance rate (elimination) of the drug.

with a high clearance rate and a small volume of distribution will have a short half-life and be eliminated from the body very quickly. A drug with a large volume of distribution and a low clearance rate will have a long half-life.

A drug's half-life is one of the major determining factors in how often a drug will be given. As a rule, a drug with a long half-life will have a long dosage interval. A drug with a short half-life will have a short dosage interval. If the clearance rate of a drug is decreased by renal or hepatic dysfunction, this will increase the half-life of the drug and necessitate an increase in the dosage interval. Individuals with an altered volume of distribution because of disease (e.g., ascites) also will have altered drug half-life. It is important to know the disease's effect on drug half-life so that changes in the dosage regimen may be made.

Routes of Administration

Drugs can enter the body through a variety of routes (Box 3-1), and these paths of administration promote the drug's absorption. The oral route is certainly the most common for the administration of drugs, but often it is appropriate to use a parenteral (nonoral) route of administration. The preferred route is determined by multiple factors including ease of administration, patient adherence, desired onset of action, local versus systemic distribution, and properties of the drug itself. An example is the destruction of insulin in the gastrointestinal tract, which necessitates its administration through a nonoral route.

Oral

The oral route is a convenient, noninvasive route used to deliver drugs that are distributed systemically. Tablets, capsules, solutions, and suspensions are dosage forms used to deliver drugs via the oral route. Tablets contain drug compressed or embedded along with inert ingredients into a compact unit and may be either uncoated or coated. Enteric coatings are used to ensure that a tablet does not dissolve in the low pH of gastric acid but rather passes into the small intestine where the tablet is dissolved and the drug absorbed. Drugs that are destroyed by gastric acid or drugs that may cause local irritation in the stomach such as aspirin are delivered in an enteric coating. Other coatings provide a controlled release of drug so that the drug is released from the tablet over an extended period of time, allowing for less frequent doses. Delayed release, extended release, and controlled release are all terms used to refer to dosage forms that are constructed to prolong the release of the drug from the tablet or capsule so that the drug may be given at extended dosage intervals. For example, Sudafed (pseudoephedrine) in conventional 30 mg and 60 mg tablets must be given every 4 to 6 hours. Pseudoephedrine is also available in 120 mg and 240 mg extended-release capsules that allow for the drug to be released over 12 hours and 24 hours, respectively.

Box 3-1   Routes of Drug Administration

- Oral
- Intravenous
- Intramuscular
- Subcutaneous
- Inhalation
- Intraarterial
- Sublingual
- Rectal
- Topical
- Intravaginal
- Intranasal
- Subarachnoid

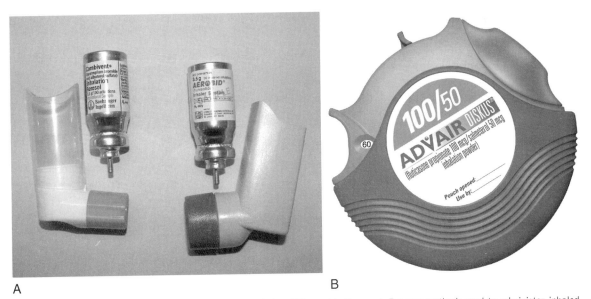

Figure 3-1 Metered-dose inhalers (A) and dry powder inhalers (B) provide the most common methods used to administer inhaled medications. (B, Courtesy GlaxoSmithKline.)

Other mechanisms allow for controlled release of the drug from a tablet, such as an osmotic delivery system used to deliver the antihypertensive drug nifedipine (Procardia XL). In such systems, the drug is contained in an osmotically active core surrounded by a semipermeable membrane. When the tablet is exposed to the water in the gastrointestinal tract, water is drawn into the core at a controlled rate resulting in a suspension of the drug that is pushed out through an orifice in the tablet.

Capsules are solid oral dosage forms that contain powdered, beaded, or liquid drug inside a shell. Some shells are formulated to dissolve in the stomach; others will dissolve in the intestines. Some capsule shells, such as those encapsulating the pseudoephedrine extended-release capsules, are designed to release the drug in a controlled fashion over an extended period.

Oral solutions, elixirs, and syrups contain drug completely dissolved in a liquid medium. Elixirs typically contain alcohol to aid in the dissolution of the drug (Key Points—Dissolution). Syrups contain high concentrations of sugar to make them more palatable. Oral suspensions are also liquids, but they contain undissolved drug dispersed or suspended throughout the liquid. All suspensions must be shaken before administration to ensure that the drug is evenly dispersed throughout the liquid. Antibiotic suspensions frequently require refrigeration and may have a short expiration date after which they must be discarded.

Inhaled

Inhaled drugs are most frequently used for their local effect on the bronchial passages. Bronchodilators and corticosteroids to treat bronchoconstriction from asthma are the drugs most frequently given via this route to treat bronchoconstriction from asthma. These drugs may be administered via metered-dose inhalers (MDIs), powder inhalers, or nebulizers. MDIs (Figure 3-1, A) and dry-powder inhalers (Figure 3-1, B) deliver a set dose of the drug with each inhalation. **Nebulizers** are machines that use compressed air to cause aerosolization of a liquid drug, which is then inhaled through a mask or a mouthpiece. Intranasal sprays and inhalers are used for a local effect on the intranasal passages. Corticosteroids are the most common drugs delivered by the intranasal route to treat allergic rhinitis.

Ophthalmic

Ophthalmic administration of drugs may be used to treat eye infections, allergies, dryness, glaucoma, and other eye disorders. The droppers used to administer drugs into the eye must be kept sterile, and therefore the eyedropper must never touch the eye. Individuals administering the drops must wash their hands thoroughly before and after administration of the drops. Warming the drops to body temperature by rolling the dropper bottle rapidly between the hands may increase the comfort of ophthalmic administration.

KEY POINTS
Dissolution

Dissolution is the process of dissolving a substance. In the context of pharmaceuticals, it is the process of a solid, oral dosage form (e.g., tablet or capsule) being dissolved in the gastrointestinal tract so that it can be absorbed. Poorly manufactured products may not dissolve at all and may be passed through the gastrointestinal tract and into the stool without allowing the expected dose of medication to be absorbed.

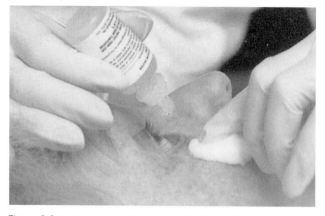

Figure 3-2 Ophthalmic solutions are applied by holding the eyedropper above the conjunctival sac laterally to allow the drops to flow toward the nasolacrimal duct. (From Potter PA, Perry AG: *Fundamental of nursing*, ed 5, St Louis, 2001, Mosby, p 311.)

Administration of the drops into the lateral area of the eye also increases comfort since the medial area, pupil, and iris are much more sensitive. Applying the drops laterally also helps bathe the eye since tears are produced laterally and flow medially to the nasolacrimal duct (Figure 3-2).

Otic

Otic administration of drugs is used primarily to treat otitis, decrease pain from otitis, and prevent recurrence of otitis in individuals whose ear canals are frequently exposed to moisture, such as swimmers. The droppers used to administer drugs into the ear canal do not need to be sterile, but every attempt must be made to avoid contact of the dropper with the ear during administration. As with ophthalmic administration, individuals administering the drops must wash their hands before and after administration. Rolling the dropper bottle rapidly between the hands or running the bottle under warm water will bring the temperature of the drops closer to body temperature, which will make the administration of the drops more comfortable for the athlete. Although it is not uncommon for ophthalmic drops to be prescribed for use in the ear, otic drops are never used in the eye (Box 3-2).

Topical

Topical administration refers to the application of a drug to the outer areas of the body for a local effect rather than a systemic effect. Creams, ointments, gels, and solutions are the most common dosage forms used for topical administration. Topical drugs may be used for a number of purposes, such as treatment of infection, treatment of inflammatory skin disorders such as dermatitis, or treatment of acne. The drug and its intended use will determine the frequency of

---

Box 3-2 Administration of Ear Drops

1. Place the athlete in a sitting or a side-lying position.
2. Straighten the ear canal by pulling up and back on the pinna.

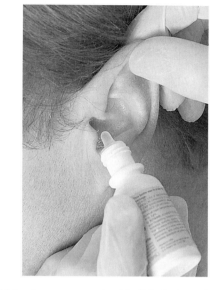

3. Hold the dropper approximately ½ inch above the ear canal (see illustration).
4. Gently massage the tragus of the ear; the athlete then remains quiet for a few minutes to allow the medication to work into the ear.

Modified from Potter PA, Perry AG: *Fundamental of nursing*, ed 5, St Louis, 2001, Mosby, p 315.

---

application, whether it should be applied in a thick layer or sparingly, and if a dressing or bandage should be used after application. The area where the drug is to be applied should be as clean and dry as possible. Individuals applying topical preparations must wash their hands before and after application of the drug; sometimes a drug necessitates wearing gloves when applying treatment.

Transdermal

Transdermal administration is the application of a drug to the skin, usually in the form of a patch. Once the drug is absorbed, it produces a systemic effect. Nitroglycerin, estrogen, testosterone, and fentanyl (i.e., a pain medication) are all available in patches for transdermal administration. The frequency with which old patches are removed and replaced with new patches will vary depending on the drug. It is important that patches be applied to hairless areas on the trunk, with the exception that estrogen patches should not be applied to the breasts. When an old patch is removed and a new one applied, the new patch is put in a different area to minimize irritation, and the old patch is then folded in on itself with the sticky side in and discarded in the trash so that the patch cannot be reapplied.

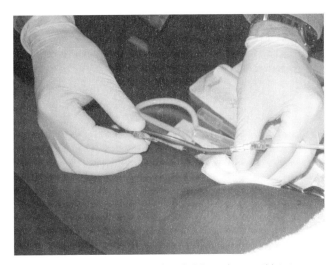

Figure 3-3 Intravenous fluids may be administered to an athlete to achieve rapid hydration.

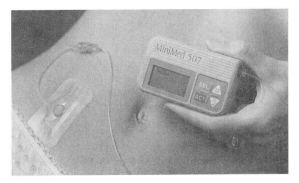

Figure 3-4 Insulin pump. (From Monahan FD, Neighbors M: *Medical-surgical nursing: foundations in clinical practice*, ed 2, Philadelphia, 1998, WB Saunders.)

Intravenous

The intravenous (IV) route, injection of a drug directly into a vein, is used in situations where immediate onset of drug action is required or where the use of other routes of administration is not possible because of patient condition or drug characteristics. The athletic trainer will see the IV route most frequently in situations where IV fluids (typically without medication added) are administered to achieve rapid hydration of an athlete who is experiencing heat-related illness (Figure 3-3). Athletic trainers must be aware of state practice laws to determine their role in administering IV fluids. Some states allow athletic trainers who have gone through IV training and certification to administer IV fluids under the supervision of a physician.

Intramuscular

The intramuscular (IM) route may be used for various reasons. In situations where a rapid, reliable onset of drug action is required but IV access is impractical, the IM route is the best alternative. Meperidine (Demerol) can be administered via IM injection for migraines. IM injection is also used for the injection of suspensions that will be slowly absorbed to deliver drug over prolonged periods. Medroxyprogesterone (Depo-Provera), a birth control injection lasting for 3 months, is given via the IM route. Last, the IM route is used to administer nearly all vaccinations.

Subcutaneous, Intrasynovial, and Intraarticular Injections

Subcutaneous injection (i.e., SQ or SC) is the injection of a drug into the subcutaneous fat and is used for rapid, reliable onset of action when IV access is impractical. It is also preferred for medications that are self-injected (e.g., insulin, epinephrine in EpiPens, and some pain medications such as morphine). Pumps are now available that provide a continuous infusion of drug into a subcutaneous catheter. Individuals with diabetes using subcutaneous insulin pumps will adjust the insulin infusion rate on the basis of their current blood sugars, activity level, and food intake to achieve much better control of blood sugars than with conventional subcutaneous injections (Figure 3-4).

Intrasynovial injection is used to place a drug, usually an antiinflammatory corticosteroid suspension, into the synovial cavity of a joint. The drug will not be systemically absorbed but will act locally to decrease inflammation.

Intraarticular injection refers to injection of the drug into the joint. As with intrasynovial injection, the drug will not be systemically absorbed but will act locally to decrease inflammation.

Iontophoresis and Phonophoresis

Drugs may also be introduced into the body through the use of electricity (iontophoresis) or ultrasound (i.e., phonophoresis). Both these delivery methods "drive" ionized medication into the subcutaneous tissues. Iontophoresis utilizes low-voltage, high-amperage direct current (DC) and requires the use of customized electrodes (Figure 3-5). The transdermal introduction has advantages over oral ingestion because it bypasses the liver, reducing metabolic breakdown of the medication, and can be concentrated in a local area. It provides advantages over injected medications since it is less painful and traumatic and does not result in high concentrations in the soft tissue, which have been associated with tendon rupture.

Iontophoresis does have disadvantages as well. It does not have the ability to reach deep tissue structures or areas of thick skin. There have also been conflicting reports about the amount of medication actually introduced into the affected tissue.[4,5]

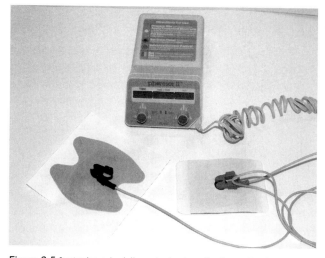

Figure 3-5 Iontophoresis delivers ionized medication using low-voltage, high-amperage direct current (DC).

Many medications may be used with iontophoresis and are usually dissolved in a carrier. Typical medications include acetic acid, dexamethasone, lidocaine, and epinephrine in varying combinations.

Phonophoresis is another method that is commonly used to deliver medications to a local area. It does not actually "drive" the ions of the medication through the skin but rather opens pathways that allow the medication to diffuse through the skin and pass deeper into the tissue. Some medications have been shown to be delivered up to 6 cm into the tissue with phonophoresis. Medications typically administered this way include corticosteroids such as hydrocortisone and dexamethasone, salicylates, and anesthetics.

Some controversy exists about the actual transmission of the medication into the skin because many medications do not transmit sound waves. Hydrocortisone had been used for many years but is increasingly being replaced by dexamethasone as the drug of choice in phonophoresis since the conductivity of dexamethasone to ultrasonic energy is considerably higher than hydrocortisone. Recently, low-frequency ultrasound has become increasingly popular as a means to deliver medications into soft tissue.

Drug Storage

The proper storage of drugs is essential to maintain drug potency. Temperature, humidity, and exposure to light must all be considered. Most drugs are best stored in a cool, dry, dark place. This means room temperatures of 65° to 80° F, with a low humidity of less than 50% and limited exposure to sunlight. Drugs requiring refrigeration are typically oral antibiotic suspensions, immunizations, insulin, and injected drugs that have been reconstituted from powders.

Whereas some refrigerated drugs may be allowed limited times at room temperature, others will lose potency rapidly if left unrefrigerated. Many emergency drugs (e.g., epinephrine, phenylephrine) will degrade rapidly on exposure to sunlight and high temperatures. Other drugs cannot tolerate freezing.

It is particularly important to consider the storage needs of all drugs during transportation. Medical kits for use at outdoor athletic events must be inspected regularly to ensure the integrity of the drug products stocked in the kit. In addition, security of the drugs must be ensured. All prescription medications must be stored in a locked cabinet or a locked portable medical treatment kit. Protocols must be followed that do not violate state practice acts or federal DEA guidelines for dispensing prescription medication. Dispensing prescription medications is not within the scope of practice for certified athletic trainers. However, some states may allow the athletic trainer to be licensed as an agent for the physician. It is important that the certified athletic trainer be assigned only duties that are allowed by applicable state law.[5]

Resources

With the ever-increasing number of pharmaceutical products on the market today and the vast volume of medical research being published, it is essential that anyone involved in health care have up-to-date resources available. The best options are electronic references that are updated frequently, such as Mosby's Drug Consult or Micromedex (Figure 3-6, *A*), but subscriptions to these services can be quite costly. Individuals who are associated with universities may have access to on-line drug information resources through their library's subscription.

Drug information programs are also available for personal digital assistants (PDAs) and handheld personal computers (Figure 3-6, *B*). Free programs such as ePocrates are adequate for most athletic trainers' needs; however, a professional edition that is more detailed can be purchased. Both desktop and PDA versions are available for many on-line drug information programs. The advantages of electronic drug references over printed references are that the medical professional may select two or more drugs and access comparative information including drug interactions. Table 3-2 lists common printed and electronic drug references.

Printed references are still a viable option as long as they are replaced annually. The *Physician's Desk Reference* (PDR) is published annually and maintains consistent popularity. The PDR contains a collection of package inserts from all prescription products available in the United States. There is a companion volume that contains

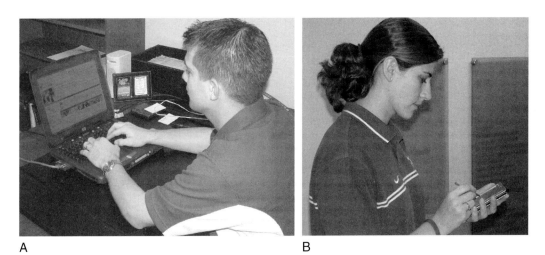

A   B

Figure 3-6 Electronic references such as Mosby's Drug Consult (A) and programs for PDAs (B) make information about medications readily available for the athletic trainer.

Table 3-2	Pharmacology References		
Topic	**Author**	**Title**	**Publisher**
Pharmacology and Pharmaceutics	JG Hardman and LE Limbird	*Goodman and Gilman's The Pharmacological Basis of Therapeutics*	McGraw-Hill Medical, New York
		American Hospital Formulary Service	American Society of Health System Pharmacists
		Drug Facts and Comparisons	Facts and Comparisons, St Louis
	AR Gennaro	*Remington's Pharmaceutical Sciences*	Mack Publishing Co, Easton, Pa
	MA Hollinger	*Introduction to Pharmacology*	Taylor & Francis, New York (2003) http://www.netlibrary.com/ EbookDetails.aspx
		Physician's Desk Reference	Thomson PDR, Stamford, Conn
Drug Therapy	BS Reiss, ME Evans, and BE Broyles	*Pharmacological Aspects of Nursing Care*	Delmar/Thomson Learning, Clifton Park, NY
	MA Koda-Kimble and LE Young	*Applied Therapeutics: the Clinical Use of Drugs*	Lippincott Williams & Wilkins, Baltimore, Md
	The Johns Hopkins Hospital, C Nechyba, and VL Gunn	*The Harriet Lane Handbook: a Manual for Pediatric House Officers*	Mosby, St Louis
	WE Benitz and DS Tatro	*The Pediatric Drug Handbook*	Year Book Medical Publishers, Chicago
		Micromedex	Thomson, Stamford, Conn
Regulations		Controlled Substances Act	usdoj.gov/dea/agency/csa.htm
		Food and Drug Administration	www.fda.gov
Antimicrobial Therapy	DN Gilbert, RC Moellering, and MA Sande	*The Sanford Guide to Antimicrobial Therapy*	Hyde Park, Vt
Electronic Sources	Gold Standard Multimedia	http://www.gsm.com	
Banned Substances	NCAA	http://www.ncaa.org/sports_sciences/ drugtesting/banned_list.html	
	USOC	http://usoc.org/inside/drugadmin.html	
	United States Anti- Doping Agency	http://www.usantidoping.org	

NCAA, National Collegiate Athletic Association; *USOC,* United States Olympic Committee.

information for over-the-counter products. The PDR is limited, however, because comparative information among various drugs and information on a drug's off-label uses (i.e., indications that are not approved by the FDA) are not included.

Popular printed drug information references include *Drug Facts and Comparisons*, which receives monthly updates; the *American Hospital Formulary Service*, which is published by the American Society of Health System Pharmacists with a new edition annually; and the *United States Pharmacopoeia Drug Information*, which contains information for the patient in nontechnical language. Information about pediatric patients is available in *The Harriet Lane Handbook: a Manual for Pediatric House Officers*. When foreign medications need to be used, the health professional may refer to *Martindale's*, which provides information in print and on-line. The ability to synthesize the drug information available and apply it to real situations requires an advanced level of training (Red Flags—Drug Expertise).

> ▶ **Red Flags for Drug Expertise** ══════
> No printed resources can replace the expertise of the pharmacist or physician when dealing with issues of drug therapy, drug interactions, or adverse reactions.

The athletic trainer's responsibility is to monitor for and prevent allergic reactions when possible, recognize and report adverse drug reactions, and realize situations in which drug interactions may occur. The athletic trainer is often asked by athletes to make recommendations regarding the use of over-the-counter or herbal supplements. In complex situations, where multiple medications or supplements are involved, it is advisable to seek an opinion from either a physician or a pharmacist.

Pharmacodynamics

Pharmacodynamics is the study of how medications work in the body: the mechanisms of action, drug interactions, side effects, adverse reactions, and allergic reactions. The sections of this chapter under Drug Categories discuss specific drug classes and the basic pharmacological considerations for each drug class. Some concepts necessary to later discussion are reviewed here.

A drug's mechanism of action may be very simple. An example is the action of magnesium hydroxide in the stomach, where it neutralizes stomach acid through a simple acid-base reaction. Another simple mechanism of action is exhibited by bulk-forming laxatives, in which insoluble fibers cause increased stool volume in the large intestine.

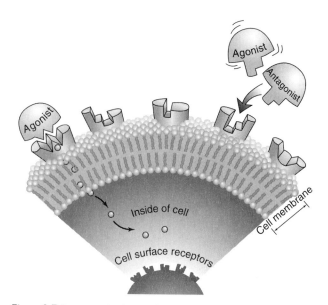

Figure 3-7 Drug-receptor interaction can take place when agonists with shapes that match an endogenous chemical fit exactly into a cell receptor or with an antagonist that binds to a receptor, thereby blocking the agonist and preventing it from stimulating the receptor. (From Gutierrez K: *Pharmacotherapeutics: clinical decision making in nursing*, Philadelphia, 1999, WB Saunders, p 62.)

Other drugs act through more complicated mechanisms. **Agonists** are drugs that exert their effect by attaching to cellular receptors in the body causing stimulation of the receptor (Figure 3-7). Agonists mimic the effects of endogenous chemicals, which normally target cellular receptors. Morphine, an opiate agonist, stimulates opiate receptors in the body that are normally the target of the body's own endorphins. Endorphins cause decreased sensitivity to pain and a sense of well-being or euphoria. Intense exercise causes the release of endorphins in the body, which explains the euphoria and pain tolerance that occur in many athletes during endurance events. Morphine, a very potent opiate agonist, is used for its therapeutic effect of decreasing an individual's sensitivity to pain. The euphoria produced by morphine is the reason for its high abuse potential.

Antagonists also act by binding to cellular receptors, but they do not cause stimulation of the receptor. An antagonist binds to the receptor and blocks other chemicals or agonists from binding to it (see Figure 3-7). Antihistamines bind to histamine receptors in the body but cause no stimulation of the receptors. Rather, antihistamines block the binding of histamine-to-histamine receptors, thereby preventing the itching, rhinitis, and edema that histamine will cause when it is released by immune system cells in response to an allergen.

The inhibition of enzyme action is another important mechanism of action for several of the drugs discussed later in this chapter. Enzymes are proteins that act as biochemical catalysts for chemical reactions that occur in the body. Some drugs exert their effect by breaking down enzymes or blocking the effect of enzymes, thereby preventing or slowing down the reactions for which these enzymes are responsible. Cyclooxygenase-1 and -2 (COX-1 and COX-2) are enzymes that are involved in the biochemical transformation of arachidonic acid into prostaglandins. Prostaglandins are chemicals that cause pain and inflammation. Antiinflammatory drugs are cyclooxygenase inhibitors that prevent COX-1 or COX-2 from facilitating the production of prostaglandins. A drug's mechanism of action often is directly related to its side effects and drug interactions. For example, beta-adrenergic agonists, which stimulate beta-adrenergic receptors, cause bronchodilation and are used to treat asthmatic attacks. Individuals who are taking beta-blockers to treat hypertension may have a decreased response to beta-agonists.

Indications

Drug indications outline conditions for which the drug shows a therapeutic effect. The indications are FDA approved, meaning the drug manufacturer has provided a body of research to the FDA supporting use of the drug for a particular indication and the FDA has approved use of the drug for that indication. FDA-approved indications are found on the package insert of the drug (Key Points—Indications and Contraindications).

> **KEY POINTS**
> **Indications and Contraindications**
>
> - Indications: those conditions for which the drug has been found to have a therapeutic effect
> - Contraindications: situations where a drug should be absolutely avoided

Contraindications

Contraindications are those situations when a specific drug must be absolutely avoided. Disease states, other medications, pregnancy, age, and gender may all be reasons for a particular drug to be contraindicated. For example, the use of tetracycline antibiotics is contraindicated in children under the age of 7 years because it will cause staining of the permanent teeth. Decongestants, which can cause profound, transient elevations in blood pressure, are contraindicated in individuals with uncontrolled hypertension (Red Flags—Contraindications).

> **Red Flags for Contraindications**
> Individuals with uncontrolled hypertension should avoid decongestants because the medication may cause profound, transient elevations in blood pressure.

Although athletic trainers do not prescribe or dispense medications, they need to be aware of contraindications to medications commonly used by athletes. They may know about an athlete's drug history. Working closely with the team physician and pharmacist will ensure the best health care for the athlete.

Warnings and precautions are statements that alert health care professionals to the serious adverse events associated with the use of a drug. Black box warnings are strong precautions that the FDA mandates be printed inside a black box at the very top of a product's package insert. As with contraindications, the athletic trainer must be familiar with the warnings and precautions for all drugs that are prescribed for the athletes. The electronic drug resources mentioned previously make this information readily accessible.

Drug interactions most commonly refer to the interaction of one drug with another drug but may also refer to interactions between drugs and foods and drugs with disease states. Drug interactions with foods occur most commonly when the minerals in a particular food inhibit the absorption of a drug. For example, the administration of fluoroquinolone antibiotics with calcium-containing foods will decrease absorption of the antibiotic because the calcium binds to the antibiotic and forms an insoluble complex (Table 3-3).

Drug-disease interactions may occur for a variety of reasons. For example, the administration of drugs that block the beta-adrenergic receptors, or beta-blockers, is not recommended in individuals with diabetes since these drugs will mask the symptoms of hypoglycemia that are mediated by the sympathetic nervous system (e.g., tremor).

Drug-drug interactions occur when one drug affects the absorption, metabolism, distribution, receptor binding, or elimination of another drug. For example, many antibiotics, such as penicillins, change the bacterial composition of the intestine, which in turn alters the metabolism of oral contraceptives. The result is that the effectiveness of oral contraceptives may be decreased in women taking certain antibiotics. Although many drug interactions are undesirable, some interactions can be used for a beneficial therapeutic effect. Histamine$_2$ (H$_2$) receptor blockers, such as famotidine (Pepcid), interact with orally administered pancreatic enzymes (Pancrease) in a way that is beneficial. Pancreatic enzymes are susceptible to acid–peptic enzyme degradation. The administration of an H$_2$ blocker raises the gastric pH and decreases the acid-peptic degradation of pancreatic enzymes, thereby decreasing the dose of pancreatic enzymes required.

Drug allergies occur when the medicine produces a response different from what is expected. Symptoms may include severe itching and hives, signs of an allergic response. Some allergic reactions may be anaphylactic in nature and may include bronchospasm and

Table 3-3 Selected Drug-Food Interactions

Drug	Food	Adverse Interaction
Calcium antagonists (felodipine, nifedipine, nitrendipine), terfenadine, caffeine	Grapefruit juice	Increased bioavailability, inhibition of first-pass metabolism, increased toxicity
Monoamine oxidase (MAO) inhibitors	Foods containing tyramine: cheese, sour cream, nuts, bananas, beer, wine, yogurt, yeast, liver, pickled herring, avocados, soup	Palpitations, headache, hypertensive crises
Digitalis	Licorice	Digitalis toxicity
Griseofulvin	Fatty foods	Increased blood levels of griseofulvin
Timed-release drug preparations	Alcoholic beverages	Increased rate of release for some
Lithium	Decreased sodium intake	Lithium toxicity
Quinidine	Antacids and alkaline diet (alkaline urine)	Quinidine toxicity
Thiazide diuretics	Carbohydrates	Elevated blood sugar
Tetracyclines	Dairy products high in calcium, ferrous sulfate, antacids	Impaired absorption of tetracycline
Vitamin B_{12} (cyanocobalamin)	Vitamin C—large doses	Precipitate B_{12} deficiency
Fenfluramine	Vitamin C addition	Antagonism of antiobesity effect of fenfluramine
Thiamine	Blueberries, fish, alcohol	Foods containing thiaminases; decreased intake, absorption, utilization
Benzodiazepines	Caffeine	Antagonism of antianxiety action

From Smith CM, Reynard AM, editors: *Essentials of pharmacology*, Philadelphia, 1995, WB Saunders.

> **Red Flags for Drug Allergies**
>
> May include the following:
> - Severe itching
> - Hives or other signs of allergic response
> - Bronchospasm
> - Shock

shock (Red Flags—Drug Allergies).[7] It is important to differentiate drug allergies from drug side effects. Drug side effects are a condition reported by the majority of people who take a particular medication, but a drug allergy is an unusual presentation seen in approximately 6% to 10% of the patients who take that medication. Because of the potential severity of drug allergy reactions, it is important to know if the athlete is allergic to any medications. Allergy to a medication is obviously a contraindication for taking that medication.

Dosages

Drug dosages take many factors into consideration. The first consideration is age. Children over the age of 12 years may generally be given dosages using guidelines for the adult. For children under 12 years of age, many drugs may be given based on age (Figure 3-8). This method of drug dosages assumes that the child is of a normal weight for age. For premature infants and underweight or overweight children, giving doses by age range is not an optimal method.

On the opposite end of the age spectrum, many drugs must be used at a decreased dose in older adults.

The two main reasons for this are (1) advanced age causes an increased sensitivity to many drugs such as central nervous system depressants, and (2) aging also is associated with diminished hepatic and renal function, which decreases the rate at which drugs are eliminated from the body and necessitates the use of smaller doses.

Dosages based on weight or body surface area are a preferable method to use when children need medications. *The Harriet Lane Handbook*, *Micromedex*, and *The Pediatric Drug Handbook* are all excellent resources on pediatric dosages. Also, a few drugs used in adults have dosages based on weight or body surface area, such as cancer chemotherapy drugs or certain antibiotics. In children and adults who are obese, it may be necessary to use an ideal body weight or adjusted body weight to calculate an appropriate drug dose.

For some drugs given by weight, the dose will be expressed in terms of milligrams, grams, or units per kilogram per dose (e.g., acetaminophen, 10 mg/kg/dose given every 4 to 6 hours). For other drugs, the dose will be published as milligrams, grams, or units per kilogram per day followed by the recommended number of divided doses per day (e.g., amoxicillin, 40 mg/kg/day divided every 8 hours, or in three divided doses). It is important to make the distinction between whether the dose is being expressed as the total daily dose or the quantity to be given in a single dose. Physicians typically express dosages on prescription pads or orders as abbreviations. Therefore the athletic trainer needs to be familiar with common medical abbreviations used in prescribing (see Appendix B).

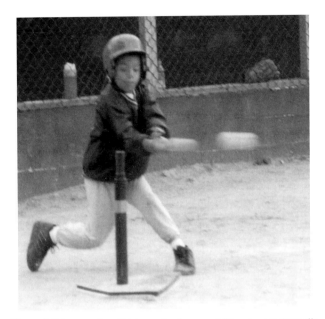

Figure 3-8 Dosages for athletes under the age of 12 years are generally determined by age if the child is normal weight for age.

The side effects or adverse reactions of a drug are the drug's nontherapeutic actions. Usually drugs of the same class will have similar side effect profiles. For example, ibuprofen (Advil, Motrin) and naproxen (Naprosyn, Aleve), both nonsteroidal antiinflammatory drugs (NSAIDs), have nearly identical side effects. Serious adverse effects of a drug should be reported to the FDA's MedWatch program at www.fda.gov. This includes any adverse effect that results in death, disability, hospitalization, life-threatening condition, or congenital anomaly. Adverse drug effects that require medical or surgical intervention to prevent permanent impairment should also be reported. The pharmacy that dispensed the medication or the office of the prescribing physician may facilitate the report. Reporting of adverse reactions is extremely important, especially in the case of newly approved drugs, because it is used to identify potentially serious adverse effects of a drug that may lead to changes in the product's labeling or even withdrawal of the drug from the market (Red Flags—COX-2 Antiinflammatory Agents).

> **Red Flags for COX-2 Antiinflammatory Agents**
>
> In 2004, a COX-2 antiinflammatory medication called rofecoxib (Vioxx) was voluntarily pulled from the market by its manufacturer amid concerns that it increased the risk of cardiovascular problems. As with any medication, potential benefits must be weighed against the drug's adverse side effects. The athletic trainer must remain abreast of drug cautions and recalls.

Many drugs are being given expedited, fast track FDA approval. Thus, compared with other drugs, fewer numbers of people will receive these fast track drugs before they are approved. Therefore serious adverse reactions or serious drug interactions may not be discovered before the drug receives FDA approval. The FDA and the drug manufacturers rely on postmarketing surveillance, including the MedWatch program, for the reporting of these adverse incidents.

Special Considerations for Athletes

Sometimes the drug of choice for an athlete with a particular condition is not viable because it may be banned during competition or is ergolytic and negatively affects athletic performance. Therefore a particular drug may not be the drug of choice but rather the most viable drug choice. For example, the athlete with seasonal allergies may benefit greatly from a decongestant and antihistamine. Until recently, pseudoephedrine, a common decongestant, was banned for certain competitions.

In 2004, the World Anti-Doping Agency (WADA) and subsequently the U.S. Anti-Doping Agency (USADA) and the National Collegiate Athletic Association (NCAA) loosened the ban for some therapeutic drugs, such as pseudoephedrine, instead placing them on a watch list.[8-11] In addition, many antihistamines are sedating and therefore have a detrimental effect on performance. Therefore the drug of choice, by default, needs to be a drug that is approved for competition and is nonsedating. Appendix G lists substances banned by the NCAA. Because the lists of the NCAA, USADA, and WADA change frequently, it is important to consult the agency websites, which are listed later in this chapter.

Potential Drug Misuse

Everyone including athletes often think that if some is good, more is better. This is extremely problematic when dealing with medication. In addition, athletes will often self-medicate with over-the-counter medications using prescription strength dosages. Warner and colleagues[12] found that 75% of high school football players surveyed were daily users of over-the-counter drugs and took NSAIDs independently without supervision. The athletic trainer must be involved in the education of the athlete about the dangers of self-medicating or taking medications in dosages other than what is indicated on the prescription or on the over-the-counter label.

Athletes may also be tempted to use medications for conditions other than originally intended or indicated to potentially improve performance. Educating athletes about the dangers of using drugs for purposes other than those prescribed is paramount to their continued safety. Although drug testing may be a deterrent for some athletes, the technology used to circumvent drug tests is typically years ahead of the technology to detect a given drug.

DRUG CATEGORIES

Antiinflammatory Agents

One of the most common conditions that athletic trainers encounter is inflammation. Following injury, irritation, or overuse, inflammation occurs to limit the spread of the damage caused by the injurious agent to adjacent tissue. It is both a chemical and a vascular response at the site of injury or exposure to the injurious agent. The process is nonspecific and is the same regardless of whether the injury or irritation is mechanical or caused by a noxious foreign substance.

Initially, a vasoconstriction occurs to prevent the loss of blood. This is followed by the release of chemical mediators such as prostaglandin, histamine, leukotrienes, and bradykinins. These mediators cause vasodilation and an increase in cell wall permeability resulting in fluid escaping from the cells into the interstitial spaces in the quickly progressing inflammatory cascade (Figure 3-9, *A* and *B*). Inflammation results in pain, redness, warmth, swelling, and loss of function. The inflammatory process is covered in detail in many therapeutic modality texts for athletic trainers.

The physician may prescribe antiinflammatory medication to limit the extent of the inflammatory process or cascade. Antiinflammatory medications are classified as steroidal or nonsteroidal antiinflammatory agents.

Steroidal Antiinflammatory Agents: Corticosteroids

Corticosteroids are defined by the *American Hospital Formulary Service Drug Information* as hormones secreted by the adrenal cortex or synthetic analogs of these hormones. Although corticosteroids and anabolic steroids, which are analogs of testosterone, both contain a steroid ring, corticosteroids have very different pharmacological actions from anabolic steroids. The actions of corticosteroids can be classified as either mineralocorticoid or glucocorticoid. Mineralocorticoid actions are those that affect electrolytes, fluid balance with net effect being sodium and fluid retention, and potassium and hydrogen excretion. Glucocorticoid actions decrease inflammation, cause immune system suppression, and stimulate gluconeogenesis. They also promote protein catabolism, redistribute peripheral fat to central areas, decrease intestinal absorption of calcium, and increase renal excretion of calcium. The pharmacological effects of the corticosteroids are most likely caused by their complex influence on various enzyme systems.

For the athletic trainer, the most important effects of corticosteroids are their antiinflammatory properties, which are beneficial in the treatment of inflammatory joint disorders and environmental allergies (Table 3-4).

Most corticosteroids used to treat joint disorders are administered in one of three ways: by intrasynovial

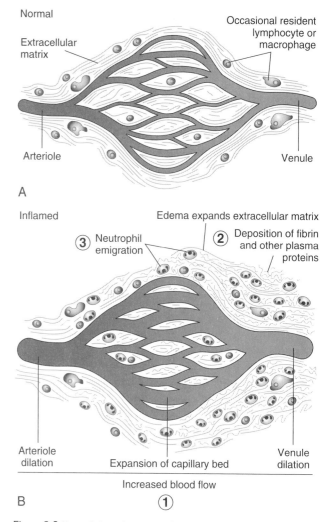

Figure 3-9 Normal tissue is compared with inflamed tissue that has been altered by the inflammatory process. **A,** Normal tissue. **B,** Changes that occur in the tissue during inflammation: *(1)* vasodilation and increased blood flow that cause erythema and warmth, followed by *(2)* the escape of plasma fluid and proteins into the interstitial spaces, and finally *(3)* neutrophil emigration and accumulation at the site of the injury and the release of chemical mediators, which result in fluid escaping from the cells into the interstitial spaces. (From Kumar V, Robbins SL, Cotran RS: *Pathologic basis of disease,* ed 7, St Louis, 2005, Eleseiver, Inc, p 50.)

injection, intraarticular injection, or iontophoresis. It is not atypical that these injections are accompanied by a short-acting anesthetic such as lidocaine (Xylocaine). Injectable corticosteroids are typically used after more conservative treatments have failed and the inflammatory process can be localized to a small area.

The immunosuppressive properties of corticosteroids make them invaluable in the treatment of allergies and inflammatory joint conditions. Prednisone (Deltasone) and methylprednisolone (Medrol) are the oral agents used most frequently in the treatment of allergic reactions and acute joint inflammation. Typically a large dose, equivalent to 30 mg of prednisone, will be given on the first day of treatment and then the dose will be reduced by 5 mg/day until the drug is completely

Table 3-4	**Corticosteroids**		
Trade Name(s)	**Generic Name**	**Route**	**Usual Dose**
Cortef, Solu-Cortef	Hydrocortisone	Intraarticular or intralesional	5-75 mg
		IM or IV	15-240 mg/day
		PO	20-240 mg/day
		Rectal	100 mg/day
Deltasone, Liquid Pred, Orasone	Prednisone	PO	5-60 mg/day
Various	Prednisolone	IM, intraarticular, IV, soft tissue, or interphalangeal	4-60 mg
		PO	5-60 mg/day
Medrol, Solu-Medrol	Methylprednisolone	IM	80-120 mg
		Intraarticular and soft tissue	4-80 mg
		Dermatological	40-120 mg/wk
		IV	10-40 mg
		PO	4-48 mg/day
Kenalog, Kenacort, Aristocort	Triamcinolone	IM	25-60 mg/day
		Intraarticular or intrabursal	2.5-40 mg/day
		Intradermal	1 mg per site
		Intralesional or sublesional	5-48 mg
		PO	8-16 mg/day
Decadron	Dexamethasone	IM	4-8 mg
		Intraarticular or soft tissue	4-16 mg
		PO	0.75-9 mg/day

Data from (A) Micromedex, 1974-2004, Thomson MICROMEDEX Healthcare Series, vol 122. Thomson Healthcare, Inc; (B) Clinical pharmacology. Gold Standard. Available at http://cp.gsm.com. Accessed May 2004; (C) Drug facts and comparisons, EFacts. Wolters Kluwer Health, Inc. Available at http://efactsweb.com. Accessed May 2004; (D) American Hospital Formulary Service accessed using Silver Platter, Drug Information Full Text, American Society of Hospital Pharmacists, Inc. Accessed May 2004.

tapered off. The initial dose and subsequent doses may be given as a single daily dose or in divided doses. The very popular Medrol Dosepak contains 4 mg methylprednisolone tablets in a six-row blister pack with complete instructions for how the drug is to be started and tapered over the course of 6 days. For inflammatory conditions of a joint, the steroid taper will be followed by a course of a nonsteroidal antiinflammatory drug, such as ibuprofen or a COX-2 inhibitor. If the condition being treated is exacerbated during the taper, then the dose of steroid will be increased and maintained for a short time before the taper is restarted.

Intranasal steroids are also used in the treatment of allergic rhinitis or allergies. They include beclomethasone dipropionate (Beconase AQ, Vancenase AQ), flunisolide (Nasalide), fluticasone propionate (Flonase), and mometasone furoate (Nasonex). These steroids are manufactured as intranasal metered-dose sprays, which provide a local antiinflammatory effect and reduce the effects of environmental allergens through immunosuppressive mechanisms.

Inhaled corticosteroids are used in the treatment of asthma (Key Points—Inhaled Corticosteroids). Beclomethasone dipropionate (Beconase, Vancenase),

fluticasone (Flovent), and triamcinolone (Azmacort) are dispensed from MDIs; the dry powder inhaler ADVAIR DISKUS dispenses a combination of two drugs: fluticason propionate and salmeterol. Inhaled corticosteroids provide a local antiinflammatory effect in the airways. They should never be used for acute exacerbations of asthma because they do not cause immediate bronchodilation.

Side Effects

The side effects of corticosteroids depend on the dose and the route of administration. They are minimal with intrasynovial injection, intraarticular injection, intranasal application, inhalation, or short-term therapy. However, tendon ruptures have occurred in patients receiving corticosteroid injections. The Achilles tendon is especially susceptible to this effect. Research supports that repeated short courses, intranasal corticosteroids, and inhaled corticosteroids may also cause decreased bone density and osteoporosis.[13,14]

For orally administered short-course tapers, the most common side effects are increased appetite, restlessness, insomnia, fluid retention, gastrointestinal disturbances, and decreased glucose tolerance. Gastrointestinal effects are diminished if doses are taken along with food. Less common but serious effects of corticosteroids are the development of and the impaired healing of peptic ulcers.

In addition, high doses or prolonged use of corticosteroids used for treatment of systemic inflammatory

KEY POINTS
Inhaled Corticosteroids

The antiinflammatory benefits of inhaled corticosteroids are not realized until after 1 to 4 weeks of therapy.

or autoimmunediseases, such as lupus, multiple sclerosis, or inflammatory bowel syndromes (e.g., Crohn's disease), may produce devastating side effects. These may include changes in physical appearance caused by changes in fat deposition, adrenal suppression, cataracts, or peptic ulcers. Long-term use of corticosteroids causes decreased bone density and osteoporosis.[13,14]

In the diabetic athlete, corticosteroids, even in short courses, must be used with caution because of their effects on glucose tolerance. Changes in insulin doses or diet may be required in diabetic individuals during treatment with corticosteroids.

Corticosteroids, including those administered intranasally, may cause a reduction in growth velocity in pediatric patients but no impact on final adult height.[15] The growth of pediatric patients receiving corticosteroids should be monitored routinely. In addition, in order to prevent decreases in bone density children older than 11 years of age should receive calcium, 1500 mg/day, and vitamin D, 800 IU/day, throughout the course of treatment with corticosteroids.[16]

Repeated intrasynovial or intraarticular injection will not result in any systemic effects but will cause damage to the joint. Intraarticular injections in major weight-bearing joints are not recommended because of the potential softening of joint cartilage.[6] Even after a single injection, if the joint is not allowed proper time to heal, damage may occur. Iontophoresis is a much less invasive way to administer corticosteroids superficially since it uses direct electrical current to introduce ions into the body.[17] Often ionized medications can be introduced through iontophoresis; however, the most common are the corticosteroids in combination with a topical anesthetic such as lidocaine. Some debate is ongoing about whether iontophoresis is as effective as intraarticular injection.[5,17]

Intranasal corticosteroids are generally very well tolerated. The most common side effects are nasal irritation, pharyngeal irritation, and dryness. Similarly, the most common side effects of inhaled corticosteroids are hoarseness, dry mouth, sore throat, and oropharyngeal fungal infections, such as *Candida albicans* or *Aspergillus niger*. After using an inhaled corticosteroid, the mouth is always rinsed to prevent oral fungal infections.

Nonsteroidal Antiinflammatory Agents

Among the most common medications used in the athletic setting are the NSAIDs (Table 3-5). NSAIDs decrease pain, inflammation, and fever (i.e., antipyretic effect). Many of these drugs are available over the counter, and thus are frequently used by both athletes and the general population (Key Points—Antiinflammatory Agents) (Figure 3-10).

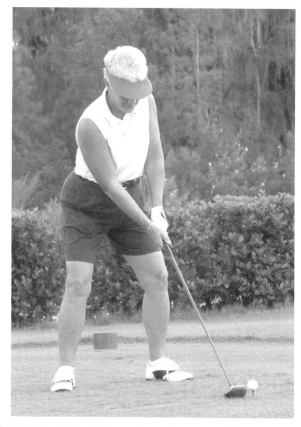

Figure 3-10 Athletes of all ages will sometimes use antiinflammatory drugs to treat both acute and chronic conditions. An athlete may use an antiinflammatory drug on a regular basis to decrease pain during activity.

KEY POINTS
Antiinflammatory Agents

It will typically take 2 weeks for the maximum antiinflammatory response to occur although some decrease of inflammation will occur after 2 to 7 days.

Drugs in this class exert their pharmacological effect through the inhibition of prostaglandin synthesis. The NSAIDs inactivate the COX-1 and COX-2 enzymes and the prostaglandin G/H synthase 1 and 2 enzymes that catalyze the formation of prostaglandins from arachidonic acid (Figure 3-11). The COX-2 inhibitors (e.g., celecoxib [Celebrex], valdecoxib [Bextra]) are selective for the COX-2 enzyme (see Red Flags—COX-2 Antiinflammatory Agents). NSAIDs are given primarily via the oral route, although ketorolac (Toradol) may be given orally (PO), IM, or IV. Lower doses are adequate for treating pain and fever (e.g., 200 to 400 mg of ibuprofen or 5 to 10 mg/kg/dose in children 6 months to 12 years of age), whereas higher doses are required for antiinflammatory effects. The best results in inflammatory conditions are obtained when scheduled doses of 600 to 800 mg every 6 to 8 hours around the clock are given for several weeks.

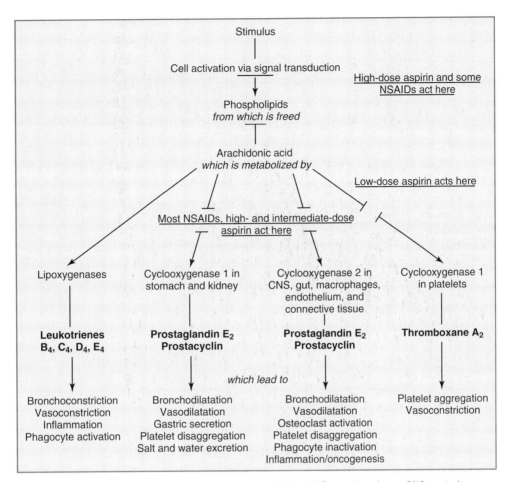

Figure 3-11 The inflammatory cascade. *NSAIDs,* Nonsteroidal antiinflammatory drugs; *CNS,* central nervous system. (From Goldman L, Bennett JC: *Cecil textbook of medicine,* ed 21, Philadelphia, 2000, WB Saunders, p 115.)

Table 3-5	Nonsteroidal Antiinflammatory Drugs (NSAIDs)		
Trade Name(s)	**Generic Name**	**Usual Dose**	**Maximum Dose per Day**
Advil, Motrin	Ibuprofen	400 mg every 4-6 hr	3200 mg
Aleve, Anaprox, Naprosyn	Naproxen	250 mg every 6-8 hr	1250 mg
Cataflam, Voltaren	Diclofenac	50 mg 3 times daily	200 mg
Lodine	Etodolac	200-400 mg every 6-8 hr	1200 mg
Indocin	Indomethacin	25-50 mg PO or rectal 2 or 3 times daily	200 mg
Orudis, Orudis KT	Ketoprofen	25-50 mg every 6-8 hr	300 mg
Toradol	Ketorolac	IV: 30 mg × 1 dose or 30 mg every 6 hr IM: 60 mg × 1 dose or 60 mg every 6 hr PO: 20 mg initially, then 10 mg every 4-6 hr	120 mg 120 mg 40 mg
Mobic	Meloxicam	7.5 mg every day	15 mg
Relafen	Nabumetone	1000-2000 mg every day or twice daily	2000 mg
Daypro	Oxaprozin	1200 mg every day	1800 mg
Feldene	Piroxicam	20 mg every day or twice daily	40 mg
Celebrex	Celecoxib	100-200 mg twice daily	400 mg
Bextra	Valdecoxib	10-20 mg once or twice daily	40 mg
Vioxx*	Rofecoxib	12-5-50 mg every day	N/A

Data from (A) Micromedex, 1974-2004, Thomson MICROMEDEX Healthcare Series, vol 122. Thomson Healthcare, Inc; (B) Clinical pharmacology. Gold Standard. Available at http://cp.gsm.com. Accessed May 2004; (C) Drug facts and comparisons, EFacts. Wolters Kluwer Health, Inc. Available at http://efactsweb.com. Accessed May 2004; (D) American Hospital Formulary Service accessed using Silver Platter, Drug Information Full Text, American Society of Hospital Pharmacists, Inc. Accessed May 2004.
PO, Oral; *IV,* intravenous; *IM,* intramuscular; *N/A,* not applicable.
*Vioxx was voluntarily taken off the market by its manufacturer, Merck, in September, 2004, because of documented increased links with heart attack and stroke. In February, 2005, the FDA ruled that, although there is an increased risk of cardiovascular events in specific populations, Vioxx is still considered an effective and safe medication.

Side Effects

The major side effects of NSAIDs are gastrointestinal and include dyspepsia, heartburn, nausea, vomiting, abdominal pain, peptic ulcer, and gastrointestinal bleeding. Prostaglandins stimulate the secretion of a protective mucosal layer in the gastrointestinal tract.

Inhibition of these prostaglandins leads to a breakdown in this mucosal layer, which leads to ulceration. Aspirin, when administered without an enteric coating, buffers, or antacids, causes increased entry of acid into the gastric mucosa leading to cellular damage at the site of dissolution. As mentioned previously, enteric-coated aspirin will undergo dissolution in the small intestine, therefore avoiding the direct effect on the gastric lining. The administration of NSAIDs with food or milk will minimize gastrointestinal adverse effects. Coadministration of aspirin and other NSAIDs along with corticosteroids increases the risk of gastrointestinal lesions. People who drink alcohol or alcoholics who are taking aspirin or NSAIDs are at higher risk of upper gastrointestinal bleeding, a risk that is elevated by increased alcohol consumption.[18,19]

Aspirin, salicylates, and to a much lesser extent NSAIDs have hematological effects that must be considered in the athlete. Aspirin inhibits platelet aggregation and decreases hepatic synthesis of blood coagulation factors. At normal doses of up to 6 g/day, aspirin rarely increases **prothrombin time** (PT), the time it takes blood to clot, by more than 2 to 3 seconds. Higher doses, fever, and increased metabolic rate may cause larger increases in PT. For athletes in contact sports, especially where the likelihood of head trauma is high, aspirin may not a good therapeutic choice. Head trauma occurring in an athlete in an anticoagulated state might increase the risk or extent of intracranial bleeding. Research is mixed on the probability of aspirin causing increased intracranial bleeding following head trauma for the patient who is receiving low-dose aspirin therapy.[20,21]

Other NSAIDs, such as ibuprofen, do inhibit platelet aggregation but to a lesser extent than aspirin. This has raised some concern that NSAIDs not be used by athletes in sports that may put the athlete at risk for head trauma. Physicians have varying views on this subject. Athletic trainers have a responsibility to know and uphold the views of the team physicians on this subject.

Renal effects of NSAIDs are also of concern. Prostaglandins play a role in maintaining renal perfusion in individuals with certain renal conditions (e.g., decreased extracellular fluid depletion). An athlete receiving long-term NSAID therapy who becomes dehydrated may be at risk for renal impairment and needs to be monitored for symptoms of **azotemia,** such as malaise, fatigue, or loss of appetite.

Other adverse effects of NSAIDs include rashes, dermatitis, photosensitivity (use sun block), dizziness, headache, nervousness, fatigue, drowsiness, fluid retention, anaphylaxis, bronchospasm, tinnitus, and visual disturbances.

Recently the safety of the COX-2 NSAIDs has been questioned with the voluntary recall of rofecoxib (Vioxx), which was shown to increase the risk of cardiovascular events. Studies involving the COX-2, celecoxib (Celebrex) have had conflicting results. A recent National Cancer Institute clinical trial investigating the use of celecoxib in the prevention of colon polyps was stopped when it was determined that celecoxib increased the risk of cardiovascular events.[22] However, a similar study in patients receiving celecoxib for a similar period of time has not shown any increased risk.[23] The nonselective NSAID naproxen recently has also been associated with an increased cardiovascular risk in a study involving patients with Alzheimer's disease. The athletic trainer and general consumer must remember that along with benefits, potential adverse effects occur with any drug. Individual patient needs and risk factors must be considered to make the best drug therapy choices. The lowest possible effective dose should always be used to minimize the chance of adverse drug events.

Contraindications

NSAIDs are contraindicated for individuals who have had a previous hypersensitivity reaction or other severe allergic reaction to aspirin or any other NSAID and for individuals who have experienced bronchospasm, angioedema, or nasal polyps when taking aspirin or other NSAIDs. Extreme caution is needed when giving aspirin or other NSAIDs to individuals with a history of gastrointestinal lesions (e.g., peptic ulcer), athletes who have sickle cell anemia, and those taking blood thinners such as enoxaparin (Lovenox) or warfarin (Coumadin).

Interactions

Because many NSAIDs are readily available over the counter, the athlete may be tempted to take NSAIDs such as ibuprofen with acetaminophen. These two drugs have different mechanisms of action, and therefore it is safe to combine them if the maximum dosage of over-the-counter NSAIDs is not providing enough analgesia. However, better prescription medications are probably available and if the athlete's discomfort is not relieved with over-the-counter medications, the team physician should be consulted about the condition. The athletic trainer also needs to educate the athlete that many products contain the same active ingredients and therefore care must be taken when combining over-the-counter medications of any kind.

Narcotic Analgesics

Analgesic agents that stimulate the opiate receptors are the narcotic analgesics (Table 3-6). Some of these agents are derived from opium (e.g., morphine, codeine, oxycodone). Others, including meperidine (Demerol), sufentanil, and fentanyl, are a group of synthetic opiate agonists that share structural similarities. A third group of related opiate agonists are methadone and propoxyphene (Darvon).

These agents stimulate opiate receptors causing analgesia, sedation, and euphoria. The analgesia is produced not by an actual decrease in the level of pain but rather by altering the way that pain is perceived. Opiate agonists cause dissociation from the pain. A person who takes an opiate agonist still has pain but does not care about it. Because these drugs also cause a feeling of euphoria, there is significant potential for addiction.

Opiates are found in combination with aspirin, ibuprofen, or most commonly acetaminophen. This is very effective because the aspirin and ibuprofen decrease the production of pain mediators (e.g., prostaglandins) and the opiate agonist minimizes the perception of pain.

Side Effects

The side effects of opiate agonists are constipation, physical dependence or addiction, sedation, drowsiness, dry mouth, blurred vision, urinary retention, nausea, vomiting, histamine release, respiratory depression, and allergic reactions. The athlete taking these medications must avoid alcohol and exercise caution if taking other drugs that cause CNS sedation (Red Flags—Narcotic Analgesics). These sedating effects are additive and can be very dangerous. Individuals taking opiate agonists also should avoid operating any machinery

Table 3-6	Narcotic Analgesics		
Trade Name(s) (Opioid/ASA or APAP)	Combination	Dosage	
Percodan Demi (2.44/325 mg)	Oxycodone with aspirin	1-2 every 6 hr	
Percodan, Roxiprin (4.88/325 mg)		1 every 6 hr	
Vicoprofen (7.5/200 mg)	Hydrocodone with ibuprofen	1 every 4-6 hr up to 5 times/day	
Tylox (5/500 mg)	Oxycodone with acetaminophen	1 every 6 hr*	
Roxilox (5/500 mg)			
Roxicet (5/325, 5/500 mg)			
Endocet (5/325, 7.5/325, 10/325 mg)			
Percocet (2.5/325, 5/325, 7.5/500, 10/325, 10/650 mg)			
Vicodin (5/500, 7.5/750, 10/660 mg)	Hydrocodone with acetaminophen	1-2 tablets every 4-6 hr*†	
Lorcet (5/500, 7.5/650, 10/650 mg)			
Lortab (2.5/500, 5/500, 7.5/500, 10/500 mg)			
Anexsia (5/325, 5/500, 7.5/325, 7.5/650, 10/660 mg)			
Norco (5/325, 10/325 mg)			
Zydone (5/400, 7.5/400, 10/400 mg)			
Maxidone (10/750 mg)			
Darvocet (50/325, 100/650 mg)	Propoxyphene with acetaminophen	1-2 tablets every 4 hr*	
MSIR (15, 30 mg), MS	Morphine sulfate	PO: 5-30 mg every 4 hr	
Contin, Avinza, Kadian		200 mg 30 mg/24 hr, maximum: 1600 mg 20 mg SC/IM: 10 mg every 4 hr IV: 2-10 mg/70 kg over 4-5 min	
Tylenol with Codeine (15/300, 30/300, 60/300 mg)	Codeine with acetaminophen	½-4 every 4 hr*	
Dolophine, Methadose	Methadone	2.5-10 mg IM, SC, or PO every 3-4 hr	
Demerol	Meperidine	50-150 mg IM, SC, or PO every 3-4 hr	

Data from (A) Micromedex, 1974-2004, Thomson MICROMEDEX Healthcare Series, vol 122. Thomson Healthcare, Inc; (B) Clinical pharmacology. Gold Standard. Available at http://cp.gsm.com. Accessed May 2004; (C) Drug facts and comparisons, EFacts. Wolters Kluwer Health, Inc. Available at http://efactsweb.com. Accessed May 2004; (D) American Hospital Formulary Service accessed using Silver Platter, Drug Information Full Text, American Society of Hospital Pharmacists, Inc. Accessed May 2004.
ASA, Aspirin; *APAP*, acetaminophen; *PO*, oral; *SC*, subcutaneous; *IM*, intramuscular; *IV*, intravenous.
*Daily dose of acetaminophen should not exceed 4000 mg.
†Daily dose of hydrocodone should not exceed 60 mg.

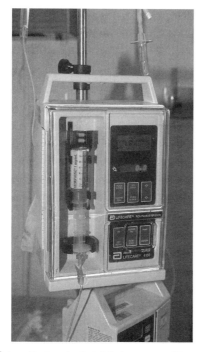

Figure 3-12 A patient-controlled infusion pump. (From Pottter PA, Perry AG: *Fundamentals of nursing*, ed 5, St Louis, 2001, Mosby.)

⚑ **Red Flags for Narcotic Analgesics**
- Alcohol and other sedating drugs must be avoided when taking narcotic analgesics because the sedating effects may be dangerous as a result of additive effects.
- Athletes should not operate motor vehicles while taking narcotic analgesics.

---

that could potentially be dangerous, such as an automobile. Obviously the athlete who is in enough pain to warrant narcotic analgesics should not participate in sports. Figure 3-12 shows a patient-controlled infusion pump, which is often used for the hospitalized athlete following surgery.

To minimize opiate agonists' constipating effects, fluid and fiber intake can be increased. It may be necessary for the athlete to take a stool softener such as docusate sodium (Colace) to alleviate the constipation. To minimize nausea and vomiting, opiate agonists are taken with food rather than on an empty stomach.

Opiate agonists can also cause the release of histamine, which may result in mild to severe itching, especially in the facial area. This itching can be alleviated by antihistamines, such as diphenhydramine (Benadryl); caution needs to be exercised because of additive sedative effects. The adverse reaction of itching is sometimes confused with an allergy, but itching alone in the absence of a rash or hives is an irritating but harmless side effect. An allergic reaction to opiate agonists will manifest itself through hives, difficulty breathing, and facial or tongue swelling. Allergic reactions to opiates are a contraindication to prescribing

these medications. There will be cross-allergenicity between those agents sharing structural similarities (e.g., codeine and morphine or methadone and propoxyphene). If an athlete reports an allergy to opiates, the athletic trainer needs to ascertain that the reaction experienced is not just itching caused by histamine release.

Narcotic analgesics have a very high potential for misuse. For this reason, the vast majority of these drugs are controlled substances. Tramadol (Ultram) is the most notable exception. Tramadol stimulates a subset of opiate receptors that do not cause physical dependence. Whereas this limits the potential for misuse of the drug, use of tramadol in individuals with a history of dependence on opioids may cause this dependence to reemerge. Although the athletic trainer must be alert for signs of dependence (e.g., drug-seeking behavior), the vast majority of individuals who take opioids for legitimate pain never experience a physical dependence (Key Points—Narcotic Analgesics).

KEY POINTS
Narcotic Analgesics

Almost all narcotic analgesics are banned by the U.S. Anti-Doping Agency (USADA) and the National Collegiate Athletic Association (NCAA). See www.usantidoping.org for the latest information.

Local Anesthetics

Local anesthetics produce their effect by reversibly blocking nerve conduction near the site of administration (Table 3-7). Blocked nerve conduction is caused by a decrease in the permeability of the nerve cell membrane to sodium ions. Small nerve fibers (e.g., C- and A-delta) are affected more than large fibers (e.g., A-alpha and A-beta). Autonomic activity is affected first, then loss of sensory functions (e.g., pain), and finally loss of motor activity. The anesthetic effects regress in the reverse order.

Although allergic reactions occur rarely, there is cross-allergenicity between the agents having the same type of linkage. There is no cross-allergenicity between agents having different linkages. Therefore an individual who is allergic to procaine (Novocain) will also be allergic to benzocaine but will not be allergic to lidocaine.

As the name implies, local anesthetics are used to produce a temporary, localized loss of sensory function. In some cases, these drugs may be used for a therapeutic effect in treating pain. In other cases, the anesthetic effect is desired for dental and surgical procedures or sutures. Local anesthetics may be administered through a variety of techniques. Topical administration, ophthalmic administration, infiltration, and

Table 3-7   Local Anesthetics

Type	Trade Name(s)	Generic Name	Route of Administration	Duration of Action
Ester	Americaine, Ora-Jel	Benzocaine	Topical	Short (oral gels have longer duration)
	Nesacaine	Chloroprocaine	Parenteral	Short
		Cocaine	Topical	Short
	Novocain	Procaine	Parenteral	Short
	Alcaine, AK-Taine	Proparacaine	Topical	Short
	Pontocaine	Tetracaine	Parenteral, topical	Long
	Cetacaine	Tetracaine/benzocaine/ butamben	Topical	Long
Amide	Marcaine, Sensorcaine	Bupivacaine	Parenteral	Long
	Nupercainal	Dibucaine	Topical	Long
	Duranest	Etidocaine	Parenteral	Long
	Chirocaine	Levobupivacaine	Parenteral	Long
	Xylocaine	Lidocaine	Parenteral, topical	Intermediate
	Carbocaine, Polocaine	Mepivacaine	Parenteral	Intermediate
	Citanest	Prilocaine	Parenteral, topical	Intermediate
	Emla	Lidocaine/prilocaine	Topical	Intermediate

Data from (A) Micromedex, 1974-2004, Thomson MICROMEDEX Healthcare Series, vol 122. Thomson Healthcare, Inc; (B) Clinical pharmacology. Gold Standard. Available at http://cp.gsm.com. Accessed October 2003; (C) Drug facts and comparisons, EFacts. Wolters Kluwer Health, Inc. Available at http://efactsweb.com. Accessed October 2003; (D) American Hospital Formulary Service accessed using Silver Platter, Drug Information Full Text, American Society of Hospital Pharmacists, Inc. Accessed October 2003.

nerve block are the most common methods of administration seen by the athletic trainer.

Infiltration anesthesia involves the injection of the local anesthetic intradermally, subcutaneously, or submucosally across the nerves supplying the area being anesthetized. Nerve block is the injection of the anesthetic agent into or around the nerve trunks or ganglia that supply the area being anesthetized. Local anesthetics for injection will often be combined with vasoconstrictors, usually epinephrine, to decrease the systemic absorption of the anesthetic and to decrease bleeding. Epinephrine is especially useful when the athlete requires sutures because it assists in controlling bleeding, but it is contraindicated in areas that have poor blood supply, such as the tips of the fingers or the nose.

Topically administered agents, such as lidocaine or EMLA cream, may be used to numb the skin before certain procedures. Benzocaine and dibucaine are used in topical preparations for the relief of sunburn pain. Benzocaine also is found in otic preparations for the relief of ear pain associated with otitis. Other topical anesthetics, such as benzocaine-containing oral gels or throat lozenges, are formulated for application to the oral mucosa to relieve minor irritations of the mouth or throat. These agents are for short-term use only. Any persistent pain in the ear, mouth, or throat should be evaluated by a physician.

Proparacaine and tetracaine are examples of topical ophthalmic anesthetic agents. Topical anesthetics should be used in the eye only to desensitize or anesthetize the eye before ophthalmic procedures such as corneal scraping or foreign body removal. They should never be used for pain control because prolonged use of topical ophthalmic anesthetics has been associated with severe keratitis and permanent corneal opacity and scarring.

Table 3-8   Side Effects of Local Anesthetics

System	Effect
CNS (initial)	Anxiety
	Restlessness
	Confusion
	Tremors
	Seizures
CNS (delayed)	Drowsiness
	Respiratory arrest
Cardiovascular	Bradycardia
	Cardiac arrhythmias
	Hypotension
	Cardiovascular collapse
	Cardiac arrest
Integumentary	Vasoconstriction occurs when coupled with epinephrine; problematic when used as local anesthetic in fingers, toes, ears, and tip of nose

CNS, Central nervous system.

Side Effects

The adverse effects associated with local anesthetics vary with the site of application. The most common adverse effect associated with the use of local anesthetic agents is a burning or stinging sensation associated with an application or injection. For the injected agents, adverse reactions usually result from high concentrations of the local anesthetic in the blood either from inadvertent IV injection or from high doses. These adverse reactions will affect the central nervous and cardiovascular systems. When anesthetic agents combined with epinephrine are used, adverse effects of the epinephrine must be considered. Table 3-8 lists side effects of local anesthetics. Anxiety, palpitation, dizziness, headache, restlessness, tremors, tachycardia, and hypertension may result from high blood levels of epinephrine.

The use of local anesthetics often presents difficult decisions for the team physician. The athlete may encourage the use of topical anesthetics to allow pain-free participation; however, the use must be strictly monitored to prevent further harm to athletes because they cannot protect themselves from further injury. Local anesthetics should only be administered when medically justifiable. The risks of participation need to be fully explained to the athlete and only allowed when there is no increased chance for injury in the anesthetized body part.[6]

Antibiotics

Antibiotics are drugs used to treat bacterial infections. The discussion of antibiotic medications or antimicrobial therapy is a very broad and complex topic. Although the coverage in this text is neither comprehensive nor exhaustive, it does include the most commonly used agents that will be encountered by the athletic trainer. For more complete information on antimicrobial therapy, the reader can refer to the recommended readings in Table 3-2.

Antibiotics may be classified in many different ways on the basis of their chemical structure, mechanism of action, or the spectrum of bacteria for which they are used. The four primary mechanisms of action are disruption of the cell wall, disruption of cytoplasmic metabolism, disruption of deoxyribonucleic acid (DNA) replication, and disruption of protein synthesis. Table 3-9 lists classes of antibiotics, common indications, dosages, and adverse reactions.

Table 3-9 Antibiotics

Aminoglycosides	Common Indication(s)	Usual Adult Dosage	Adverse Reactions
Gentamicin (Garamycin) 0.3% ophthalmic ointment 0.3% ophthalmic solution 0.1% topical cream 0.1% topical ointment	Ocular bacterial infections Dermatological infections	Ophthalmic ointment: 1/2 inch to affected eye(s) 2-3 times daily Solution: 1-2 drops into affected eye(s) every 4 hr Topical cream and ointment should be applied 3-4 times daily to affected area(s)	Ointment: stinging, blurred vision Solution: stinging
Tobramycin (Nebcin, Tobrex) 0.3% ophthalmic ointment 0.3% ophthalmic solution	Ocular bacterial infections Dermatological infections	Ointment: 1/2 inch to affected eye(s) 2-3 times daily Solution: 1-2 drops into affected eye(s) every 4 hr	Ointment: stinging, blurred vision, hypersensitivity: tearing, itching, edema, conjunctival erythema Solution: stinging, hypersensitivity: tearing, itching, edema, conjunctival erythema

Macrolides	Common Indication(s)	Usual Adult Dosage	Adverse Reactions
Erythromycin E-mycin Erythrocin	Sexually transmitted diseases Lyme disease Diphtheria, pertussis Legionnaire's disease Penicillin-sensitive sensitive infections in individuals with penicillin allergy	250 mg PO 4 times daily 333 mg PO 3 times daily 500 mg PO 2 times daily	Nausea, vomiting, diarrhea, abdominal pain, cramping, stomatitis, heartburn, anorexia, melena, pruritus ani, reversible mild acute pancreatitis, pseudomembranous colitis Hepatic dysfunction, reversible cholestatic hepatitis (estolate) Mild allergic reaction: rash, urticaria
Clarithromycin (Biaxin)	Upper and lower respiratory tract infections Skin and skin structure infections Otitis media *Helicobacter pylori* infections (peptic ulcer) Pharyngitis, tonsillitis Lyme disease	250-500 mg PO 2 times daily	Nausea, vomiting, diarrhea, abdominal pain, cramping, stomatitis, heartburn, anorexia, melena, pruritus ani, reversible mild acute pancreatitis, pseudomembranous colitis Mild allergic reaction: rash, urticaria Abnormal taste, headache, behavioral changes, hallucinations, insomnia, tinnitus, tremor, vertigo
Azithromycin (Zithromax)	Mild to moderate upper and lower respiratory tract infections Uncomplicated skin and skin structure infections STDs Acute otitis media Pharyngitis, tonsillitis Pelvic inflammatory disease	500 mg on the first day of treatment followed by 250 mg daily for 4 days A single 1 g dose may be used in the treatment of STDs	Nausea, vomiting, diarrhea, abdominal pain, cramping, stomatitis, heartburn, anorexia, melena, pruritus ani, reversible mild acute pancreatitis, pseudomembranous colitis

Table 3-9   Antibiotics—cont'd

Cephalosporins	Approved Uses	Dosage Range	Adverse Reactions
First Generation Cephalexin (Keflex)	Mild to moderate respiratory tract infections Skin and skin structure infections Acute bacterial otitis Pharyngitis, tonsillitis Mild to moderate urinary tract infections	250-500 mg every 6 hr Uncomplicated urinary tract infections: 500 mg every 12 hr	Gastrointestinal reactions (including pseudomembranous colitis) Headache, rash Hypersensitivity reactions: rash, urticaria, pruritus, fever, chills, arthralgia, edema, hypotension, Stevens-Johnson syndrome, and rarely anaphylaxis Renal dysfunction, nephropathy, increases in serum hepatic enzyme concentrations, increased serum bilirubin, hepatic dysfunction, dizziness, malaise, fatigue, cough, rhinitis, superinfections
Cefadroxil (Duricef)	Mild to moderate respiratory tract infections Skin and skin structure infections Acute bacterial otitis Pharyngitis, tonsillitis Mild to moderate urinary tract infections	500 mg twice daily Uncomplicated urinary tract infections: 1 or 2 g single dose Other urinary tract infections: 1 g twice daily	Same as above
Second Generation Cefuroxime (Ceftin)	Mild to moderate respiratory tract infections Acute otitis media Uncomplicated UTI Uncomplicated gonorrhea Early Lyme disease	250-500 mg every 12 hr Uncomplicated UTI: 125-250 mg every 12 hr Uncomplicated urethral, endocervical, or rectal gonorrhea: single 1 g dose	Same as above Decreased hemoglobin and hematocrit in 10% of individuals
Third Generation Cefdinir	Mild to moderate upper and lower respiratory tract infections Acute otitis media Streptococcal pharyngitis and tonsillitis Uncomplicated skin and skin structure infections	600 mg once daily 300 mg twice daily	Gastrointestinal reactions (including pseudomembranous colitis) Headache, rash Hypersensitivity reactions: rash, urticaria, pruritus, fever, chills, arthralgia, edema, hypotension, Stevens-Johnson syndrome, and rarely anaphylaxis Renal dysfunction, nephropathy, increases in serum hepatic enzyme concentrations, increased serum bilirubin, hepatic dysfunction, dizziness, malaise, fatigue, cough, rhinitis, superinfections
Cefixime	Uncomplicated UTI Acute otitis media Streptococcal pharyngitis and tonsillitis Respiratory tract infections	400 mg once daily 200 mg twice daily	Same as above

Quinolones	Approved Uses	Dosage Range	Adverse Reactions
Ciprofloxacin (oral: Cipro, ophthalmic: Ciloxan, otic: Cipro HC)	UTI Acute sinusitis, lower respiratory tract infections Skin and skin structure infections Bone and joint infections Salmonella Uncomplicated Gonorrhea Infectious diarrhea, travelers' diarrhea Otic: otitis externa, chronic otitis media Ophthalmic: bacterial conjunctivitis, corneal ulcers	Oral: 250-750 mg every 12 hr Ophthalmic: 1-2 drops every 2-4 hr Otic: 3-5 drops twice daily	Bone marrow depression, eosinophilia, hemolysis in individuals with G6PD deficiency, ECG changes, CNS disturbances, nausea, vomiting, diarrhea, taste disturbances, tendon rupture

PO, Oral; *STDs*, sexually transmitted diseases; *UTI*, urinary tract infection; *ECG*, electrocardiogram; *CNS*, central nervous system: *IV*, intravenous.   *Continued*

Table 3-9   Antibiotics—cont'd

Quinolones	Approved Uses	Dosage Range	Adverse Reactions
Levofloxacin (oral: Levaquin, ophthalmic: Quixin)	Acute sinusitis, lower respiratory tract infections (e.g., community-acquired pneumonia) Skin and skin structure infections Urinary tract infections, acute pyelonephritis Travelers' diarrhea Ophthalmic: bacterial conjunctivitis, corneal ulcers	Oral: 250-500 mg once daily; single-dose therapy may be used for STDs Ophthalmic: 1-2 drops every 2-4 hr	Bone marrow depression, eosinophilia, hemolysis in individuals with G6PD deficiency, ECG changes, CNS disturbances, blood glucose disturbances, nausea, diarrhea, taste disturbances, nephrotoxicity; rash, hypersensitivity reactions, Stevens-Johnson syndrome, arthralgias, tendon rupture Ophthalmic: ocular pain, burning, dryness, transient decreased vision
Ofloxacin (oral and otic: Floxin, ophthalmic: Ocuflox)		Oral: 300-400 mg twice daily; 400 ng single dose used for STDs Ophthalmic: 1-2 drops every 2-4 hr Otic: 10 drops 1-2 times daily	Blood dyscrasias, hemolysis in individuals with G6PD deficiency, CNS disturbances, nausea, vomiting, diarrhea, taste disturbances, vaginitis, dysuria, skin eruptions, rash, eczema, photosensitivity, arthralgia, myalgia, tendon rupture, hypersensitivity Otic: dizziness or vertigo Ophthalmic: burning, redness, itching, blurred vision, dryness

Penicillins (Drug)	Therapeutic Uses	Usual Adult Dosage	Adverse Effects
Natural penicillins (penicillin VK)	Upper and lower respiratory tract infections Skin and skin structure infections Lyme disease	250-500 mg every 6 hr for 7-14 days	Mild to severe allergic reactions: rash, urticaria, pruritus, Stevens-Johnson syndrome, fever, chills, malaise, arthralgia, myalgia, lymphadenopathy, splenomegaly, angioedema, anaphylaxis Gastrointestinal disturbances: nausea, vomiting, diarrhea
Aminopenicillins (ampicillin)	Upper and lower respiratory tract infections Gastrointestinal tract infections Skin and skin structure infections, genitourinary tract infections Otitis media	250-500 mg PO every 6 hr	Same as the natural penicillins Mild, nonallergic maculopapular rash (especially in viral infection) Candidal or bacterial superinfections
Aminopenicillins (amoxicillin)	Upper and lower respiratory tract infections Gastrointestinal tract infections Skin and skin structure infections, genitourinary tract infections Otitis media	250-500 mg every 8 hr	Same as the natural penicillins Mild, nonallergic maculopapular rash (especially in viral infection) Candidal or bacterial superinfections
Penicillinase-resistant penicillins (dicloxacillin)	Skin and skin structure infections Acute or chronic osteomyelitis	250-500 mg PO every 6 hr for at least 14 days Osteomyelitis may require up to 2 mo of oral therapy after initial course of therapy with an IV penicillinase-resistant penicillin	Same as the natural penicillins Prolonged therapy: hematological, renal, and hepatic adverse events

Tetracycline	Therapeutic Uses	Usual Adult Dosage	Adverse Effects
	Rocky Mountain spotted fever Q fever Urogenital chlamydial infections Psittacosis *Mycoplasma pneumoniae* ("walking") pneumonia Nongonococcal urethritis, gonorrhea, syphilis Anthrax Acne Lyme disease, *Helicobacter pylori* gastrointestinal infections, cholera, leprosy	Doxycycline: 100 mg twice daily Minocycline: 100 mg twice daily Tetracycline: 250-500 mg orally 1-2 times daily	Gastrointestinal reactions: nausea, vomiting, diarrhea, anorexia, abdominal discomfort Rash, discoloration of the nails Jarisch-Herxheimer reaction: headache, fever, malaise, myalgia, Tetracycline and doxycycline: photosensitivity Minocycline: lightheadedness, dizziness, vertigo, ataxia, drowsiness, headache, fatigue, nausea, vomiting

Data from (A) Micromedex, 1974-2004, Thomson MICROMEDEX Healthcare Series, vol 122. Thomson Healthcare, Inc; (B) Clinical pharmacology. Gold Standard. Available at http://cp.gsm.com. Accessed October 2003; (C) Drug facts and comparisons, EFacts. Wolters Kluwer Health, Inc. Available at http://efactsweb.com. Accessed October 2003; (D) American Hospital Formulary Service accessed using Silver Platter, Drug Information Full Text, American Society of Hospital Pharmacists, Inc. Accessed October 2003.
PO, Oral; *STDs*, sexually transmitted diseases; *UTI*, urinary tract infection; *ECG*, electrocardiogram; *CNS*, central nervous system: *IV*, intravenous.

Antibiotics that disrupt cell wall synthesis are **bactericidal.** They bind to enzymes in the cytoplasmic membrane that are essential to cell wall synthesis. Beta-lactam antibiotics (cephalosporins, penicillins, carbapenems, vancomycin) act through this mechanism. Polymyxin B, which is found in many topical antibiotic creams and ointments, exerts its bactericidal effect through cell wall disruption.

A few antibiotics exert their effect by interfering with cellular metabolism. Sulfonamides, such as sulfamethoxazole, a component of co-trimoxazole (Bactrim, Septra), interfere with the early stages of folic acid production in organisms that synthesize their own folic acid.

Antibiotics that disrupt protein synthesis do so by binding irreversibly to ribosomal subunits. Aminoglycosides, macrolides, clindamycin, and tetracyclines fall into this category. Aminoglycosides are bactericidal (Key Points—Antibiotic Actions). Macrolides and tetracyclines are **bacteriostatic.**

KEY POINTS
Antibiotic Actions

- Bactericidal antibiotics cause bacterial cell death.
- Bacteriostatic antibiotics inhibit further replication of the bacteria but do not cause cell death.
- Bacteriostatic antibiotics may be bactericidal at high concentrations or against highly susceptible organisms.

The physician determines which antibiotic is appropriate to use in a particular situation, ideally on the basis of a culture of body fluids or tissues from the infected area. For practical reasons, culture is reserved for those situations where the infection is of a serious nature or resistant to empirical therapy. In most situations, choosing antibiotic therapy empirically will suffice (Box 3-3).

Patient age, history of allergic reactions, and adverse reactions to previous antibiotic therapy must be considered. Antibiotics with a broad spectrum of action are reserved for infections where resistant organisms or multiple organisms may be the cause of the infection. It is imperative that antibiotics be used appropriately to achieve complete eradication of the infecting organism or organisms. Incomplete courses of antibiotic therapy, inappropriate use of broad-spectrum antibiotics, and the use of antibiotics to treat viral infections all contribute to bacterial resistance.

If antibiotic therapy is discontinued prematurely, then not only is there a chance the infection will recur

but also the infecting organisms are likely to show resistance to the antibiotic used. The reason for this resistance is that the bacteria most susceptible to the antibiotic will be eradicated first and the bacteria with some level of resistance to the antibiotic will linger longer and will be the organisms that cause a recurrence of the infection in the event the antibiotic is stopped before all infecting organisms are eradicated.

When antibiotic therapy is initiated unnecessarily (e.g., to treat viral infections), then bacteria in the body are being exposed to antibiotics unnecessarily. Exposure of bacteria to any antibiotic allows the organism an opportunity to develop adaptive resistance mechanisms to the agent. The more often that bacteria are exposed to an antimicrobial agent, the greater the likelihood that resistance will develop. Antibiotic use must be minimized in order to prevent the development of resistant bacteria (Key Points—Viral Infections).

KEY POINTS
Viral Infections

Viruses are not susceptible to antibiotic therapy; therefore antibiotics are not used to treat a viral infection, such as the common cold.

The use of broad-spectrum antibiotics is reserved for those situations where the infecting bacteria have exhibited resistance to other antimicrobials either through culture results or treatment failure (Box 3-4). Broad-spectrum antibiotics are the most powerful tools in the antimicrobial arsenal. They should be used only in situations where no other agents will work. By minimizing unnecessary exposure of bacteria to antibacterial agents, subsequent development of resistant bacterial colonies will be decreased.

Side Effects

Adverse reactions associated with antibiotics include nausea, vomiting, diarrhea, and abdominal pain (Table 3-10). Specific side effects for various antibiotics are also discussed individually with common uses and dosages. A more serious gastrointestinal adverse effect associated with the use of certain antibiotics is antibiotic-associated pseudomembranous colitis and diarrhea. The seriousness of this infection ranges from mild to life threatening. Pseudomembranous colitis may respond to discontinuation of the antibiotic or may require additional antibiotic therapy and supportive treatment to resolve.

Box 3-3 Empirical Therapy
Empirical therapy relies on an understanding of organisms and knowledge about the common causes of the specific disease and infection. Practitioners choose antibiotic therapy based on their experience rather than on culture results.

Box 3-4 Broad-Spectrum Antibiotics
Broad-spectrum antibiotics are antibiotics that exhibit activity against a wide variety of organisms, including drug-resistant strains.

Table 3-10	Common Adverse Effects of Antibiotics					
Gastrointestinal	Dermatological	Central Nervous System	Systemic	Gynecological	Cardiovascular	Metabolic
Nausea	Rash	Headache	Fever	Vaginal candidiasis	Tachycardia	Hepatic dysfunction
Vomiting	Pruritus	Behavioral changes	Chills		Hypotension	
Diarrhea	Urticaria		Malaise	Decreased effectiveness of birth control pills		
Abdominal pain		Hallucinations	Arthralgia			
Cramping		Insomnia	Lymphadenopathy			
Heartburn		Tremor				
Anorexia		Vertigo				
		Tinnitus				

Antibiotic therapy commonly contributes to the overgrowth of nonsusceptible bacteria or fungi, often described as a superinfection. It is common for women taking antibiotics to develop vaginal fungal infections as a result of the disruption of normal vaginal flora. The physician may choose to prescribe an antifungal agent for use as needed whenever antibiotic therapy is prescribed in women who commonly experience such infections.

Rashes, pruritus, urticaria, and other dermatological reactions are also common with various antibiotics. These rashes may or may not be associated with a hypersensitivity or allergic reaction. Amoxicillin frequently causes rashes in the presence of certain viral infections, but these rashes are not due to an allergic reaction to the drug. A very serious, sometimes fatal dermatological reaction to antibiotics, **Stevens-Johnson syndrome,** is a severe form of erythema multiforme that includes involvement of the oronasal mucosa, eyes, and viscera; malaise; headache; fever; and arthralgia.

Aminoglycosides

Aminoglycoside antibiotics are used primarily via the IV, topical, and ophthalmic routes. They are active against aerobic gram-negative and aerobic gram-positive bacteria. The athletic trainer will see these drugs used most frequently for the treatment of eye infections and sometimes for skin infections. When used for eye infections, the most common adverse effects are transient burning or stinging.

Macrolides

Macrolide antibiotics are administered primarily via the PO, IV, and topical routes. Athletic trainers will see these drugs used most frequently as oral preparations for the treatment of infection. Some athletes may be using erythromycin topical preparations (A/T/S, Benzamycin) for the treatment of acne.

Erythromycin is used in the treatment of several sexually transmitted diseases, Lyme disease, diphtheria, **pertussis, Legionnaire's disease,** and penicillin-sensitive infections in individuals with penicillin allergy.

Clarithromycin (Biaxin) is used in the treatment of upper and lower respiratory tract infections, skin and skin structure infections, otitis media, *Helicobacter pylori* infections associated with peptic ulcer disease, pharyngitis, tonsillitis, otitis media, and Lyme disease.

Azithromycin (Zithromax) is used in the treatment of mild to moderate upper and lower respiratory tract infections, uncomplicated skin and skin structure infections, sexually transmitted diseases, acute otitis media, pharyngitis, tonsillitis, and pelvic inflammatory disease. The major advantage of azithromycin over other antibiotics is its once-daily dosage frequency and 5-day duration of therapy. Several sexually transmitted diseases may be treated with a single, 1 g dose of azithromycin.

Table 3-10 gives the most common adverse effects of macrolides. Less common are heartburn, anorexia, melena, pruritus ani, and reversible mild acute pancreatitis. Prolonged or repeated erythromycin therapy has been associated with pseudomembranous colitis. These adverse gastrointestinal effects occur less frequently with clarithromycin and azithromycin than with erythromycin. Azithromycin does interact with aluminum- and magnesium-containing antacids, which decrease the rate of absorption of azithromycin.

Erythromycin and clarithromycin also have a significant interaction with warfarin (i.e., similar to heparin). Patients stabilized on warfarin have experienced prolonged prothrombin time and bleeding when erythromycin or clarithromycin therapy was initiated. Prothrombin time needs to be monitored closely in individuals receiving warfarin and one of these macrolides simultaneously.

Hepatic dysfunction may occur in patients receiving erythromycin. Erythromycin estolate can cause hepatotoxicity or reversible cholestatic hepatitis in adults who have received the drug for 10 days or longer. The estolate salt of erythromycin should not be used in adults.

Penicillins

Penicillins may be administered by PO, IM, or IV routes. These drugs were the magic bullet against bacterial infection in the early twentieth century but can be

Penicillinase is an enzyme produced by bacteria that reacts with the penicillin molecule and causes the drug to completely lose its antimicrobial activity.

rendered ineffective by some enzymes (Box 3-5). The athletic trainer most often will see these agents being given via the PO route. The penicillins that will be addressed here are the orally administered agents penicillin V, dicloxacillin, ampicillin, and amoxicillin. Penicillin V is classified as a natural penicillin exhibiting activity against *Streptococcus pneumoniae*; group A, B, C, G, H, K, L, and M streptococci; nonenterococcal group D streptococci; and numerous other bacteria as well.

Penicillin V is used principally for the treatment of upper and lower respiratory tract infections and skin and skin structure infections caused by susceptible organisms (e.g., group A beta-hemolytic streptococci) and Lyme disease. It may also be used for the treatment of upper and lower respiratory tract infections caused by susceptible strains of *Streptococcus pneumoniae*. The prevalence of *Streptococcus pneumoniae* resistance to penicillin was 18% during the 2001 to 2002 respiratory season.[24] For this reason, the prevalence and pattern of penicillin resistance of *Streptococcus pneumoniae* in the local community must be considered before using penicillin for empirical therapy.

Penicillin G or some other form of IM penicillin may be used in the treatment of sexually transmitted diseases caused by susceptible organisms (e.g., syphilis).

Side Effects

The most common adverse reaction to penicillins is an allergic reaction ranging from mild to severe (see Table 3-10). The most serious reaction to penicillins, occurring in 0.05% of people receiving the drug, is anaphylaxis, which is fatal in 5% to 10% of cases. Anaphylactic reactions usually occur within 30 minutes of administration of the drug.

A highly significant drug interaction with penicillins, and many other antibiotics, is an interaction with oral contraceptive agents. Use of penicillins and many other antibiotics concomitantly with estrogen-containing oral contraceptives may decrease the efficacy of the contraceptive and increase the incidence of breakthrough bleeding (Red Flags—Contraceptives).

Dicloxacillin is classified as penicillinase-resistant penicillin. It is used mainly in the treatment of skin

> ▶ **Red Flags for Contraceptives**
>
> Many antibiotics interact with oral contraceptives and decrease the efficacy of the contraceptive. This can increase the incidence of breakthrough bleeding. The female athlete taking oral contraceptives and receiving antibiotic therapy should use a second form of birth control during sexual intercourse to prevent pregnancy.

and skin structure infections caused by staphylococci (e.g., cellulitis). Dicloxacillin may also be used in the treatment of acute or chronic osteomyelitis after an initial course of IV therapy with penicillinase-resistant penicillin (e.g., nafcillin).

The adverse reactions associated with the use of dicloxacillin are the same for the natural penicillins. Prolonged therapy with penicillinase-resistant penicillins (e.g., osteomyelitis therapy) has been associated with adverse hematological, renal, and hepatic events.

Amoxicillin and ampicillin are classified as aminopenicillins. Aminopenicillins have the same spectrum of antimicrobial activity as the natural penicillins with enhanced activity against gram-negative bacteria. Aminopenicillins are used in the treatment of upper and lower respiratory tract infections, gastrointestinal tract infections, skin and skin structure infections, genitourinary tract infections, and otitis media caused by susceptible organisms.

The aminopenicillins exhibit the same adverse reactions as the natural penicillins (see Table 3-10). In addition to hypersensitivity reactions, ampicillin and amoxicillin frequently cause a mild **maculopapular rash,** more intense at pressure areas (e.g., knees, elbows), that resolves in 1 to 2 weeks even if drug therapy continues. This rash, which is not an allergic reaction, occurs more frequently when aminopenicillins are used in individuals with viral disease and will resolve in 1 to 7 days if the drug is discontinued. This amoxicillin rash must be differentiated from a true allergic reaction, and individuals experiencing it must not be labeled as penicillin allergic. Prolonged therapy with aminopenicillins needs to be accompanied by periodic monitoring of renal, hepatic, and hematological function. The drug interactions of the aminopenicillins are the same as those for the natural penicillins.

Cephalosporins

Cephalosporin antibiotics may be administered by PO, IV, or IM routes. The agents in this class that will be discussed are cefadroxil (Duricef), cephalexin (Keflex), cefuroxime (Ceftin), cefdinir (Omnicef), and cefixime (Suprax).

Cefadroxil (Duricef) and cephalexin (Keflex) are classified as first-generation cephalosporins. First-generation cephalosporins are active against gram-positive cocci including *Staphylococcus aureus, Staphylococcus epidermidis*, group A beta-hemolytic streptococci, group B streptococci, and *Streptococcus pneumoniae*. Cefadroxil and cephalexin are used in the treatment of mild to moderate respiratory tract infections, skin and skin structure infections (Figure 3-13), acute bacterial otitis, pharyngitis, and tonsillitis caused by susceptible bacteria. They also are used in the treatment of mild to moderate urinary tract infections caused by susceptible gram-negative organisms.

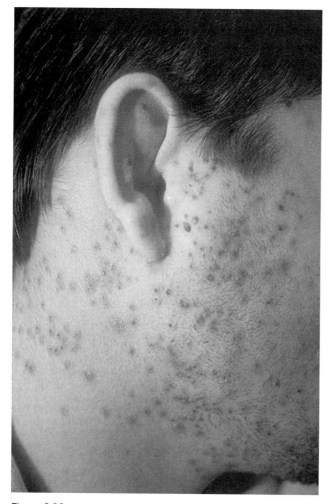

Figure 3-13 An athlete with a staphylococcus infection of the skin is typically treated with a first-generation cephalosporin, such as cephalexin (Keflex).

ated with decreased hemoglobin and hematocrit in 10% of patients.[25]

Fluoroquinolones

Ciprofloxacin (Cipro) is a broad-spectrum fluoroquinolone antibiotic active against most gram-negative aerobic bacteria and many gram-positive aerobic bacteria with the exception of streptococci.

Ciprofloxacin is used orally in the treatment of urinary tract infections, acute sinusitis, lower respiratory tract infections, skin and skin structure infections, or bone and joint infections. Oral ciprofloxacin has also been used in the treatment of salmonella infections, uncomplicated gonorrhea, and infectious diarrhea and in the prevention or empirical treatment of travelers' diarrhea. Ciprofloxacin and hydrocortisone otic drops (Cipro HC) are used in the treatment of otitis externa and chronic otitis media. Ciloxan, ophthalmic ciprofloxacin, is used in the treatment of bacterial conjunctivitis and corneal ulcers caused by susceptible bacteria.

Levofloxacin (Levaquin) is a fluoroquinolone with a similar antimicrobial spectrum to ciprofloxacin but with increased activity against gram-positive organisms, including *Streptococcus pneumoniae*. Levofloxacin is used in the treatment of acute sinusitis, lower respiratory tract infections (e.g., community-acquired pneumonia), skin and skin structure infections, and urinary tract infections. Oral levofloxacin has also been used in the treatment of travelers' diarrhea.

The adverse reactions for ciprofloxacin (Cipro) and levofloxacin (Levaquin) are similar to other antibiotics (see Table 3-10). Tendon ruptures have been reported in individuals receiving fluoroquinolones, however; and in the athlete, this association is of particular concern. Any athlete taking a fluoroquinolone who experiences pain or inflammation of a tendon needs to discontinue use of the drug immediately. The risk of rupture may increase in athletes taking fluoroquinolones and corticosteroids simultaneously.

The safe use of fluoroquinolones in children under the age of 18 years has not been established. Although altered skeletal growth in human children has not been reported, fluoroquinolones cause arthropathy in young animals. Therefore fluoroquinolones are avoided in children and adolescents whose skeletal growth is incomplete.

Aluminum, magnesium, calcium, iron, and zinc decrease the absorption of orally administered fluoroquinolones; therefore antacids and multivitamin or mineral supplements containing these minerals should be avoided during fluoroquinolone therapy. If concomitant use is unavoidable, then the minerals or antacids should not be ingested within 2 to 4 hours of the fluoroquinolone (Red Flags—Minerals and Antacids).

Cefuroxime (Ceftin) is classified as a second-generation cephalosporin and is used in the treatment of mild to moderate respiratory tract infections caused by susceptible bacteria, acute bacterial otitis media, uncomplicated urinary tract infections, uncomplicated gonorrhea, and early Lyme disease.

Cephalosporins should be used with caution in individuals with a history of penicillin hypersensitivity because there is a partial cross-allergenicity between penicillins and cephalosporins. Hypersensitivity reactions occurring with cephalosporins are rash, urticaria, pruritus, fever, chills, arthralgia, edema, hypotension, Stevens-Johnson syndrome, and, rarely, anaphylaxis. Other adverse reactions reported with cephalosporins include renal dysfunction, nephropathy, hepatic dysfunction, dizziness, headache, malaise, fatigue, cough, rhinitis, and superinfections. Cefixime causes adverse events in 50% of individuals, most commonly gastrointestinal (30%), headache (15%), and hypersensitivity reactions (up to 7%). Cefuroxime use has been associ-

Fluoroquinolones cause blood glucose disturbances, both hypoglycemia and hyperglycemia, in individuals taking either oral antidiabetic agents or insulin. These agents must be used with caution in individuals receiving oral hypoglycemic agents or insulin to treat diabetes.

Ciprofloxacin may cause adverse events including nausea, vomiting, dizziness, headache, tremor, agitation, confusion, seizures, tachycardia, and respiratory failure.

Levofloxacin occasionally causes anemia, leukopenia, thrombocytopenia, eosinophilia, fever, chills, rash, and itching. Levofloxacin, whose use has been associated with seizures, may lower the seizure threshold and must be used with caution in individuals with a history of seizure. The risk of seizure is increased if NSAIDs and levofloxacin are being used concomitantly.

Tetracyclines

Tetracyclines are antibiotics with activity against most *Rickettsia, Chlamydia, Mycoplasma,* and spirochetes. Many gram-negative bacteria are susceptible to tetracyclines. Most gram-positive bacteria are susceptible to the tetracyclines, although staphylococci and streptococci are becoming increasingly resistant.

Tetracyclines are used in the treatment of rickettsial infections, including Rocky Mountain spotted fever and Q fever; urogenital chlamydial infections; psittacosis; *Mycoplasma pneumoniae* pneumonia; nongonococcal urethritis; infections caused by uncommon gram-negative bacteria (e.g., brucellosis); gonorrhea; anthrax; acne; syphilis; Lyme disease; *Helicobacter pylori* gastrointestinal infections; cholera; and leprosy. Tetracyclines may also be used for the prevention of malaria. The athletic trainer most often will see the oral tetracyclines doxycycline (Vibramycin), minocycline (Minocin), and tetracycline (Sumycin) used for the treatment of acne.

Common adverse reactions associated with tetracyclines are similar to other antibiotics (see Table 3-10). Dysphagia, sore throat, and black hairy tongue have also been reported. Photosensitivity reactions can be striking and appear almost immediately to a few hours after ingestion (Red Flags—Photosensitivity). Other dermatological reactions such as rash and discoloration of the nails may occur occasionally. A Jarisch-Herxheimer reaction has occurred when tetracyclines were used to treat spirochetal infections, Lyme disease, or brucellosis. This reaction consists of headache, fever, malaise, myalgia, and arthralgia and typically occurs within 12 to 24 hours after initiation of tetracycline therapy.

Minocycline use is associated with a high incidence of vestibular symptoms (up to 90%). These symptoms include lightheadedness, dizziness, vertigo, ataxia, drowsiness, headache, fatigue, nausea, and vomiting.

Tetracyclines will bind to orally administered aluminum, calcium, and magnesium ions resulting in decreased gastrointestinal absorption of the tetracyclines. Antacids containing these minerals should not be taken within 2 hours of the tetracycline. Iron more significantly decreases the absorption of tetracyclines and should not be ingested within 3 hours of tetracyclines. Antidiarrheals containing kaolin, pectin, or bismuth subsalicylate also impair absorption of tetracyclines and should not be used concurrently.

Oral tetracyclines can reduce the effectiveness of oral contraceptives. Concurrent use has resulted in pregnancy and breakthrough bleeding. Women taking oral contraceptives and tetracyclines need to use a second form of birth control during sexual intercourse to avoid pregnancy.

Antivirals

The agents discussed here are used to treat herpes and influenza infections, but antivirals used in the treatment of human immunodeficiency virus (HIV) infection are not covered.

Acyclovir and valacyclovir (i.e., a pro-drug of acyclovir) are agents used in the treatment of herpesvirus, which causes infections of the skin and mucous membranes. Genital herpes infections are contracted through sexual contact, but there are many ways in which herpesvirus may be spread through nonsexual contact. Wrestlers may experience herpes infections of the skin that are contracted through skin-to-skin contact with infected wrestlers (see Chapter 13 for a discussion of viral skin infections).

Acyclovir (Zovirax) is most frequently administered as a topical agent that is applied five or six times per day directly on the herpes lesions. Before valacyclovir became available, oral acyclovir was the only oral drug that could treat herpes infections. Unfortunately, the frequency of oral administration of acyclovir is five or six times per day, which makes it extremely inconvenient. Valacyclovir (Valtrex) oral tablets are administered only one to three times daily. For treatment of acute, localized herpes lesions, the dose of valacyclovir is 1 g every 8 hours for 7 days.

Frequently, wrestlers are given valacyclovir prophylaxis throughout the wrestling season to prevent the occurrence of cutaneous herpes infections. The dose for prophylaxis is 500 mg twice daily.

For athletes with genital herpes, the treatment dose of valacyclovir is 1 g twice daily for 10 days. For the treatment of cold sores, two 2 g doses are given separated by an interval of 12 hours. Regardless of the condition, treatment is most effective if it is started within 48 hours of the onset of symptoms.

Side Effects

Oral acyclovir and valacyclovir are generally well tolerated. The most common adverse effects are gastrointestinal in nature and include nausea, vomiting, or diarrhea. Malaise and headache also occur in around 10% of patients. Occasionally, dermatological reactions such as rash, pruritus, or urticaria may be seen. It is extremely rare to see any adverse reaction from topical acyclovir, although 30% of individuals using topical acyclovir in the treatment of genital lesions will experience burning and pain on application.

Antifungals

Discussion of antifungal agents is limited to agents that are used in the treatment of dermatological and vaginal fungal infections. The most common fungal conditions are tinea pedis, tinea corporis, and tinea cruris, which are generally caused by *Trichophyton* species or *Epidermophyton floccosum* (see Chapter 13 for descriptions of these conditions).

Antifungal agents exert their fungicidal effect through a variety of mechanisms: alteration of the fungal cell wall permeability, inhibition of transmembrane transport, interference with fungal cellular metabolism, and growth inhibition. Topical fungal infections are common, and the athlete can often safely self-medicate with over-the-counter agents. These products include miconazole products, such as Desenex and Micatin, or clotrimazole products, such as Lotrimin. Terbinafine creams, such as Lamisil, and tolnaftate-containing products, such as Tinactin, are also popular. Over-the-counter antifungal medications are available in sprays, powders, and creams. The typical rule of thumb is that sprays and powders are used prophylactically, and the creams are used for active fungal infection. Topical

antifungal agents are sometimes combined with corticosteroids (e.g., Lotrisone), which relieve the itching and burning that may be caused by the fungal infection. Caution is necessary when using these combination products because the corticosteroid may inhibit the activity of some antifungal agents against certain pathogens.

If the infection has not resolved by the end of the duration of therapy recommended for the particular antifungal being used, if the infection is recurring, or if a more hasty recovery is needed, such as in returning a wrestler to competition, then oral antifungals may be prescribed by the physician.

Vaginal fungal infections are caused by *Candida albicans* or other species of *Candida*. Many women experience vaginal candidiasis during antibiotic therapy because of suppression of the normal vaginal flora that allows for overgrowth of *Candida*. These infections may be safely self-medicated in otherwise healthy individuals. Any athlete who is diabetic or immunocompromised should consult a physician rather than self-medicate. If vaginal candidiasis occurs during a woman's menstrual period, she should either delay therapy until after the flow has stopped or begin treatment but avoid the use of tampons. Several products for the treatment of vaginal candidiasis have a petroleum base that may interact with the rubber or latex used in condoms or contraceptive diaphragms. Condoms or diaphragms should not be used within 72 hours of a dose of these products. As with topical fungal infections, if relief of vaginal candidiasis is not achieved by the end of the duration of therapy recommended for the product being used, then the advice of a physician is needed.

Oral candidal infections, which may also occur during antibiotic therapy, should be treated under the advice of a physician using either clotrimazole or nystatin. Table 3-11 lists various antifungal agents, their uses, and the adverse effects associated with each.

Two oral antifungal agents, griseofulvin and ketoconazole, are used in the prevention and treatment of topical fungal infections in wrestlers. These athletes are at risk for developing fungal infections from skin-to-skin contact with other wrestlers or contact with wrestling mats. Griseofulvin (Fulvicin, GrisPEG) comes in two different forms: microsize and ultramicrosize. The difference between these two is the particle size in the drug, which affects absorption. The microsize drug has a particle size of 4 μm; anywhere from 25% to 70% of an oral dose is absorbed. Absorption is increased by administering the drug with a high fat meal. The ultramicrosize drug has a particle size of 1 μm and is nearly completely absorbed. The griseofulvin microsize is given as a 500 to 1000 mg dose once daily. The griseofulvin ultramicrosize is given as a 330 to 750 mg dose once daily.

Table 3-11   Antifungal Agents

Antifungal Agent	Trade Name(s)	Use(s)	Duration of Therapy	Adverse Effects
Butenafine 1% cream	Mentax	Tinea pedis, tinea corporis, tinea cruris, tinea versicolor	Tinea pedis: 4 wk Tinea corporis, tinea cruris, tinea versicolor: 2 wk	Burning, stinging, local irritation
Butoconazole 2% vaginal cream*	Femstat-3, Mycelex-3	Vulvovaginal candidiasis	3 days	Burning, itching
Ciclopirox 0.77% gel, cream, lotion	Loprox	Tinea pedis, tinea cruris, tinea corporis, tinea versicolor	Tinea versicolor: 2 wk All other conditions: 4 wk	Pruritus, transient burning
Clotrimazole 1% cream, solution, lotion, lozenges	Mycelex, Lotrimin, Gyne-Lotrimin, Lotrisone (with betamethasone)	Tinea pedis, tinea cruris, tinea corporis Vulvovaginal and oral candidiasis	Tinea cruris: 2 wk Tinea corporis and tinea pedis: 4 wk Vulvovaginal candidiasis: 7 days Oral candidiasis: 14 days	Erythema, pruritus, burning, stinging, peeling, contact dermatitis
Econazole 1% cream	Spectazole	Tinea corporis, tinea cruris, tinea pedis, tinea versicolor	Tinea cruris, tinea corporis, tinea versicolor: 2 wk Tinea pedis: 1 mo	Burning, stinging, pruritus, erythema
Ketoconazole 2% cream and shampoo	Nizoral	Tinea corporis, tinea cruris, tinea pedis, tinea versicolor	Tinea corporis, tinea cruris, tinea versicolor: 2 wk Tinea pedis: 6 wk	Irritation, pruritus, stinging, contact dermatitis
Miconazole 1% and 2% aerosol, cream, lotion, powder, solution, vaginal cream, vaginal suppositories (100 mg and 200 mg)*	Desenex, Lotrimin AF, Micatin, Ting, Monistat, Femizol-M Nystat-Rx,	Tinea pedis, tinea cruris, tinea corporis, tinea versicolor Vulvovaginal candidiasis	Tinea cruris, tinea corporis, tinea versicolor: 2 wk Tinea pedis: 1 mo Vulvovaginal candidiasis: 3-7 days	Irritation, burning, contact dermatitis
Nystatin oral suspension, tablets, lozenges, cream, ointment, powder	Mycostatin, Nystex, Nystop, Mycolog with triamcinolone, Mycogen with triamcinolone	Vulvovaginal and oral candidiasis	Vulvovaginal candidiasis: 14 days Oral candidiasis: 14 days	Irritation
Oxiconazole 1% cream and lotion	Oxistat	Tinea corporis, tinea cruris, tinea pedis, tinea versicolor	Tinea corporis, tinea cruris, tinea pedis: 2-4 wk Tinea versicolor: 2 wk	Pruritus, burning, contact dermatitis
Sulconazole 1% cream or solution	Exelderm	Tinea corporis, tinea cruris, tinea pedis, tinea versicolor	Tinea corporis, tinea cruris, tinea versicolor: 3 wk Tinea pedis: 4-6 wk	Pruritus, erythema, burning, irritation, stinging, tingling
Terbinafine 1% cream or solution	Lamisil	Tinea corporis, tinea cruris, tinea pedis, tinea versicolor	Tinea corporis, tinea cruris, tinea versicolor: 1 wk Tinea pedis: 2 wk	Burning, pruritus, erythema, skin discoloration
Terconazole 0.4% and 0.8% cream, supositories (80 mg)*	Terazol	Vulvovaginal candidiasis	Vulvovaginal candidiasis: 3-7 days	Itching, burning, pruritus, irritation, abdominal pain, dysmenorrheal, fever, chills, headache
Tioconazole 6.5% ointment*	Monistat-1, Vagistat-1	Vulvovaginal candidiasis	Vulvovaginal candidiasis: single dose, improvement in 3 days	Burning, vaginitis, pruritus, headache, abdominal pain, dysuria, nocturia, pharyngitis, rhinitis
Tolnaftate 1% powder, cream, solution	Tinactin, Aftate, Zeasorb-AF	Tinea corporis, tinea cruris, tinea pedis, tinea versicolor	Tinea corporis, tinea cruris, tinea pedis, tinea versicolor: 4-6 wk	Slight local irritation

Data from (A) Micromedex, 1974-2004, Thomson MICROMEDEX Healthcare Series, vol 122. Thomson Healthcare, Inc; (B) Clinical pharmacology. Gold Standard. Available at http://cp.gsm.com. Accessed October 2004; (C) Drug facts and comparisons, EFacts. Wolters Kluwer Health, Inc. Available at http://efactsweb.com. Accessed October 2004; (D) American Hospital Formulary Service accessed using Silver Platter, Drug Information Full Text, American Society of Hospital Pharmacists, Inc. Accessed October 2004.
*These products contain a petroleum base that may interact with the latex or rubber of condoms or contraceptive diaphragms. Do not use condoms or a contraceptive diaphragm within 72 hours following a dose of these products.

The most common side effects of griseofulvin therapy are headache, which often resolves with continued therapy, fatigue, dizziness, insomnia, gastrointestinal disturbances, rash, urticaria, and photosensitivity. Griseofulvin rarely causes proteinuria, hepatotoxicity, and leukopenia, but because of the serious nature of these disorders, it is recommended that hepatic function, renal function, and white blood cell (WBC) counts be monitored periodically throughout the course of therapy (Red Flags—Antifungal Agents).

> ### ▶ Red Flags for Antifungal Agents
> - Athletes should avoid alcohol when taking oral antifungals because the medication increases the alcohol's effects and causes adverse effects.
> - Hepatic and renal functions as well as white blood cell (WBC) counts are monitored periodically throughout the course of oral antifungal therapy.

Griseofulvin may cause tachycardia and flushing when taken concurrently with alcoholic beverages. Griseofulvin may also potentiate the effects of alcohol; therefore it may be wise to advise athletes to avoid ingestion of alcohol during treatment.

Griseofulvin may decrease the effectiveness of warfarin. In individuals taking warfarin and griseofulvin concurrently, prothrombin time (PT) and international normalized ratio (INR) should be monitored. The dose of warfarin also may need to be adjusted during therapy with griseofulvin.

Griseofulvin also may decrease the effectiveness of oral contraceptives and cause amenorrhea or breakthrough bleeding. Another form of contraception other than birth control pills must be used during therapy. Griseofulvin also has significant teratogenic potential, which makes the requirement for an alternative form of birth control even more urgent. Because griseofulvin has caused sperm abnormalities in mice studies, it is recommended that men wait at least 6 months after the discontinuation of griseofulvin therapy before fathering a child.[26]

Ketoconazole (Nizoral) is prescribed in a 200 to 400 mg single daily dose. The most common side effect of ketoconazole is gastrointestinal disturbance, which may be lessened by administration with food. Gynecomastia with breast tenderness has also been reported in males taking ketoconazole. This condition may resolve with continued therapy, but some cases may require discontinuation of the drug. Because of the unusual nature of this reaction, all men receiving ketoconazole should be advised of this reaction and encouraged to continue therapy.

Rarely, ketoconazole can cause hepatotoxicity. More frequently, increases in liver function tests (LFTs) will be transient. The hepatotoxicity usually resolves on discontinuation of the drug and usually occurs very early in the course of therapy. Individuals receiving ketoconazole should have LFTs performed before the initiation of therapy, every 2 weeks thereafter for the first 2 months of therapy, and then every month until therapy is discontinued.

Ingestion of alcohol during treatment with ketoconazole may result in an Antabuse-like reaction consisting of flushing, rash, nausea, vomiting, and headache. Although this reaction is not dangerous, it is quite uncomfortable. Individuals receiving ketoconazole therapy are cautioned not to ingest alcohol within 48 hours of a dose of ketoconazole.

The absorption of ketoconazole is significantly decreased by drugs that decrease gastric acidity. For this reason, ketoconazole should not be administered within 2 hours of antacids, H_2 antagonists (Zantac, Pepcid), or proton-pump inhibitors (Prilosec, Prevacid).

Ketoconazole may increase the anticoagulant effect of warfarin. PT and INR should be monitored when the two drugs are used together and the dose of warfarin adjusted accordingly. When ketoconazole is administered with phenytoin or theophylline, metabolism of the latter two drugs may be altered. Serum levels need to be monitored and doses adjusted accordingly.

Ketoconazole may cause increased plasma concentrations of systemically administered corticosteroids. In addition, ketoconazole may potentiate the adrenal suppression caused by corticosteroids. For these reasons, the dose of corticosteroids may need to be decreased when administered with ketoconazole.

Bronchodilators

Bronchodilators are beta-adrenergic agonists (Table 3-12). These agents stimulate the beta-adrenergic receptors in the bronchi and bronchioles to cause a widening of these airways and allow for improved airflow. In the athlete, exercise-induced asthma is the most common cause of airway constriction requiring treatment with bronchodilators. Albuterol is the agent used to treat exercise-induced bronchospasm. Albuterol is available as a metered-dose inhaler (MDI),

Table 3-12	Bronchodilators
Drug	**Administration**
Albuterol (Ventolin, Proventil)	Metered-dose inhaler, oral tablets, oral solution, solution for nebulization
Levalbuterol (Xopenex)	Solution for nebulization
Racemic epinephrine (S-2 Inhalant)	Solution for nebulization

Data from (A) Micromedex, 1974-2004, Thomson MICROMEDEX Healthcare Series, vol 122. Thomson Healthcare, Inc; (B) Clinical pharmacology. Gold Standard. Available at http://cp.gsm.com. Accessed October 2003; (C) Drug facts and comparisons, EFacts. Wolters Kluwer Health, Inc. Available at http://efactsweb.com. Accessed October 2003; (D) American Hospital Formulary Service accessed using Silver Platter, Drug Information Full Text, American Society of Hospital Pharmacists, Inc. Accessed October 2003.

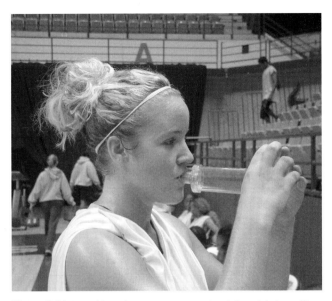

Figure 3-14 An athlete demonstrates a metered-dose inhaler with a spacer.

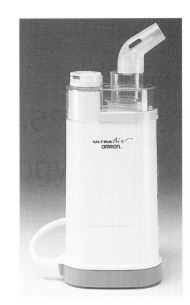

Figure 3-15 A nebulizer contains a pump and compressor that deliver a mist of medication through a face mask or tube. (From Monahan FD, Neighbors M: *Medical-surgical nursing: foundations in clinical practice*, ed 2, Philadelphia, 1998, WB Saunders.)

which offers the most convenient dosing, but proper technique must be used for the drug to be maximally effective (see Figure 3-1, *A*).

Proper technique for using an inhaler is discussed in Chapter 4 as well as on the DVD that accompanies the text. A spacer that holds the puff of medicine between the inhaler device and the athlete can be used to increase the ease of use. When a spacer is used, the actuation of the inhaler does not have to be timed to the inhalation of the drug; the inhaler delivers the drug into the spacer (Figure 3-14). The athlete then inhales the drug slowly and often more completely through the spacer as a separate step.

Nebulizers are machines that use air pressure to aerosolize the drug and then deliver the quickest onset and maximized amount of drug. They are expensive and bulky to transport, but the drug can be delivered simply by placing a mask over the mouth and nose (Figure 3-15).

Side Effects

The main adverse effects of bronchodilators are tremor, nervousness, dizziness, headache, nausea, and tachycardia. A paradoxical bronchospasm also has been reported in 8% of individuals using bronchodilators. It is usually associated with the first use of a new MDI canister and may be related to exposure to the propellant. To avoid this reaction, a new MDI can be actuated into the air a few times before its first use. Nebulized albuterol caused coughing in 4% of individuals in various clinical trials. Side effects that occurred in less than 3% of individuals but that may be significant in the athlete include muscle cramping, muscle spasm, and dilated pupils.

Levalbuterol (Xopenex) is the R-enantiomer of albuterol. It is only available as a solution for nebulization. Levalbuterol is considerably more expensive than albuterol, but it is associated with a lower rate of adverse effects. For treating exercise-induced asthma in the athlete, albuterol, the less expensive alternative, is adequate.

Antihistamines

Antihistamines are drugs used to treat allergies. When the body's immune system reacts to an allergen, histamine is released by the mast cells and basophils. Histamine binds to histamine receptors in the nose, eyes, respiratory tract, and skin causing the classic allergic signs (e.g., rhinitis, sneezing, watery eyes, itching, dermatitis). Antihistamines are antagonists that block the histamine receptors and prevent histamine from binding to the cell's receptors.

The histamine antagonists are classified into two groups on the basis of their likelihood of causing sedation. The first-generation, or sedating, antihistamines are older agents with a much higher incidence of anticholinergic adverse effects, including sedation (Table 3-13). They are used in the treatment of seasonal allergies and some cold symptoms. The sedating properties associated with these drugs also make them useful in the short-term treatment of insomnia. In addition, some antihistamines, such as meclizine (Antivert) and hydroxyzine (Atarax, Vistaril), are used in the treatment of nausea, vertigo, motion sickness, and hives. Sedating antihistamines are commonly used

Table 3-13 Sedating Antihistamines

Antihistamine (Sedating)	Trade Name(s)	Usual Adult Dose
Azatadine	Optimine, 1 mg Rynatan and Trinalin, 1 mg, with pseudoephedrine, 120 mg	1-2 mg twice daily
Brompheniramine	Numerous	4 mg every 4 hr *or* 6-12 mg every 12 hr (extended release)
Dexbrompheniramine with pseudoephedrine	Drixoral	6 mg every 12 hr (extended release)
Carbinoxamine with pseudoephedrine	Rondec, Cardec	4 mg 4 times daily *or* 8 mg every 12 hr (extended release)
Chlorpheniramine	Chlor-Trimeton, numerous others	4 mg every 4-6 hr *or* 8-12 mg twice daily (extended release) *or* 16 mg once daily (extended release)
Clemastine	Tavist	1.34 mg every 12 hr
Diphenhydramine	Benadryl, various others	25-50 mg every 4-6 hr
Promethazine	Phenergan	6.25 mg every 4-6 hr
Triprolidine	Actifed	2.5 mg every 4-6 hr

Data from (A) Micromedex, 1974-2004, Thomson MICROMEDEX Healthcare Series, vol 122. Thomson Healthcare, Inc; (B) Clinical pharmacology. Gold Standard. Available at http://cp.gsm.com. Accessed October 2003; (C) Drug facts and comparisons, EFacts. Wolters Kluwer Health, Inc. Available at http://efactsweb.com. Accessed October 2003; (D) American Hospital Formulary Service accessed using Silver Platter, Drug Information Full Text, American Society of Hospital Pharmacists, Inc. Accessed October 2003.

Table 3-14 Nonsedating Antihistamines

Antihistamine (Nonsedating)	Trade Name(s)	Usual Adult Dose	Drug Interactions	Adverse Effects
Cetirizine	Zyrtec	5-10 mg once daily		Somnolence, fatigue, dizziness, dry mouth
Desloratadine	Clarinex, Clarinex Reditabs	5 mg daily		
Fexofenadine	Allegra	60 mg twice daily *or* 180 mg once daily	Aluminum- and magnesium-containing antacids decrease absorption and peak plasma levels; do not take fexofenadine within 2 hr of antacids	Headache, insomnia, dizziness, back pain
Loratadine	Claritin, Alavert	10 mg once daily		Headache, sedation, insomnia, nervousness, dry mouth, abdominal pain

Data from (A) Micromedex, 1974-2004, Thomson MICROMEDEX Healthcare Series, vol 122. Thomson Healthcare, Inc; (B) Clinical pharmacology. Gold Standard. Available at http://cp.gsm.com. Accessed October 2003; (C) Drug facts and comparisons, EFacts. Wolters Kluwer Health, Inc. Available at http://efactsweb.com. Accessed October 2003; (D) American Hospital Formulary Service accessed using Silver Platter, Drug Information Full Text, American Society of Hospital Pharmacists, Inc. Accessed October 2003.

to treat allergy symptoms associated with seasonal allergies and are usually formulated in combination with decongestants.

Nonsedating, or second-generation, antihistamines are used to treat and prevent seasonal allergies and to treat chronic idiopathic urticaria. These antihistamines are often the drug of choice for the athlete because they are nonsedating (Table 3-14). The nonsedating antihistamines currently available by prescription are cetirizine (Zyrtec), fexofenadine (Allegra), and desloratadine (Clarinex). Loratadine (Claritin, Alavert) is now available as an over-the-counter product. Cetirizine and fexofenadine are also formulated in combination with the decongestant pseudoephedrine (Zyrtec-D, Allegra-D).

The adverse effects most often associated with the first-generation sedating antihistamines are those caused by CNS depression, such as drowsiness, muscular weakness, and dizziness. Therefore antihistamines should be used with caution in athletes participating in events where coordination and alertness are needed to prevent injury. The incidence of injury may be increased and performance decreased even with a mild sedation effect from the antihistamine. Anyone taking antihistamines should avoid alcohol intake because of the additive effect on CNS depression.

Additional adverse effects seen with first-generation antihistamines are gastrointestinal in nature and include nausea, vomiting, diarrhea, or constipation. These antihistamines also cause anticholinergic side effects, such as dry mouth, blurred vision, urinary retention, impotence, nervousness, and irritability.

Antihistamines must be used with caution in individuals with hyperthyroidism and hypertension (see Chapter 11). Although there is some controversy over the potential for antihistamines to induce asthma attacks by virtue of their drying effect on bronchial tissues, antihistamines are contraindicated in individuals who experience acute asthmatic attacks. The drug interactions of the sedating antihistamines are primarily with other CNS depressants, which will cause an additive CNS depressant effect.

Decongestants

Decongestants are drugs that primarily stimulate the alpha-adrenergic receptors and to a lesser extent the beta-adrenergic receptors (Table 3-15). The beneficial result of this alpha-adrenergic stimulation is

Table 3-15   Decongestants

Generic Name	Trade Name(s)	Usual Adult Dose	Adverse Effects
Naphazoline	Privine	2 drops every 3-6 hr	Rebound congestion, burning, stinging, nasal dryness, sneezing, headache, hypertension, palpitations, tachycardia, reflex bradycardia, nervousness, nausea, dizziness, weakness, sweating
Oxymetazoline	Afrin Allerest Cheracol Dristan Genasal Neo-Synephrine Maximum Strength	2-3 drops/sprays every 10-12 hr for no more than 3 days	Rebound congestion, burning, stinging, rhinorrhea, nasal dryness, sneezing, hypertension, nervousness, nausea, dizziness, headache, insomnia, palpitations, tachycardia, reflex bradycardia
Phenylephrine	Neo-Synephrine Alconefrin Nostril Mild Vicks Sinex	2-3 drops or 1-3 sprays every 4 hr	Rebound congestion, burning, stinging, sneezing, rhinorrhea, nasal dryness, palpitation, tachycardia, PVCs, headache, pallor, tremors, sweating, hypertension, nausea, dizziness, nervousness
Propylhexedrine	Benzedrex	2 inhalations every 2 hr	Rebound congestion, burning, stinging, nasal dryness, sneezing, headache, hypertension, nervousness, tachycardia
Tetrahydrozoline	Tyzine	2-4 drops/sprays every 4-6 hr	Rebound congestion, burning, stinging, nasal dryness, sneezing, headache, hypertension, weakness, sweating, palpitation, tremor
Xylometazoline	Otrivin	2-3 drops/sprays every 8-10 hr for no more than 3-5 days	Rebound congestion, burning, stinging, nasal dryness, sneezing, hypertension, nervousness, nausea, dizziness, headache, insomnia, palpitations, tachycardia, arrhythmia
Ophthalmic Decongestants			
Naphazoline	Allerest Clear Eyes Naphcon VasoClear Comfort Vasocon	1-3 drops every 3-4 hr	Blurred vision, mild stinging or irritation, pupil dilation, headache, hypertension, palpitations, tachycardia, reflex bradycardia, nervousness, nausea, dizziness, weakness, sweating
Oxymetazoline	OcuClear Visine LR	1-2 drops every 6 hr	
Phenylephrine	Isopto Frin Ocu-Phrin Prefrin Relief Zincfrin Vasosulf	1-2 drops every 3-4 hr	Headache, blurred vision, irritation, pupil dilation, palpitation, tachycardia, PVCs, headache, pallor, tremors, sweating, hypertension, nausea, dizziness, nervousness
Tetrahydrozoline	Collyrium Fresh Extra Murine Plus Visine	1-2 drops up to 4 times daily	Irritation, blurred vision, pupil dilation, rebound congestion, headache, hypertension, weakness, sweating, palpitation, tremor

Data from (A) Micromedex, 1974-2004, Thomson MICROMEDEX Healthcare Series, vol 122. Thomson Healthcare, Inc; (B) Clinical pharmacology. Gold Standard. Available at http://cp.gsm.com. Accessed October 2003; (C) Drug facts and comparisons, EFacts. Wolters Kluwer Health, Inc. Available at http://efactsweb.com. Accessed October 2003; (D) American Hospital Formulary Service accessed using Silver Platter, Drug Information Full Text, American Society of Hospital Pharmacists, Inc. Accessed October 2003. PVC, Premature ventricular contraction.

vasoconstriction in the nasal mucosa that shrinks swollen nasal passages, thereby relieving nasal congestion. The decongestants are used orally either alone or in combination with other agents used to treat cold and allergy symptoms (e.g., antihistamines).

Topical decongestants can also be applied directly to the nasal mucosa (e.g., Afrin) to provide relief from congestion without systemic side effects. Ophthalmic decongestants (e.g., Visine) are applied to the eye to produce vasoconstriction of the conjunctival vasculature reducing redness of the eyes.

Pseudoephedrine (Sudafed) is the oral decongestant most commonly used alone or in combination products. Pseudoephedrine is a naturally occurring substance found in plants of the genus *Ephedra* and is an isomer of ephedrine. The usual adult dose of pseudoephedrine is 30 to 60 mg every 4 to 6 hours. Sustained-release products of pseudoephedrine are available as 120 mg tablets given every 12 hours and 240 mg tablets given every 24 hours. The side effects associated with the use of pseudoephedrine include mild CNS stimulation such as nervousness, dizziness, weakness, insomnia, and headache. Whereas pseudoephedrine causes minimal blood pressure changes in individuals with normal blood pressure, it should be used with caution in individuals with high blood pressure because alpha-adrenergic stimulation causes vasoconstriction and may raise blood pressure.

Pseudoephedrine can be used to make methamphetamine, a CNS stimulant with high addictive potential. For this reason, federal law limits the quantity of pseudoephedrine that can be sold by retail distributors. It is also vital that the athletic trainer be aware that as CNS stimulants, oral decongestants are listed in the NCAA bylaws (Section 31.2.3.1) as banned drugs (see Appendix G). As mentioned previously, for athletes susceptible to drug testing, the drug of choice for allergic rhinitis should not contain pseudoephedrine.

Phenylephrine (Neo-Synephrine) is used as a topical decongestant in nasal drops and sprays. It is also listed on the NCAA list of banned drugs because of its stimulant properties. Phenylephrine nasal drops or sprays for adults are available as 0.25% or 0.5% solutions that are applied to the nasal mucosa every 4 to 6 hours. Adverse effects of phenylephrine nasal solutions include transient burning, stinging, sneezing, rhinitis, and nasal dryness. Prolonged use of phenylephrine nasal solutions should be avoided because it may result in chronic or rebound swelling of the nasal mucosa, which resolves within 1 week of discontinuing the drug.

Oxymetazoline (Afrin, Dristan) and xylometazoline (Otrivin) are long-acting topical decongestants found in nasal sprays and drops. These long-acting agents should not be used for more than 3 days because significant rebound congestion frequently occurs and may promote overuse of these drugs.

Ophthalmic decongestants, such as tetrahydrozoline (Visine), provide relieve of conjunctival redness and minor eye irritation. Prolonged use of ophthalmic decongestant solutions must be avoided, however, because rebound **hyperemia** may result and promote overuse of the products. It is also important that use of ophthalmic decongestants not mask an underlying condition that may need medical attention. If ocular pain, redness, or irritation occurs or if visual changes are experienced during the use of these products, the athlete must discontinue use immediately and seek medical attention.

Individuals with glaucoma should not use ophthalmic decongestants without consulting a physician or optometrist. Also, most manufacturers recommend that contact lenses be removed before using any ophthalmic decongestant product. Whereas allergic reactions to the ophthalmic decongestants themselves are extremely rare, allergic reactions to the preservatives used in these products are common.

Supplements

No U.S. federal agency, not even the FDA, regulates the ingredient content of food supplements and herbal products. The assumption is that these products contain the ingredients or the quantities of each ingredient that are listed on the label and that the ingredients listed are safe. This puts the person using these products at risk because there has been no regulatory follow-up to make sure the products actually provide what is listed and, further, are safe for human consumption. In Canada, however, the Natural Health Products Directorate enforces the natural health products regulations ensuring all Canadians ready access to natural products that are safe, effective, and of high quality.

Ephedra (ma huang) and ephedrine, substances closely related to pseudoephedrine, are used in weight loss products, "thermogenics," and other products sold for their "energy-producing" properties. Many products sold as nutritional supplements and herbal products for weight loss or energy may contain ephedra or ephedrine. These two substances are also stimulants on the United States Anti-Doping Agency (USADA)[11] and National Collegiate Athletic Association (NCAA)[8] banned drug lists.

Both ephedra and ephedrine can cause hypertension, increased cardiac workload, and arrhythmias, especially in high doses (>150 mg per 24 hours). The use of these agents has been associated with hemorrhagic stroke. Other problems associated with the use of food supplements or herbal products containing ephedra or ephedrine is the lack of consistency and reliability of active ingredient content in these products.

WEB RESOURCES

Anaphylaxis.com
http://www.anaphylaxis.com
Provides information on allergic reactions and anaphylaxis; a step-by-step guide on the use of the EpiPen is available

U.S. Anti-Doping Agency (USADA)
http://usantidoping.org
U.S. antidoping organization for Olympic, Paralympic, and Pan-American games participation

World Anti-Doping Agency
http://www.wada-ama.org/
Regulates all international and Olympic competitions to ensure fair play and standards regarding drug use and testing; lists banned substances and describes drug testing policies and procedures

Health Canada Online
www.hc-sc.gc.ca
The federal department in Canada responsible for establishing and enforcing policies concerning the health care of the citizens of Canada

Canadian Inter-University Sport (CIS)
www.universitysport.ca
The Canadian equivalent to the U.S. National Collegiate Athletic Association; rules and regulations pertaining to intercollegiate athletes at Canadian universities are presented

National Collegiate Athletic Association (NCAA)
www.ncaa.org
A comprehensive site including rules and regulations for compliance in all matters concerning intercollegiate athletics; also gives information on drug testing and banned substances

Medline Plus, sponsored by the National Library of Medicine
http://www.nlm.nih.gov/medlineplus/druginformation.html
Health information provided for the consumer and the health care professional on thousands of prescription and over-the-counter medications

National Center for Drug Free Sport
http://www.drugfreesport.com/home.asp
Provides educational information on banned substances and nutritional supplements

Drug Information Online
http://www.drugs.com/
Searchable database that provides information on prescription and over-the-counter medications for patients and health professionals

Canadian Adverse Drug Reaction Database
http://www.cbc.ca/news/adr/database/
A complete reference of all adverse drug reaction (ADR) reports currently held in Health Canada's database

---

Caffeine is another CNS stimulant that is banned in high doses from international competitions. A concentration of caffeine in the urine of greater than 12 µg/ml of urine is considered banned. The athlete electing to have a couple cups of coffee before competition will not risk such high urinary concentrations, but the athlete who takes a supplement containing guarana or a caffeine pill may be over the banned urinary concentration because these supplements do not metabolize at the same rate and produce higher urine concentrations than the amount of caffeine found in coffee or soft drinks.

Other supplements, such as anabolic steroids, are typically not used therapeutically and are not covered in this chapter. The NCAA and USADA are good sources of information on additional banned substances in athletes.

SUMMARY

This chapter describes the basic principles of pharmacology including pharmaceuticals and pharmacokinetics. Although dispensing medications is not within the scope of practice of the certified athletic trainer, it is imperative that the athletic trainer understands the range of common medications that athletes may be using as well as potential interactions with other medications or foods and possible adverse reactions. It also is important for the athletic trainer to be familiar with the basic drug classifications used in the athletic

population along with the indications, contraindications, and typical patterns of use.

In addition, the athletic trainer must know how to access current drug information and should have a good working relationship with the team physician and pharmacist to ensure the best treatment for physically active individuals.

REFERENCES

1. Health Canada: Health Canada online. Available at http://www.hc-sc.gc.ca/english/about/org.html. Accessed September 2004.
2. Food and Drug Administration: U.S. food and drug administration. Available at http://www.fda.gov. Accessed February 2004.
3. Nickell R: Prescription drugs need careful handling, *NATA News*, p 45, April 2004.
4. Prentice WE: *Rehabilitation techniques in sports medicine*, ed 3, Boston, 1999, McGraw-Hill.
5. Chantraine A, Ludy JP, Berger D: Is cortisone iontophoresis possible? *Archives of Physical Medicine and Rehabilitation* 67(1):38-40, 1986.
6. National Collegiate Athletic Association: *Sports medicine handbook 2004-2005*, ed 17, Indianapolis, 2004, NCAA.
7. Hillman SK: *Introduction to athletic training*, Champaign, Ill, 2000, Human Kinetics.
8. National Collegiate Athletic Association: *NCAA drug testing program 2003-2004*. Indianapolis, 2003, NCAA. Available at http://www2.ncaa.org/legislation_and_governance/eligibility_and_conduct/drug_testing.html. Accessed February 2005.

9. World Anti-Doping Agency: The 2005 prohibited list, international standard. Available at http://www.wada-ama.org. Accessed September 2004.

10. United States Anti-Doping Association (USADA): Guide to prohibited classes of substances and prohibited methods of doping. Available at http://www.usantidoping.org. Accessed September 2004.

11. United States Anti-Doping Agency (USADA): *Guide to prohibited classes of substances and prohibited methods of doping,* Colorado Springs, Col, 2003, USADA.

12. Warner DC, Schnepf G, Barrett MS, et al: Prevalence, attitudes, and behaviors related to the use of nonsteroidal anti-inflammatory drugs (NSAIDs) in student athletes, *Journal of Adolescent Health* 30(3):150-153, 2002.

13. Medici TC, Grebski E, Hacki M, et al: Effect of one year treatment with inhaled fluticasone propionate or beclomethasone dipropionate on bone density and bone metabolism: a randomized parallel group study in adult asthmatic subjects, *Thorax* 55:375-382, 2000.

14. Adler RA, Rosen CJ: Glucocorticoids and osteoporosis, *Endocrinology and Metabolism Clinics of North America* 23(3):641-654, 1994.

15. Allen DB: Safety of inhaled corticosteroids in children, *Pediatric Pulmonology* 33(3):208-220, 2002.

16. Lukert BP, Raisz LG: Glucocorticoid-induced osteoporosis: pathogenesis and management, *Annals of Internal Medicine* 112:352-364, 1990.

17. Costello C, Jeske A: Iontophoresis: applications in transdermal medication delivery, *Physical Therapy* 75(6):554-563, 1995.

18. Kaufman DW, Kelly JP, Wiholm BE, et al: The risk of acute major upper gastrointestinal bleeding among users of aspirin and ibuprofen at various levels of alcohol consumption, *American Journal of Gastroenterology* 94(11):3189-3196, 1999.

19. Blot WJ, McLaughlin JK (affiliation: International Epidemiology Institute): Over the counter non-steroidal anti-inflammatory drugs and risk of gastrointestinal bleeding, *Journal of Epidemiology and Biostatistics,* 2000.

20. Spektor S, Agus S, Merkin V, Constantini S: Low-dose aspirin prophylaxis and risk of intracranial hemorrhage in patients older than 60 years of age with mild or moderate head injury: a prospective study, *Journal of Neurosurgery* 99(4):661-665, 2003.

21. Mina AA, Knipfer JF, Park DY, et al: Intracranial complications of preinjury anticoagulation in trauma patients with head injury, *Journal of Trauma* 53(4):668-672, 2002.

22. United States Food and Drug Administration (FDA): Halting clinical trials of the Cox-2 inhibitor Celebrex. December 17, 2004. Available at http://www.fda.gov. Accessed February 6, 2005.

23. United States Food and Drug Administration (FDA): Alert for Practitioners. December 17, 2004. Available at http://www.fda.gov/cder. Accessed February 6, 2005.

24. Karlowsky JA, Thornsberry C, Jones ME: Factors associated with relative rates of antimicrobial resistance among Streptococcus pneumoniae in the United States: results from the TRUST Surveillance Program (1998-2002), *Clinical Infectious Diseases* 36:963-970, 2003.

25. *American Hospital Formulary Service Drug Information.* Bethesda, Md, 2004, American Society of Health-System Pharmacists, Inc.

26. *Mosby's Drug Consult.* St Louis, 2004, Mosby. II-1312-1313.

CHAPTER 4

Respiratory Disorders

Arnold Ramirez

OBJECTIVES

At the completion of this chapter, the reader should be able to do the following:

1. Describe the basic anatomy and physiology of the respiratory system.
2. Define common normal and abnormal respiratory patterns.
3. Perform a basic evaluation of the respiratory system including auscultation and percussion.
4. Identify characteristics of normal and abnormal breath sounds.
5. Recognize common pathological conditions including signs and symptoms, differential assessment, referral, standard medical treatment, and implications for participation in athletics.

INTRODUCTION

Respiratory disorders can be very alarming to the athlete and the medical professional. Not only do respiratory conditions affect athletic performance, but acute respiratory distress can be life threatening. Great strides have been made in the recognition and treatment of common respiratory anomalies, such as asthma. Only a few years ago, it was uncommon for an athlete with these conditions to be able to compete at the highest level. Advances in medication allow athletes with respiratory conditions to participate at all competitive levels. Because so many more athletes with respiratory conditions are participating in athletics, athletic trainers must be competent in the recognition, evaluation, and referral of conditions that can affect otherwise healthy individuals.

This chapter describes the evaluation techniques, including percussion and auscultation, used with an athlete who exhibits a respiratory condition. Normal and abnormal breathing patterns are reviewed as part of a differential diagnosis of respiratory conditions. Common respiratory disorders are considered in relation to their signs, symptoms, and need for medical attention. Asthma and pneumonia as well as influenza, bronchitis, and upper respiratory infection are also discussed. Respiratory health is integral to physical activity and must be properly assessed, with referral of the athlete to a physician if warranted.

OVERVIEW OF ANATOMY AND PHYSIOLOGY

The pulmonary system is primarily involved in the exchange of oxygen and carbon dioxide, which are vital in the production of the energy involved in metabolism at the cellular level. This process known as respiration can be divided into two distinct but simultaneous steps: ventilation and oxygenation. During **ventilation,** air moves through the respiratory tract. **Oxygenation** describes the actual exchange of gases in the alveolar-capillary beds.

The body organs involved in respiration are divided into the upper and lower respiratory tracts. The upper respiratory tract consists of the following:

- Nasal passages
- Paranasal sinuses
- Pharynx including nasopharynx and oropharynx
- Larynx or voice box

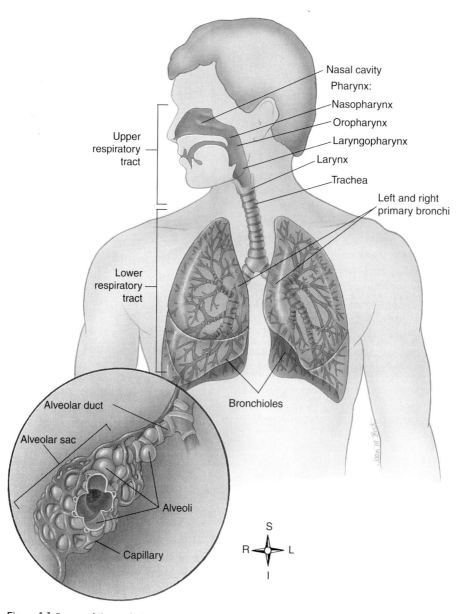

Figure 4-1 Organs of the respiratory system with a detailed view of the alveolar sac. (From Thibodeau GA, Patton KT: *Anatomy and physiology,* ed 5, St Louis, 2003, Mosby.)

The upper respiratory section of the tract is primarily responsible for warming, humidifying, and filtering the air as it reaches the lower respiratory tract.[1] As air is pulled from the external environment into the nasal passages, secretions from the paranasal sinuses add moisture. Cilia, tiny hairlike projections that line the upper airway, filter out fine particles of debris as the air moves into the lower respiratory tract.

The lower respiratory tract comprises the trachea and lungs, which include the bronchi, bronchioles, and terminal alveoli (Figure 4-1). The tracheobronchial tree is a tubular system supported by cartilaginous rings that divides from the trachea into a right and left bronchi at approximately T4 or T5. These main bronchi then divide further into three branches on the right and two on the left. This tubular system serves as a passageway for air as it reaches the bronchioles and, finally, the terminal alveoli where the exchange of oxygen and carbon dioxide from the surrounding capillary beds takes place. The right lung is divided into three separate lobes: upper, middle and lower, whereas the left has only an upper lobe and a lower lobe (Figure 4-2).

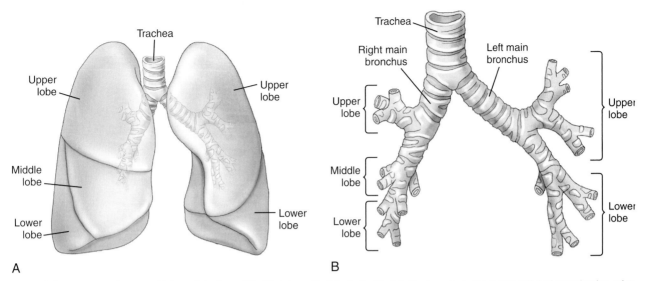

Figure 4-2 The bronchial tree and lobes of the lung. (Modified from Epstein O, Perkin GD, Cookson J, de Bono DP: *Clinical examination,* ed 3, St Louis, 2003, Mosby, pp 96-97.)

EVALUATION OF THE RESPIRATORY SYSTEM

History and Inspection

An athlete may present with an acute or chronic respiratory condition while complaining of shortness of breath, abnormal breathing pattern, or cough. The first step in evaluation is to take a thorough history, which includes questions about how long the problem has existed, what exacerbates the symptoms, and the severity of the symptoms. In an athlete experiencing an acute respiratory attack, the history is abbreviated to only those questions necessary to determine the immediate course of action. A more thorough history is taken once the immediate emergency is controlled. If a cough is present, the examiner asks the patient to describe the characteristics of the cough. Is it "hacking," "dry," or "barking"? If shortness of breath is the complaint, the examiner attempts to discover its severity (e.g., how long the athlete has felt short of breath, and what activity precipitated it) and to find out whether the athlete has chest pain with breathing and, if so, when it starts and how long it lasts. Also, the examiner asks the athlete about any past history of respiratory infections, smoking, and environmental exposure to potential allergens.

The chest is examined after the history is taken. In the athletic training clinic, a chest examination is usually performed on a male athlete who has removed his shirt and on a female athlete dressed in a sports bra and shorts. The examiner inspects the chest for shape and configuration including any skeletal deformities. Congenital deformities, such as scoliosis or kyphosis, as well as other chest deformities may be present and affect not only the shape of the chest but also the efficiency of the respiration (Box 4-1).

The athletic trainer also inspects the chest for potential bruising of the ribs or chest wall, with special attention to the effort and posture of the athlete when breathing, and notes the rate and rhythm of respirations.

Respiratory Patterns

Breathing involves several simultaneous processes. Chemoreceptors in the medulla oblongata of the brain sense changes in pH and carbon dioxide levels. Decreases in pH as well as corresponding increases in carbon dioxide result from normal cellular metabolism and stimulate an increase in ventilation to remove these by-products. Neural control of breathing comes from the phrenic nerve, which arises from cervical nerve roots C3, C4, and C5 and innervates the diaphragm as well as the nerves that innervate the intercostal muscles (Key Points—Neural Control of Breathing). As the diaphragm and intercostal muscles contract, the thoracic

---

KEY POINTS
Neural Control of Breathing

Neural control of breathing comes from the phrenic nerve, which arises from cervical nerve roots C3, C4, and C5, and innervates the diaphragm and the nerves that innervate the intercostal muscles.

C3
C4 } Keep the diaphragm alive
C5

| **Box 4-1** | Common Chest Shapes |

A. Normal Adult
The thorax in the normal adult is elliptical in shape and is narrower anterior to posterior than it is across the transverse axis.

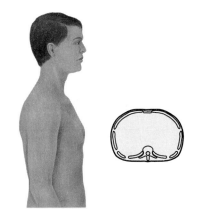

C. Pectus Excavatum (Funnel Breast)
Pectus excavatum, a congenital shape, is usually not symptomatic but presents as a depression at the junction of the xiphoid with the sternum.

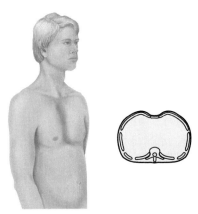

B. Barrel Chest
A barrel chest presents as a rounded shape that is the same diameter from anterior to posterior as it is transversely. Barrel chest is associated with chronic emphysema and asthma but may also be present in the normal, older adult.

D. Pectus Carinatum (Pigeon Chest)
Pectus carinatum presents as a forward protrusion of the sternum. It is less common than pectus excavatum, and minor conditions require no treatment.

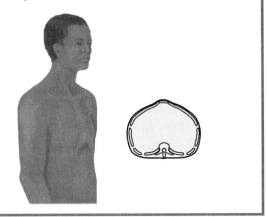

Modified from Jarvis C: *Physical examination & health assessment*, ed 4, Philadelphia, 2004, WB Saunders, p 470.

cavity expands. This generates negative pressure, which causes movement of air into the lungs during inspiration. When alveolar pressure equalizes with atmospheric pressure, intercostal stretch receptors fire and inspiration ceases. The elastic recoil of the thoracic cage results in the passive process of expiration. Accessory muscles of breathing, which include the abdominal, the sternocleidomastoid, and the scalene muscles, are relatively quiet during normal breathing but become active as the work of normal breathing increases.

Normal respiration is unlabored, with 12 to 20 breaths/min. When breathing becomes disordered, several patterns can emerge (Table 4-1). The term **dyspnea** refers to the subjective sensation of difficulty breathing or shortness of breath. When patients have dyspnea, it is important to determine its severity. For example, does the difficulty occur at rest or only with exertion? Certain situations may produce dyspnea,

Table 4-1	Classification of Breathing Terms
Classification	**Description**
Tachypnea	Rapid breathing: >24 breaths/min
Hyperpnea	Tachypnea with very large breaths
Bradypnea	Slow breathing: <12 breaths/min
Hypopnea	Shallow, slow breaths
Orthopnea	Shortness of breath when lying down

such as eating, being exposed to cold **ambient temperatures,** or lying down at night. A condition known as **paroxysmal nocturnal dyspnea** is found in patients with underlying congestive heart failure and causes the individual to be short of breath when lying down at night. Dyspnea may accompany other symptoms in various disease processes, such as fever in infections such as pneumonia, wheezing in asthma, or chest pain in acute myocardial infarction.

Tachypnea refers to breathing that has become more rapid than 24 breaths per minute. This can be seen in a number of respiratory conditions that require the body to increase ventilation. Pulmonary embolism will cause tachycardia. Conditions that limit diaphragmatic excursion, such as an enlarged liver or spleen, also cause tachycardia. **Hyperpnea** refers to a type of tachypnea in which breaths are unusually large and deep resulting in hyperventilation. This can be seen following normal exercise and in anxiety but is also associated with certain metabolic and central nervous system disorders. One example of hyperpnea is known as **Kussmaul breathing** and is found in patients with **diabetic ketoacidosis (DKA).**

When breathing slows to fewer than 12 breaths a minute, it is called **bradypnea.** Electrolyte and acid-base disturbances can produce this pattern, but well-conditioned athletes with higher levels of cardiorespiratory fitness can develop this slowed breathing pattern as well. When breathing becomes slow and shallow it is called **hypopnea** and is seen as an adaptive response to pleuritic painful situations, such as rib fractures. The absence of spontaneous respiration is known as **apnea.** A condition called obstructive sleep apnea occurs primarily in obese patients during rapid-eye-movement sleep. Periods of apnea can also be found in a respiratory pattern called **Cheyne-Stokes respiration** or periodic breathing. This breathing pattern can be normal in children and infants during sleep, but it also occurs pathologically in brain-damaged individuals. Figure 4-3 is a visual representation of the respiratory patterns.

As mentioned earlier, disordered breathing may have a cardiac origin. The symptom of **orthopnea,** which describes a type of dyspnea that begins or increases as the patient lies down, results from the pulmonary edema from congestive heart failure. The severity of orthopnea is often gauged by the number of pillows needed for the patient to sleep. Dyspnea that reliably occurs with exertion may be attributed to cardiac **angina** rather than a respiratory condition. It is important for the athletic trainer to consider the possibility of cardiac involvement when abnormal breathing or chest pain occurs.

Palpation and Percussion of the Chest

The next step of the evaluation is to palpate the chest for symmetrical expansion. The athletic trainer places the hands on the posterior chest wall with the thumbs placed on either side of the spine at the level of T9 or T10 (Figure 4-4, *A*).[2] The examiner asks the athlete to inhale deeply and then watches the hands move apart symmetrically with the chest wall. Next, one feels for **tactile fremitus.** This is a palpable vibration that

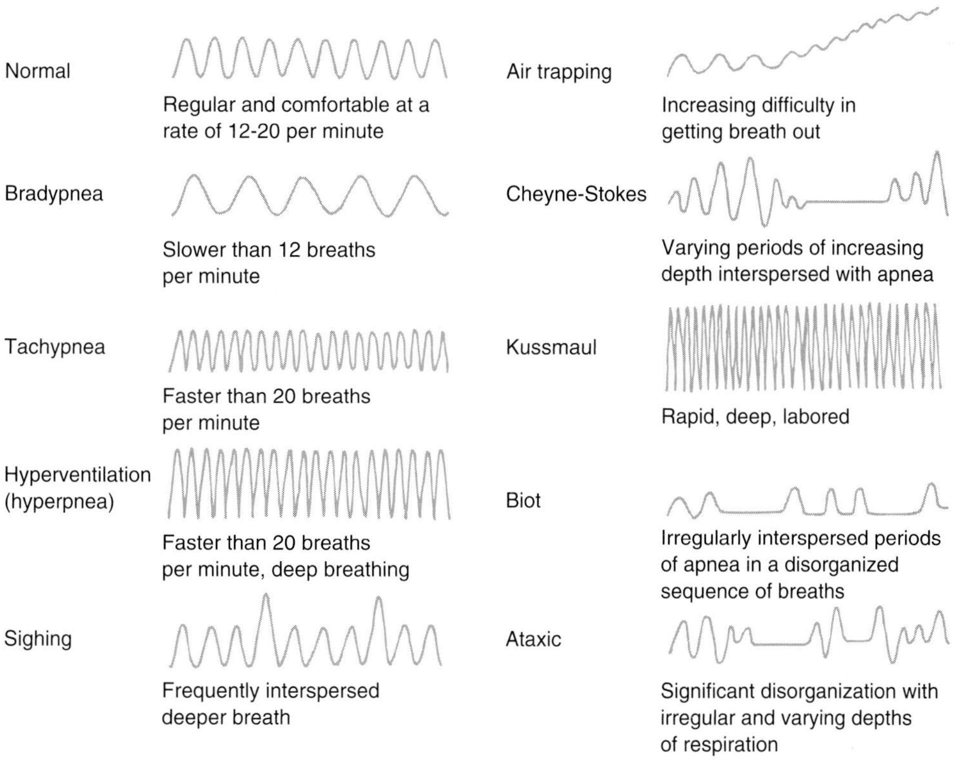

Normal		Air trapping
Regular and comfortable at a rate of 12-20 per minute		Increasing difficulty in getting breath out
Bradypnea		Cheyne-Stokes
Slower than 12 breaths per minute		Varying periods of increasing depth interspersed with apnea
Tachypnea		Kussmaul
Faster than 20 breaths per minute		Rapid, deep, labored
Hyperventilation (hyperpnea)		Biot
Faster than 20 breaths per minute, deep breathing		Irregularly interspersed periods of apnea in a disorganized sequence of breaths
Sighing		Ataxic
Frequently interspersed deeper breath		Significant disorganization with irregular and varying depths of respiration

Figure 4-3 Normal and disordered breathing patterns. (From Seidel HM, Ball JW, Dains JE, Benedict GW: *Mosby's guide to physical examination*, ed 5, St Louis, 2003, Mosby, p 372.)

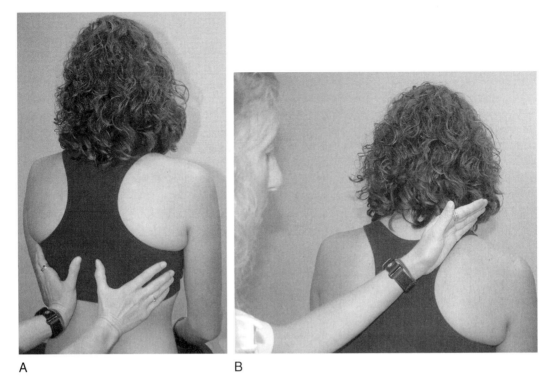

Figure 4-4 A, The examiner places the hands on the athlete's back with the thumbs at T9-T10. As the athlete takes a deep breath, it is easy to visualize the symmetry of chest expansion by watching the movement of the hands. **B,** The examiner uses the ulnar surface of the hand (palmar surface may also be used) to feel for the tactile fremitus while the patient says, "99." Compare the vibration from side to side.

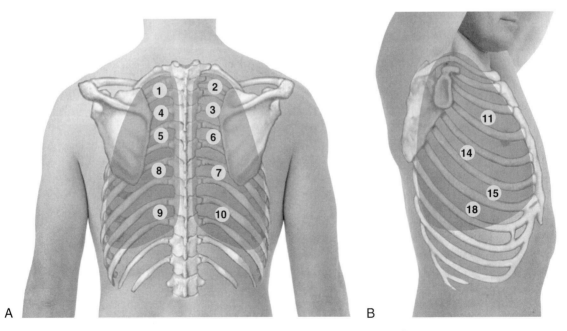

Figure 4-5 Suggested percussion and auscultation sequence. **A,** Posterior chest. **B,** Right lateral thorax.

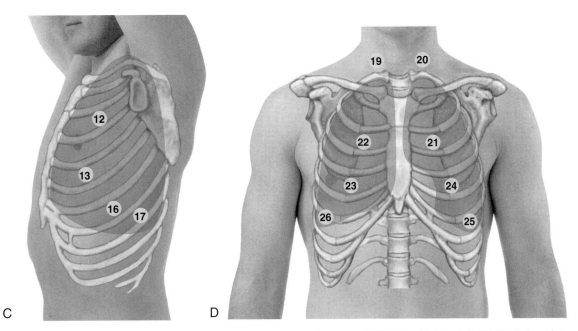

Figure 4-5 Cont'd., C, Left lateral thorax. D, Posterior thorax. (From Seidel HM, Ball JW, Dains JE, Benedict GW: *Mosby's guide to physical examination*, ed 5, St Louis, 2003, Mosby, p 380.)

is generated from the larynx and transmitted through the patient's bronchi and lungs to the chest wall. Use the palmar or ulnar surface of the hand to feel the vibrations while the patient speaks the words "ninety-nine" (Figure 4-4, *B*). The intensity of the fremitus is not as important as the symmetry between lungs. Fremitus will decrease over the scapula and will also decrease as the hand is moved distally to the lower posterior chest. Decreased fremitus occurs when anything obstructs the transmission of the vibrations to the chest wall. Examples of obstructions include pleural effusion, pneumothorax, or emphysema, all of which will be discussed in detail later in this chapter.

After palpation, the chest is percussed using either direct or indirect percussion techniques (see Chapter 2). The examiner uses a systematic sequence of percussion alternating from one side of the chest to the other to compare sounds (Figure 4-5) and starting at the apices of the lungs at the top of the shoulders (see Figure 2-19). The predominant sound found at the top of theshoulders will be resonant. Progressing inferiorly, the examiner percusses the chest at approximately 5 cm intervals in the intercostal interspaces. In a healthy adult lung, resonance will be the predominate sound. Hyperresonance is found when too much air is present, such as in pneumothorax or emphysema. A dull note will occur over bone (e.g., over the scapula) or where there is abnormal density in the lungs, which is seen in pneumonia or pleural effusion.[2] Dullness will also be found when percussing the

inferior posterior chest wall over the liver and abdominal viscera (Figure 4-6).

Characteristics of Normal and Abnormal Breath Sounds

Auscultation with a stethoscope is an important technique when assessing the condition of the lungs and pleura. Characteristic qualities, such as intensity, pitch, quality, and duration in both inspiration and expiration, help the medical professional assess breath sounds.

The diaphragm of the stethoscope is used on bare skin to auscultate the lungs (see Chapter 2 for basic auscultation skill review). The examiner must listen systematically at each position throughout inspiration and expiration[1,2] and evaluate lungs in the anterior, posterior, and lateral aspects to ensure that each lobe of the lungs is properly examined. Figure 4-7 shows the surface markings of the lobes of the lung. The examiner is always mindful of which lobe is being examined: the front of the chest provides access to primarily the upper lobes whereas auscultation of the back exposes mainly the lower lobes of the lungs. One useful technique involves listening in the same sequence that is used in percussion from left side to right at symmetrical locations to make comparisons as the examiner moves downward from the apex to the base of the lungs. When the athletic trainer listens to the lungs, three different sounds can be appreciated in

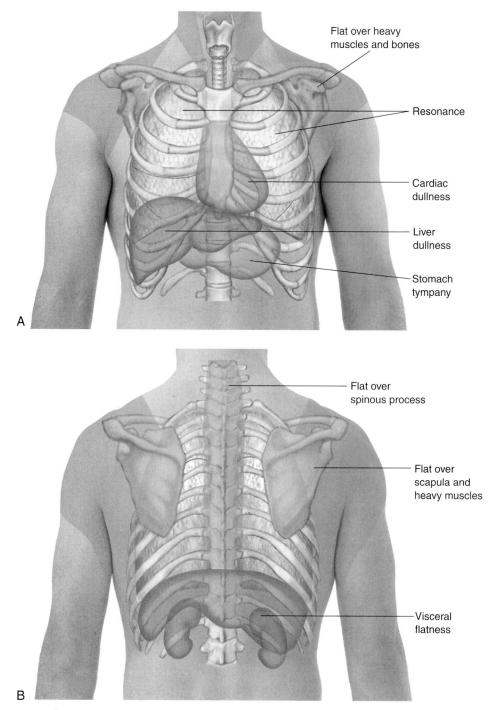

Figure 4-6 Percussion tones throughout the chest. **A,** Anterior view. **B,** Posterior view. (From Seidel HM, Ball JW, Dains JE, Benedict GW: *Mosby's guide to physical examination,* ed 5, St Louis, 2003, Mosby, p 378.)

normal individuals depending on the position of the stethoscope (Figure 4-8).

Bronchial breath sounds are loud, high pitched, and predominantly expiratory. These sounds represent air moving through large airways and sound more tubular. They are normally heard only over the trachea in the anterior chest midline. **Bronchovesicular** breath

sounds are heard when air moves through medium-sized airways, such as the main stem bronchi, and can be heard both anteriorly and posteriorly, toward the center of the thorax. These sounds are of medium pitch and moderate intensity. Inspiratory and expiratory phases are approximately equal. **Vesicular breath sounds** predominate in most of the peripheral lung

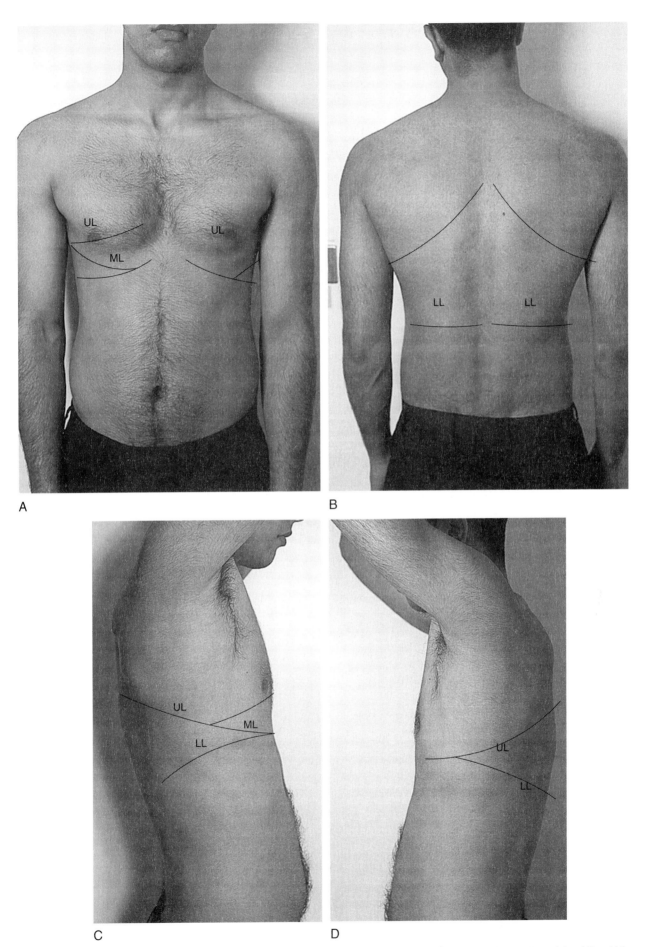

Figure 4-7 Surface markings of the lobes of the lung. **A,** Anterior. **B,** Posterior. **C,** Right lateral. **D,** Left lateral. *UL,* Upper lobe; *ML,* middle lobe; *LL,* lower lobe. (From Epstein O, Perkin GD, Cookson J, de Bono DP: *Clinical examination,* ed 3, St Louis, 2004, Mosby, p 97.)

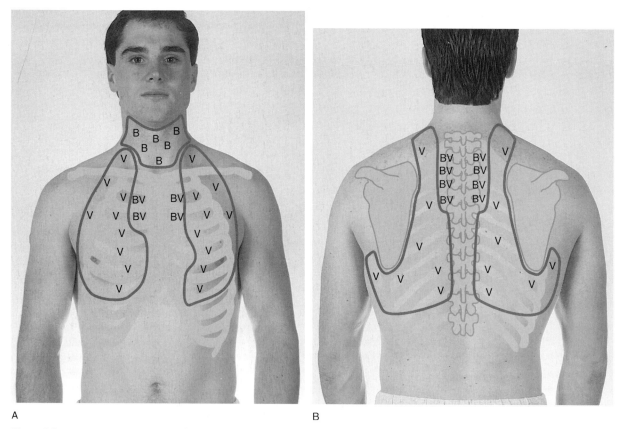

A   B

Figure 4-8 Normal auscultation sounds. **A,** Anterior. **B,** Posterior. *B,* Bronchial (tracheal); *BV,* bronchovesicular; *V,* vesicular. (From Jarvis C: *Physical examination & health assessment*, ed 4, Philadelphia, 2004, WB Saunders, p 456.)

tissue and represent the air as it moves into the smaller airways, such as the bronchioles and lung **parenchyma.** These sounds are soft, low-pitched noises that involve mostly inspiration.

When disease affects the lungs, normal breath sounds are altered depending on the condition (Table 4-2). Fluid in the pleural space may make breath sounds distant or even absent; however, fluid within the lung parenchyma, such as in pulmonary edema or pneumonia, may accentuate breath sounds since sound is transmitted quicker through liquids than through air. Similarly, consolidated masses within the lungs, such as pneumonia, will transmit louder sounds. Most of the abnormal breath sounds heard will be superimposed on normal breath sounds and are called **adventitious breath sounds** (Figure 4-9).

Crackles or rales are adventitious sounds that occur as a result of disruption of airflow in the smaller airways, usually by fluid. They are brief discontinuous noises that can be either low or high pitched depending on the location within the respiratory tree. They commonly resemble the noise made when several strands of hair are rubbed together between the thumb and index finger held close to the ear.

Wheezes are also adventitious sounds that represent airway obstruction from mucus, spasm, or even a foreign body. These sounds are usually more pronounced during expiration and can be either high-pitched, musical noises in the smaller airways (e.g., asthma) or low pitched in the larger airways (e.g., bronchitis). Such low-pitched, sonorous wheezes are also referred to as **rhonchi.** The stridor sound is also caused by airway obstruction and can often be confused with wheezes. The obstruction in stridor generally occurs in the central airways, such as the trachea or larynx, and is more pronounced during inspiration as opposed to the expiratory predominant wheeze.[1,2] **Croup** is a condition that classically can produce **stridor. Pleural rubs** are sounds that occur outside the respiratory tree and result from friction between visceral and parietal pleura in conditions that cause inflammation of the pleura, such as **pleurisy** or pleuritis. Usually low pitched, they can be heard in both inspiration and expiration and can resemble the sound made when two balloons are rubbed together.

Abnormalities can also be detected by listening to the transmission of speech while auscultating the lungs. Transmitted speech is normally muffled and best heard toward the midline. In pneumonia, when there is consolidation, changes in vocal resonance occur. **Bronchophony** occurs when speech becomes clearer and louder. In the extreme, namely, **whispered**

Table 4-2   Physical Findings Associated with Common Respiratory Conditions

Condition	Inspection	Palpation	Percussion	Auscultation
Asthma	Tachypnea Dyspnea	Tachycardia	Occasional hyperresonance	Prolonged expiration Wheezes Diminished lung sounds
Bronchitis	Occasional tachypnea Occasional shallow breathing Often no deviation from normal	Tactile fremitus	Resonance	Occasional crackles Occasional expiratory wheezes
Pneumonia	Tachypnea Shallow breathing Flaring of nostrils	Increased fremitus in presence of consolidation	Dullness if consolidation is great	Variety of crackles Bronchial breath sounds Egophony, bronchophony
Pneumothorax	Tachycardia Cyanosis Respiratory distress Tracheal deviation	Diminished to absent fremitus Tachycardia	Hyperresonance	Diminished to absent breath sounds Sternal and precordial clicks and crackling Diminished to absent whispered voice sounds

Modified from Seidel HM, Ball JW, Dains JE, Benedict GW: *Mosby's guide to physical examination*, ed 5, St Louis, 2003, Mosby, pp 397-398.

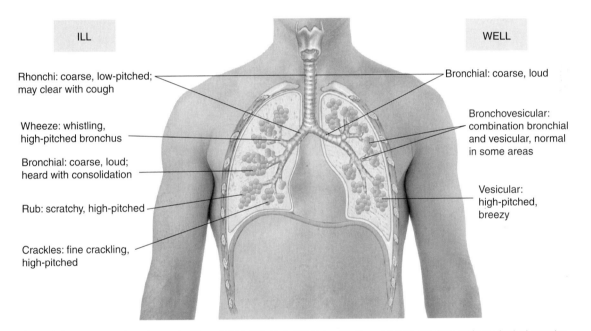

Figure 4-9 Adventitious breath sounds. (From Seidel HM, Ball JW, Dains JE, Benedict GW: *Mosby's guide to physical examination*, ed 5, St Louis, 2003, Mosby, p 384.)

pectoriloquy, whispered speech can be heard clearly through the stethoscope. Consolidation of lung tissue will also produce **egophony,** in which a spoken "e" is heard as "a." Conversely, any obstruction of the respiratory tree causes diminished vocal resonance.

The athletic trainer must become familiar with normal breath sounds through auscultation, thus better realizing when adventitious sounds are present in the lungs. Box 4-2 summarizes the steps in the evaluation of an athlete's respiratory system. In addition, the athletic trainer needs to be vigilant in recognizing the signs and symptoms of respiratory disorders (Red Flags—Respiratory Disorders).

The following sections will discuss the pathological conditions of the respiratory system beginning with

> ### Red Flags for Respiratory Disorders
> - Labored breathing with the use of accessory muscles (not associated with exercise)
> - Adventitious breath sounds
> - Hemoptysis
> - Orthopnea
> - Dyspnea of rapid onset
> - Prolonged cough
> - Deviated trachea

the signs and symptoms of each disorder and including differential diagnosis, referral and diagnostic tests, treatment, implications for return to participation, and prevention.

| **Box 4-2** | Evaluation of the Chest and Lungs |

History
- Determine onset and duration of symptoms.
- Ask about cough, shortness of breath, and chest pain.
- Obtain history of previous respiratory infections.
- Obtain smoking and environmental exposure history.
- Obtain family history.

Inspection
- Check rate, rhythm, and effort of respirations.
- Assess skin color and condition.
- Check posture associated with breathing (note use of accessory muscles).

Palpation
- Palpate any point tenderness or masses.
- Confirm symmetrical expansion.
- Palpate for tactile fremitus.

Percussion
- Percuss over lungs starting at the apex.

Auscultation
- Assess breath sounds comparing side to side over all lobes of lung.
- Auscultate both anterior and posterior chest.
- Listen for normal breath sounds, and note any abnormal breath sounds.
- Listen for sounds with speaking, such as egophony and bronchophony

| **Box 4-3** | Common Triggers for Asthma |

- Allergens
- Stress
- Anxiety
- Smoke
- Cold temperatures
- Exercise

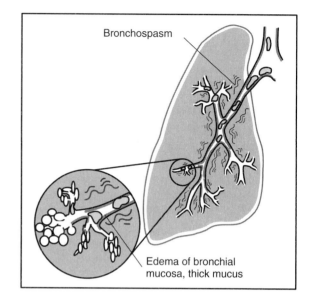

Figure 4-10 Asthma causes bronchospasm and edema of the bronchial mucosa in response to hypersensitivity to certain inhaled allergens. (From Jarvis C: *Physical examination & health assessment*, ed 4, Philadelphia, 2004, WB Saunders, p 478.)

PATHOLOGICAL CONDITIONS

Asthma

Asthma is a pulmonary disorder characterized by reversible airway obstruction that results from hyperreactivity and is also referred to as "twitchy" airways. Allergens, stress or anxiety, smoke or other environmental pollutants, cold ambient temperatures, and even exercise commonly trigger this hyperreactivity (Box 4-3). Asthma generally has two components that lead to the obstruction: inflammation and spasm. Inflammation, characterized by mucosal edema and increased secretions along with bronchospasm of smooth muscle, results in an increase in airway resistance and impeded airflow (Figure 4-10).

Asthma often begins in childhood and has varying degrees of severity and progression. Some individuals require the use of daily oral or inhaled medicines, whereas others need only sporadic or intermittent treatment. Despite the various presentations of asthma, it can be life threatening if not treated promptly and adequately.

Signs and Symptoms

Patients with asthma experience episodic, paroxysmal attacks of shortness of breath and wheezing as well as other symptoms, such as chest tightness and a dry cough. These episodes can be transient, lasting a few minutes to hours, or prolonged over several days. Severe attacks can be associated with much respiratory distress and tachypnea. Wheezing may be audible by an unaided ear in some cases. Mild cases may present as only a chronic cough (cough variant asthma).

On examination, both the respiratory rate and heart rate may be elevated depending on the severity of the condition. Use of accessory muscles of respiration especially may also be seen during respiratory distress. On auscultation, wheezes are usually present, particularly during expiration. In addition, there is prolongation of the expiratory phase as airway resistance is increased. Breath sounds can be diminished.

Referral and Diagnostic Tests

If the patient history and exam suggest asthma, response to empirical treatment with beta-agonist medications such as albuterol is often diagnostic (see Chapter 3 for a review of medications). A decrease in the predicted forced expiratory volume within the first second (FEV_1) measured by spirometry, particularly in response to **cholinergics** such as methacholine (i.e., methacholine challenge test), is considered the gold standard for diagnosis. A peak flow meter provides a quick record of pulmonary function and can be used to help assess the severity of the asthma or the effectiveness of medication (Box 4-4).

Box 4-4 Use of a Peak Flow Meter

1. Stand or sit up straight.
2. Place the mouthpiece onto the peak flow meter.
3. Slide the indicator to the base of the meter.
4. Exhale completely.
5. Take a deep breath.
6. Place the mouthpiece in mouth and seal lips tightly around the mouthpiece.
7. Blow out as hard and fast as you can one time.
8. Reset the indicator.
9. Repeat steps 4-7.
10. Record the higher of the two numbers.
11. Assess forced expiratory volume.

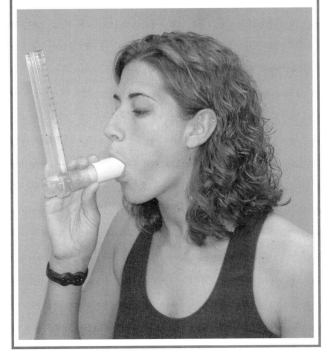

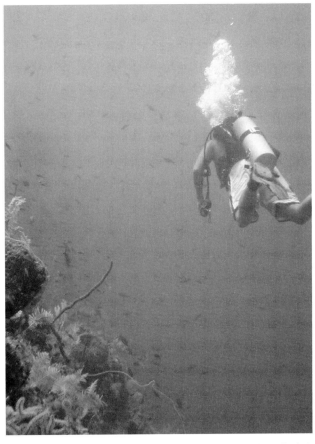

Figure 4-11 Scuba divers with asthma must work directly with their physician to determine if it is safe for them to dive because of the potential for increased risk from barotraumas such as pulmonary embolism. (Courtesy Bill Dent.)

Differential Diagnosis

Asthma always needs to be differentiated from other upper and lower respiratory diseases, including laryngeal dysfunction, croup, infiltrative lung disease, and even foreign body aspiration.[3] The examiner must always consider cardiac failure, chronic obstructive pulmonary disease, or airway tumors as differential diagnoses in older patients, especially smokers.

Treatment

Inhaled beta-agonist medications, both long and short acting, are the mainstays in the treatment of asthma. Other medications used to treat asthma include oral and inhaled steroids, mast cell stabilizers such as cromolyn, leukotriene modifiers, and theophylline. Treatment recommendations generally follow a step-wise approach in the use of both "rescue" and maintenance medications as the severity of the disease dictates.[4] In addition to pharmacotherapy, attention needs to be given to the avoidance of known triggers and the treatment of concomitant allergies.

Prognosis and Return to Participation

In general, athletes with mild asthma may participate in most sports. However, because cold ambient temperatures are known to exacerbate the symptoms of asthma, many athletes with asthma prefer sports that involve competition in warm, temperate climates, such as track and field. Individuals with moderate to severe asthma are unlikely to be involved in vigorous athletic activities since the disease often will limit performance. Athletes with acute exacerbations of the disease should refrain from activity until the acute attack resolves and they no longer require rescue medications, such as albuterol, on a regular basis. Although no absolute contraindication exists to participation in sports in individuals with asthma,[5,6] some controversy does exist regarding individuals with asthma and scuba diving because of a theoretical increased risk for barotrauma such as arterial gas embolism (Figure 4-11). No studies have conclusively demonstrated such a risk, and most experts agree that decisions regarding diving participation by persons with asthma must be made on an individual basis.[5,6]

Exercise-Induced Asthma

As previously discussed, exercise, and in particular aerobic exercise, can stimulate airway hyperreactivity. Symptoms of exercise-induced asthma (EIA) usually occur 10 to 15 minutes after the onset of exercise and are defined by a fall in FEV_1 of 15% or more during exercise spirometry. Recent research shows that the prevalence of EIA in athletes varies from 10% to 50% depending on the population studied[7] and occurs in about 80% to 90% of patients with intrinsic asthma.[5] EIA is more common in winter sport athletes who compete in cold ambient temperatures.

Signs and Symptoms

EIA should be suspected in any athlete who complains of shortness of breath, chest congestion, or tightness with exertion. Other subtle clues might be a dry cough that develops after practice or exercise (i.e., locker-room cough) or simply unusual fatigue compared with similarly trained athletes. Athletes will often complain that they feel out of shape despite regular training.

Referral and Diagnostic Tests

The physical exam is usually normal. Some athletes with EIA may experience symptoms that develop several hours after exercise. This late-phase response is due to the activity of inflammatory mediators.

Differential Diagnosis

In athletes suspected of having EIA, other etiologies, such as acute sinusitis, otitis media (middle ear infection), bronchitis, or even pneumonia, need to be excluded, particularly in the context of other constitutional symptoms, such as fever, chills, or night sweats. If fatigue is the only presenting symptom, deconditioning may also be a cause. In addition, environmental allergies can account for many of the nonspecific symptoms that mimic EIA. More serious cardiac causes, such as arrhythmias and pericarditis, might also need to be excluded.[7] Most commonly, response to an empirical trial of a beta-agonist medication before exercise will establish the diagnosis.

Treatment

The treatment of choice in EIA is an inhaled beta-agonist from a metered-dose inhaler (e.g., albuterol)

Box 4-5   Use of a Metered-Dose Inhaler
1. Remove dust cap and shake the inhaler system before each use.
2. Inspect mouthpiece for contamination or foreign objects.
3. Breathe out through the mouth, exhaling as completely as possible.
4. Hold the inhaler system upright with mouthpiece in mouth, with lips closed tightly around mouthpiece.
5. Breathe in slowly while pressing down on the metal cartridge.
6. Hold breath as long as possible.
7. Release pressure while still holding breath.
8. Remove mouthpiece.
9. Wait for the container to repressurize, shake, and then repeat steps 3 through 8 when more than one inhalation is prescribed.
10. Rinse mouth with water after prescribed number of inhalations.
11. Clean the inhaler system every few days by removing metal cartridge and rinsing the plastic inhaler and cap with running warm water. Replace cartridge and cap.

taken 15 to 30 minutes before the onset of exercise (see Figure 3-1, *A*). Inhaled cromolyn delivered through a metered-dose inhaler can also be used 15 to 30 minutes before exercise and is used mostly in pediatric populations (see Box 4-5 for proper use of an inhaler). Emerging studies show promise using long-acting beta-agonists such as salmeterol and leukotriene inhibitors such as montelukast (Singulair).[8-10] Other nonpharmacological strategies include pre–warm-up bursts of physical activity at 80% to 90% of the individual's maximum workload to induce a refractory period that lasts up to 3 hours after the initial attack of EIA[11] (Figure 4-12).

Prognosis and Return to Participation

Athletes with controlled EIA need not be excluded nor discouraged from participating in sports. Effective strategies, both pharmacological and nonpharmacological, exist that can allow an athlete to compete even at an elite level.

Bronchitis

Bronchitis is a term that refers to any inflammatory condition of the bronchial passages. Generally, it can present in one of two ways: acute or chronic.

In acute bronchitis, the inflammation most commonly results from self-limited viral infections (Figure 4-13). Acute bronchitis is rarely caused by bacterial infections in healthy individuals. It is seen more commonly in smokers and in patients with **chronic obstructive pulmonary disease (COPD)** who have underlying impairment of bronchial ciliary motility. Acute bronchitis can also occur as a noninfectious condition in response to environmental allergens.

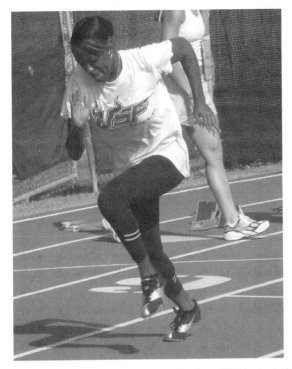

Figure 4-12 Athletes with exercise-induced asthma (EIA) who include pre–warm-up bursts of physical activity at 80% to 90% of their maximum workload may induce a refractory period.

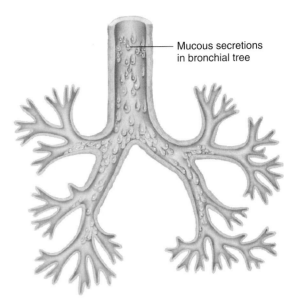

Mucous secretions in bronchial tree

Figure 4-13 Acute bronchitis. (From Seidel HM, Ball JW, Dains JE, Benedict GW: *Mosby's guide to physical examination*, ed 5, St Louis, 2003, Mosby, p 400.)

Chronic bronchitis occurs mainly in smokers as a subset of one of two forms of COPD, the other being **emphysema.** Patients with chronic bronchitis tend to be older and have the typical "smoker's cough." In severe forms, patients may even be somewhat cyanotic. Acute exacerbations of chronic bronchitis are often bacterial and require the use of antibiotic therapy. Because chronic bronchitis is rare in the athletic population, the remainder of the discussion will focus on the assessment and evaluation of acute bronchitis.

Signs and Symptoms

The most common sign seen in an individual who presents with acute bronchitis is a productive cough. Sputum is usually clear but can have a yellowish tinge. Chest congestion or tightness may be present along with some mild shortness of breath. If the cause is infectious, constitutional symptoms, such as fever, chills, or night sweats, may be present although transient. The physical exam is often normal, but occasionally rhonchi and crackles can be heard.

Referral and Diagnostic Tests

Although no diagnostic tests other than the clinical exam are used to make the diagnosis of bronchitis, specific tests may help to exclude other causes. Chest radiographs as well as a complete blood count (CBC) to look for elevations in white blood cells (WBCs)

are useful in diagnosing pneumonia. Computerized tomography (CT) of the sinuses may reveal an underlying sinusitis, and an empirical trial of an antihistamine can help distinguish allergic causes. Since most cases of bronchitis are self-limited, if symptoms do not resolve, referral for medical evaluation is indicated.

Differential Diagnosis

Bronchitis must be differentiated from underlying pneumonia, which can present similarly. The respiratory symptoms tend to be more severe with pneumonia, and the constitutional symptoms, such as chills and fever, are more self-limited in cases of acute infectious bronchitis. Underlying allergic rhinitis as well as sinusitis may also present with a persistent cough secondary to postnasal drainage. In athletes with intermittent bouts of bronchitis, the diagnosis of asthma, either intrinsic or exercise induced, needs to be considered.

Treatment

Treatment in most cases is supportive. Mucolytics, cough suppressants, and nonsteroidal antiinflammatory drugs (NSAIDs) are helpful in reducing the severity of symptoms. Fluids to keep secretions loose are also essential (Box 4-6).

Box 4-6   Supportive Treatments for Viral Bronchitis
• Rest
• Antiinflammatory, antipyretic medications
• Cough suppressants
• Mucolytics
• Fluids

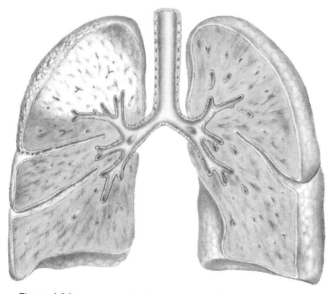

Figure 4-14 Pneumonia (in the right upper lobe). (From Seidel HM, Ball JW, Dains JE, Benedict GW: *Mosby's guide to physical examination*, ed 5, St Louis, 2003, Mosby, p 404.)

Prognosis and Return to Participation

Acute viral cases of bronchitis may last 7 to 10 days. Athletes with acute bronchitis may be allowed to play as tolerated so long as the fever has resolved. Because a small increase in expectorated secretions is possible, attention to fluid status and adequate hydration is essential in minimizing the risk for dehydration.

Pneumonia

Pneumonia is a diagnosis given to any condition that results in inflammation of the lung parenchyma. Usually the cause is infectious and can result from a viral, bacterial, or fungal pathogen. By far, the more common forms are viral or bacterial (Figure 4-14). Fungal infections typically occur in the immunocompromised patient. Patients with pneumonia generally appear ill although some forms of "walking pneumonia" caused by atypical bacteria such as *Mycoplasma pneumoniae* may not be severe. In general, community-acquired pneumonia is easily treatable once properly identified, although hospitalization is sometimes needed in severe cases.

Signs and Symptoms

Patients with pneumonia often have constitutional symptoms that persist if not treated adequately. They may complain of shortness of breath or pleuritic chest pain. A productive cough with dark, discolored sputum is not unusual. If the pneumonia affects the lower lobes of the lungs, diaphragmatic irritation and abdominal pain may be the presenting symptoms.

At physical examination, the respiratory rate may be mildly elevated and breathing may be labored. If there is consolidation, dullness to percussion over the affected lung field may be appreciated as well as changes in vocal resonance, such as bronchophony or egophony, on auscultation of the involved areas. Pooling of secretions in pneumonia concentrated in the lower lobe can produce adventitious rales at the lung bases along with an occasional wheeze.

Referral and Diagnostic Tests

It is virtually impossible to distinguish viral versus bacterial pneumonia on the basis of the clinical exam. Because of the morbidity associated with pneumonia, it is often treated empirically with antibiotics. The athletic trainer refers any athlete who exhibits resting labored breathing with chest pain or cough and presents with signs of consolidation to a physician. Additional diagnostic tests, such as a chest radiograph, are often ordered by the physician and can aid in confirming the diagnosis. Certain microorganisms, such as viruses and atypical bacteria, may not consolidate, and a normal chest radiograph will result (Figure 4-15). Sputum cultures taken to isolate specific organisms are usually done when empirical treatment fails. In general, the athletic trainer should refer athletes suspected of having pneumonia to the team physician as soon as possible for further evaluation.

Differential Diagnosis

Pneumonia can present similarly to other infections of the upper respiratory tract, such as bronchitis and sinusitis. Bronchitis is often confused with pneumonia, particularly when the pneumonia is not severe. Tuberculosis is also a possibility in a patient who presents with pneumonia of the upper lung lobes. Occasionally pneumonia results from an obstruction by a foreign body or mass in the airway.

Treatment

Treatment for pneumonia with first-line antibiotics such as Zithromax (azithromycin) or Biaxin (clarithromycin) is usually successful. Attention to proper hydration and supportive care with mucolytics and cough suppressants (Robitussin-DM Liquid [guaifenesin and dextromethorphan]) are also helpful. The athletic trainer refers athletes who do not improve within 2 to 3 days after initiating therapy back to the team physician for

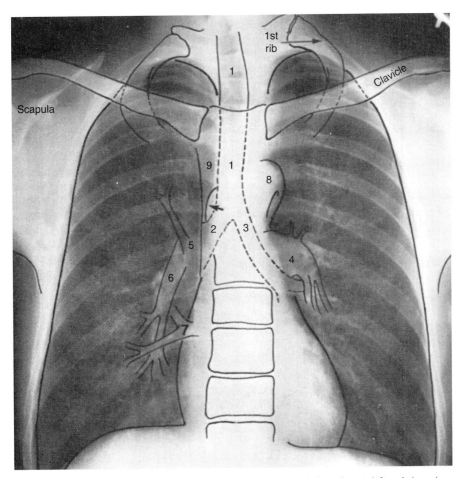

Figure 4-15 Normal radiograph of the chest. *1,* Trachea; *2,* right main bronchus; *3,* left main bronchus; *4,* pulmonary artery; *5,* right upper lobe vein; *6,* right pulmonary artery; *7,* right lower and middle lobe veins; *8,* aortic arch; *9,* superior vena cava. (From Fraser RS et al, editors: *Fraser and Parés diagnosis of diseases of the chest,* ed 4, Philadelphia, 1970, WB Saunders.)

reevaluation and encourage older adult and high-risk patients to ask their physician about the pneumococcal vaccine, which confers protection against the most common strains of pneumonia.

Prognosis and Return to Participation

As with any acute infection, participation is restricted until the athlete is no longer febrile. In addition, in cases of bacterial pneumonia it is recommended that definitive treatment with antibiotics be initiated before an athlete returns to activity. Because of the respiratory compromise that often accompanies acute pneumonia, athletes may not feel well enough to return to sport for about 7 to 10 days.

Pleurisy

Pleurisy is a descriptive term for any inflammation of the pleura (i.e., the lining of the lungs) that causes subsequent pain. It is also known as pleuritis or pleuritic

chest pain. Pleurisy may develop in the presence of lung inflammation, such as pneumonia or tuberculosis, but it can also develop in association with rheumatic diseases, chest trauma, cancer, and asbestos-related diseases. This condition often results in fluid accumulation at the site of pleural inflammation, known as a pleural effusion. The fluid that collects between the lining of the lung and the chest wall may alleviate the chest pain despite worsening of the illness. Large accumulations of fluid can compromise breathing and cause coughing, dyspnea, tachypnea, cyanosis, and **retractions.**

Signs and Symptoms

The hallmark of pleurisy is chest pain at the site of inflammation associated with breathing or any movement of the chest wall, such as coughing, sneezing, or laughing. Pain may be referred to the shoulder, and symptoms of coexisting respiratory infection, such as fever, cough, and malaise, may occur. The normally smooth pleural surfaces, now roughened by inflammation, rub together with each breath and can produce a rough, grating sound called a friction rub. This can be heard easily with a stethoscope or an unassisted ear held to the patient's chest.

Other physical exam findings include rales or rhonchi if there is an accompanying pneumonia or bronchitic condition. If a pleural effusion is present, the examiner also can appreciate decreased breath sounds.

Referral and Diagnostic Tests

A diagnosis of pleurisy is based primarily on the clinical exam. The athletic trainer should refer any athlete with nontraumatic chest pain associated with breathing to the team physician for the evaluation of secondary causes and underlying pathology that is necessary to initiate adequate treatment. Laboratory tests including a CBC can help differentiate bacterial versus viral infections. A chest radiograph may reveal an underlying pneumonia or mass, which may or may not be a malignancy. Chest CT can also be useful to further clarify underlying lung disease, and an ultrasound of the chest can detect fluid associated with pleurisy. If fluid is present, an invasive procedure called a **thoracentesis** may be performed diagnostically to analyze the fluid or therapeutically to alleviate the symptoms associated with a pleural effusion.

Differential Diagnosis

When the diagnosis of pleurisy is possible, the health care professional should always consider primary processes, such as pneumonia, tuberculosis, malignancies including mesothelioma, and autoimmune conditions, in particular systemic lupus erythematosus.

Treatment

Treatment of pleurisy is directed at the underlying illness. Bacterial infections are treated with appropriate antibiotics. Viral infections normally run their course without medications. NSAIDs are helpful in alleviating pain and inflammation associated with pleurisy.

Recovery depends on the nature of the underlying illness but is generally good with treatment. Recuperation from pleurisy caused by malignant disease depends on the type and extent of the illness. Early treatment of bacterial respiratory infections can prevent pleurisy. No treatments are available for viral respiratory infections with the exception of several drugs for influenza type A.

Prognosis and Return to Participation

An individual with pleurisy may return to activity once a work-up has been completed to rule out a primary condition such as pneumonia and if the individual remains **afebrile.** In addition, the athlete refrains from activity if there continues to be any evidence of respiratory compromise at rest or with exertion. When an athlete returns to activity, workloads should be increased gradually over a period of weeks to ensure safe return to competition.

Influenza

Generally known as the "flu," influenza is a common viral infection. Outbreaks in the United States usually occur during the fall and winter months. Various strains of the influenza virus can cause outbreaks in epidemic proportions and lead to thousands of hospitalizations each year. Individuals most susceptible to severe complications are considered high risk and include older adults, individuals who live in close quarters (i.e., students), and people with compromised immune systems, diabetes, or chronic heart, lung, or kidney disease. Influenza is transmitted from person to person via contagious droplets that are spread when an infected person sneezes or coughs (Figure 4-16).

Signs and Symptoms

Whereas milder forms of influenza can be confused with other viral upper respiratory infections, such as the common cold, patients with influenza are generally sicker than those with a regular cold. The onset of symptoms is rapid and can include high fever, headache, muscle aches, cough, chest pain, shortness of breath, fatigue, loss of appetite, nasal congestion, and sore throat. One clue that aids diagnosis is the reported contact with others who have been diagnosed with influenza. Complications may include secondary bacterial infections, such as sinusitis or pneumonia. The influenza virus also can cause pneumonia and encephalitis, an infection of the brain.

Referral and Diagnostic Tests

The athletic trainer should refer athletes who have had close contact with a person diagnosed with influenza and are symptomatic to the team physician for further evaluation and diagnosis. Diagnosis is usually made on clinical grounds, but occasionally antigen testing on secretions from a nasopharyngeal swab is used for definitive results. Laboratory tests including CBCs can be used to delineate viral versus bacterial infection, and blood and sputum cultures obtained in severe illness can isolate pathogens and determine the presence of bacteremia. Chest radiographs will be ordered if pneumonia is suspected on the clinical exam.

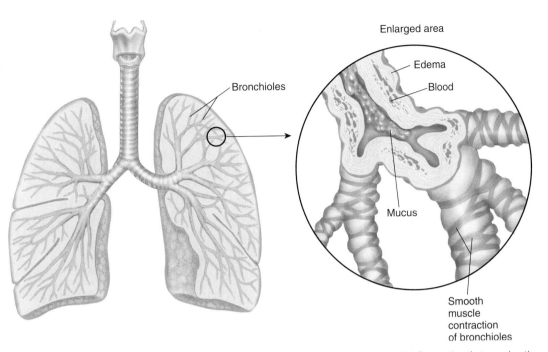

Figure 4-16 Influenza causes inflammation of the lungs; the enlarged area shows the interstitial inflammation that can clog the bronchiolar and alveolar tissues. (From Seidel HM, Ball JW, Dains JE, Benedict GW: *Mosby's guide to physical examination*, ed 5, St Louis, 2003, Mosby, p 405.)

Differential Diagnosis

Influenza must be differentiated from sinusitis, bronchitis, upper respiratory infection, and pneumonia. Fever is a hallmark with influenza whereas the patient with sinusitis is typically afebrile.

Treatment

Treatment for influenza is frequently supportive and includes bed rest, analgesics for muscle aches and pains, and increased intake of fluids for mild illness in generally healthy people. The athlete should be sent home to rest and, if possible, should avoid contact with teammates to limit the spread of the disease. If influenza is diagnosed within 48 hours of symptom onset, in particular among high-risk groups, several antiviral medications are available that may shorten the duration of symptoms by approximately 1 day. These medications include amantadine or rimantadine (active against influenza A only) and oseltamivir or zanamivir (active against influenza A and B). In most individuals who are otherwise healthy, influenza fully resolves within 7 to 10 days. Among individuals in high-risk groups, influenza may be quite severe and can lead to complications.

Prognosis and Return to Participation

Athletes recovering from the flu are usually fit to return to activity in 1 to 2 weeks and must be afebrile and have no respiratory compromise at rest, such as shortness of breath or pleuritic chest pain.

Prevention

The best approach in the management of influenza is prevention. Depending on the supply of vaccine, the athletic trainer should encourage all athletes to be immunized yearly against the common strains of the influenza virus. Immunization typically begins in late October and early November. Those at high risk are generally immunized first. The vaccine has a success rate that ranges from 60% to 70% in preventing influenza in individuals with normal immune systems and can be given to children as young as 6 months of age.[12] Other means of prevention, especially for the athletic population, include hand washing and not sharing drinking receptacles or athletic towels.

Upper Respiratory Infections

Upper respiratory infection (URI) is a diagnosis typically given to any number of self-limited viral infections affecting the upper respiratory tract including the nasopharynx, trachea, and bronchi. Common pathogens include the **rhinovirus** that produces the "common cold," **adenovirus,** and parainfluenza virus.[13,14] These viruses are highly transmissible through contact with infected respiratory droplets via cough or sneeze, and therefore whole households are usually affected.

Signs and Symptoms

URI symptoms are generally mild; although the symptoms are an annoyance, patients can go about their daily activities normally. These symptoms may include fever, which usually resolves in 24 to 48 hours, cough, nasal congestion, sore throat, and runny nose. The sore throat and fever are usually the first presenting symptoms with cough usually the last to resolve. Secondary bacterial infections such as otitis media (i.e., middle ear infection) and sinusitis may result if mucosal inflammation persists. Viral URI symptoms often last 7 to 10 days.

Referral and Diagnostic Tests

When symptoms include high fever, dark purulent nasal discharge, or last longer than 7 to 10 days, athletes should be referred to the team physician for evaluation of other causes including a secondary bacterial infection.

Differential Diagnosis

Viral URIs are diagnosed clinically and many times to the exclusion of other more severe infections such as influenza and bacterial infections. Diagnostic testing is usually not indicated nor useful.

Treatment

The athletic trainer should assure athletes with a URI that the condition is self-limited. Treatment is mainly supportive. Medicines such as over-the-counter cough suppressants, decongestants, antihistamines, and expectorants can alleviate symptoms. The athletic trainer can encourage patients to keep hydrated so that secretions remain loose. This is particularly important in athletes where fluid losses associated with exertion may exacerbate symptoms.

Prognosis and Return to Participation

Athletes may participate in sport as long as they are afebrile and able to drink plenty of fluids.

Prevention

Hand washing and not sharing drinking containers and towels are particularly important in the prevention of transmission of URIs.

Tuberculosis

Pulmonary tuberculosis (TB) is a highly contagious bacterial infection caused by the organism

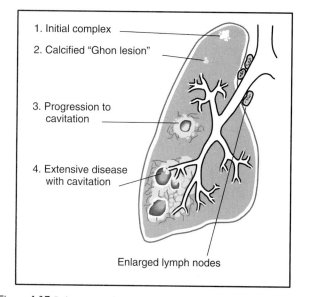

1. Initial complex
2. Calcified "Ghon lesion"
3. Progression to cavitation
4. Extensive disease with cavitation

Enlarged lymph nodes

Figure 4-17 Pulmonary tuberculosis (TB) is a highly contagious bacterial infection caused by the organism *Mycobacterium tuberculosis*. (From Jarvis C: *Physical examination & health assessment*, ed 4, Philadelphia, 2004, WB Saunders, p 480.)

Mycobacterium tuberculosis. The infection primarily involves the lungs, but it can spread to other organs. TB can develop after inhaling droplets sprayed into the air from a cough or sneeze by someone infected by the disease. It is characterized by the development of granulomas (granular tumors) in the infected tissues. The primary stage of the infection is usually asymptomatic and is otherwise known as latent TB.

In the United States, the majority of people will recover from latent TB without further evidence of the disease. Those most at risk for developing active TB have compromised immune systems. Individuals with human immunodeficiency virus (HIV) infection are documented with up to 162 cases of TB per 1000 person-years, and those recently infected are susceptible to 12.9 cases per 1000 person-years within the first year.[15] TB may occur within weeks after the primary infection, or it may lie dormant for years before causing active disease. The risk of contracting TB increases with the frequency of contact with people who have the disease, when living in crowded or unsanitary conditions, and under conditions of poor nutrition (Figure 4-17).

Signs and Symptoms

Patients are asymptomatic in cases of latent TB. For those with active pulmonary TB, the symptoms may be mild and insidious. Fatigue, fever, weight loss, and cough are common.[16,17] The cough may produce sputum containing blood (i.e., **hemoptysis**). Other symptoms include chest pain, shortness of breath, and wheezing. Auscultation of the lungs may reveal crackles or wheezing. A pleural effusion may also be found. Enlargement or tender lymph nodes may be present in the neck and other areas. Often, active TB produces some degree of hypoxia and, if present for some time, results in clubbing of the fingers or toes.

Referral and Diagnostic Tests

Latent TB infections are identified solely on the basis of a positive skin test involving a subcuticular injection of a purified protein derivative (PPD), which causes local induration and erythema of the skin when an infection with *Mycobacterium tuberculosis* is present. Active TB is diagnosed when patients with a positive PPD test have symptoms consistent with pulmonary TB and radiographic evidence of infection. A chest radiograph typically demonstrates granulomatous disease with a predilection for the upper lung fields. Definitive diagnosis of active disease is made with sputum cultures demonstrating acid-fast bacilli.

Differential Diagnosis

Differential diagnosis includes community-acquired bacterial pneumonia, fungal pneumonias, primary as well as metastatic lung malignancies, interstitial lung disease, and opportunistic infections of HIV disease.[17] Any athlete with a persistent cough and constitutional symptoms should be referred to the team physician for follow-up evaluation (Key Points—Constitutional Symptoms).

> ## KEY POINTS
> **Constitutional Symptoms**
>
> - Fever >100° F
> - Chills
> - Night sweats

Treatment

Despite the low conversion rate to active TB, latent TB is usually treated by **chemoprophylaxis** with medications such as isoniazid and rifampin for several months under the supervision of a physician. Because of the emerging multidrug-resistant strains of *Mycobacterium tuberculosis*, the treatment of active TB involves the concomitant use of several antibiotics (up to four) to treat the infection.

Prognosis and Return to Participation

Hospitalization may be indicated to prevent the spread of the disease to others until the contagious period has resolved through the patient's receiving drug therapy. Normal activity can be continued after the contagious period.

Any athlete suspected of having TB must be suspended from activity and referred to a physician immediately. All active cases of tuberculosis need to be reported to the local health department for tracking and surveillance.

Lung Cancer

Lung cancer is by far one of the most common cancers in the United States and is the leading cause of death from cancer. This disease primarily affects smokers although there is increased risk among those exposed to secondhand smoke. Each of the various types of lung cancer affects different types of cells within the lung. Some are more aggressive than others, and some are more responsive to therapy. In general, the prognosis is poor for all types because most lung cancers are not detected until the later stages, usually after there is involvement of or spread to other organs including the brain.

Signs and Symptoms

Symptoms of lung cancer develop slowly over time and are often overlooked until the later stages of the disease. Constitutional symptoms predominate including fever, fatigue, weight loss, and loss of appetite. Cough is usually present with or without bloody sputum. There may be chest pain and shortness of breath. Pneumonia can develop as a secondary consequence. The physical exam is usually nonspecific; however, a pleural effusion can sometimes be detected.

Referral and Diagnostic Tests

Chest radiographs can detect possible malignancies that can be more clearly visualized by CT scans if necessary. Definitive diagnosis is made when cells obtained by bronchoscopy or biopsy are found to be malignant. Other laboratory test abnormalities that may suggest lung cancer include elevated serum (blood) calcium and alkaline phosphatase, decreased serum sodium (i.e., hyponatremia), and abnormal serum levels of carcinoembryonic antigen (CEA).

Differential Diagnosis

The primary diagnostic dilemma in lung cancer is to determine whether the malignancy is primary or has metastasized from another site. Histological analysis of tissue biopsies can usually reveal the source. Clinical presentation of lung cancer can be similar to many chronic lung diseases, including tuberculosis, interstitial lung disease, and COPD. On radiographs, lung cancers may resemble benign granulomas, consolidated pneumonias, or even lung abscesses.

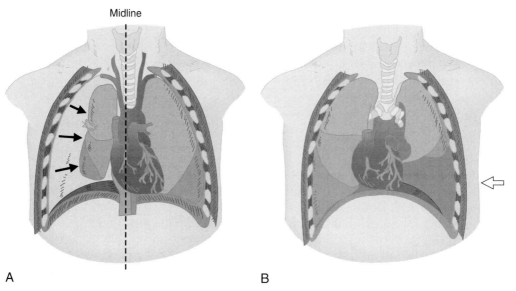

Figure 4-18 A, Pneumothorax. B, Hemothorax. (From Black JM, Hawks JH: *Medical-surgical nursing: clinical management for positive outcomes,* ed 7, St Louis, 2005, Mosby, p 1903.)

Treatment

Treatment of lung cancer depends on its type and stage at diagnosis. Options may include radiation therapy, chemotherapy, or surgical excision. In the most advanced cases, **palliative therapy** is the only viable option.

Prognosis and Return to Participation

The overall survival depends on the stage of the disease. For limited disease, cure rates may be as high as 25%, whereas cure rates for advanced stages are less than 5%.[3]

Spontaneous Pneumothorax and Hemothorax

A **pneumothorax** is a condition that results when gas or air is trapped in the chest wall between the parietal and visceral pleura and causes the lung to collapse (Figure 4-18, *A*). It is deemed spontaneous if the pneumothorax occurs in the absence of a traumatic injury to the chest or lungs. Pneumothorax tends to be more common in tall, thin men in the second and third decades of life and is usually the result of a rupture of a small **bleb** or an air- or fluid-filled sac called a **bulla.** Other lung diseases commonly associated with spontaneous pneumothorax include tuberculosis, pneumonia, asthma, cystic fibrosis, lung cancer, and certain forms of interstitial lung disease (Box 4-7).

A more serious condition known as a hemothorax occurs when blood collects in the pleural space (Figure 4-18, *B*). This condition usually is a result of trauma to

Box 4-7   Some Causes of Pneumothorax
• Apical blebs
• Chronic bronchitis and emphysema
• Staphylococcal pneumonia
• Asthma
• Trauma

the chest wall. In athletes, rib fractures that bleed into the plural space are a common cause. Hemothorax may also result from malignancies.

Signs and Symptoms

A spontaneous pneumothorax is characterized by the sudden onset of pleuritic chest pain and shortness of breath. Patients are usually tachypneic and have a cough that exacerbates the chest pain. Mild respiratory distress may be apparent, and there may be little chest wall motion on the affected side with breathing. A common sign of pneumothorax is a shift of the trachea away from the affected lung as air pressure pushes the lung toward the midline (Figure 4-19). Physical examination of the lungs with a stethoscope reveals decreased or absent breath sounds over the pneumothorax. A hemothorax is also characterized by pleuritic chest pain and dyspnea that worsens rapidly as the chest wall fills with blood. Dullness to percussion in dependent areas can also be appreciated on exam.

Referral and Diagnostic Tests

Any athlete suspected of a pneumothorax or hemothorax should be immediately referred to a medical facility.

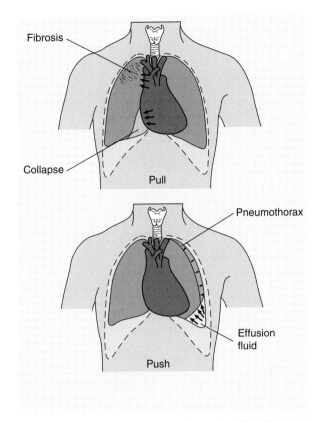

Figure 4-19 A common sign of a pneumothorax is a shift of the trachea away from the affected lung as air pressure pushes the lung toward the midline. (From Epstein O, Perkin GD, Cookson J, de Bono DP: *Clinical examination*, ed 3, St Louis, 2003, Mosby, p 118.)

Generally a chest radiograph is conclusive in the diagnosis of a pneumothorax, although small pneumothoraces may be overlooked without clinical suspicion. In some cases air continues to be trapped in the chest cavity through a one-way valve mechanism and can result in a dangerous life-threatening condition known as a **tension pneumothorax.** This condition requires immediate attention and needle decompression of the chest. The diagnosis of a hemothorax is definitively made when blood is aspirated by thoracentesis.

Differential Diagnosis

A small pneumothorax can easily be missed clinically and sometimes is overlooked as pleurisy, EIA, bronchitis, or a simple URI. Larger pneumothoraces are associated with some degree of respiratory compromise and can present a clinical picture similar to conditions such as a pulmonary embolism or foreign body aspiration.

Treatment

The physician's treatment objective is to remove the air from the pleural space, allowing the lung to reexpand. Small pneumothoraces may resolve without treatment.

Aspiration of air, using a catheter linked to a vacuum bottle, may reexpand the lung. The placement of a chest tube between the ribs into the pleural space allows the evacuation of air from the pleural space when simple aspiration is not successful or the pneumothorax is large. Reexpansion of the lung may take several days with the chest tube left in place. Hospitalization is required for chest tube management. Surgery may be indicated for recurrent episodes.

If a hemothorax is suspected, immediate hospitalization for decompression and drainage of blood is required. Exploration for an active bleeding site is mandatory, and other coexisting traumatic injuries to the chest are possible.

Prognosis and Return to Participation

Individuals diagnosed with a pneumothorax or hemothorax cannot participate in athletics until the condition has resolved radiographically and the athlete is clinically asymptomatic. Because the recurrence rate of a spontaneous pneumothorax can be as high as 50%,[18] the physician will encourage patients to discontinue smoking and avoid flying in unpressurized aircraft. Moreover, those with increased risks such as scuba divers and athletes competing at high altitude need to be counseled carefully and possibly encouraged to discontinue their activities.

SUMMARY

The athletic trainer must remember that chest pain and dyspnea may indicate a respiratory condition but also can point to a cardiovascular problem. The ability of the athletic trainer to perform a thorough examination of the respiratory system will help differentiate between a less serious condition and one that needs immediate attention. It takes considerable practice to recognize characteristics of normal and abnormal breath sounds. The DVD that accompanies this textbook provides opportunities for the reader to listen to normal and abnormal lung sounds and practice identifying them. There are also many websites that include both audio and animated replication of normal and abnormal breath sounds.

In addition, the athletic trainer needs to be familiar with the signs and symptoms, differential diagnoses, and common treatments of respiratory conditions such as asthma, bronchitis, pneumonia, upper respiratory infections, and influenza. Understanding common treatments, implications of illness and treatment on participation in sports, and prevention techniques allows athletic trainers to provide the best medical care and follow-up for their athletes. Awareness of conditions that less commonly affect athletes, such as hemothorax or pneumothorax, emphysema, tuberculosis, and lung cancer, is important because the athletic trainer is often the first person an athlete seeks help from when experiencing respiratory system problems. The athletic trainer who recognizes an abnormal condition can quickly refer an athlete who otherwise might not seek further medical assistance.

REFERENCES

1. Seidel HM, Ball JW, Dains JE, Benedict GW: *Mosby's guide to physical examination*, ed 5, St Louis, 2003, Mosby.
2. Jarvis C: *Physical examination & health assessment*, ed 4, Philadelphia, 2004, WB Saunders.
3. Williams CT: Chest pain. In Noble J, editor: *Textbook of primary care medicine*, ed 3, St Louis, 2001, Mosby, pp 163-168.
4. National Asthma Education and Prevention Program: Expert panel report: guidelines for the diagnosis and management of asthma update on selected topics—2002, *Journal of Allergy and Clinical Immunology* 110(5 Suppl): S141-S219, 2002.
5. American Academy of Pediatrics: Medical conditions affecting sports participation, *Pediatrics* 107(5):1205-1209, 2001.
6. Koehle M, Lloyd-Smith R, McKenzie D, Taunton J: Asthma and recreational SCUBA diving: a systematic review, *Sports Medicine* 33(2):109-116, 2003.
7. Storms WW: Review of exercise-induced asthma, *Medicine and Science in Sports and Exercise* 35(9):1464-1470, 2003.
8. Edelman JM, Turpin JA, Bronsky EA, et al: Oral montelukast compared with inhaled salmeterol to prevent exercise-induced bronchoconstriction. A randomized, double-blind trial. Exercise Study Group, *Annals of Internal Medicine* 132(2):97-104, 2000.
9. Malonne H, Lachman A, Van den Brande P, et al: Impact of montelukast on symptoms in mild-to-moderate persistent asthma and exercise-induced asthma: results of the ASTHMA survey. Adding Singulair treatment to handle symptoms in mild to moderate asthmatics, *Current Medical Research and Opinion* 18(8):512-519, 2002.
10. Steinshamn S, Sandsund M, Sue-Chu M, Bjermer L: Effects of montelukast on physical performance and exercise economy in adult asthmatics with exercise-induced bronchoconstriction, *Scandinavian Journal of Medicine and Science in Sports* 12(4):211-217, 2002.
11. McKenzie DC, McLuckie SL, Stirling DR: The protective effects of continuous and interval exercise in athletes with exercise-induced asthma, *Medicine and Science in Sports and Exercise* 26(8):951-956, 1994.
12. Ferri F: *Ferri's clinical advisor instant diagnosis and treatment*, St Louis, 2004, Mosby.
13. O'Bryan TA, Joshi N: Common cold. In Noble J, editor: *Textbook of primary care medicine*, ed 3, St Louis, 2001, Mosby, pp 306-309.
14. Bickley L: *Bates' guide to physical examination and history taking*, ed 8, New York, 2003, Lippincott Williams & Wilkins.
15. American Thoracic Society: Targeted tuberculin testing and treatment of latent tuberculosis infection, *MMWR Recommendations and Reports* 49(RR-6):1-51, 2000.
16. Rosenzweig D: Tuberculosis and nontuberculous mycobacterial disease. In Noble J, editor: *Textbook of primary care medicine*, ed 3, St Louis, 2001, Mosby, pp 669-677.
17. Beers MH, Berkow R, editors: *The Merck manual of diagnosis and therapy*, ed 17, Whitehouse Station, NJ, 1999, Merck Research Laboratories.
18. Sadikot RT, Greene T, Meadows K, Arnold AG: Recurrence of primary spontaneous pneumothorax, *Thorax* 52(9): 805-809, 1997.

CHAPTER 5

Cardiovascular Disorders

Bryan W. Smith

OBJECTIVES

At the conclusion of this chapter, the reader should be able to do the following:
1. Understand the anatomy and physiology of the cardiovascular system.
2. Understand cardiovascular adaptations to exercise.
3. Identify various cardiac arrhythmias.
4. Identify signs and symptoms for cardiovascular abnormalities.
5. Know when to refer an athlete to a physician for further cardiovascular evaluation.

INTRODUCTION

Cardiovascular disorders in the athlete have taken on particular importance because of their potential to cause catastrophic consequences during exercise. Although these tragedies bring notable publicity, many individuals with varying cardiac conditions can safely participate in a variety of physical activities. Therefore the athletic trainer must be knowledgeable about and able to distinguish between the normal physiological changes of the heart seen with exercise training and the pathological cardiac conditions that can result in exercise-related sudden death.

Vascular conditions such as hypertension and deep vein thrombosis (DVT) result in significant morbidity and can precipitate potentially fatal conditions such as myocardial infarction and pulmonary embolus. Early referral for diagnosis and treatment can limit harmful complications. Hematological conditions ranging from anemia to sickle cell trait are also discussed in this chapter. Prompt referral of the athlete to a physician for these conditions can enhance athletic performance as well as save a life.

OVERVIEW OF ANATOMY AND PHYSIOLOGY

The heart is a strong muscular organ made up of four chambers, two atria and two ventricles, that are responsible for pumping the blood that circulates through the body. Blood from the right side of the heart flows to the lungs, and simultaneously blood from the left side of the heart flows to the body. The two sides of this muscular pump are separated by the septum and work in a parallel manner. The right side atrium and ventricle pump the pulmonary circuit. The left side atrium and ventricle pump the systemic circuit.

Four valves help to direct the flow. The tricuspid valve separates the right atrium and ventricle; the mitral valve lies between the left atrium and left ventricle. Another set of valves connects the ventricles to the distal circulation.

On the right side of the heart, the pulmonary valve is connected to the pulmonary artery, whereas on the left side, the aortic valve controls flow to the aorta (Figure 5-1). Blood flow returning to the heart from the

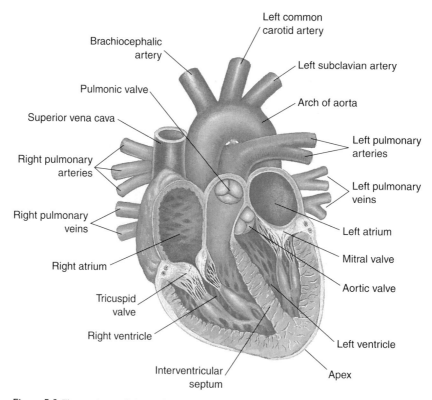

Figure 5-1 The anatomy of the cardiac chambers. (From Seidel H, Ball J, Dains J, Benedict G: *Mosby's guide to physical examination,* ed 5, St Louis, 2003, Mosby, p 415.)

body enters the corresponding atrium: pulmonic blood into the left atrium via the pulmonary vein and systemic blood into the right atrium via the superior and inferior vena cava (Figure 5-2).

The heart is positioned in the chest like an acorn, pointing inferiorly and to the left. The anterior surface of the heart is made up primarily of the right ventricle. A sliver of the left ventricle makes up the left border and the apex or inferior end of the anterior cardiac surface. Many times the heartbeat can be palpated at this apical end located in the fifth rib interspace at the nipple line.

The systemic vasculature is a pipeline that delivers blood to the organs and tissues throughout the body. Arteries carry blood to the tissues via a high-pressure system, and veins return blood to the atria under much lower pressure. With each contraction of the ventricle, a pressure wave (i.e., the pulse) is created moving through the arteries.

Pulse palpation can provide much useful clinical information. The intensity, contour, and regularity of the pulse are just as important as the rate. The pulse diminishes with inspiration, but this may not be perceptible. Weak, decreased pulses may indicate shock, heart failure, or a mechanical obstruction such as **aortic stenosis.** Strong, bounding pulses are common after exercise but at rest may be a sign of anemia, **hyperthyroidism,** or anxiety. A double peak pulse is called a **bisferiens pulse** and can be detected in **hypertrophic cardiomyopathy** or aortic regurgitation.

Understanding how the cardiovascular system responds to exercise requires understanding basic cardiovascular physiology at rest. The right and left sides of the heart work together pumping 5 to 6 L of blood per minute at rest (i.e., cardiac output). The heart pumps in a rhythmical cycle. Both ventricles contract during systole and relax during diastole. During the relaxed stage, they are passively filled with blood by atrial contraction. Pressures are rising and falling during this cardiac cycle, which permits the heart valves to open and close (see Figure 5-2).

Cardiac muscle is unique because it is able to contract within itself and operates on a serial electrical system, free from stimuli external to the heart. An electrical impulse begins at the sinoatrial (SA) node within the walls of the upper right atrium. This impulse travels through both atria to the atrioventricular (AV) node in the atrial septum. After a brief delay, the electrical impulse is promulgated to the bundle of His along the ventricle septum to the Purkinje fibers through the inferior and lateral ventricles[1] (Figure 5-3). An **electrocardiogram** (ECG) records this electrical activity as

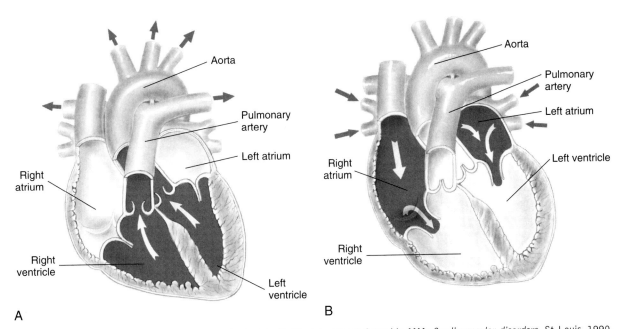

Figure 5-2 The flow of blood through the heart. **A,** Systole. **B,** Diastole. (From Cannobio MM: *Cardiovascular disorders,* St Louis, 1990, Mosby.)

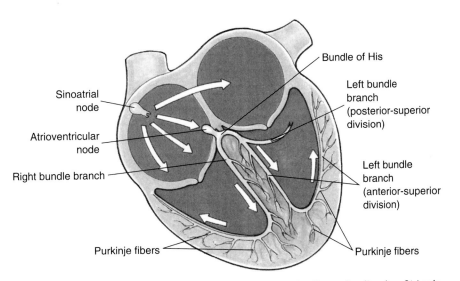

Figure 5-3 Electrical activity of the heart. (From Cannobio MM: *Cardiovascular disorders,* St Louis, 1990, Mosby.)

two phenomena: depolarization (the spread of electricity through the cardiac muscle) and repolarization (the return of the stimulated heart to rest) (Box 5-1).[1]

When the ventricles begin to contract, the pressure increases and that closes the mitral and tricuspid valves. A sound is produced, which is called the first heart sound, or S_1. As the pressure continues to rise, it forces the opening of the aortic and pulmonic valves. Once the blood is expelled, the ventricular pressure drops and the aortic and pulmonic valves close. The sound of this closure is the second heart sound, or S_2.

Because of pressure differences between the right and left sides of the heart, this sound splits into two components during inspiration but is one sound during expiration.

As the ventricles relax, the pressure drops and allows the mitral and tricuspid valves to open. The rush of blood into the ventricles can cause a sound in children and young adults that is called S_3. There is a fourth heart sound, S_4, that marks atrial contraction and immediately precedes S_1 of the next cardiac cycle. In older adults, S_3 and S_4 can be pathological heart sounds.

Box 5-1	Electrical Activity of the Heart Recorded on an ECG

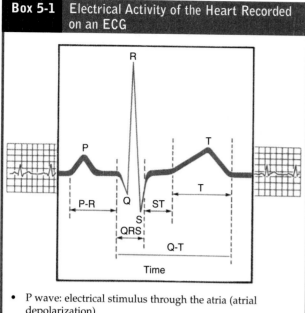

- P wave: electrical stimulus through the atria (atrial depolarization)
- PR interval: time between stimuli of atria and ventricles
- QRS complex: stimuli traveling through ventricles (ventricular depolarization)
- ST segment and T wave: ventricular repolarization (relaxing)
- U wave: final stage of ventricular repolarization

From Berne RM, Levy MN: *Cardiovascular physiology*, ed 7, St Louis, 1996, Mosby.

Other pathological sounds, such as snaps and clicks, may also be heard (Figure 5-4).

Another sound that is frequently heard is a murmur caused by turbulent blood flow or valvular vibration. Heart murmurs can be benign or pathological. Pathological conditions include leaky (i.e., regurgitation) or stiff (i.e., stenosis) valves, holes between chambers (i.e., septal defects), and metabolic conditions, such as anemia. Murmurs can occur during or throughout systole, diastole, or both. They can be localized to a particular valvular area, or they may be diffuse. The sound, called a **bruit,** can transmit into the carotid vasculature. Besides location and radiation, murmurs can vary in intensity, pitch, and quality. They can be loud or soft, harsh or blowing, and high or low pitched in character. Respiration or positioning of the patient can alter the murmur. For examples of cardiac sounds, please refer to the accompanying DVD.

Benign murmurs are common in children and young adults. A common cause of a benign murmur is increased venous return and subsequent flow through the pulmonic valve. These types of murmurs are most commonly heard at the upper left sternal border or pulmonic area and vary with position (i.e., the loudest when supine, the quietest when standing). Quite often they are found incidentally on examination. Over time, they may disappear.

When the left ventricle contracts, a volume of blood called stroke volume is ejected into the aorta and peripheral circulation. Blood pressure describes the pressure that the blood is subjected to with each contraction.

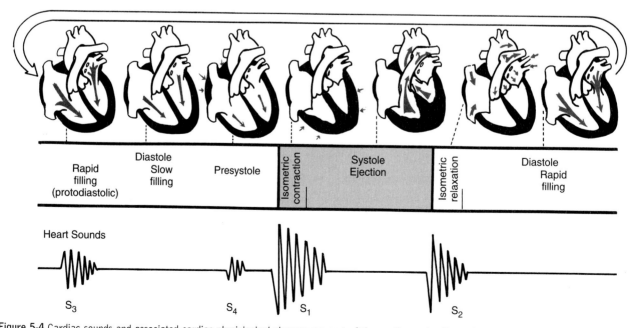

Figure 5-4 Cardiac sounds and associated cardiac physiological changes are part of the cardiac cycle. (From Jarvis C: *Physical examination & health assessment,* ed 4, Philadelphia, 2004, WB Saunders, p 489.)

It has a peak, which is the systolic measurement, and a trough, which is the diastolic measurement. The difference between the systolic and diastolic pressures is known as the pulse pressure. The average blood pressure in adults is 120/80 mm Hg.

High blood pressure, or hypertension, is defined as either systolic or diastolic pressure at or above 140/90 mm Hg. Conversely, hypotension, or low blood pressure, is defined as either systolic or diastolic pressure at or below 90/60 mm Hg. Children have lower blood pressure than adults. In fact, a blood pressure of 120/80 in an 8-year-old child would suggest hypertension.[1] During dehydration from illness or heat, a drop in blood pressure caused by the decreased plasma volume can occur. A fall in systolic blood pressure of 20 mm Hg or more when accompanied by symptoms such as lightheadedness or fainting is called orthostatic hypotension. When this happens, the patient's blood pressure is checked in supine, sitting, and standing positions.

Blood volume is just one factor that influences blood pressure. Cardiac output, peripheral resistance, blood viscosity, and the elasticity of the large arteries can cause variations in systolic pressure, diastolic pressure, or both. Because of the potential variability in blood pressure, proper measurement is important. Making sure the patient is calm and relaxed, using the proper size cuff, supporting the patient's arm, and keeping the blood pressure cuff level with the heart are all important points to remember when measuring blood pressure. Chapter 2 gives instructions on how to take blood pressure.

CARDIOVASCULAR ADAPTATIONS TO EXERCISE

Review of Exercise Physiology

Exercise is usually defined in metabolic characteristics: dynamic or aerobic exercise versus static or anaerobic exercise.[2] Most exercise is a composite of both types. Endurance running and swimming are examples of dynamic exercise whereas sprint running and power weightlifting are examples of static exercise.

In immediate outcomes, dynamic exercise results in increased cardiac output. Both components of cardiac output, stroke volume and heart rate, are increased. Enhanced cardiac contractility and increased venous return to the heart increase stroke volume. Blood flow is redistributed to the heart and skeletal muscles at the expense of the viscera while remaining constant to the brain. Vascular resistance is decreased because of vasodilation in the skeletal muscle, but blood pressure does not decrease because of the increased cardiac output.[2,3] Pulse pressure is widened during dynamic exercise.

KEY POINTS
Measuring Heart Rate

Heart rate can be easily measured by counting the pulse for 15 seconds and multiplying by four. If the heart rate at rest is less than 60 beats/min, which is common in well-trained athletes, it is termed **bradycardia**. A resting heart rate of 100 beats/min or greater is referred to as **tachycardia**. Heart rhythm irregularities may also be palpated and are called palpitations.

Maximal dynamic exercise results in a four- to six-fold increase in cardiac output, a three-fold increase in heart rate, and a two-fold increase in stroke volume.[2]

Heart rate and blood pressure increase in static exercise (Key Points—Measuring Heart Rate). The pressure increase can be dramatic with systolic pressure exceeding 250 mm Hg.[2] A high blood pressure is required to maintain blood flow to exercising muscles whose vessels are being occluded because of the intense muscle contraction. Stroke volume, ejection fraction, and systemic vascular resistance remain unchanged. The higher pressures result in a higher cardiac workload compared with dynamic exercise.

Over the long term, dynamic exercise training results in increased cardiac output. The maximal heart rate cannot change with training so increased cardiac output is the result of increased stroke volume. The heart adapts to the dynamic work by increasing in size or hypertrophy. With this hypertrophy comes ventricular cavity dilation caused by the chronic volume loading. The increased diastolic volume permits greater stroke volume for less work. These changes can occur in athletes across the life span, including master-level athletes.[2]

Because stroke volume is increased at rest while cardiac output is maintained, a decreased resting heart rate occurs. This decrease in heart rate also occurs at submaximal workloads. Therefore highly aerobically trained athletes have decreased resting heart rates, or bradycardia, when compared with their less trained counterparts.

Blood pressure during ongoing dynamic exercise training in elite athletes has been commonly thought to decrease. This has not been supported in many research studies.[2] Scientific evidence, however, supports lowered blood pressure in sedentary adults after engaging in dynamic exercise training.[4]

Long-term, static exercise training also causes cardiovascular adaptations. In untrained subjects, small decreases are found in heart rate and blood pressure.[2] Heavy weight training has been commonly believed to cause hypertension, but this has not been shown in body builders.[2] In individuals with hypertension, however, chronic heavy weight training is not recommended. Pressure overload from chronic resistance training can cause cardiac hypertrophy without the

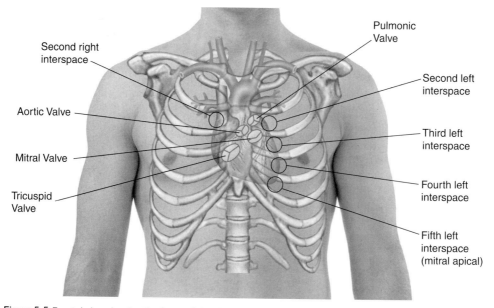

Figure 5-5 Frontal view showing the five traditional designated areas for auscultation of the heart. (From Seidel H, Ball J, Dains J, Benedict G: *Mosby's guide to physical examination,* ed 5, St Louis, 2003, Mosby, p 433.)

chamber enlargement seen with dynamic exercise. Septal and posterior left ventricular wall thickening may also be seen.

Athlete's Heart

The term **athlete's heart** refers to the physiological and morphological adaptations mentioned previously, which an athlete's cardiovascular system may undergo as a result of ongoing exercise training.[5] Some of these adaptations can be confused with pathological cardiac conditions. Just as it is important to allow healthy individuals the privilege of sports participation, it is more important to distinguish athlete's heart from pathological disease and minimize the risk of sudden cardiac death.

Both long-term dynamic and static exercise training can result in cardiac hypertrophy; these changes can occur after just a few weeks of training. Because heart wall thickness can be quite variable, sometimes as thick as 16 mm,[6] one way to evaluate whether the cardiac changes are pathological is to detrain the athlete. If the wall thickness shrinks, the change is felt to be the benign effects of the athlete's heart. A hypertrophic ventricle that does not diminish in size with detraining indicates possible cardiac disease or an idiopathic anomaly.

PREPARTICIPATION EXAMINATION

As discussed in Chapter 1, the preparticipation examination (PPE) sheds light on any medical problems that may affect athletic participation. The American

Academy of Family Physicians (AAFP) recommends an initial evaluation for first-time participation in school or college athletics, with annual follow-up questions in certain areas. One of the areas of concern on both the initial and subsequent annual evaluation is cardiac health.[7] Appendix A gives the recommended questions for PPEs, including those related to potential cardiac problems. These questions are designed to alert the physician to potential life-threatening anomalies related to the heart and especially sudden death events (Red Flags—Potential Cardiac Problems). Any athlete who complains of symptoms consistent with these questions should be referred to a physician before continuing activity, regardless of whether the athlete has already passed a PPE screening.

Red Flags for Potential Cardiac Problems

Questions for preparticipation evaluation:
1. Have you ever passed out during or after exercise?
2. Have you ever been dizzy during or after exercise?
3. Have you ever had chest pain during or after exercise?
4. Do you get tired more quickly than your friends do during exercise?
5. Have you ever had racing of your heart or skipped heartbeats?
6. Have you had high blood pressure or high cholesterol?
7. Have you ever been told you have a heart murmur?
8. Has any family member or relative died of heart problems or sudden cardiac death before the age of 50 years?
9. Have you had a severe viral infection (e.g., myocarditis or mononucleosis) within the past month?
10. Has a physician ever denied or restricted your participation in sports for any heart problems?

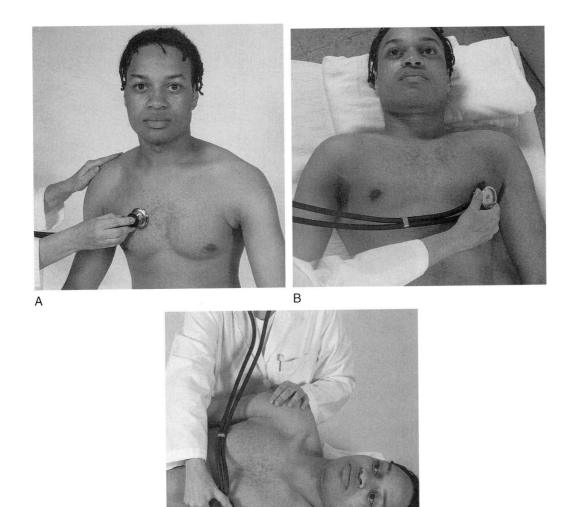

Figure 5-6 Cardiac auscultation. **A,** The athlete sitting. **B,** The athlete supine. **C,** The athlete lying lateral recumbent. (From Jarvis C: *Physical examination & health assessment,* ed 4, Philadelphia, 2004, WB Saunders, pp 509, 511.)

GENERAL EVALUATION OF THE CARDIOVASCULAR SYSTEM

When assessing an athlete for cardiac sounds, the patient needs to be in a still and quiet environment. The most important aspect of cardiac auscultation is to develop a routine and listen to five specific areas of the chest (Figure 5-5) while the athlete is in one position (e.g., sitting) and then repeat the sequence of auscultation while the athlete is supine and again with the athlete lying in a lateral recumbent position (Figure 5-6). The five auscultatory areas are as follows[1]:

1. Aortic valve: second right intercostal space at right sternal border
2. Pulmonic valve: second left intercostal space at left sternal border

3. Second pulmonic valve: third intercostal space at left sternal border
4. Tricuspid valve: fourth intercostal space along lower left sternal border
5. Mitral valve: fifth intercostal space at apex of heart

The diaphragm of the stethoscope is warmed before being placed on the athlete's bare chest if the examination is not caused by an emergent situation. When auscultating, the athletic trainer explains what is being done before placing the stethoscope and always follows proper draping protocol when working with female athletes. Cardiac sounds can be assessed on a woman wearing a sports bra if the stethoscope is placed on the skin under the clothing.

Accurate cardiac auscultation takes time. The examiner pauses at each auscultatory area to completely hear and isolate the sounds of each valve opening and closing. This skill requires patience, practice, and a quiet area. The examiner listens for the normal rate and rhythm of the heart in each auscultatory area and then specifically listens for the sounds associated with systole (i.e., contraction of the ventricles) followed by diastole (i.e., relaxation of the ventricles). Diastole is a longer interval than systole.[1] When auscultating in each area, the examiner should make sure to also listen for adventitious or extra sounds or noises. The DVD that accompanies this text includes both normal and abnormal cardiac sounds for instructional purposes. The examiner should be aware that if athletes are asked to hold their breath during expiration, S_1 may be more predominant; holding their breath on inspiration will cause S_2 to be more distinct.

The physical examination of the athlete can be variable and nonspecific. In many high-performance athletes, particularly those who practice endurance sports, an increase in parasympathetic tone may cause a resting bradycardia. Resting heart rates have been recorded as low as 25 beats per minute in elite endurance athletes. Resting blood pressure usually is not changed, but it may be lowered. Third and fourth heart sounds may be present and are of no clinical significance as an isolated finding. Palpation may reveal a left ventricular impulse that is displaced to the left and prolonged. Because of the cardiac hypertrophy, 3% to 50% of high-performance athletes may have a mild mid-systolic heart murmur.[6] These benign flow murmurs are best heard in the supine position and often disappear on standing.

The ECG in an individual with athlete's heart can mimic many pathological conditions. The increased vagal tone and resultant bradycardia seen in trained athletes are associated with a greater incidence of benign arrhythmias, such as **premature atrial complex** (PAC) and **premature ventricular complex** (PVC), than in the general population.[5] Conduction blocks and **junctional rhythms** also are more common.[8] Complete, or third-degree, **atrioventricular (AV) blocks,** however, are rare and need to be investigated for pathology. High voltage on the ECG is common and can skew determining hypertrophy. The most common change seen in the athletic heart is early repolarization of the ventricles. On the ECG, this is evidenced by characteristic ST- and T-wave changes.[8]

PATHOLOGICAL CONDITIONS OF THE CARDIAC SYSTEM

This section reviews various pathological cardiac conditions that may be seen in athletes. Rare congenital cardiac conditions are beyond the scope of this chapter. The most recent recommendations for determining eligibility for competition by athletes with cardiovascular abnormalities were presented at the 26th Bethesda Conference in January of 1994.[9,10]

Sudden Cardiac Death

Sudden cardiac death is a rare event in the young athlete. In U.S. society, athletes are viewed as physically invincible because of the incredible physical feats displayed in the athletic arena. Any time a tragedy of this proportion occurs, the public's reaction is one of disbelief and medical knowledge is called into question. Studies that have tracked these deaths during sports used the National Federation of State High School Association (NFHS) and National Collegiate Athletic Association (NCAA) governing organizations as well as newspaper clipping services for data collection. Approximately 90% of the data collected involved male athletes, with an equal distribution between Caucasians and African-Americans.[11,12] Sudden death cases in young women are rare, and the disproportionate number of football and basketball cases may call the previously used reference sources into question. One explanation for the rising incidence of sudden death among women may be the growing numbers of young women involved in a wider variety of sports.

The prevalence of cardiac sudden death in young athletes (those less than 35 years old) is estimated to be between 1 in 100,000 and 1 in 300,000.[11,12] This is much higher than statistics reported in a more general population of active individuals, which show 1 in 735,000 U.S. Air Force recruits experiencing sudden cardiac death over a 20-year period.[13] In contrast, Thompson and colleagues found the incidence of sudden death in joggers ranging from 30 to 65 years of age to be 1 in 7620.[14] These data indicate that active people are not immune to cardiovascular events that may result in death.

Causes

The most common cause of sudden cardiac death in the young athlete is hypertrophic cardiomyopathy, which accounts for up to 50% of the cases. Other significant causes of sudden cardiac death in a young athlete are coronary artery anomalies, increased cardiac mass, aortic rupture, myocarditis, and aortic stenosis.[11,12,15] Rare causes include dilated cardiomyopathy, atherosclerotic coronary artery disease, mitral valve prolapse, isolated arrhythmias such as **long QT syndrome** and **Wolff-Parkinson-White syndrome,** and **arrhythmogenic right ventricular dysplasia** (ARVD).[11,12] In the Veneto region of Italy, researchers have found ARVD to be the most common cause of sudden cardiac death in the athlete.[16,17] This research suggests that a specific population may have different genetic subtraits.

In the older athlete, coronary artery disease is by far the most common cause of sudden death. Rarely is sudden death in the older athlete caused by hypertrophic cardiomyopathy, mitral valve prolapse, or acquired valvular conditions.[18]

Traumatic sudden cardiac death has not captured as much attention because its epidemiology is harder to track. However, it is a growing problem that strikes without warning. In 2001, the U.S. Commotio Cordis Registry reported 128 cases of traumatic sudden cardiac death,[19] and most of the cases involved youngsters.

Commotio cordis refers to trauma to the chest wall that interrupts the electrical impulse in the heart. If the cardiac rhythm is not promptly normalized, the individual dies. Typically the ribs or sternum is not broken, although some contusions may be found. Research has found a window of time in the cardiac cycle during which a blow over the center of the heart can induce ventricular fibrillation.[20,21]

Although children with thin chest walls are most vulnerable to commotio cordis (Figure 5-7), deaths have been reported in teenagers. Sports such as baseball, hockey, lacrosse, and softball, which have hard projectiles that can strike the chest, have been associated with the greatest number of deaths

> ▶ **Red Flags for Traumatic Sudden Cardiac Death**
>
> Sports with projectile implements that can hit the chest at an inopportune time in the cardiac rhythm cycle have been known to cause commotio cordis in young athletes. These sports include the following:
> - Baseball
> - Softball
> - Hockey
> - Lacrosse
> - Soccer
> - Football
> - Karate

(Red Flag—Traumatic Sudden Cardiac Death). Commotio cordis also has occurred in sports such as soccer, football, and karate where the blow came from a soft projectile or a collision. It appears the timing of the incident rather than the degree of impact of the object is the causative factor. Commotio cordis is the only significant cause of traumatic sudden cardiac death in athletes.

Prevention

Because death can be the outcome, prevention has become the focus of attention for commotio cordis. Changes in practice have ranged from protective padding to softer balls that are used in Little League

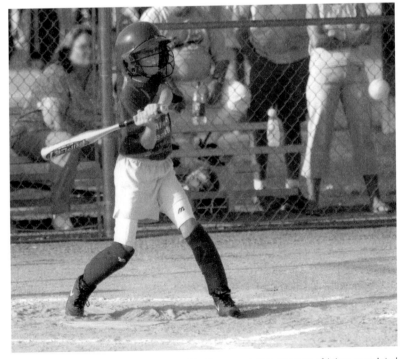

Figure 5-7 A child is much more susceptible than an adult to the type of injury associated with commotio cordis because of a thinner and less developed chest wall. (Courtesy Mike Hanley.)

and softball. Because this may not completely resolve the problem, another solution is defibrillation in conjunction with cardiopulmonary resuscitation (CPR). Defibrillation stops the heart rhythm so it can "reboot" into a normal rhythm.

The American Heart Association estimates that 100,000 deaths could be prevented each year with prompt defibrillation.[22] If defibrillation is performed within 3 minutes, the likelihood of survival is high. For every minute of delay the chance of survival drops by as much as 10%.

The advent of the automated external defibrillator (AED) has provided greater public access to lifesaving technology (Figure 5-8). These devices can be operated by trained laypeople and are increasingly affordable in all sectors. The AED is portable, rechargeable, simple to operate, and easy to maintain. The American Red Cross, American Heart Association, and National Safety Council offer AED certification courses in addition to CPR courses for the lay public. Athletic trainers are required to be certified in AED use and need to have ready access to an AED in order to provide rapid cardiac assessment and care to those in fibrillation (Key Points—AED Certification). When working with

---

KEY POINTS
Automated External Defibrillator (AED) Certification

The Board of Certification (BOC) requires proof of current certification in AED use for every practicing certified athletic trainer at each Continuing Education Unit (CEU) reporting period.

---

adolescents, athletic trainers need to consult the team physicians to make sure AED usage is appropriate

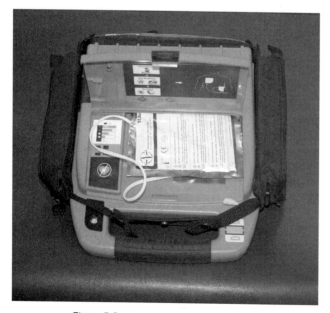

Figure 5-8 Automated external defibrillator.

because the AED currently is limited to children over 8 years old or those who weigh more than 55 pounds.

Hypertrophic Cardiomyopathy

Hypertrophic cardiomyopathy (HCM) is the leading cause of cardiac sudden death in athletes in the United States under the age of 35 years (Figure 5-9). The disorder is characterized by an abnormally hypertrophied but nondilated left ventricle in the absence of physiological conditions such as physical training or pathological conditions such as aortic stenosis or hypertension that would result in left ventricular hypertrophy.[23] Numerous genetic mutations have been identified, and an autosomal dominant transmission of this disorder has been described.[23]

The prevalence of HCM is estimated at 1 in 500 in the general population, but no consensus exists about whether this disorder is more prevalent in males or females or in certain racial groups.[24] The incidence of sudden death from HCM is two to three times higher in children and adolescents compared with adults.[25]

The walls of the left ventricle thicken in a variable pattern in HCM. As often as 25% of the time, physical obstruction of blood flow results during systole. Up to 80% of individuals with HCM have abnormally small coronary arteries that may cause myocardial ischemia.[23] Cellular abnormalities include myositic disorganization and death with resultant fibrotic scarring.

Although outflow obstruction can occur, the presence of left ventricular diastolic dysfunction is more common. Either outflow obstruction or diastolic dysfunction can impair exercise performance even in the least symptomatic individual.[26,27] Both decreased wall distensibility and incomplete myocardial relaxation contribute to altered left ventricular filling,[23] which leads to left atrial dilation and potential development of emboli. Regional myocardial ischemia likely occurs because of the abnormally small coronary arteries and inadequate capillary density.[23] Adding random fibrosis of the cardiac musculature produces a combination of ischemia, fibrosis, and impaired vasodilator reserve that can lead to arrhythmia and sudden death.

Signs and Symptoms

Symptoms of HCM are fatigue, dyspnea, exertional angina, and syncope or near syncope. These symptoms may not correlate with the degree of ventricular hypertrophy or be predictive for sudden death.[12] Physical exam can provide valuable information, but the findings are not consistent. On palpation, an increased left ventricular impulse may be felt. Pulses may be **bifid** in character and exhibit a brisk upstroke. On cardiac auscultation, a classic, harsh precordial ejection murmur

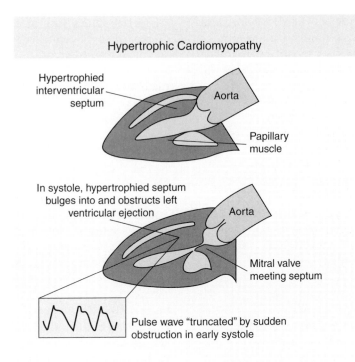

Figure 5-9 Hypertrophic cardiomyopathy is characterized by a jerky or rapid pulse, which may be the result of dynamic left ventricular outflow obstruction. (From Epstein O, Perkin GD, Cookson J, deBono DP: *Clinical examination,* ed 3, St Louis, 2003, Mosby, p 148.)

may be heard at the left lower sternal border toward the apex. An example of this can be found on the accompanying DVD. The murmur increases with standing or Valsalva's maneuver and diminishes with squatting; however, a murmur is not always present.

Referral and Diagnostic Tests

Athletes with symptoms of exertional angina, syncope, or near syncope should be referred immediately to a sports medicine physician or cardiologist for evaluation (Red Flags—Hypertrophic Cardiomyopathy). Fatigue

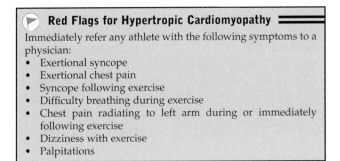

> **Red Flags for Hypertropic Cardiomyopathy**
> Immediately refer any athlete with the following symptoms to a physician:
> * Exertional syncope
> * Exertional chest pain
> * Syncope following exercise
> * Difficulty breathing during exercise
> * Chest pain radiating to left arm during or immediately following exercise
> * Dizziness with exercise
> * Palpitations

and dyspnea uncharacteristic for a particular athlete warrant concern and certainly physician referral when accompanied by a heart murmur.

Standard laboratory tests, such as a resting 12-lead ECG or chest radiograph, have limited utility in screening for HCM. The most useful diagnostic test is echocardiography. Increased left ventricular wall thickness (>15 mm) is the most helpful diagnostic parameter. The majority of male athletes and all female athletes have ventricular wall thickness of 12 mm or less.[6,28] Therefore the range from 13 to 15 mm may pose a diagnostic dilemma because it is possible to have physiological hypertrophy in this wall thickness range; however, this hypertrophy has only been reported in male cyclists and rowers.[6] Another sign of HCM that can be seen on an echocardiogram is a ventricular septum/free wall thickness ratio greater than 1:3. Asymmetrical wall thickening and decreased left ventricular diastolic cavity dimension (<45 mm) may also be present. In addition, the echo may reveal abnormal diastolic filling with decreased early filling and increased late filling and abnormal ultrasonic myocardial reflex activity in the athlete with HCM.[29]

Discontinuing athletic activities over a few weeks to 1 month for the athlete with these symptoms may distinguish whether the problem is the athlete's heart or HCM.[30] Hypertrophy of the ventricular wall will not resolve in an individual with HCM.

As a diagnostic tool for HCM, echocardiography is the gold standard. Its value as a screening tool, however, is limited by its relative expense. The cost to prevent one death from HCM by using echocardiography as a preparticipation screening tool would exceed $100 million.[31] In the future genetic markers may hold the greatest promise as effective screening tests.

Differential Diagnosis

The clinical symptoms alone of exertional angina, syncope, and near syncope point to numerous conditions that potentially can cause sudden death. They also can be related to benign conditions, such as dehydration or vasovagal syncope, or noncardiac conditions, such as asthma or gastroesophageal reflux disease. The potential for a serious, life-threatening condition, however, warrants an immediate referral.

Prognosis and Implications for Participation

On the basis of the Bethesda Conference recommendations, athletes with hypertrophic cardiomyopathy should be restricted from participation in all competitive sports with the possible exception of low-intensity (class IA) sports such as golf, bowling, and billiards (Table 5-1).[32,33] Even though HCM is the leading cause of cardiac sudden death in young athletes, current screening methods and stratification risks for sudden death are limited. This necessitates medical disqualification of athletes with HCM from competition at the present time.

Prevention

Detection of HCM is difficult without sophisticated and expensive laboratory testing. In seeking a secondary tool, the individual's medical history would seem to be invaluable. A comprehensive medical history can reveal an autosomal dominant transmission pattern, family history of cardiac disease, or record of other premature sudden death in family members. Unfortunately, a medical history has not been as useful as expected because of the variability of expression of the trait. Nonetheless, the athletic trainer should ask about a family history of cardiovascular disease in every athletic preparticipation exam as discussed previously.

Table 5-1 Classification of Sports Based on Peak Static and Dynamic Components During Competition			
Classification	**A. Low Dynamic**	**B. Moderate Dynamic**	**C. High Dynamic**
I. Low static	Billiards Bowling Cricket Curling Golf Riflery	Baseball* Softball* Fencing Table tennis Volleyball	Badminton Cross-country skiing (classic technique) Tennis (singles) Field hockey* Orienteering Racquetball/squash Race walking Distance running Soccer* Tennis

II. Moderate static	Archery
	Auto racing*†
	Diving*†
	Equestrian*†
	Motorcycling*†
		American football*†
		Field events (jumping)
		Figure skating*
		Rodeo*†
		Sprint running
		Surfing
		Synchronized
		  swimming†
		Rugby*
			Basketball*
			Ice hockey*
			Cross-country skiing
			  (skating technique)
			Lacrosse*
			Mid-distance running
			Swimming
			Team handball

III. High static	Bobsledding/luge*† Field events (throw) Gymnastics*† Karate/judo* Sailing Rock climbing Water skiing*† Weight lifting*† Wind surfing*†	Body building*† Downhill skiing*† Wrestling*	Boxing* Canoeing/kayaking Cycling*† Decathlon Rowing Speed skating*† Triathlon*†

Modified from Mitchell JH, Haskell W, Snell P, Van Camp SP: Task force 8: classification of sports, *Journal of the American College of Cardiology* 45(8):1364-1367, 2005.
*Danger of body collision.
†Increased risk if syncope occurs.

Coronary Artery Abnormalities

Congenital coronary anomalies are a much less frequent cause of sudden death than HCM in athletes. They are characterized by either an aberrant (i.e., deviating or abnormal) coronary artery takeoff or the complete absence of a coronary artery. Most reports rank coronary anomalies as the second leading cause of sudden death in athletes,[11,12] with the majority of events happening during or just following strenuous exercise.

Myocardial bridging refers to a coronary artery that is surrounded by myocardium for a portion of its course. This tunneling is seen in up to 25% of hearts at the time of **necropsy** following sudden death and usually involves the left anterior descending artery. Rarely does a congenital aberration result in clinical pathology, but the vascular compression from the ventricle during systole has been reported as an exercise-related cause of sudden death.[34]

Acquired coronary artery abnormalities that have been associated with exercise-related sudden death are atherosclerotic coronary artery disease, Kawasaki's disease, and coronary artery vasospasm.

Signs and Symptoms

Symptoms preceding death from coronary artery anomalies are infrequent but include anginal chest pain with exertion, exertional syncope, or near syncope with exertion. If there is any symptom with myocardial bridging, it is usually angina because of **myocardial ischemia.**[35]

Referral and Diagnostic Tests

Any athlete presenting with unexplained exertional chest pain or an exertional syncopal episode must be referred immediately to a physician. An echocardiogram may demonstrate the anomalous takeoff. However, **cardioangiography** is usually required for a conclusive diagnosis (Figure 5-10).

Treatment

Currently no medical treatment exists that can permit continued athletic competition. The individual may benefit from **beta-blocker** medication for everyday living. Surgery is sometimes an option. In myocardial bridging, surgical resection may resolve the symptoms.

Prognosis and Return to Participation

It is recommended that the athlete with an anomalous coronary artery retire from competitive sports

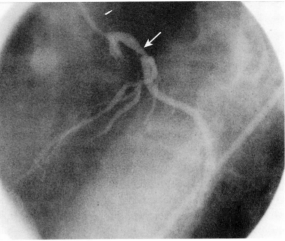

Figure 5-10 Cardioangiography shows left main coronary stenosis *(arrow).* (From Epstein O, Perkin GD, Cookson J, deBono DP: *Clinical examination,* ed 3, St Louis, 2003, Mosby, p 163.)

participation.[36] If possible, surgery to re-create the abdominal artery should be performed, and if after 6 months the athlete is nonischemic at maximal exercise testing, then sports participation may be permitted.[36]

If there is no evidence of myocardial ischemia following surgery in a patient with myocardial bridging, the patient may participate in all sports.[37] Any evidence of ischemia, however, will restrict the athlete to low-intensity sports, such as golf or bowling.[33,37]

Special Concerns in the Mature Athlete

Whereas atherosclerotic coronary disease resulting in myocardial infarction is the overwhelming cause of sudden death in athletes over 35 years of age, it is much less common in younger populations. The tragic death of Olympic skater Sergei Greneko at 29 years of age, however, demonstrates that it can occur. Usually, major risk factors for coronary artery disease are present, such as family history, hypercholesterolemia, and hypertension.

Coronary artery vasospasm is a rare cause of exercise-related sudden death. Although most individuals who experience vasospasm are shown to have evidence of atherosclerosis, there are reports of individuals with vasospasm and normal coronary arteries.[38] Cocaine use can be an inciting factor regardless of evidence of atherosclerosis.

Diagnosis of a myocardial infarction (MI) is beyond the scope of this chapter. Common symptoms of an MI are crushing substernal chest pain that can radiate into the left arm, neck, and jaw; **diaphoresis;** nausea;

vomiting; and dyspnea. Sometimes the symptoms are quite nonspecific and easily mistaken for indigestion. Quite often a history of angina can be elicited from the patient.

While waiting for emergency transport, the patient may take an aspirin or his prescribed nitroglycerin if available. Obviously, the patient is given nothing by mouth if unconscious or unable to swallow. Oxygen can also be given if available. The athletic trainer must be prepared to perform CPR and defibrillate.

The older athlete with coronary artery disease faces several factors that are considered when determining the level of risk for sudden death. They include resting ventricular function, exercise-induced ischemia, exercise-induced ventricular arrhythmia, and degree of coronary artery stenosis.[37] Evidence of abnormalities places the athlete at significant risk and requires restriction to low-intensity competitive sports, such as golf or bowling.[33,37] Reevaluation is recommended every 6 months. The athlete with minimal risk who has evidence of coronary artery disease may be advised to avoid intensely competitive activities whereas other activity recommendations are individualized on an annual basis.[37]

For an individual with coronary artery vasospasm, the risk of athletic participation is uncertain. Caution and frequent reevaluation for clearance to participate are the best advice because spontaneous remission can occur.[37]

Special Concerns in the Adolescent Athlete

Kawasaki's disease is a rare, inflammatory condition of unknown origin that usually occurs in young childhood. Cardiac complications sometimes include coronary artery **aneurysm,** a sac filled with fluid or clotted blood that results from **dilation** of the wall and that can cause stenosis of the coronary artery.

Athletes with a history of Kawasaki's disease who have no evidence of cardiac involvement or have achieved complete resolution of cardiac involvement may participate in all sports.[37] Minor residual abnormalities following resolution of coronary aneurysms may limit an athlete to participation in sports such as golf, bowling, baseball, volleyball, and doubles tennis.[33,37] Unresolved aneurysms or stenosis places the athlete at significant risk for sudden death, and only sports such as golf and bowling are recommended.[33,37] Athletes with evidence of myocardial ischemia are restricted from all competitive sports.[37]

No guidelines are available for the young athlete with coronary artery disease. Any decision to permit athletic participation must be based on the extent of increased risk for a cardiac event to occur.[37] An athlete with these conditions needs to be under appropriate medical and surgical management.

Marfan Syndrome

Marfan syndrome is an autosomal dominant, heritable disorder of connective tissue. Aortic dissection and rupture along with severe aortic regurgitation account for the majority of deaths in adolescents and adults with Marfan syndrome.[39] Maron and colleagues[12] have reported that approximately 5% of sudden death events in young athletes are due to aortic rupture secondary to Marfan syndrome.

The prevalence of Marfan syndrome is estimated to be 1 in 10,000.[40] There is no racial or ethnic predilection; males and females are equally affected (Figure 5-11). The syndrome does not skip generations, but at least 25% to 35% of the cases occur sporadically without a family history.[40]

Signs, Symptoms, and Diagnostic Tests

Multiple variations can be seen in organ systems affected by Marfan syndrome (Box 5-2). The most commonly affected organ systems are the musculoskeletal, cardiovascular, and ocular. It can be very difficult to make a definitive diagnosis, particularly if there is no family history. The accompanying box contains the requirements for diagnosis (Key Points—Diagnostic Criteria for Marfan Syndrome). Conclusive diagnosis usually

---

KEY POINTS
Diagnostic Criteria for Marfan Syndrome

Negative Family History (Primary Relative)
- Skeletal involvement
- Involvement of two other organ systems
- At least one major manifestation
- Absence of homocystinuria

Positive Family History (Primary Relative)
- Involvement of two organ systems
- At least one major manifestation (depends on family phenotype)
- Absence of homocystinuria

---

requires confirmation by several specialists under the direction of a primary care physician. Many common clinical manifestations worsen with growth, such as pectus deformities and scoliosis; diagnosis is sometimes delayed until adolescence or early adulthood when scoliosis becomes obvious. Rarely, a spontaneous, nontraumatic pneumothorax can be a diagnostic tip-off.

A 4-year, prospective study to develop a screening protocol for Marfan syndrome in athletes was conducted at the University of California–Los Angeles (UCLA). Otis and coworkers[41] evaluated female athletes taller than 5'10" and male athletes taller than 6', using

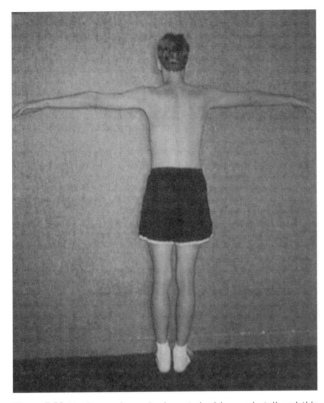

Figure 5-11 Marfan syndrome is characterized by overly tall and thin physical stature with hypermobile joints, sternal deformity, and arm span that exceeds the person's height. (From Jarvis C: *Physical examination & health assessment,* ed 4, Philadelphia, 2004, WB Saunders, p 203.)

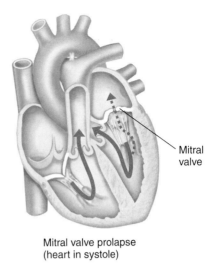

Mitral valve prolapse
(heart in systole)

Figure 5-12 Mitral valve prolapse. (From Seidel H, Ball J, Dains J, Benedict G: *Mosby's guide to physical examination,* ed 5, St Louis, 2003, Mosby.)

| Box 5-2 | Most Commonly Affected Organ System Manifestations of Marfan Syndrome |

Skeletal
Anterior chest deformity
Scoliosis
Thoracic lordosis
Tall stature
High arched palate
Hypermobile joints

Ocular
Superior lens dislocation
Flat cornea
Elongated globe
Retinal detachment
Myopia

Cardiovascular
Ascending aorta dilatation
Aortic dissection
Aortic regurgitation
Mitral regurgitation secondary to mitral valve prolapse
Calcification of the mitral annulus
Mitral valve prolapse
Abdominal aortic aneurysm
Dysrhythmia
Endocarditis

echocardiography and **slit lamp** examination when any of the following criteria were positive:

- Arm span greater than height
- Moderate kyphoscoliosis
- Heart murmur or mid-systolic click
- Family history of Marfan syndrome or sudden death before 40 years of age
- Pectus deformity
- Decreased upper body length/lower body length ratio

No cases of Marfan syndrome were identified in more than 1000 athletes who participated. Arm span and body ratio, which are commonly employed as crude clinical screens, were not discriminating.

Numerous cardiovascular manifestations have been documented in individuals with Marfan syndrome (see Box 5-2). Before the advent of echocardiography, such abnormalities were estimated to occur in 40% to 60% of patients.[42] It is now well established that more than 95% of patients with Marfan syndrome have cardiovascular abnormalities. Because it is impossible to determine whether a person has a potentially lethal cardiac abnormality without special studies, the athletic trainer needs to promptly refer anyone suspected of having Marfan syndrome to a physician for assessment.

The mitral valve can have multiple abnormalities in an athlete with Marfan syndrome that may lead to mitral valve prolapse (Figure 5-12) and to moderate or severe **mitral regurgitation** (Figure 5-13) in more than 25% of cases.[43] Regurgitation is evidenced on exam by **apical systolic murmurs.** The more redundant the mitral valve, the more prevalent ventricular and supraventricular dysrhythmias become.[43]

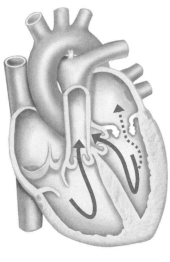

Mitral regurgitation
(heart in systole)

Figure 5-13 Mitral valve regurgitation. (From Seidel H, Ball J, Dains J, Benedict G: *Mosby's guide to physical examination,* ed 5, St Louis, 2003, Mosby.)

Aortic root and sinus dilation may be present at the time of birth, whereas dilation of the ascending aorta usually does not begin until the child is older.[44] The rate of dilation is unpredictable, so it is wise to assess any enlargement beyond the time of long bone epiphyseal closure ascribed to pathological dilation.[44] The aortic root must dilate 50 to 55 mm in order to produce audible aortic regurgitation characterized by a diastolic murmur at the upper right sternal border. Prophylactic surgical repair of the aortic root is usually recommended when the root diameter reaches 55 mm.[40,43]

The most dramatic cardiovascular manifestation is aortic dissection, which occurs in about two thirds of cases.[45] Once thought to be caused by cystic medial necrosis, it is believed to be the result of separation and fragmentation of elastic components of the aorta.[45] The greater the degree of aortic dilation, the greater the risk of dissection.

With the many potential manifestations seen with Marfan syndrome, a multidisciplinary approach to management is usually optimal. Musculoskeletal manifestations may require surgical intervention if cardiopulmonary compromise or progressive spinal curvature beyond 45 degrees occurs.

Ocular screening is conducted annually, but rarely is lens surgery necessary for the characteristic upwardly dislocated lens seen in 60% to 80% of patients.[46] An athlete should not be barred from participation because of dislocated lenses, but contact sports are restricted because of an increased risk for retinal detachment.[46]

Prognosis and Return to Participation

Athletes with Marfan syndrome are restricted from participation in sports that risk body collision.[36] Similarly, individuals with aortic regurgitation and aortic dilation should not participate in competitive sports[47]; but athletes with aortic root dilation can participate in competitive sports such as golf, bowling, and billiards.[33,36] And athletes without a family history of sudden death and no evidence of mitral regurgitation or aortic root dilation may participate in class IA and IIA sports such as archery, golf, bowling, and billiards (see Table 5-1).[33,36] Brisk walking for aerobic exercise also is acceptable. Serial 6-month echocardiographic evaluation is required for continued sports participation.[36]

Prevention

Prompt cardiovascular management is critical because more than 95% of the time aortic dissection and rupture are the cause of death for a Marfan syndrome patient. An annual evaluation is the minimal requirement and includes a complete cardiac examination with echocardiography. **Endocarditis** antibiotic prophylaxis is instituted for any mitral or aortic valve defect.

Magnetic resonance imaging or transesophageal echocardiography is used to evaluate or monitor aortic dissection.[48] More frequent examination is required when the aortic diameter increases. Quarterly monitoring of the aorta once the root has reached 50 mm is suggested because the risk for dissection significantly increases at this point.[47] Research suggests that prophylactic beta-blocker therapy may slow the rate of aortic dilation.[49] Once the aortic root diameter has reached 55 to 60 mm, surgical evaluation for aortoplasty, graft repair, or aortic valve replacement is advised.[40,43] Anticoagulants may be required depending on the procedure performed.

Special Concerns in the Preadolescent and Adolescent Athlete

In children, mitral regurgitation may be a more significant problem than aortic root dilation. If mitral regurgitation is severe, mitral valve repair may be necessary, although the long-term results are not known. Mitral valve repair obviates the need for anticoagulation. This can allow the child to engage in mild to moderate physical activity. Competitive sports as well as activities with the danger of body collision need to be avoided.[9,43] Depending on the situation, the child may need to be excused from all physical education activities.

Myocarditis

Myocarditis is an inflammatory process of the cardiac **myocytes** often resulting from enteroviral infections, most commonly coxsackievirus B. It traditionally has been regarded as an important cause of unexplained sudden death in young individuals. Cardiac dysfunction arises from inflammation of the myocardium with necrosis or degeneration of adjacent myocytes.[32] Healed or active areas of such inflammation may be a pathological substrate for cardiac arrhythmias, and physical activity may trigger a catastrophic event.[32]

Signs and Symptoms

Early in the course of the illness, the patient may experience what is thought to be a generalized viral illness with fever, body aches, nausea, vomiting, and diarrhea. However, the illness may be subclinical, and the patient can be asymptomatic aside from some mild fatigue. In this previously healthy person symptoms of unexplained **congestive heart failure** (CHF) can herald myocarditis. These symptoms may include increased fatigue, dyspnea, pitting edema, syncope, **palpitations,** and exercise intolerance. Sometimes the patient is asymptomatic, and sudden death may be the initial presentation (Red Flags—Myocarditis).

> ### ⚑ Red Flags for Myocarditis
> * Body aches
> * Fever
> * Nausea
> * Vomiting
> * Diarrhea
> * Mild fatigue
> * Dyspnea
> * Pitting edema
> * Syncope
> * Palpitations
> * Exercise intolerance

The patient experiencing congestive heart failure gains weight, exhibits tachycardia, and is hyperventilating. Auscultation often reveals a prominent S_3 heart sound and rales in the lung bases.

Referral and Diagnostic Tests

An athlete who is having difficulty recovering from what appears to be a routine viral illness needs to be referred to a physician. Clinical tests such as a chest radiograph, ECG, and echocardiogram may demonstrate arrhythmias or acute CHF. Nuclear imaging can be used to pinpoint areas of acute inflammation. For cases in which the diagnosis is in question, endomyocardial biopsy is considered.

Differential Diagnosis

Pericarditis is an inflammation of the pericardium surrounding the heart and may present with similar symptoms. It is usually caused by a virus as well and can be seen in collagen vascular diseases.

Treatment

Treatment using diuretics and antiarrhythmic drugs is usually directed at the CHF. Immunosuppressive therapy is controversial and still under study.

Prognosis and Return to Participation

More than 30% of individuals with myocarditis return to full activity. One third will experience residual problems, and the final third will need cardiac transplantation. Athletes suspected of having myocarditis need to refrain from all sports activity for 6 months (a convalescent period) and then undergo an evaluation of cardiac status and ventricular function at rest and with exercise.[32] If cardiac function and dimensions have returned to normal and there are no clinically relevant arrhythmias, the athlete may return to competition.[32] Insufficient data are available to justify performance of an endomyocardial biopsy as a precondition of return to activity following the 6-month recuperative period.

Prevention

Although the incidence of myocarditis is relatively small, the prognostic outcome for the majority of cases is poor. It is important for all health care providers to discourage ill athletes from participation in sports practice and events, particularly those with febrile illnesses. Such care not only will reduce the spread of infection but also may decrease the risk of contracting myocarditis.

Congenital Aortic Stenosis

Congenital aortic valve stenosis (AS) occurs in approximately 2% of the population. It is most commonly related to a bicuspid valve malformation. The pathophysiology arises from impaired left ventricular outflow with compensatory hypertrophy of the interventricular septum and left ventricular (LV) free wall (Figure 5-14). Other causes of aortic stenosis are rheumatic heart disease and atherosclerosis.

Signs and Symptoms

Patients may also develop significant myocardial ischemia and LV dysfunction from the increased pressure workload of the heart. This can result in hypotension and exertional syncope, which may be accompanied by lethal arrhythmias.

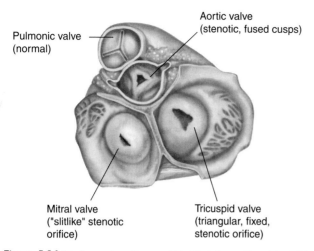

Pulmonic valve (normal)

Aortic valve (stenotic, fused cusps)

Mitral valve ("slitlike" stenotic orifice)

Tricuspid valve (triangular, fixed, stenotic orifice)

Figure 5-14 Cardiac valve disease. (Modified from Cannobio MM: *Cardiovascular disorders,* St Louis, 1990, Mosby.)

Referral and Diagnostic Tests

Patients with fatigue, dizziness, chest pain, syncope, or pallor on exertion require medical follow-up. AS can be readily identified on clinical exam by its characteristic loud crescendo-decrescendo systolic murmur heard at the upper right sternal border (i.e., aortic area).

Differential Diagnosis

Other cardiac and noncardiac conditions that may present in this fashion include hypertrophic cardiomyopathy. However, the characteristic murmur is definitive.

Prognosis and Return to Participation

Untreated athletes with mild AS can participate in all sports if they have a normal ECG, exercise tolerance, and no history of exercise-associated chest pain, syncope, or arrhythmia with symptoms.[30] Athletes with moderate AS can participate in low-static, low-to-moderate dynamic exercises and moderate-static, low-dynamic exercises (classes IA, IB, and IIA; see Table 5-1) if they have mild or no LV hypertrophy by echocardiography, no LV strain on ECG, a normal exercise test, and absence of exercise-associated symptoms.[33,36] However, athletes with severe AS are not candidates for competitive sports.[36]

Patients undergoing surgical repair may display regression of hypertrophy and improvement in exercise capacity.[50] However, residual outflow obstruction, aortic valve insufficiency, ventricular arrhythmias, and LV dysfunction may be present.[48] Athletes with mild, moderate, or severe residual stenosis are managed as outlined above.

Mitral Valve Prolapse

Mitral valve prolapse (MVP) is one of the most common cardiac abnormalities and is seen in as many as 6% to 8% of individuals, predominantly women. Although MVP is frequently mentioned as a cause of exercise-induced sudden death, reports of sudden death are rare. The etiology of MVP is unknown.

Signs and Symptoms

Symptoms include chest pain, heart palpitations, and uncharacteristic shortness of breath. Occasionally, patients complain of syncope or near syncope.

Referral and Diagnostic Tests

Any of the previously mentioned symptoms warrant referral to a physician. Diagnosis can frequently be made on the auscultative findings of a mid- to late-systolic apical click along with a systolic murmur. Patient positioning is important because both the click and the murmur vary with the patient's position. Squatting accentuates the click, and standing or Valsalva's maneuver increases the murmur. Echocardiography can confirm the diagnosis and record the degree of mitral regurgitation. Athletes who complain of palpitations or syncope require Holter monitoring.[51] A **Holter monitor** is a portable device that records the ECG over a 24-hour period. It has leads with electrodes that are attached to the patient's chest, and it feeds information to a small receiver, which is the size of a portable hand-held radio or pager.

Treatment

No treatment is needed in asymptomatic individuals, and athletic participation is unrestricted. Symptomatic individuals may need antiarrhythmic treatment. Antibiotic prophylaxis for dental procedures is recommended for any athlete with MVP with evidence of mitral regurgitation.

Prognosis and Return to Participation

Arrhythmias are closely associated with MVP and are generally the cause of palpitations reported by patients. Although numerous arrhythmias have been associated with MVP, ventricular arrhythmias are of the most concern because, although they are rare, they have been assumed to be the cause of sudden death.[52]

Participation in all competitive sports is allowed if the athlete with MVP does not show evidence of any of the conditions noted in Red Flags—Mitral Valve Prolapse.[32]

If any of these conditions are detected, the athlete may only participate in class IA sports, such as golf and bowling (see Table 5-1).[32,33]

Arrhythmias

The electrical pathway that synchronizes and controls the contraction of the atria and the ventricles can malfunction without warning. Most of these malfunctions are innocent, but some are pathological. Arrhythmias can recur frequently or disappear for years, and they vary with activity. Most benign arrhythmias in the athlete are due to increased vagal tone and disappear with exercise. Pathological arrhythmias can compromise blood flow and blood pressure. Some can result in sudden death. It is now well understood that a subset of arrhythmias and heart blocks is inherently safe in athletic participation if certain criteria are met.

As discussed earlier, the electrical activity of the heart is generated via the SA node that the ECG depicts as two events, depolarization (contraction) and repolarization (relaxation).

Arrhythmias are divided into two groups depending on the structures they impact: supraventricular and ventricular. Wolff-Parkinson-White syndrome and long QT syndrome are associated with sudden death and discussed below. Other abnormal arrhythmic conditions are beyond the scope of this chapter (Red Flags—Arrhythmic Conditions).

A patient with a suspected rhythm or conduction disturbance needs to have a 12-lead ECG, echocardiography, stress test, and prolonged ambulatory ECG recordings (using a Holter monitor) as warranted. If this evaluation reveals no evidence of structural heart disease and the patient has no symptoms, the 26th Bethesda Conference deems a number of conditions acceptable for full participation in sports (Box 5-3).[10]

Wolff-Parkinson-White Syndrome

Wolff-Parkinson-White (WPW) syndrome manifests by ventricular preexcitation and tachycardia as a result of electrical conduction over accessory pathways. Occurring in 0.1% to 3% of the population, it is characterized by a short PR interval (<0.12 second) and a prolonged QRS complex (>0.12 second) with a distinctive early depolarization, the delta wave.

It is fortunate that the incidence of WPW in athletes is very low and it is rarely provoked by exercise testing.[53] The occurrence of sudden death as the initial manifestation of WPW is rare but well documented and appears to be confined to those patients with accessory pathways that have short refractory periods.[54] In individual patients, the occurrence of secondary ventricular fibrillation after a paroxysmal WPW tachycardia has been occasionally reported.[53]

Referral and Diagnostic Tests

Those athletes with symptoms of palpitations, near syncope, or syncope must have an assessment of functional capabilities and electrophysiological properties of the accessory pathway in addition to a standard evaluation.[54]

Treatment

Surgical treatment for symptomatic WPW is typical. If a short refractory period is found, **radiofrequency**

Box 5-3   Arrhythmic Conditions Requiring No Limitation of Activity in Asymptomatic Patients Without Structural Heart Disease

- Sinus bradycardia
- Sick sinus syndrome
- Sinus tachycardia
- Premature atrial contractions (PACs)
- Sinus arrhythmia
- First-degree heart block
- Sinus arrest
- Second-degree heart block, type I (Mobitz I)
- Sinus node exit block
- Sinus node reentry
- Wandering pacemaker
- Atrial tachycardia
- Premature ventricular contractions (PVCs)

catheter ablation is often considered. This technique, carried out via a catheter inserted by way of the lower extremity veins, simply destroys the accessory pathway of the ventricle, thereby allowing the normal electrophysiological characteristics of the heart to proceed.

Prognosis and Return to Participation

Asymptomatic athletes over age 20 years without structural disease are unrestricted for athletic participation.[10] Younger patients may require more in-depth evaluation before undertaking moderate- to high-intensity competitive sports.[53] Athletes with atrial fibrillation or flutter with a resting rate below 240 beats/min without syncope or near syncope are at low risk for sudden death and can participate fully.[51] Those patients with higher rates or symptoms are limited to class IA activities and should consider ablation.[10,33] Following ablation, asymptomatic athletes with no inducible arrhythmia, normal AV conduction, and no spontaneous recurrence of tachycardia for 3 to 6 months are cleared for full participation.[10]

Long QT Syndrome

A ventricular repolarization abnormality (i.e., QT prolongation) that can be idiopathic or acquired characterizes long QT syndrome. Affected individuals may be at high risk for syncope and fatal ventricular arrhythmias. The idiopathic form is inherited in both an autosomal dominant manner (i.e., Jervell and Lange-Nielsen syndrome) and an autosomal recessive manner (i.e., Romano-Ward syndrome). Acquired forms of the disorder are usually the result of drug or electrolyte abnormalities.

The prevalence of long QT syndrome is rare in the general population and unknown in athletes. Most patients are identified from a family history of an affected patient having syncope or sudden death.[55] Evaluation for long QT syndrome particularly in a child is prompted by unexplained seizures or syncope.[56]

Signs and Symptoms

Patients experience a varied clinical course from no symptoms to syncope with sudden death. Syncope is almost always due to a transient malignant arrhythmia, usually a **torsades de pointes** (Key Points—Torsades de Pointes) type of polymorphic ventricular tachycardia.[57]

KEY POINTS
Torsades de Pointes

Torsades de pointes is an extremely rapid ventricular tachycardia determined by a changing QRS complex as seen on an electrocardiogram (ECG), which may be self-limited or progress to ventricular fibrillation.

Referral and Diagnostic Tests

Any athlete with exertional syncope or near syncope needs a prompt physician evaluation. The diagnosis of long QT syndrome uses an electrocardiogram; the corrected QT interval (QTc) must meet specific criteria to be considered prolonged but is affected by gender, age, and heart rate.[55] Borderline prolongation must be interpreted carefully, looking for reproducibility and other evidence of abnormal repolarization, such as prominent U waves and alterations in the T wave.[55] In 10% to 15% of athletes, QT interval is prolonged, particularly in endurance athletes, but no relationship between QT prolongation and ventricular arrhythmias in athletes has been observed.[58] Tests such as Holter monitoring, echocardiography, and exercise stress testing may be useful for confirming the diagnosis in equivocal cases.[55,57]

Treatment, Prognosis, and Return to Participation

Beta-blockers are the most effective antiarrhythmic agent for long QT syndrome. In acquired long QT syndrome, identifying and correcting the agent or abnormality may be all that are necessary for resolution.

Athletes with prolonged QT syndrome are at risk for sudden death with activity and need to be restricted from all competitive sports.[10]

Syncope

Syncope, or fainting, can be a challenging and frustrating condition for the practitioner as well as the patient to encounter. The many causes of syncope range from benign conditions, such as vasovagal reaction, to life-threatening conditions, such as hypertrophic cardiomyopathy. In many cases, no definitive cause can be established.

Signs and Symptoms

The most frequent cause of syncope in young individuals is neurocardiogenic (i.e., vasovagal). Symptoms are a prodrome of nausea, dizziness, blurred vision, and diaphoresis. The mechanism of neurocardiogenic syncope is believed to be the result of activated cardiac mechanoreceptors set off by forceful systolic contraction, causing an increased vagal stimulation with resultant bradycardia and hypotension.[59] An example of physical activity as a causative agent is jumping up from a supine position. Decreased venous return from abrupt postural changes in susceptible individuals as well as intense catecholamine release as seen in anxious, fearful, or panic situations can result in **neurocardiogenic syncope.** Athletic trainers may see a **vasovagal** response in the athlete who reacts to pain or observes an injection or minor surgery. These are all anxiety-producing situations, and the athlete (or coach) can be apparently healthy one minute and suddenly collapsed on the floor the next. These causes are different from syncope caused by an organic or physiological abnormality. Nevertheless, the immediate treatment is similar.

Referral and Diagnostic Tests

Any case of exertional syncope or near syncope, including postexercise events, requires a physician evaluation. A thorough history and physical examination are essential in the athlete with syncope. The history of the syncopal event may dictate what laboratory tests are indicated to confirm the diagnosis. Standard laboratory tests include orthostatic vital signs, hemoglobin and hematocrit, blood glucose, electrolytes, and a resting ECG. Situations that call for a more extensive cardiac assessment are exercise-induced syncope without definitive etiology, a family history of premature sudden cardiac death, or physical exam findings of a significant heart murmur or Marfan stigmata.[60,61] An athlete with a history suggestive of neurological syncope or an abnormal neurological exam receives an extensive neurological assessment as well.

Most cases of neurocardiogenic syncope do not require an extensive work-up if the athlete is young and the history is consistent for vasovagal reaction. However, Hargarten states that in individuals who have significant coronary risk factors, vasovagal reaction is a diagnosis of exclusion.[61] Objective testing for neurocardiogenic syncope uses upright, tilt-table testing. This test was developed in the mid-1980s and involves placing the patient in a supine position and measuring blood pressure and heart rate. Then the patient is tilted upright usually at an angle of 60 degrees. After passive tilting for 10 to 15 minutes without response, isoproterenol may be infused intravenously to promote a syncopal event. The test usually lasts 60 minutes. A positive test is defined as syncope or presyncope in association with hypertension or bradycardia.[59,62]

Tilt-table testing can be used in both children and adults. In cases of unexplained syncope, more than one half of patients have a positive tilt test.[59] However, this test has poor reproducibility.[59,63] Fouad-Tarazi states that the tilt test alone cannot conclusively classify the type of syncope.[63] Kapoor recommends testing only when the work-up has been negative and the patient has recurrent or disabling symptoms.[59]

Treatment

Immediate treatment for an athlete who has sustained syncope is to evaluate airway, breathing, circulation (i.e., ABC) status. If the athlete is pale and sweating and has good airway, breathing, and circulation, the immediate treatment is to raise the feet, thereby assisting the venous return to the vital organs, particularly the heart and brain. Further assessment continues as the athlete regains consciousness and can assist with the medical history. Besides the aforementioned cardiac anomalies, the athlete may simply have skipped a meal, been dehydrated, or be exhausted.

Secondary treatment for syncope depends on its etiology. If the syncope is cardiac in origin (e.g., long QT syndrome), beta-blocker medication and disqualification from sports are in order. In other cardiac conditions, such as WPW syndrome, ablation of the extra electrical pathway cures the problem and the athlete can return to full athletic participation. If the syncope is neurological in origin (e.g., epilepsy), medical treatment may permit full to modified athletic participation. If the cause of the syncope is asthma related, medical treatment may permit full to modified athletic participation. If the syncope is vasovagal, correcting the problem can be as easy as improving nutrition or hydration or adding some salt to the diet to maintain electrolyte balance in sweating athletes.

Prognosis and Return to Participation

In the athlete, syncope is a serious condition that requires a thorough evaluation. Straightforward episodes of vasovagal or **orthostatic syncope** dictate a cost-effective assessment. Questionable cases necessitate excluding cardiac or neurological etiologies. Return to participation is dictated by the etiology of the syncope and how well the underlying problem can be controlled or eliminated. Vasovagal syncope is not cause for any athletic restriction.

Prevention

Prevention depends on what is causing the syncope. Maintaining proper nutrition and hydration can usually prevent vasovagal syncope. When exercising in the heat, the athlete who does not usually salt food might benefit from some added salt to the diet because electrolytes lost in sweat could be the culprit causing the syncope.

PATHOLOGICAL CONDITIONS OF THE VASCULAR SYSTEM

Hypertension

Systemic hypertension is the most common cardiovascular disorder among athletes. The majority of the time there is no identifiable cause. The elevated blood pressure (>140/90 mm Hg in adults) results from increases in total peripheral resistance mediated by changes in plasma epinephrine and norepinephrine along with the **renin-angiotensin system.**[64]

Untreated hypertension can lead to serious consequences, such as heart disease, atherosclerosis, renal disease, visual changes, and neurological impairment. Therefore hypertension should be identified as soon as possible and treated appropriately.

Signs and Symptoms

Although most cases are asymptomatic, hypertension is more likely to occur in people with a family history of the disease. It is also more common in individuals who are obese and in African-Americans. Symptoms on presentation can include headaches, malaise, visual problems, or exercise intolerance.

Referral and Diagnostic Tests

Annual blood pressure screening is an essential part of early diagnosis. Usually, three separate measurements that demonstrate an elevated blood pressure are needed to confirm the diagnosis (see Chapter 2). New and more stringent diagnostic guidelines were issued in 2003 (Table 5-2). Proper conditions and equipment minimize false-positive measurements. Clinical findings that may be detected in those with hypertension include cardiac hypertrophy, tachycardia, decreased pulses, bruits, retinal changes, thyroid abnormalities, and tremors.

When evaluating a patient with suspected hypertension, the examiner obtains a thorough history of diet, exercise, weight, and drug use.[64] High sodium intake can contribute to hypertension. It is important to consider exercise history as well because even an athlete can overtrain, resulting in blood pressure changes or deconditioning between seasons. Both situations cause susceptibility if there is a familial tendency toward hypertension. Body weight is often elevated, which is commonly seen in specific sports (linemen in

football, throwers in track and field), and can contribute to the problem. Many drugs can contribute to or exacerbate hypertension. Common offenders include caffeine, nasal decongestants, nicotine, appetite suppressants, and nonsteroidal antiinflammatory drugs.[64] In addition, many drugs banned for those participating in athletic competition, such as ephedrine, cocaine, steroids, erythropoietin, and amphetamines, elevate blood pressure.[64]

Assessment includes an ECG to evaluate for cardiac hypertrophy. The physician orders urine tests for blood and protein and blood work that specifically checks lipid levels, electrolytes, and liver and kidney function. Thyroid function is assessed as needed. If there are cardiac concerns, an exercise stress test may be indicated in addition to the ECG.

Treatment

Treatment can follow nonpharmacological and pharmacological categories and generally is based on a step approach. Strategies such as smoking cessation, diet and weight control, alcohol moderation, and an exercise prescription all have a role in the management of hypertension.[64] For most people, medications are needed to effectively lower and maintain blood pressure. This may be especially true in athletes, as they are already exercising, rarely smoke, and typically have their weight under control. With this in mind, lifestyle changes are encouraged and may limit the number of medications required for blood pressure control.

The several classes of hypertension drugs act in different ways. For the active athlete, **angiotensin-converting enzyme (ACE) inhibitors** are the drugs of choice because they have fewer side effects with exercise. Commonly prescribed diuretics increase the chance for dehydration and heat illness. Beta-blockers restrict exercise capacity, exacerbate asthma, and are banned in certain competitive sports.

Prognosis and Return to Participation

In terms of athletic participation, patients with mild to moderate hypertension, ranging from 140 to 179 systolic/90 to 109 diastolic, can participate in all sports if there is no evidence of end-organ damage or heart disease. Activities are focused on dynamic exercise, but static activities are not prohibited.[64,65] Blood pressure needs to be under control or in the mild range (<140/90 mm Hg to 159/99 mm Hg) before an athlete engages in highly competitive sports or highly strenuous physical training. Blood pressure for a hypertensive individual should be checked every 2 to 4 months.[65]

Patients with severe hypertension (>180/110 mm Hg) are restricted from strenuous exercise until their blood pressure can be controlled.[64,65] Dynamic physical

Table 5-2	American Heart Association Recommended Blood Pressure Levels*	
Blood Pressure	**Systolic (mm Hg)**	**Diastolic (mm Hg)**
Normal	<120	<80
Prehypertension	120-139	80-89
High Blood Pressure (Hypertension)		
Stage 1 (mild)	140-159	90-99
Stage 2 (moderate)	≥160	≥100
Severe	>180	>110

Modified from American Heart Association: What is high blood pressure? Available at www.americanheart.org/presenter.jhtml?identifier=2112. Accessed October 2004.
*A physician should evaluate low or high readings.

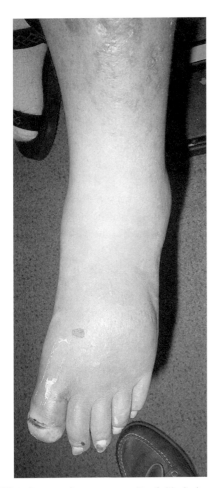

Figure 5-15 A foot swollen as a result of blocked venous return caused by a deep vein thrombosis (DVT). (From Jarvis C: *Physical examination & health assessment*, ed 4, Philadelphia, 2004, WB Saunders, p 558.)

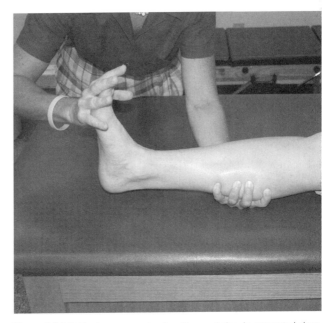

Figure 5-16 Patient assessment using Homans' sign in suspected deep vein thrombosis (DVT) of the lower leg.

activities, however, are encouraged because little data suggest strenuous dynamic exercise in persons with severe hypertension will lead to progression of the hypertension or exercise-induced sudden death.[64,65]

Deep Vein Thrombosis

Deep vein thrombosis (DVT) is a condition in which a blood clot becomes lodged in a large vein. This results in venous blockage with stasis distal to the clot. Most of these clots occur in the lower legs (Figure 5-15). However, a DVT can occur in any limb. For instance, subclavian vein thrombosis, although rare, has been reported in baseball pitchers.

Many factors contribute to the formation of a DVT. In an active population, a DVT is usually caused by trauma to the extremity from injury or surgery. Hip or knee replacement surgery carries a 50% incidence of postoperative DVT without prophylaxis.[66] Other less

common causes are prolonged sitting on a plane, in a bus, or in a car, hypercoagulability disorders such as **Factor V Leiden anticoagulant gene mutation,** pregnancy, and **polycythemia.** Women who use oral contraceptives, particularly women who smoke, also have an increased risk of blood clots.

Signs and Symptoms

The symptoms of DVT are often nonspecific; some DVTs are actually asymptomatic. The key symptoms are limb pain and swelling. In the leg, these symptoms are worsened by standing and walking. On examination, there is usually distal edema of the affected extremity. This can be confirmed by comparison with the contralateral extremity. In the lower leg, the examiner tests for Homans' sign (Figure 5-16), realizing the test is not specific for a DVT nor is it commonly present with DVT.[66] Measuring the patient's temperature can be important because fever may be the clue to a DVT proximal to the knee, which is closely associated with **pulmonary embolus.** DVT is generally confirmed through Doppler ultrasound testing (Figure 5-17) but may require invasive **contrast venography.**

Differential Diagnosis

It is possible to confuse a DVT with a more superficial **thrombophlebitis, postphlebitic syndrome,** ruptured Baker's cyst, or even cellulitis. Even the common problem of calf muscle strain may be confused with a DVT. Usually the mechanism of injury can help differentiate a strain from a DVT. Anytime the patient has had

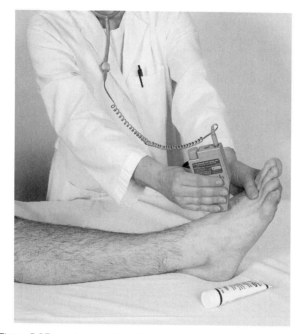

Figure 5-17 An ultrasonic Doppler stethoscope is used to determine the integrity of the dorsalis pedis vessels. (From Jarvis C: *Physical examination & health assessment,* ed 4, Philadelphia, 2004, WB Saunders, p 550.)

recent surgery, traveled long distances sitting down, or been subject to a known trauma, a DVT is highly possible (Red Flags—Deep Vein Thrombosis).

Red Flags for Deep Vein Thrombosis

Indicators of a deep vein thrombosis include the following:
- Recent surgery
- Recent travel or prolonged sitting
- Limb pain
- Limb swelling
- Pain and swelling increasing with use of limb
- Edema of affected limb
- Possible fever
- Use of oral contraceptives

Treatment

Treatment requires anticoagulation, which can be started on an outpatient basis but may require hospitalization. After adequate anticoagulation is reached with heparin, the patient usually must keep taking other anticoagulants such as warfarin (Coumadin) for 3 months or more.[66,67] Anticoagulation medications must be monitored and adjusted following blood tests every week or so until the medication level is stabilized in the patient. Another more expensive injectable drug, enoxaparin (Lovenox), is also available and requires less monitoring than other anticoagulants. Note that mixing alcoholic beverages with anticoagulant medications is dangerous; alcohol can increase the blood-thinning properties of the drugs. Serious, if not

deadly, ramifications can be caused by such combinations, and they need to be fully explained to the patient. Patients also need to be aware that antiinflammatory medications alter the blood-clotting process and may exacerbate bleeding time. While patients are taking anticoagulants, collision or contact sports are not advised. In addition to medications, the patient's diet needs to include adequate but not excessive vitamin K.

Prevention

Simple prevention is difficult with the exception that all individuals need to avoid prolonged sitting, such as when traveling by plane or automobile. Also, as women age they may need to consider an alternate form of contraception than birth control pills. Postsurgical and hypercoagulability situations require subspecialty care. Prompt recognition of symptoms by the athletic trainer is essential to initiate proper care of DVTs and prevent catastrophic results.

Pulmonary Embolus

A pulmonary embolus (PE) can be a catastrophic complication of a DVT. PE occurs when a blood clot becomes lodged in one of the pulmonary blood vessels. If the vessel is large enough, gas exchange can be interrupted long enough for death to occur before the clot can be dissolved (Figure 5-18).

Signs and Symptoms

Symptoms are not specific and can lead to a delay in diagnosis. Common symptoms include acute dyspnea and chest pain (Red Flags—Pulmonary Embolus).

Red Flags for Pulmonary Embolus

Indicators of a pulmonary embolus include the following:
- Dyspnea
- Chest pain
- History of recent surgery
- Recent travel or prolonged sitting
- Fatigue
- Exercise intolerance
- Tachycardia
- Tachypnea
- Low-grade fever
- Hemoptysis

If the embolism is large, the patient may experience a sense of impending doom. Fatigue and exercise intolerance may occur. Common clinical findings include tachycardia and tachypnea. Low-grade fever may develop, and hemoptysis may occur. There may be

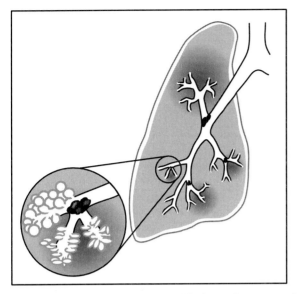

Figure 5-18 Pulmonary embolisms cause life-threatening emergencies when they occlude pulmonary vessels. (From Jarvis C: *Physical examination & health assessment,* ed 4, Philadelphia, 2004, WB Saunders, p 481.)

signs of a DVT although many instances of PE occur without warning.

Referral and Diagnostic Tests

Anytime a PE is suspected because of acute dyspnea or chest pain, the patient needs emergent medical attention. A high index of suspicion is often necessary to diagnose a PE because standard tests are going to be of limited value. Special hospital studies, such as a **ventilation-perfusion scan** or pulmonary arteriography, are performed to confirm the diagnosis.

Differential Diagnosis

Because the symptoms of a PE are nonspecific, many serious conditions need to be considered in the differential diagnosis. Cardiovascular conditions range from angina and pericarditis to aortic aneurysm and myocardial infarction. Pulmonary conditions include pneumonia, pneumothorax, and pleuritis. Gastrointestinal conditions, such as ulcers, gastritis, and esophageal rupture, can produce atypical chest pain and warrant consideration.

Treatment

As in a DVT, anticoagulation treatment is warranted and hospitalization is required in the early stages of treatment. At least 3 months of anticoagulation therapy is needed. Continuation of therapy depends on the risk factors for recurrence. Athletic participation is limited in the same manner as for a DVT.

Prevention

In most cases, the cause of the PE is not determined. For individuals with a defined cause such as hypercoagulability, long-term anticoagulation may be necessary. A person who is at risk for PE but cannot take anticoagulation therapy may need to have a filtering device inserted into the vena cava, where it will catch clots, to keep a life-threatening clot from reaching the lungs. In both instances, athletic participation is significantly restricted depending on the activity and the level of participation.

Peripheral Arterial Disease

Peripheral arterial disease (PAD), which is also referred to as peripheral vascular disease, is a condition primarily caused by atherosclerosis. It usually presents after the age of 50 years and is more common in older adults. Risk factors include smoking, hypertension, diabetes, and **hyperlipidemia.**

Signs and Symptoms

The hallmark of PAD is intermittent **claudication,** which leads to cramping, weakness, pain, or numbness in the affected muscles.[68] Most commonly, this is in the lower leg and provoked by exercise of a given intensity and duration. In the beginning, the symptoms are relieved by rest. However, as PAD progresses, pain can also occur at rest.

The key signs are diminished or absent pulses, arterial bruits, dry skin, and ulcerations on the heels and toes. When the lower extremities are elevated, pallor can develop within minutes with return of color delayed more than 15 minutes after lowering the limbs.[68]

Referral and Diagnostic Tests

Clinical suspicion for PAD warrants referral to a physician for assessment. The athletic trainer becomes suspicious when an athlete complains of cramping or weakness in the lower extremities that worsens with exercise. One way to test for PAD is to measure the ankle or brachial index. This is a hospital test that determines the ratio of ankle to brachial systolic blood pressures. The gold standard test is invasive angiography.

Differential Diagnosis

PAD could be mistaken for many common problems, such as shin splints, muscle cramps, or arthritis. Lumbar spinal stenosis causes pseudoclaudication, for which symptoms occur with walking or prolonged standing and are relieved by sitting and flexing the spine.

Individuals with these conditions do not have any pulse abnormalities or skin changes from arterial insufficiency. Claudication can occur from vein damage too. This causes venous stasis, edema, and rest pain. Other arterial diseases, such as arteritis and **Raynaud's disease,** can mimic PAD. Neurological causes of peripheral pain, such as lumbar disk disease or diabetic peripheral neuropathy, may be confused with PAD. Another condition to rule out is compartment syndrome of the lower leg, which has both acute and exertional onset.

Treatment

Treatment centers on correcting the contributing factors such as smoking, hypertension, and hyperlipidemia. To decrease the risk of stroke or heart attack, a daily aspirin is recommended. Regular exercise with breaks when the symptoms occur may be more beneficial than any medication. Initiating a walking program and gradually adding other physical activities such as biking or swimming are excellent exercise programs for the patient with PAD.

Prognosis, Return to Participation, and Prevention

Progressive deterioration occurs in up to 20% of patients.[68] In these patients, surgical referral for arterial bypass is an important consideration. Treating or resolving the risk factors can decrease the potential for deterioration. Return to participation depends on the type and level of activity. Risk factor modification is the best preventive strategy for patients with a propensity for PAD.

Anemia

Anemia refers to a decreased number of red blood cells or a decreased hemoglobin concentration in the blood. It is a common medical condition or can be a sign of a chronic disease such as cancer. The size of the red blood cell differentiates anemias into three general categories: microcytic, normocytic, and macrocytic.

Microcytic anemias include iron deficiency, **thalassemia,** lead poisoning, **sideroblastic** anemia, and anemias of chronic disease. Normocytic anemias include blood loss, hemolysis, chronic disease, dilutional pseudoanemia, and sickle cell disease. Macrocytic anemias include nutritional anemias related to deficiency of vitamins B_{12} and folate, drug-induced **aplastic** and hemolytic anemias, malignancy, and other hemolytic anemias, such as enzyme deficiencies or red blood cell membrane defects.

In the athlete, decreased hemoglobin is usually the result of iron deficiency, exertional hemolysis, or dilutional pseudoanemia.[69] These disorders are more common in endurance athletes, particularly female athletes. Because many other conditions can result in anemia, and the treatments can vary, it is important to be certain of the diagnosis.

Iron deficiency anemia is the most common true anemia seen in athletes. Whereas it is rare in male athletes unless they experience a gastrointestinal bleed, as many as 5% of female athletes have iron deficiency anemia and up to 20% of female athletes are iron deficient.[69] This is due to menstrual blood loss combined with inadequate dietary iron intake.

Dilutional pseudoanemia has been labeled sports anemia. It is not a true anemia. It is a physiological adaptation to an acute decrease in plasma volume with exercise resulting in plasma volume expansion and dilution of hemoglobin concentration from 5% to 20%.[69]

Signs and Symptoms

Anemia can produce symptoms of weakness, fatigue, dizziness, and headache. Frequently, athletes are asymptomatic if the anemia developed slowly. Decreased performance typically brings the anemia to the athlete's attention. Clinical findings include tachycardia, **orthostatic hypotension,** dyspnea, tachypnea, and pallor. Mouth and tongue abnormalities suggest nutritional deficiencies. Less common clinical findings, such as jaundice and hepatosplenomegaly, indicate serious pathology and require urgent medical referral.

Craving ice or constantly eating crunchy, raw vegetables may suggest iron deficiency anemia. Nonsteroidal antiinflammatory drugs (NSAIDs) can cause gastrointestinal irritation with resultant blood loss, and continual alcohol use can cause similar findings.

Antibiotic use (e.g., penicillin, sulfa, cephalosporin) can trigger hemolytic anemia as well as acute illnesses such as infectious mononucleosis or mycoplasma pneumonia (see Chapter 3).

Referral and Diagnostic Tests

An athlete who presents with symptoms of fatigue and loss of energy and who bruises easily should be referred to a physician for a complete blood count (CBC) as well as other tests. Initial tests also include a peripheral blood smear. The CBC measures hemoglobin concentration. The typical cutoff criterion for anemia is below 14 g/dl for men and below 12 g/dl for women.

As previously mentioned, the size of the red blood cell classifies the anemia into one of three general categories: microcytic, normocytic, and macrocytic. The mean corpuscular volume (MCV), which is one of the tests contained in the CBC, allows for this classification.

Microcytic anemia is defined by an MCV of less than 75 fl. An MCV of 75 to 95 fl defines normocytic anemia; and an MCV of greater than 95 fl defines a macrocytic anemia. The degree of abnormality in the MCV can provide a clue to the diagnosis. Although both iron deficiency and thalassemia conditions have a low MCV, an MCV of less than 60 fl is more suggestive of thalassemia than iron deficiency anemia. Table 2-5 gives normal values for the CBC.

Looking at the size, shape, and color of the red blood cell provides valuable information to determine the type of anemia. Using the previous example of iron deficiency and thalassemia, the peripheral blood smear for both conditions will show microcytic cells. The cells in iron deficiency are hypochromic compared with the normochromic cells seen in thalassemia.

Many other tests can be ordered to determine the presence of anemia. Box 5-4 lists the tests for anemia.

Differential Diagnosis

Dilutional pseudoanemia can be indistinguishable from very mild iron deficiency anemia.[69] Because lead poisoning and sideroblastic anemia are extremely rare in the athlete, a microcytic anemia is usually a choice between iron deficiency and thalassemia.

Other conditions to consider are exertional hemolysis and systemic illnesses such as infectious mononucleosis. The symptoms of hypothyroidism or depression also can mimic those of anemia.

Treatment

Iron deficiency anemia is not difficult to treat; however, before treatment one must identify and correct any source of abnormal blood loss. The patient takes 325 mg of ferrous sulfate three times per day for optimal treatment for iron deficiency anemia. When an individual cannot tolerate that dosage because of gastrointestinal irritation (i.e., constipation), taking one dose with dinner is acceptable. A response is expected within 2 weeks showing a weekly increase in hemoglobin. When the hemoglobin is back to normal (i.e., typically 3 to 6 weeks), daily iron therapy is continued for another 3 to 6 months to reestablish iron stores.

In cases where it is difficult to decide between dilutional pseudoanemia and iron deficiency anemia, an empirical trial of iron therapy is tried. If after 1 to 2 months of therapy the hemoglobin has increased, then the patient has iron deficiency anemia. In thalassemia minor, no treatment is required. In fact, iron therapy can be harmful.

Prognosis and Return to Participation

Dilutional pseudoanemia does no harm, and competition is not restricted. Because iron deficiency anemia can impair athletic performance, training and competition are limited to what the athlete can tolerate. Full training and competition are dictated by the athlete's degree of anemia and the demands of the sport.

Prevention

Prevention of iron deficiency anemia focuses on consuming adequate amounts of iron in the diet (Box 5-5). The best source of iron is lean red meat. Although some vegetables, such as spinach and beans, contain iron, these sources are not as bioavailable. Also, some foods, such as breads, pastas, and cereals, are iron fortified. To enhance absorption, advise the

---

Box 5-4   Tests to Determine the Presence of Anemia

1. Stool Blood: can be done in the physician's office or the patient can collect stool on special cards at home; can determine microscopic blood in the stool, which indicates a gastrointestinal source
2. Serum Ferritin: a measure of tissue iron stores, which are low (<12 ng/dl) in iron deficiency anemia; normal to elevated in other microcytic anemias; serum ferritin can be low and the individual not anemic; although some authorities think that decreased ferritin is associated with decreased exercise performance, scientific evidence does not support this claim
3. Serum Iron: decreased in iron deficiency anemia and in anemia of chronic disease; elevated in thalassemia and sideroblastic anemia
4. Total Iron-Binding Capacity (TIBC): increased in iron deficiency anemia and may be normal or increased in thalassemia; decreased in anemia of chronic disease and can be decreased in sideroblastic anemia
5. Reticulocyte Count: a marker of red blood cell production; should be elevated in anemia but it is inappropriately low in iron deficiency anemia
6. Hemoglobin Electrophoresis: can be ordered to identify genetic hemoglobinopathies, such as thalassemia or sickle cell disease
7. Vitamin B_{12} or Folate: may be decreased in the malnourished athlete (e.g., eating disorder) with macrocytic anemia
8. Bone Marrow Biopsy: invasive test reserved to determine very serious anemias, such as aplastic anemia that can be caused by drugs such as nonsteroidal antiinflammatory drugs (NSAIDs) or antibiotics

---

Box 5-5   Foods Rich in Iron

- Organ meat (e.g., liver, heart, kidney)
- Lean red meat
- Dark poultry
- Shellfish (e.g., oyster, clams, shrimp)
- Eggs
- Legumes (e.g., beans, dried peas, lentils)
- Leafy green vegetables
- Iron-fortified cereals

athlete to avoid coffee or tea and to drink orange juice or other drinks with vitamin C. In addition, cooking in cast iron cookware can provide some iron leaching into the food.

Hemolysis

Exertional hemolysis is defined as the intravascular breakdown of red blood cells as a result of the rigors of physical activity. Initially reported in runners, it was called *foot strike hemolysis* because it was believed to occur from the physical pounding of the soles of the feet. However, the process has been seen in a variety of sports from weight lifting to swimming.

The hemolysis may result in anemia and decreased iron stores. The hemoglobin released in the plasma binds to haptoglobin, which carries it to the liver for salvage. When hemoglobin stores are saturated, it may be secreted into the urine with iron. It would be rare for hemolysis to present with signs and symptoms because it is typically displayed as asymptomatic microscopic hematuria.

Signs and Symptoms

In an athlete with substantial hemolysis, symptoms of mild anemia, such as fatigue and weakness, may be present. It is more likely that the athlete will be asymptomatic. In anemia, dark-colored urine suggests **hemoglobinuria.** In **hemolysis,** it is more likely that the urine will have a combination of myoglobin from muscle breakdown along with some hemoglobin, particularly if the inciting activity is intense or prolonged.

Referral and Diagnostic Tests

A physician orders the following diagnostic tests to confirm hemolysis: CBC usually shows normal to mildly decreased hemoglobin and red cell concentrations, MCV is elevated but rarely exceeds 105 fl,[69] blood smear is normal, reticulocyte count is elevated, and the serum haptoglobin concentration is low. Examination of the urine may detect the presence of hemoglobin.

Differential Diagnosis

Because clinically significant exertional hemolysis is extremely rare, its diagnosis is one of exclusion. Pathological causes of hemolytic anemia including red cell trauma from other sources such as cardiac valvular disease, enzyme defects, toxin and metabolic disorders, and paroxysmal nocturnal hemoglobinuria need to be excluded.

Treatment

In most cases of exertional hemolysis, there is no anemia. Therefore no treatment is needed as long as the individual has adequate iron stores.

Prognosis and Return to Participation

Excellent prognosis and full return to participation are the norm for athletes who have exertional hemolysis. Prevention is important in the rare case of a problem.

Prevention

Prevention of hemolysis depends on the mechanism of injury. If excessive impact is to blame, then steps need to be taken to reduce the impact. Examples are better-cushioned shoes, softer running surfaces, and altering the activity with cross training.

Sickle Cell Anemia or Trait

Sickle cell anemia is caused by a genetic defect in the hemoglobin of the affected person. The altered hemoglobin, called hemoglobin S, causes a chronic hemolytic anemia characterized by decreased red blood cell survival, microvascular occlusions from sickling in which the cells stick together, and increased susceptibility to certain infections (Figure 5-19). These complications result in significant morbidity and a decreased life expectancy.

Most individuals with sickle cell anemia in the United States are of African-American descent. In the athlete with sickle cell, average hemoglobin concentration is 50% to 66% of normal counts, which is prohibitive for binding oxygen to the red blood cells. Only in very rare instances would a person with sickle cell anemia be able to participate in sports, and that would be restricted to the least physically demanding.

On the other hand, individuals with sickle cell trait are not prohibited from athletic participation. Those with the trait are not anemic and have a normal life expectancy. Approximately 1 in 12 African-Americans has sickle cell trait. In contrast, only 1 in 10,000 Caucasian Americans carries the trait.

Unfortunately, there have been some rare deaths in athletes with sickle cell trait associated with extreme environmental conditions, such as altitude or hot, humid conditions, in combination with high-intensity workouts. The causes of death have been unclear, although sickling has been postulated as a potential culprit. Ischemia resulting from sickling may cause **rhabdomyolysis, lactic acidosis,** and shock.[69]

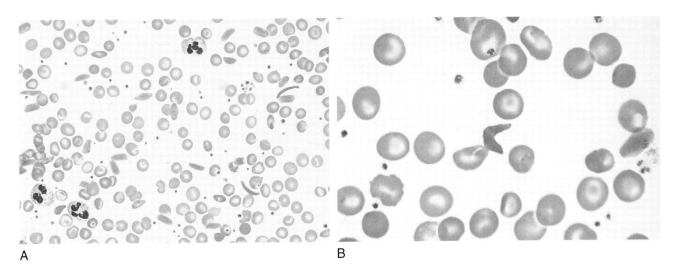

Figure 5-19 A peripheral blood smear from a patient with sickle cell anemia. **A,** Sickle cells at low magnification. **B,** An irreversibly sickled cell at higher magnification in the center of the slide. (From Kumar V, Cotran RS, Robbins SL: *Basic pathology,* ed 7, Philadelphia, 2003, WB Saunders. Courtesy Dr. Robert W. McKenna, Department of Pathology, University of Texas Southwestern Medical School, Dallas.)

People with sickle cell trait are prone to heat illness because they have an inability to concentrate their urine, which makes them prone to dehydration. It is not known if this has been a factor in these rare deaths.

Signs and Symptoms

The signs and symptoms for sickle cell anemia or trait often present in specific environments. Early, preseason practice in a hot, humid environment or events in high altitude tend to lead to attacks in a previously undiagnosed athlete. In addition, intensive exercise such as sprinting and intervals can be the trigger (Red Flags—Sickle Cell Anemia or Trait). Often the athlete develops

---

⟩ Red Flags for Sickle Cell Anemia or Trait

Indicators of sickle cell anemia or trait in an African-American athlete include the following:
- Heat intolerance
- Severe muscular cramping
- Hyperventilation
- Tachycardia
- Hypotension
- Symptomatic indicators in high altitude environments
- Symptomatic indicators after intense exercise

---

excruciating, cramping pain in the lower legs, buttocks, and low back and collapses with impaired consciousness, hyperventilation, tachycardia, and hypotension. This is an emergency situation.

Referral and Diagnostic Tests

Sickle cell trait collapse requires emergency transport to a hospital equipped to handle such an emergency.

If prompt diagnosis and management are not undertaken, the athlete may go into shock, experience multisystem organ failure, and die. Diagnosis of sickle cell trait can be made with a Sickledex test, with confirmation by hemoglobin **electrophoresis.**

Differential Diagnosis

The collapse of an athlete from sickle cell anemia or trait, if not witnessed, can be confused with heat stroke, malignant hyperthermia, syncope, or cardiac arrest.

Treatment, Prognosis, and Return to Participation

Recognition, emergent first aid (i.e., ABCs, oxygen), and triage to the hospital emergency department for appropriate care are necessary and may decrease the likelihood of the patient going into acute renal failure or multisystem organ failure.

If the athlete survives an episode of complete sickle cell anemia or trait collapse, restriction from similar exercise settings or environmental conditions is warranted. This may mean that the athlete is disqualified from that competitive sport.

Prevention

The athletic trainer should always stress proper hydration for an athlete who has sickle cell trait. Those involved with the athlete, including peers, parents, and coaches, need to understand the warning signs for collapse and consequences of inaction. Health care professionals need to offer informed screening for sickle cell trait, which is relatively inexpensive.

SUMMARY

Conditions that affect the cardiovascular system can have catastrophic sequelae in athletes. Appreciating the anatomy and physiology of the cardiovascular system is one method of understanding the demands placed on this system. Another is to understand the various cardiac arrhythmias and abnormalities, their effect on the human body, and the implications of both on strenuous activity. This chapter highlights some cardiovascular abnormalities that are problematical in regard to athletic participation, how to recognize them, and when to refer an athlete who exhibits them to a physician.

The preparticipation examination is critical in identifying underlying cardiovascular problems. The initial exam offers the best place to seek additional medical evaluation. Many athletes with cardiovascular conditions have long and productive careers within safe parameters because of early discovery and proper treatment of their particular circumstance.

REFERENCES

1. Seidel H, Ball J, Dains J, Benedict G: *Mosby's guide to physical examination*, ed 5, Philadelphia, 2003, Mosby.
2. Booher M, Smith B: Physiological effects of exercise on the cardiopulmonary system, *Clinics in Sports Medicine* 22:1-22, 2003.
3. Charlton G, Crawford M: Cardiovascular response to exercise, *Cardiology Clinics* 15:345-354, 1997.
4. Pescatello L, Kulikowich J: The aftereffects of dynamic exercise on ambulatory blood pressure, *Medicine and Science in Sports and Exercise* 33:1855-1861, 2001.
5. Smith B, Ciocca M: The athletic heart syndrome. In Garrett WJ, Kirkendall D, Squire D, editors: *Principles and practice of primary care sports medicine*, Philadelphia, 2002, Lippincott Williams & Wilkins, pp 251-259.
6. Pellicca A, Maron B, Spataro A, et al: The upper limit of physiologic cardiac hypertrophy in highly trained elite athletes, *New England Journal of Medicine* 324:295-301, 1991.
7. American Medical Society for Sports Medicine: Preparticipation exam. Available at http://www.amssm.org/. Accessed September 2004.
8. Huston T, Puffer J, Rodney W: The athletic heart syndrome, *New England Journal of Medicine* 311:24-32, 1985.
9. Cheitlin M, Douglas P, Parmley W: 26th Bethesda Conference: recommendations for determining eligibility for competition in athletes with cardiovascular abnormalities. Task force 2: acquired valvular heart disease, *Medicine and Science in Sports and Exercise* 26:S254-S260, 1994.
10. Zipes D, Garson AJ: 26th Bethesda Conference. Revised eligibility recommendations for competitive athletes with cardiovascular abnormalities. Task force 6: arrhythmias, *Journal of the American College of Cardiology* 24(4):892-899, 1994.
11. Van Camp S, Bloor C, Muller F, Cantu R, Olsen H: Nontraumatic sports death in high school and college athletes, *Medicine and Science in Sports and Exercise* 27:641-647, 1995.
12. Maron B, Shirani J, Poliac L, et al: Sudden death in young competitive athletes, *JAMA* 276:199-204, 1996.
13. Phillips M, Robinowitz M, Higgins J, et al: Sudden cardiac death in Air Force recruits, *JAMA* 247:2696-2700, 1986.
14. Thompson P, Funk E, Carlton R, Sturner W: Incidence of death during jogging in Rhode Island from 1975 through 1980, *JAMA* 247:2535-2538, 1982.
15. Wen D: Preparticipation cardiovascular screening of young athletes. An epidemiologic perspective, *Physician and Sportsmedicine* 32(6):23-30, 2004.
16. Thiene G, Nava A, Corrado D, et al: Right ventricular cardiomyopathy and sudden death in young people, *New England Journal of Medicine* 318:129-133, 1988.
17. Corrado D, Thiene G, Nava A, et al: Sudden death in young competitive athletes: clinicopathologic correlations in 22 cases, *American Journal of Medicine* 89:588-596, 1990.
18. Hosey R, Armsey T: Sudden cardiac death, *Clinics in Sports Medicine* 22:51-66, 2003.
19. Maron B, Gorham T, Kyle S, et al: Clinical profile and spectrum of commotio cordis, *JAMA* 287:1142-1146, 2002.
20. Link M, Wang P, Pandian N, et al: An experimental model of sudden death due to low-energy chest-wall impact (commotio cordis), *New England Journal of Medicine* 338:1805-1811, 1998.
21. Link M, Maron B, VanderBrink B, et al: Impact directly over the cardiac silhouette is necessary to produce ventricular fibrillation in an experimental model of commotio cordis, *Journal of the American College of Cardiology* 37:649-654, 2001.
22. Cantwell J: Automatic external defibrillators in the sports arena: the right place, the right time, *Physician and Sportsmedicine* 26(12):33-36, 1998.
23. Maron B, Bonow R, Cannon R, et al: Hypertrophic cardiomyopathy: interrelations of clinical manifestations,

pathophysiology, and therapy (first of two parts), *New England Journal of Medicine* 316:780-789, 1987.

24. Maron B, Gardin J, Flack J, et al: Prevalence of hypertrophic cardiomyopathy in a general population of young adults: echocardiographic analysis of 4111 subjects in the CARDIA study, *Circulation* 92:785-789, 1995.

25. McKenna W, Franklin R, Nihoyannopoulos P, et al: Arrhythmia and prognosis in infants, children and adolescents with hypertrophic cardiomyopathy, *Journal of the American College of Cardiology* 11:147-153, 1988.

26. Nihoyannopoulos P, Karatasukis G, Frenneaux M, et al: Diastolic function in hypertrophic cardiomyopathy: relation to exercise capacity, *Journal of the American College of Cardiology* 19:536-540, 1992.

27. Klues H, Leuner C, Kuhn H: Left ventricular outflow tract obstruction in patients with hypertrophic cardiomyopathy: increase in gradient after exercise, *Journal of the American College of Cardiology* 19:527-533, 1992.

28. Pelliccia A, Maron B, Culesso F, et al: Athlete's heart in women: echocardiographic characterization of highly trained elite female athletes, *Journal of the American Medical Association* 17:211-215, 1996.

29. Maron B: Structural feature of the athlete heart as defined by echocardiography, *Journal of the American College of Cardiology* 7:190-203, 1986.

30. Maron B, Pellicca A, Spataro A, Granata M: Reduction in left ventricular wall thickness after deconditioning in highly trained Olympic athletes, *British Heart Journal* 69:125-128, 1993.

31. Feinstein R, Colvin E, MK O: Echocardiographic screening as part of a preparticipation examination, *Clinics in Sports Medicine* 3:149-152, 1993.

32. Maron B, Isner J, McKenna W: Hypertrophic cardiomyopathy, myocarditis, and other myopericardial diseases and mitral valve prolapse, *Medicine and Science in Sports and Exercise* 26:S261-S267, 1994.

33. Mitchell JH, Haskell W, Snell P, Van Camp SP: Task force 8: classification of sports, *Journal of the American College of Cardiology* 45(8):1364-1367, 2005.

34. Morales A, Romanelli R, Boucke R: The mural left anterior descending coronary artery, strenuous exercise and sudden death, *Circulation* 62:230-237, 1980.

35. Betriu A, Tabau J, Sanz G, et al: Relief of angina by periarterial muscle resection of myocardial bridges, *American Heart Journal* 100:223-226, 1980.

36. Graham T, Bricker J, James F, Strong E: Congenital heart disease, *Medicine and Science in Sports and Exercise* 26:S246-S253, 1994.

37. Thompson P, Klocke F, Levine B, Van Camp S: Coronary artery disease, *Medicine and Science in Sports and Exercise* 26:S271-S275, 1994.

38. Yasue H, Omotu A, Takizawa M, et al: Circadian variation of exercise capacity in patients with Prinzmetal's variant angina: role of exercise-induced coronary arterial spasm, *Circulation* 59:938-948, 1979.

39. Pyeritz R, Francke U: Conference report: the second international symposium on the Marfan syndrome, *American Journal of Medical Genetics* 47:127-135, 1993.

40. Pyeritz RL: The Marfan syndrome, *American Family Physician* 34(6):83-94, 1986.

41. Otis C, Child J, Perloff J, Malotte K: Protocol for screening athletes for Marfan syndrome: report of four-years experience, *Medicine and Science in Sports and Exercise* 25:S180, 1993.

42. Pyeritz R, McKusick V: The Marfan syndrome: diagnosis and management, *New England Journal of Medicine* 300:772-777, 1976.

43. Gerry LJ, Morris L, Pyeritz R: Clinical management of the cardiovascular complications of the Marfan's syndrome, *Journal of the Louisiana State Medical Society* 143(3):43-51, 1991.

44. El Habbal M: Cardiovascular manifestations of Marfan's syndrome in the young, *American Heart Journal* 123:752-757, 1992.

45. Marsalese D, Moodie D, Vacante M: Marfan's syndrome: natural history and long-term follow-up cardiovascular involvement, *Journal of the American College of Cardiology* 14:422-428, 1989.

46. Maumenee I: The eye in the Marfan syndrome, *Transactions of the American Ophthalmological Society* 79:684-742, 1981.

47. Pyeritz R: Predictors of dissection of the ascending aorta in Marfan syndrome, *Circulation* 86:11-351, 1991.

48. Nienaber C, von Kodolitsch Y, Brockhoff C, et al: Comparison of conventional and transesophageal echocardiography with magnetic resonance imaging for anatomical mapping of thoracic aortic dissection, *International Journal of Cardiac Imaging* 10(1-14), 1994.

49. Shores J, Berger K, Murphy E, Pyeritz R: Progression of aortic dilatation and the benefit of long-term beta-adrenergic blockage in Marfan's syndrome, *New England Journal of Medicine* 330:1335-1341, 1994.

50. Cullen S, Celermajer D, Deanfield J: Exercise in congenital heart disease, *Cardiology of the Young* 1:129-135, 1991.

51. Washington R: Mitral valve prolapse in active youth, *Physician and Sportsmedicine* 21(1):136-144, 1993.

52. McFaul R: Mitral valve prolapse in young patients, *Physician and Sportsmedicine* 15(6):194-198, 1987.

53. Zehender M, Meinertz T, Keul J: ECG variants and cardiac arrhythmias in athletes: clinical relevance and prognostic importance, *American Heart Journal* 119(6):1378-1391, 1990.

54. Wiederman C, Becker A, Hopferwieser T: Sudden death in a young competitive athlete with Wolff-Parkinson-White syndrome, *European Heart Journal* 8(651-655), 1987.

55. Moss A, Robinson J: Clinical features of the idiopathic long QT syndrome, *Circulation* 85:1140-1144, 1992.

56. Singh B, Shahwan S, Habbab M, et al: Idiopathic long QT syndrome: asking the right question, *Lancet* 341:741-742, 1993.

57. Schwart P, Zaza A, Localti E, Moss A: Stress and sudden death: the case of the long QT syndrome, *Circulation* 83:1171-1180, 1991.

58. Palatini P, Maraglino G, Sperti G: Prevalence and possible mechanisms of ventricular arrhythmias in athletes, *American Heart Journal* 110:561-567, 1985.

59. Kapoor W: Evaluating unexplained syncope with upright tilt testing, *Cleveland Clinic Journal of Medicine* 62:305-310, 1995.

60. Cantwell J, Varughese A, Pettus C: Cardiovascular syncope, *Physician and Sportsmedicine* 20(1):81-92, 1992.

61. Hargarten K: Syncope: finding the cause in active people, *Physician and Sportsmedicine* 20(5):123-141, 1992.

62. Strieper M, Auld D, Hulse J, Campbell R: Evaluation of recurrent pediatric syncope: role of tilt table testing, *Pediatrician* 93:660-662, 1994.

63. Fouad-Tarazi F: Using the tilt test to diagnose the cause of syncope, *Cleveland Clinic Journal of Medicine* 62:339-341, 1995.

64. MacKnight J: Exercise considerations in hypertension, obesity, and dyslipidemia, *Clinics in Sports Medicine* 22:101-121, 2003.
65. Kaplan N, Deveraux R, Miller HJ: Systemic hypertension, *Medicine and Science in Sports and Exercise* 26:S268-S270, 1994.
66. Tanaka D: Deep venous thrombosis. In Rakel R, editor: *Saunders' manual of medical practice,* Philadelphia, 1996, WB Saunders, pp 283-285.
67. Dunn A, Coller B: Outpatient treatment of deep venous thrombosis: translating clinical trials into practice, *American Journal of Medicine* 106:660-669, 1999.
68. Goerdt C: Peripheral arterial disease. In Rakel R, editor: *Saunders' manual of medical practice,* Philadelphia, 1996, WB Saunders, pp 286-287.
69. Eichner E: Hematology. In McKeag D, Van Camp S, editors: *Manual of sports medicine,* Philadelphia, 1998, Lippincott-Raven, 1998, pp 255-259.

CHAPTER
6

Gastrointestinal Disorders

Daniel J. Van Durme

OBJECTIVES

At the completion of this chapter, the reader should be able to do the following:

1. Describe the basic anatomy of the abdomen and gastrointestinal system.
2. Perform a basic examination of the gastrointestinal system, including history, inspection, auscultation, percussion, and palpation.
3. Recognize conditions of the gastrointestinal system that require referral.
4. Describe appropriate initial management of common disorders of the gastrointestinal tract.
5. Recognize conditions of the gastrointestinal system that may preclude the athlete from participation and which symptoms are self-limiting.

INTRODUCTION

Athletic trainers hear complaints about abdominal pain or discomfort every day. Nausea, diarrhea, and constipation account for some of these complaints; heartburn and gastroesophageal reflux account for others. The stress of hectic schedules and travel involved in athletic competition and the consumption of greasy or spicy foods are certainly among the causes. Often gastrointestinal disorders are transient, and although they may affect performance or the ability to compete, they are not serious conditions. Fortunately, because of working closely with the athletes, the athletic trainer can identify more serious gastrointestinal conditions that require further medical evaluation and treatment.

This chapter reviews the anatomy and physiology of the gastrointestinal system and procedures to evaluate

the abdominal area, including auscultation, palpation, and percussion. This chapter also presents common disorders of the gastrointestinal system, including the signs and symptoms, diagnostic tests, and differential diagnoses. In addition, treatment of selected conditions and implications for athletic participation are discussed.

OVERVIEW OF ANATOMY AND PHYSIOLOGY

The gastrointestinal system is primarily composed of a long tube between the mouth and the anus that serves to process food and fluids (Figure 6-1). From ingestion of solids and liquids through the absorption and balancing of electrolytes and finally waste production and excretion, the alimentary tract performs several vital functions. For athletes, it is unlikely that sports will cause significant gastrointestinal problems, but rather that gastrointestinal problems are common and can affect athletic performance.

The major organs of the gastrointestinal tract start with the esophagus that connects the mouth to the stomach via a muscular band called the gastroesophageal junction or lower esophageal sphincter. The mouth and teeth, although part of the gastrointestinal tract, are discussed in Chapter 10. Within the pouch of the stomach hydrochloric acid and enzymes such as pepsin and gastric lipase serve to break down food for later absorption in the intestines. The stomach empties through another muscular ring, the pyloric sphincter, into the duodenum, the first portion of the small intestine.

The small intestine is about 21 feet long; comprises the duodenum, jejunum, and ileum; and serves as the organ

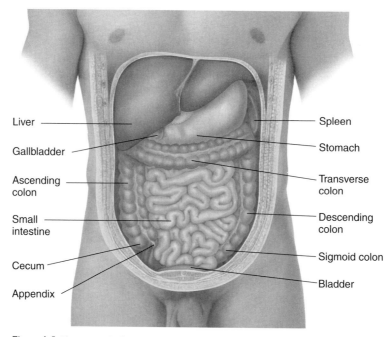

Figure 6-1 The anatomical structures of the abdominal cavity. (From Seidel HM, Ball JW, Dains JE, Benedict GW: *Mosby's guide to physical examination*, ed 5, St Louis, 2003, Mosby, p 526.)

responsible for completing the digestive breakdown with enzymes produced by the pancreas and liver. Nutrients are absorbed throughout the length of the small intestine as it coils back and forth and joins the large intestine in the lower right portion of the abdomen. This connection also has the ileocecal valve, which is designed to prevent fecal material in the large intestine from backing up into the small intestine. There is a small blind pouch called the cecum at this end of the large intestine, and the small wormlike (vermiform) appendix originates from the base of the pouch. The large intestine or colon serves to absorb water and produce neutralizing mucus as it ascends up the right side of the abdomen (i.e., ascending colon), traverses across the upper abdomen (i.e., transverse colon), and then descends down the left side (i.e., descending colon). The colon also hosts extensive bacteria that further decompose food residue. As the colon comes to an end in the lower right side of the abdomen it goes through an S-shaped curve called the sigmoid colon. This in turn empties into the rectum, and together they serve as the primary storage location for solid or semisolid waste. Finally, the rectum ends with the sophisticated musculature of the anal canal and then the anus.

Among the many important organs in the abdomen, the gastrointestinal tract includes the liver, gallbladder, pancreas, and spleen (Figure 6-2, *A*) as well as the kidneys and related structures (Figure 6-2, *B*). Each of these essential organs helps digestive and absorptive functions of the gastrointestinal system.

The liver is a large organ located under the right diaphragm that has several crucial functions in metabolism, storage of vitamins and iron, filtering toxins from the blood, and producing critical blood proteins. Bile is produced in the liver and stored in the saclike gallbladder, where it is periodically released into the duodenum to help in the absorption of fats. The pancreas sits below the stomach and assists digestion by producing several enzymes that are also released into the duodenum. In addition, the pancreas produces the essential hormones of insulin and glucagon that are released into the blood stream for maintaining blood sugar (i.e., glucose) levels.

Most abdominal organs and the inner lining of the abdominal cavity are covered with a protective membrane called the peritoneum. When this gets inflamed or irritated by blood or infection, the entire abdomen can become very tender and the muscles of the abdominal wall may become rigid. Individual sensory nerves do not innervate each organ within the peritoneum, which is why abdominal pain is not necessarily specific to the origin (location) of pathology.

The rectus abdominis and the internal and external oblique muscles serve to protect the organs of the abdominal cavity (Figure 6-3). Just like muscles elsewhere in the body, they can be injured by overuse, acute strain, or contusions. For an athlete with abdominal pain, distinguishing whether the pain is from the internal organs or the overlying muscles is important. Sometimes this distinction can be difficult, or there may be problems with both.

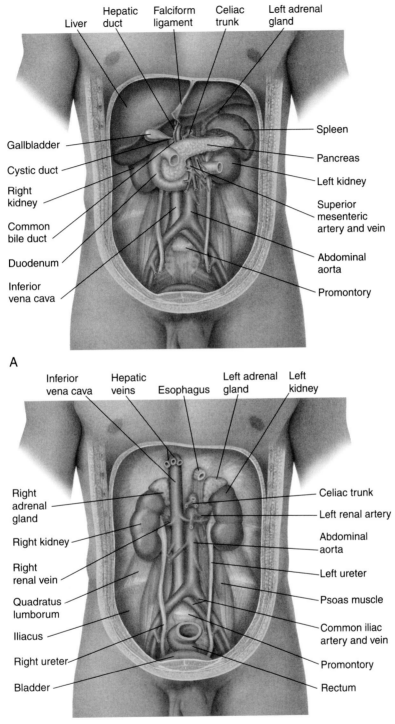

Figure 6-2 Structures of the abdominal cavity. **A,** The anatomical relationship of the pancreas, spleen, gallbladder, and related structures. **B,** The anatomical relationship of the kidneys and related structures. (From Seidel HM, Ball JW, Dains JE, Benedict GW: *Mosby's guide to physical examination,* ed 5, St Louis, 2003, Mosby, p 527.)

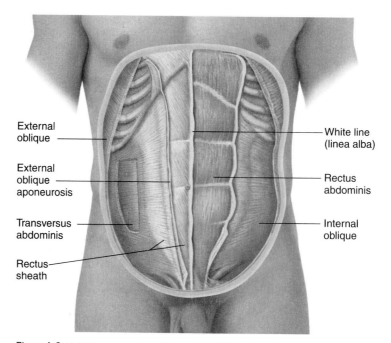

Figure 6-3 Abdominal musculature. (From Seidel HM, Ball JW, Dains JE, Benedict GW: *Mosby's guide to physical examination*, ed 5, St Louis, 2003, Mosby, p 526.)

When referring to the abdomen, clinicians will typically divide it into quadrants. The midline extends from the center of the sternum through the pubic bone, and the horizontal line extends through the umbilicus (Figure 6-4). This creates right and left upper and lower quadrants, commonly referred to as RUQ, LUQ, RLQ, and LLQ. This distinction becomes important and helpful in diagnosing many conditions.[1] **Appendicitis,** for example, will typically cause RLQ pain, whereas constipation can cause LLQ pain (Box 6-1).

PATHOLOGICAL CONDITIONS

General Evaluation of Abdominal Pain

The athlete with abdominal pain may not have a problem with the gastrointestinal tract at all. Many possible conditions, including diseases of the heart, lungs, kidneys, and musculoskeletal system, can present as "abdominal pain" (Box 6-2). For female athletes, it is important to obtain an appropriate menstrual cycle history. Pain that is perceived as being abdominal may be from the reproductive system, such as ovarian cysts, menstrual cramps, pelvic infections, or complications of pregnancy. Box 6-3 gives several key questions to ask in the evaluation of abdominal conditions.

As with other conditions, the examiner must determine whether there was any trauma involved and the details of that injury. A past medical history or family history of gastrointestinal problems can also help in

the diagnosis, as can social history factors, such as alcohol intake.[2] Signs or symptoms that may indicate a severe or life-threatening condition constitute red flags with abdominal pain (Red Flags—Abdominal Pain).

> **⚑ Red Flags for Abdominal Pain**
> - Vomiting bright red blood or black material that looks like coffee grounds
> - Fever of 38.3° C (101° F) or more, accompanied by severe abdominal pain
> - Persistent vomiting, such that the person is unable to keep any fluids down for more than 24 to 36 hours (in younger athletes the time window is shorter)

Beyond the obvious issues such as unstable vital signs or altered mental status that are always red flags, these findings are serious enough that a physician should be contacted immediately, or the patient should go to an emergency department.

Physical examination of the abdomen involves the skills of inspection, auscultation, palpation, and percussion. Inspection consists of carefully examining the abdomen when the athlete is lying comfortably supine. Initially, the examiner notes the presence of scars that may indicate prior surgery and thus could decrease the concern about acute appendicitis or gallstones and looks for obvious bruising or contusions as well as swelling or distention. A yellowish tint can indicate jaundice from liver disease, or a faint bluish discoloration around the umbilicus may indicate intraabdominal bleeding. The examiner watches the movement of the abdomen as the patient breathes in

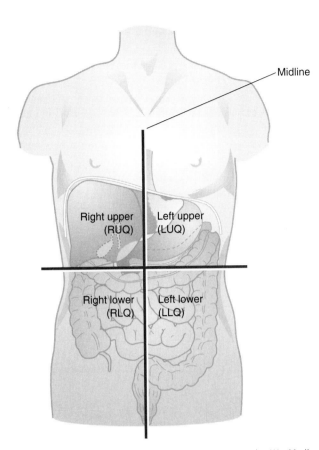

Figure 6-4 Abdominal quadrants. (From Black JM, Hawks JH: *Medical-surgical nursing: clinical management for positive outcomes,* ed 7, St Louis, 2005, WB Saunders, p 681.)

Box 6-2	Differential Diagnosis for Gastrointestinal Disorders

- Muscle contusions
- Gastroenteritis
- Appendicitis
- Peptic ulcer disease
- Cholecystitis
- Splenic rupture
- Diverticulitis
- Pelvic inflammatory disease
- Pancreatitis
- Other conditions: myocardial infarction, pneumonia, pericarditis, pneumothorax, kidney disease, reproductive system problems

Box 6-3	Key Questions to Evaluate Abdominal Pain

- **Onset of pain:** sudden or gradual?
- **Duration of pain:** present for hours? days? weeks?
- **Temporal factors:** constant pain or intermittent?
- **Relationship to meals:** better with food or worse?
- **Quality of pain:** burning, cramping, stabbing?
- **Radiation of pain:** does it seem to spread up or down?
- **Severity of pain:** may use pain scale.
- **Aggravating or alleviating factors:** better lying down or sitting up? Have over-the-counter medicines, such as antacids or others, been tried?
- **Associated symptoms:** nausea, vomiting, diarrhea, constipation, fever?
- **Last bowel movement?**
- **Medications or supplements that may cause symptoms?**

Box 6-1	Common Causes of Abdominal Pain in Different Anatomical Locations

Right Upper Quadrant (RUQ)
Cholecystitis
Duodenal ulcer
Hepatitis
Pneumonia

Left Upper Quadrant (LUQ)
Abdominal aortic aneurysm
Gastric ulcer
Pneumonia
Splenic laceration or rupture

Periumbilical
Abdominal aortic aneurysm
Diverticulitis
Early appendicitis
Intestinal obstruction

Right Lower Quadrant (RLQ)
Appendicitis
Ectopic pregnancy
Hernia
Ovarian cysts
Pelvic infection
Renal stone

Left Lower Quadrant (LLQ)
Constipation
Diverticulitis
Ectopic pregnancy
Hernia
Ovarian cysts
Pelvic infection

Modified from Seidel HM, Ball JW, Dains JE, Benedict GW: *Mosby's guide to physical examination,* ed 5, St Louis, 2003, Mosby, p 558.

and out for asymmetry that can indicate intraabdominal masses or hernia.

In distinguishing abdominal muscle pain from problems of the abdominal organs, it is helpful to have the athlete tense the muscles by doing a partial sit-up. As the athlete's head is raised from the table, the muscles are held taut and muscle pain is aggravated, indicating a problem that is muscular in origin.

Auscultation is always performed before palpation in the examination of the abdomen. In the examination of the heart and lungs, palpation is done before auscultation; however, palpation of the abdomen may create abdominal sounds that were not there before palpation. Auscultation should reveal the normal clicks and gurgling of bowel sounds that may be heard anywhere from a few times to dozens of times every minute. Chapter 2 covers use of the stethoscope and basic auscultation techniques. The athletic trainer needs to be alert to abnormal sounds, such as high-pitched tinkling sounds or rushing water sounds, as well as the potentially absent sounds that can indicate intraabdominal pathology (Figure 6-5). Some athletes may have quieter abdomens; bowel sounds are not considered absent until the examiner has listened continuously for 5 minutes with no sound heard.

Percussion is a skill that requires considerable practice and is not covered in detail in this book. It may be used to assess the size and density of abdominal organs or to detect the presence of air or fluid in the abdominal cavity. Generally the examination follows a standard sequence for abdominal percussion (Figure 6-6) or percussion to determine size of the liver (Figure 6-7). As indicated in Chapter 2 percussion may be direct or indirect.

The athletic trainer should practice percussing normal tympanic and dull sounds of the four quadrants exhibited by various positions of percussion. Tympany is the predominant sound throughout the abdomen and hollow organs because of the air contained in the stomach and intestines (Table 6-1). A dull sound is present over hollow organs and solid masses.

Examiners use indirect percussion to tell when they are directly over solid organs or hollow organs of the abdomen. A change in sound from tympanic to dull is easier to detect so examiners usually start over an area known to be normally tympanic. Percussion is most

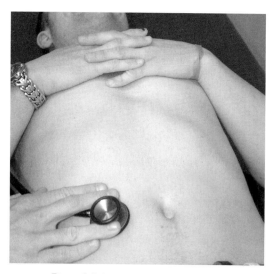

Figure 6-5 Auscultation of the abdomen.

Table 6-1	Percussion Sounds in the Abdomen	
Sound	**Description**	**Location**
Tympany	Musical note of higher pitch than resonance	Over air-filled viscera
Hyperresonance	Pitch lies between tympany and resonance	Base of left lung
Resonance	Sustained note of moderate pitch	Over lung tissue and sometimes over the abdomen
Dullness	Short, high-pitched note with little resonance	Over solid organs adjacent to air-filled structures

From Seidel HM, Ball JW, Dains JE, Benedict GW: *Mosby's guide to physical examination*, ed 5, St Louis, 2003, Mosby, p 542.

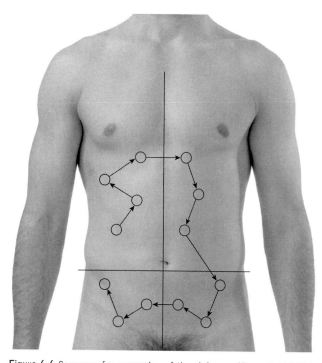

Figure 6-6 Sequence for percussion of the abdomen. (From Seidel HM, Ball JW, Dains JE, Benedict GW: *Mosby's guide to physical examination*, ed 5, St Louis, 2003, Mosby, p 543.)

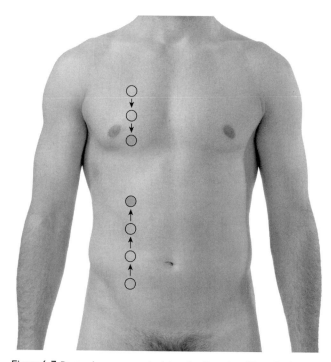

Figure 6-7 Percussion sequence to determine liver size. (From Seidel HM, Ball JW, Dains JE, Benedict GW: *Mosby's guide to physical examination*, ed 5, St Louis, 2003, Mosby, p 543.)

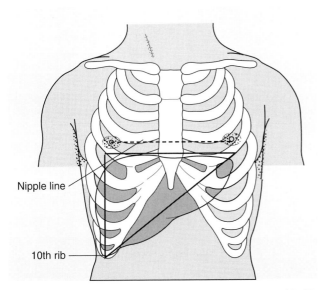

Figure 6-8 The surface anatomy of the liver. (From Epstein O, Perkin GD, Cookson J, de Bono DP: *Clinical examination*, ed 3, St Louis, 2003, Mosby, p 195.)

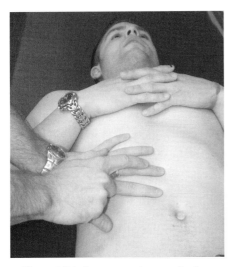

Figure 6-9 Indirect percussion over the liver.

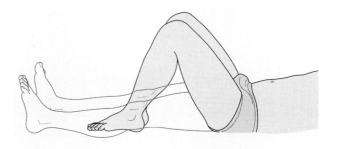

Figure 6-10 Patient position for palpation of the abdomen: flexing the hips and the knees may aid in palpation of the abdomen. (From Epstein O, Perkin GD, Cookson J, de Bono DP: *Clinical examination*, ed 3, St Louis, 2003, Mosby, p 193.)

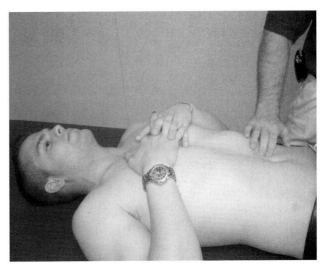

Figure 6-11 Light palpation of the abdomen: the athletic trainer uses light and superficial palpation to assess for muscular tenderness, rigidity, or superficial masses. Pain or resistance to this light palpation generally indicates either injury or inflammation of the abdominal musculature or peritoneal lining.

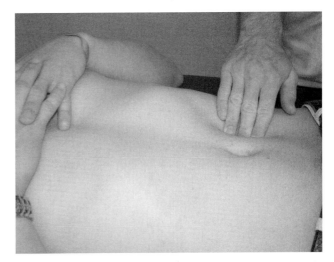

Figure 6-12 Deep palpation of the abdomen: if the athlete tolerates light palpation of the abdomen, the athletic trainer can press firmly and deeply to athlete's tolerance (3 cm to 4 cm) and try to feel the edges of the abdominal organs.

commonly performed to tell the size of the liver and spleen. It is important to understand the surface anatomy of the liver (Figure 6-8) in order to assess the liver through indirect percussion (Figure 6-9).

The athlete lies supine during palpation. If the athlete has difficulty relaxing the abdominal muscles to allow the examiner to adequately palpate deeply, the knees may be bent slightly to encourage relaxation of the abdominal muscles (Figure 6-10). Palpation attempts to assess masses or areas of tenderness at both the superficial and deep levels.[1]

Initially the abdomen is palpated lightly (pressing only about 1 cm deep) in all quadrants to assess for muscular tenderness or rigidity as well as any superficial masses (Figure 6-11). The palmar aspect of the

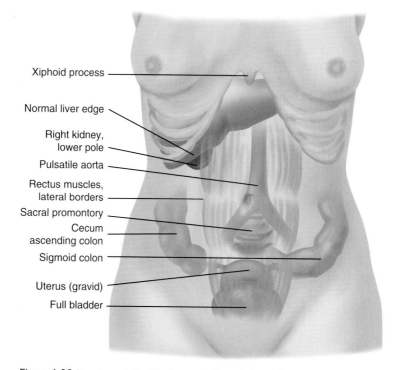

Xiphoid process

Normal liver edge

Right kidney,
lower pole

Pulsatile aorta

Rectus muscles,
lateral borders

Sacral promontory

Cecum
ascending colon

Sigmoid colon

Uterus (gravid)

Full bladder

Figure 6-13 Structures felt with deep palpation of the abdomen. (From Jarvis C: *Physical examination & health assessment*, ed 4, Philadelphia, 2004, WB Saunders, p 581.)

fingers is used in a steady, even fashion, avoiding any sharp or sudden jabbing motions. The pain or resistance to even this light palpation generally indicates either injury or inflammation of the abdominal musculature or peritoneal lining.

If significant tenderness is not present with light palpation, the examiner presses more firmly and deeply and continues to press as deeply as the patient will comfortably allow, generally to a depth of at least 3 or 4 cm (Figure 6-12). In this manner, the examiner may be able to feel the edges of the liver in the RUQ or an enlarged spleen in the LUQ (Figure 6-13). Tenderness in the RLQ with deep palpation may indicate appendicitis or pelvic or ovarian problems in a female athlete.

To more adequately palpate the liver, the athletic trainer stands on the right side of the patient with the left hand placed under the patient. The left hand presses up at the eleventh or twelfth rib, causing the liver to be lifted toward the anterior abdominal wall. The right hand simultaneously palpates the liver (Figure 6-14). The edge of the liver should be smooth and firm. Palpation of the liver does not normally cause pain, so the athletic trainer should be suspicious if direct palpation of the liver is painful for the athlete.

The athletic trainer pays special attention to the spleen while palpating the LUQ. The same basic technique may be used as when palpating the liver, namely,

to reach across the patient with the right hand, placing it beneath the costovertebral angle (Figure 6-15). The fingers of the left hand are placed just below the patient's left costal margin. The patient takes a deep breath while the athletic trainer moves the fingers of the left hand toward the spleen. The breath may move an enlarged spleen up to meet the fingers of the left hand; however, a normal-sized spleen is typically not palpable. Pain with palpation of the spleen is an indication for the athletic trainer to refer the athlete to a physician.

Evaluation of the Athlete with Acute, Traumatic Abdominal Pain

As with any traumatic injury, an assessment of the specific mechanism of injury is important. A sharp blow with the end of a hockey stick is obviously more likely to cause damage than a blow with an elbow. Fortunately, the abdominal organs are generally well protected and most trauma results only in contusions to the muscles. After confirming that there is no damage to the underlying organs, these injuries can be treated just like any other muscle contusion.

The spleen is the most commonly injured solid abdominal organ.[3] The spleen that is not enlarged is generally well protected by the lower ribs on the left.

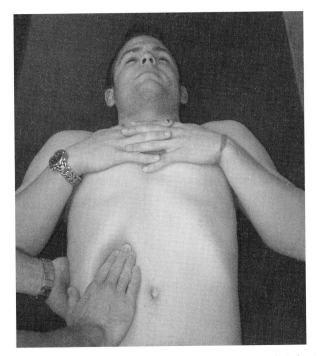

Figure 6-14 Palpation of the liver: the left hand presses upward at about the eleventh or twelfth rib. The athletic trainer asks the athlete to breathe regularly and then tries to feel the edge of the liver with the right hand as the athlete breathes. Often the liver is not palpable except in a very thin person or if it is enlarged.

When trauma results in rib fracture, however, the ribs can lacerate the spleen. The spleen can become enlarged (i.e., **splenomegaly**) from various causes; most commonly the enlargement resulting from infectious mononucleosis is temporary and lasts a few weeks. This enlargement will cause the spleen to extend downward beyond the protection of the ribs and make it vulnerable to direct trauma that can cause splenic contusion or laceration. (See Chapter 12 for more information on mononucleosis.)

Less commonly, the liver can also be lacerated or contused by direct trauma. The pancreas is deep enough in the abdomen that contusion is rare, but it should be suspected if there is persistent abdominal pain with radiation through to the back. Injury to the hollow organs (i.e., stomach, intestines) is rare and generally occurs only when there is enough force to cause crushing damage against the spine.

When an athlete sustains an injury to the abdomen, the athletic trainer initially assesses the overall status and vital signs. Unfortunately, sideline evaluations can be normal or reveal only vague, nonspecific findings even in athletes with significant injuries. If there is diffuse abdominal tenderness or rigidity, pain in the back without trauma to the back, low blood pressure, or rapid heart rate or if the mechanism of injury suggests injury to the liver or spleen, then the athlete must be seen by a physician before resuming play (Key Points—Abdominal Exam).

KEY POINTS
Abdominal Exam

History
    Pain: onset, duration, quality, severity, radiation
    Associated symptoms: nausea, vomiting, diarrhea,
        constipation, fever, fatigue, painful urination
    Aggravating or alleviating factors
    Medications
    Appetite and food intolerance
    Bowel habits
Observation
    Shape and symmetry
    Assessment of skin and scars
Auscultation: Do before palpation in the abdomen!
    Bowel sounds
    Vascular sounds
Percussion
    The four quadrants
    Liver span and spleen
Palpation
    Light palpation to assess tenderness in all four quadrants
    Deeper palpation for masses in all four quadrants
    Palpation of spleen, liver, kidneys, and McBurney's point

---

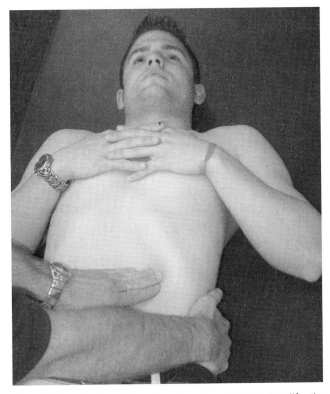

Figure 6-15 Palpation of the spleen: when the athletic trainer lifts the athlete upward with the right hand, the spleen will lift up toward the left fingers as they palpate the abdominal surface. The athletic trainer can feel the spleen just below the left costal margin.

Nausea, Vomiting, and Diarrhea

Nausea, vomiting, and diarrhea can be the result of any one of numerous conditions, including self-limited viral illness, food poisoning, side effects of medications, dietary indiscretions, or stress. They may also be signs of more serious conditions, such as appendicitis, pancreatitis, or **pelvic inflammatory disease.** In most cases, however, nausea, vomiting, and diarrhea are self-limiting conditions that can be managed with over-the-counter medicines and common sense.

An important consideration is the severity and duration of symptoms of nausea, vomiting, or diarrhea in terms of the athlete's hydration status. With mild or intermittent symptoms, most people will still take in enough oral fluids that they can go for several days without significant concerns about dehydration. However, when symptoms are more severe, then intravenous fluids may be needed to treat dehydration that develops over 36 hours or longer. When these symptoms have been present for more than 36 hours or are accompanied by significant pain or fever, referral is made to a physician.

The character of the vomited material must be determined. Undigested food or minimal amounts of yellow to green stomach acid or bile are common and not worrisome. If the athlete has been persistently vomiting bilious material; blood; dark, coffee-ground material; or foul-smelling, stool-like material, then urgent referral is needed.

Similarly, for the athlete with diarrhea, it is important to get a description of the character of the stool. Loose or watery brown stools are most common and reflect a more benign process. If the diarrhea is bloody, is maroon in color, or seems to be more like mucus than water, then referral is needed.

Treatment

The athlete who feels nauseated or queasy but has not been vomiting and has little or no pain or fever safely and effectively can take over-the-counter **antiemetic agents** containing a high-concentration carbohydrate and phosphoric acid solution, such as Emetrol, Nausetrol, or Naus-A-Way. When used as directed on the label, these agents can safely treat the symptoms and will not mask a more serious condition. If they fail, numerous prescription medicines can be used, including promethazine (Phenergan) and prochlorperazine (Compazine).

Once the athlete has started to vomit, the stomach must be given enough time to settle down between vomiting spells. A common scenario is the person who vomits, then feels better, and decides to drink some water or other fluids in order to both quench thirst and avoid dehydration. If this happens too soon after the last vomiting spell, the hypersensitive stomach will start the vomiting again. This behavior of drinking too quickly is very common in the person who "just can't

stop vomiting." After any spell of vomiting, the person should not drink anything at all, not even a sip of water, for about 1 hour (sometimes 2 hours). Once the stomach has remained quiet for that time, then one of the over-the-counter or prescription antinausea (or antiemetic) medicines listed previously can be used. The athlete who is able to tolerate these medicines can slowly advance to sips of water or electrolyte solutions (e.g., Gatorade, Powerade, Pedialyte). Finally, the athlete can add more carbohydrates to the diet in the form of grains and fruits as tolerated. The BRAT (i.e., bananas, rice, applesauce, toast) diet has long been used in children with nausea, vomiting, and diarrhea. These foods are tolerated well by both children and adults and may be helpful in quieting the gastrointestinal tract while recovering from nausea, vomiting, and diarrhea. Acidic, spicy, or greasy foods should be avoided for 1 or 2 days to be certain the athlete can tolerate these items and that they do not trigger a recurrence of vomiting.

For the treatment of diarrhea, loperamide (Imodium) obtained over the counter can be very effective in the control of diarrheic episodes but may have side effects of drowsiness and dizziness that may impair performance. Loperamide can decrease stool frequency and volume to allow the athlete to continue a somewhat normal routine. Use of antidiarrheals when invasive pathogens are suspected is controversial because they can delay clearance of pathogens from the bowel, thereby prolonging the disease. However, in the afebrile athlete with a nonbloody stool they can be a very effective and safe method of treatment.[4] The athlete needs to hydrate as discussed previously with electrolyte solution and water and adhere to a bland diet until symptoms subside.

Prognosis and Return to Participation

The decision of when to return to participation depends on the sport in question and the severity and duration of symptoms. It is unlikely that mild illnesses that cause nausea, vomiting, or diarrhea in the absence of fever will be significantly aggravated by athletic activity; rather, the performance may be significantly impaired by the illness. A mild case of nausea, vomiting, or diarrhea may have little impact on most sports. For sports in which stamina plays a larger role, such as cross-country running, the athlete may see a significant impairment of performance with mild to moderate symptoms that may have little to no effect on the athlete for whom performance time is relatively short, such as in weightlifting or gymnastics. A good rule of thumb for most athletes with afebrile illnesses is to avoid activities when there are symptoms below the neck (e.g., chest congestion, vomiting, diarrhea) and play as tolerated when symptoms remain above the neck (e.g., headache, sore throat, earache).

Viral Gastroenteritis

Viral **gastroenteritis,** or acute gastroenteritis, is a very common condition caused by any one of several viruses including adenovirus, astrovirus, echovirus, and Norwalk agent.[5] These viruses cause a self-limited inflammation of the stomach and intestines and usually are completely resolved within 2 to 3 days. The infections are contagious and can spread through a family or college dormitory or by food handlers.[5]

Signs, Symptoms, Treatment, and Referral

Signs and symptoms of viral gastroenteritis include watery diarrhea, nausea with or without vomiting, and fever. The affected athlete may also have diffuse aches, pains, and chills. Management includes general supportive measures and attention to hydration as noted previously. Over-the-counter loperamide (Imodium) is very effective for diarrhea but may have side effects of drowsiness and dizziness that can significantly affect performance. Referral is considered if there is no response to over-the-counter medicines, if symptoms persist for more than 48 hours, or if the athlete has an accompanying high fever.

Prognosis and Return to Participation

The athlete can return to participation whenever symptoms are resolved and hydration is adequate. With usual good hygiene, the risk of spread to fellow athletes is extremely low.

Food Poisoning or Bacterial Diarrhea

The term food poisoning is often overused. People who experience the sudden onset of gastrointestinal symptoms often will attribute it to something they ate or drank. Although bacterial contamination of foods can occur, the diagnosis of food poisoning generally only is suspected when multiple people who ate the same food get ill at about the same time. Sampling and culturing the person's stool can confirm the diagnosis. Food poisoning typically occurs when food is improperly handled, cooked, stored, or refrigerated. In some cases the problem is the bacterium itself, and in other cases it may be from the toxin or toxins produced by the bacterium. The most common causes are *Campylobacter, Salmonella,* and *Staphylococcus* species, but several other bacteria can also cause problems, including *Shigella* species, *Bacillus cereus, Yersinia,* and *Escherichia coli.*[6]

Signs and Symptoms

Bacterial diarrhea is typically more severe and lasts longer than viral gastroenteritis. It may cause higher fevers or severe abdominal cramps and is more likely to result in weight loss and dehydration. Depending on the bacterium, the onset may occur 4 to 6 hours after eating the contaminated food (e.g., *Staphylococcus*) or 3 to 10 days later (e.g., *Salmonella*). This variable duration obviously makes it difficult to pinpoint a specific food.

Treatment, Prognosis, and Return to Participation

Initial management of the diarrhea can include over-the-counter medicines as for viral gastroenteritis. If the athlete is significantly ill or there is blood in the stool, then referral is needed for thorough evaluation and treatment. This may include stool specimens and antibiotics. If several athletes become ill at the same time, then it may be important to trace back to a shared meal as the source. If the problem was simply poor refrigeration of a single food, then the problem may resolve on its own. However, the problem may be an infected food worker who may continue to spread the infection until treated. The athlete may return to participation when symptoms have been completely resolved and strength and hydration are back to normal.

Parasitic Infection

Parasitic infections of the gastrointestinal tract are less common than bacterial or viral infections but may still cause significant problems. The most common parasites are single-celled organisms called protozoa. *Giardia* is a common water-borne protozoan that is found worldwide, especially in people who drink from more remote streams when hiking or camping. *Entamoeba* species are parasitic protozoa that are also found worldwide but are much more common in tropical regions.[7] In addition, tapeworms, roundworms, and flukes can be parasitic in humans. These infestations are uncommon, and discussion is beyond the scope of this text.

Giardia-induced diarrhea is characterized by the significant gas that typically results. The diarrhea may be acute or chronic and intermittent. It is often explosive diarrhea, with patients complaining of dull abdominal cramping and bloating with gas and flatulence. *Entamoeba* may cause a variety of symptoms from chronic intermittent diarrhea, abdominal pain, and weight loss to profound bloody diarrhea and fever.[8]

Prognosis and Return to Participation

Parasitic infections must be recognized by the athletic trainer as different from self-limited viral and bacterial diarrhea and promptly referred for the appropriate antibiotic treatments. The treating physician is the one to make decisions about return to participation.

Stress-Induced Gastrointestinal Symptoms

It is well known that stress can cause a wide variety of gastrointestinal symptoms from diffuse abdominal pains and cramps to heartburn, nausea, vomiting, diarrhea, constipation, and anorexia.[9] The diagnosis of stress-induced or functional gastrointestinal problems is a diagnosis of exclusion. The athlete is thoroughly evaluated for other causes of the symptoms, and only when these have been excluded can the problem be considered stress induced. Even highly stressed athletes can get other easily treatable conditions so the athletic trainer must not be too quick to attribute symptoms to stress.

Treatment

If the athlete has been thoroughly evaluated and other causes have been ruled out, the athletic trainer can play an important role in the management of stress-induced gastrointestinal symptoms. Primarily, it is important to understand and to remind the athlete that the symptoms are not imaginary. Recent medical research has increasingly helped in understanding the vital connection between the mind and the body: biochemicals of the brain can get out of balance causing major depression or symptoms of anxiety. These conditions in turn can affect the rest of the body and impair healing or worsen other chronic illnesses. Stress does cause very real symptoms of stomach pain, nausea, or even vomiting or diarrhea.

Prognosis and Return to Participation

The athletic trainer can assist in management through close communication with the team physician and allowing the athlete to have time off as needed or to play through the symptoms as needed in each specific case.

Constipation

Constipation is commonly misunderstood as a simple decrease in the frequency of bowel movements, with many people feeling that they must have a bowel movement every day or there is something wrong. A better definition is a subjective discomfort from a difficulty in passing stool or a change in the consistency such that stools are excessively hard or small. People have a wide range of tolerance, but constipation can cause significant abdominal pain, cramps, and general discomfort.[10]

An initial evaluation to determine the cause of the constipation is helpful. Hundreds of medications, such as narcotic or nonsteroidal antiinflammatory pain relievers and antidepressant medicines, can cause temporary or persistent constipation.

Treatment

Treatment is best directed at increasing fluid and fiber intake. Fiber intake may be dietary by means of whole grains and vegetables or over-the-counter fiber supplements, such as Metamucil or Citrucel. These fiber supplements can be taken indefinitely as needed. The stronger over-the-counter agents, such as milk of magnesia or magnesium citrate, are effective but may be too strong for some people and lead to temporary diarrhea. These medications are for short-term use because long-term use can lead to a form of dependence.

Referral

Referral to a physician is indicated if the athlete fails to respond to over-the-counter agents or if the problem persists over a period of weeks and the athlete is unable to participate without restriction.

Acid-Related Disorders

Heartburn and Gastroesophageal Reflux Disease

The terms *heartburn* and *esophageal reflux*, or **gastroesophageal reflux disease** (GERD), are generally interchangeable and refer to a very common condition in which stomach acid travels up through the lower esophageal sphincter into the esophagus or even into the back of the throat. The numerous causes include family history, obesity, tight-fitting clothing, and certain medications. Behavioral factors include overeating in general and especially exercising or lying down with a full stomach. Certain foods are also well-known triggers for some people, including high-fat foods, citric acid–based or tomato-based foods, mints, alcohol, carbonated beverages, and caffeine-containing foods, including chocolate.

Signs and Symptoms

In addition to the heartburn sensation, signs and symptoms of GERD include chest pain (potentially severe), belching, regurgitation of food and acid, chronic cough, and laryngitis. It is essential to remember that not all people will feel a heartburn sensation with this condition. Some people experience only a chronic cough or frequent asthmatic attacks from acid that goes up the esophagus and then into the airways.

In some cases, after persisting for years, heartburn and GERD can cause significant damage to the esophagus, including an increased risk for esophageal cancer. These complications are rare in people under the age of 40 years. Nonetheless, any athlete who does not respond to over-the-counter medicines or who needs these medicines on a daily basis for weeks should be referred for further evaluation.

Treatment

Management of GERD is initially directed toward appropriate lifestyle management. The athlete may need to do some self-assessment to determine how much of which foods and behaviors will cause symptoms and adjust accordingly. Although over-the-counter medicines can be very effective, it is rather foolish to take a pill when simple avoidance of the offending agent will handle the problem. The over-the-counter medications work by decreasing the acidity of the stomach and thus diminishing the symptoms and not by stopping the reflux itself. Several effective agents include antacids (e.g., Maalox, Mylanta, Rolaids, Tums) and H_2 blockers (e.g., cimetidine [Tagamet HB], famotidine [Pepcid AC], ranitidine [Zantac]). The most effective and most expensive over-the-counter agent is the proton-pump inhibitor omeprazole (Prilosec). Taken before known triggering behaviors or foods these agents can prevent symptoms, or they can be taken as needed after symptoms start.[2,11]

Prognosis and Return to Participation

Heartburn and GERD are rarely severe enough to interfere with athletic activity. Athletes should be reminded not to eat for 2 to 3 hours before activity to avoid triggering symptoms during their sport.[12]

Gastritis and Peptic Ulcer Disease

Gastritis is a diffuse or patchy inflammation of the lining of the stomach. **Peptic ulcer disease** (PUD) is a more serious condition in which there is a deeper ulcer in the stomach (i.e., gastric ulcer) or, much more commonly, in the duodenum (i.e., duodenal ulcer). Although gastritis can have several causes, in otherwise healthy and younger athletes it is usually from either (1) processes of erosion and then ulcer caused by nonsteroidal antiinflammatory drugs (NSAIDs) or alcohol or (2) infectious processes caused by the bacterium *Helicobacter pylori*. PUD may also be caused by

Helicobacter pylori.[13] These conditions are more common in people over the age of 40 years but may be seen in those as young as teenagers.

Signs and Symptoms

Symptoms with gastritis are generally mild to moderate persistent mid-abdominal pain, loss of appetite, and nausea. Eating often aggravates the pain. The patient with PUD will have similar symptoms but will often have more severe pain that is worse a couple of hours after eating but gets better with food. Pain can wake the patient from sleep. Both these conditions can lead to gastrointestinal bleeding. Gastritis is less likely to bleed, but PUD can sometimes cause severe and dangerous bleeding. The bleeding may present as black and tarry stools or as blood with vomiting. Occasionally, a patient may have bleeding gastritis or PUD with no apparent gastrointestinal distress, and thus any black or tarry stools are cause for concern and prompt referral.

Although the over-the-counter antacids, H_2 blockers, and proton-pump inhibitors discussed previously can all provide substantial relief of symptoms for gastritis or PUD, the athlete should see a physician regularly because of the potential of severe complications. Testing for and treating potential *Helicobacter pylori* infection can bring about a cure and thus avoid the long-term need for acid suppression (Box 6-4).

Prognosis and Return to Participation

Symptoms will rarely interfere with athletic activity, and the athlete can fully participate in sports.

Box 6-4   Diagnostic Tests for Gastrointestinal Disorders

Tests may include the following:
Radiological studies
    Radiograph of abdomen
    Upper gastrointestinal series (barium swallow)
    Ultrasound
    Computerized tomography (CT) scan
Endoscopy
    Upper endoscopy (esophagogastroduodenoscopy [EGD])
    Lower endoscopy (colonoscopy or flexible sigmoidoscopy)
Laboratory testing
    Complete blood count (CBC)
    Chemistry panel (sodium, potassium, blood urea nitrogen [BUN], creatinine)
    Serology for *Helicobacter pylori*
    Liver enzymes (alanine transaminase [ALT], aspartate transaminase [AST], gamma-glutamyltransferase [GGT], bilirubin)
    Pancreatic enzymes (amylase, lipase)
Stool studies
Evaluation for red blood or white blood cells
    Stool cultures
    Microscopic evaluation for parasites

Irritable Bowel Syndrome

Irritable bowel syndrome (IBS) is a common chronic condition of unknown cause, most typically affecting people in their twenties. It is a disorder of gastrointestinal motility with abnormal cycles of muscle contraction and relaxation. It can run in families and is often triggered by stress.

Signs and Symptoms

Each of the four primary types of IBS has different symptoms. Some people have diarrhea-predominant IBS, some have the constipation-predominant type, and some have diarrhea alternating with constipation. Finally, some people have neither significant constipation nor diarrhea but instead have persistent upper abdominal bloating and generalized discomfort. Abnormalities associated with bowel movements are most characteristic with abdominal pain that is relieved by a bowel movement and changes in the frequency and form of the stool. Athletes may complain of urgency with bowel movements and a sense of incomplete evacuation. Patients may complain of occasional mucus mixed with stool or abdominal distention and nausea.

Referral and Diagnostic Tests

No specific test exists for IBS, and thus any athlete with these symptoms is referred for evaluation for other causes of symptoms, including inflammatory bowel diseases (see subsequent sections), tumors, or infections.

Treatment

Control of IBS symptoms consists of constant vigilance toward a high-fiber diet and stress management. Diarrhea and constipation can each be managed with over-the-counter medicine, but athletes must be cautious to avoid inadvertently causing themselves to cycle back and forth between the two. Prescription medicines can sometimes be used to control cramping and pain.[14] Behavioral modification can be very helpful as an adjunct to medical treatment.[15]

Prognosis and Return to Participation

The athlete with IBS can fully participate in sports depending on the severity of symptoms. Although some athletes may cope better with symptoms during critical games or performances, others may become incapacitated at these times. Professional assessment and management of stress, including techniques such as biofeedback, can be very helpful for these athletes.

Appendicitis

Appendicitis is the most common cause for urgent abdominal surgery in the United States, with about 7% of the population requiring an appendectomy at some time in their life.[16] It is caused by an acute obstruction and inflammation of the appendix (Key Points—Signs and Symptoms of Appendicitis).

KEY POINTS
Signs and Symptoms of Appendicitis*

- Diffuse epigastric or periumbilical pain early
- Pain localization to right lower quadrant (RLQ) within 12 to 18 hours
- Point of maximum tenderness at McBurney's point
- Low-grade fever
- Nausea or vomiting

*Athletes with these symptoms need to be referred to a physician or hospital immediately.

Signs and Symptoms

Numerous signs and symptoms point toward appendicitis, and the diagnosis is usually suspected on the basis of several symptoms and confirmed at surgery.[17] The pain of appendicitis generally starts as a nonspecific discomfort located around the umbilicus or in the midline epigastric region. As it progresses, the pain will usually begin to localize to the RLQ and be improved when the patient flexes the hip. A patient typically progresses from anorexia with the complete loss of appetite to abdominal pain to nausea and mild vomiting. Patients may have a slight fever and either constipation or diarrhea.

As the pain progresses, the athlete will often lie motionless with the right thigh drawn up, and attempts to straighten the thigh will increase the pain. The athlete's abdomen may be very tender to even light touch around McBurney's point in the RLQ, halfway between the anterior superior iliac spine (ASIS) and the umbilicus, and may be significantly rigid (Figure 6-16).

Referral and Diagnostic Tests

Appendicitis is a surgical emergency because of the risks of rupture of the appendix and severe intraabdominal infection that can result.[18] Any athlete with sudden and severe RLQ pain and tenderness associated with anorexia, nausea, or vomiting should be sent to the emergency department of the closest hospital. Although some cases may progress over a few days, it is more typical to see progression over several hours. Athletes at away games who are more than a couple hours from home may need to be seen in the emergency department at an away hospital and should not wait until they

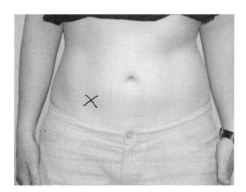

Figure 6-16 McBurney's point: tenderness at this point (*X*), halfway between the umbilicus and the anterior superior iliac spine (ASIS), generally indicates appendicitis when accompanied by fever and nausea.

get home. Other conditions can mimic appendicitis; some of these are fairly benign, but others can also be serious, such as acute pelvic inflammatory disease.

Treatment

Even with advanced diagnostics such as computerized tomography (CT) scans, it is not always possible to diagnose appendicitis until surgery, and it is expected and understood that some cases of suspected appendicitis will have a normal appendix surgically removed.

Prognosis and Return to Participation

The timing of the return to participation is best deferred to the surgeon. It depends on the sport in question, the type of surgical procedure (open versus laparoscopic), and the extent of potential surgical complications.

Cholecystitis and Cholelithiasis

Inflammation of the gallbladder is called **cholecystitis** and is most commonly caused by gallstones, or **cholelithiasis.** Gallstones are common, occurring in about 8% to 10% of the U.S. population. They are more common over the age of 30 years, in women, and in American Indians and Hispanics.[6]

Signs and Symptoms

Gallstones often cause no symptoms at all, but they are the underlying cause of more than 90% of the cases of cholecystitis. Symptoms are generally caused by a stone blocking the bile duct that drains the gallbladder. The patient may have intermittent RUQ pain, nausea, vomiting, or simply indigestion. Frequently symptoms are worse after eating a high-fat meal. Symptoms may be mild and minimally distressful or sudden and very severe. If the duct is blocked for a

prolonged time, the athlete may develop jaundice or severe pain and fever. On examination of the abdomen, the patient typically has tenderness in the RUQ and may exhibit a sudden stopping or arrest of inspiration when the examiner deeply palpates over the liver and the patient takes a deep breath. This is called Murphy's sign.

Referral and Diagnostic Tests

Any patient with significant RUQ pain and tenderness needs to be seen by a physician. Typical evaluation will include an ultrasound of the gallbladder, which is highly accurate at diagnosing gallstones and can also indicate thickening of the wall of the gallbladder with cholecystitis.

Treatment

Gallstones and cholecystitis are treated surgically by removal of the gallbladder (i.e., cholecystectomy). This procedure can usually be done by laparoscopic surgery with a short overnight hospital stay and return to most activities within a few days. Sometimes, an open surgery is needed and the patient may be hospitalized for several days and recover slowly over weeks.

Prognosis and Return to Participation

Overall, prognosis is excellent for cholecystitis and cholelithiasis. Return to play after surgery depends on the type of surgery, and the decision is best left to the surgeon. For many patients, however, the symptoms of gallstones may be fairly mild and intermittent and the patient can simply remain on a very low-fat diet to get through the season and have elective surgery after the season.

Crohn's Disease and Ulcerative Colitis

Crohn's disease and **ulcerative colitis** are severe inflammatory diseases of the small intestines and colon. Although these conditions can occur in families, the underlying cause is unknown. Each condition has certain specific characteristics; for example, Crohn's disease more commonly affects the small intestines and ulcerative colitis is more likely to have symptoms beyond the gastrointestinal tract.[19] This text will discuss both conditions together.

Signs and Symptoms

Crohn's disease and ulcerative colitis typically present with chronic abdominal pain, cramping, and weight loss. The diarrhea is often bloody and can lead to anemia. Some patients also develop other symptoms beyond the gastrointestinal tract, including arthritis and eye and skin conditions.

Referral and Diagnostic Tests

Any athlete with bloody diarrhea or persistent gastrointestinal symptoms needs to be referred to a physician. Evaluation will routinely include direct visualization of the colon by means of colonoscopy and frequently a biopsy of a small piece of the bowel wall to make the diagnosis. Laboratory testing can also reveal anemia and other evidence of inflammation that accompany these conditions.

Treatment

Ulcerative colitis and Crohn's disease require regular and close management by a physician. Although several prescription medications can help to control symptoms, the medicines have significant side effects. In addition, even when symptoms seem controlled the athlete needs to be monitored for potential complications, including an increased risk for colon cancer.

Prognosis and Return to Participation

Athletic performance will vary depending on the severity of disease and degree of control with medications. The disease state may or may not interfere with participation depending on whether it is currently flaring up or well controlled. In addition, the medications used to treat the disease can cause problems and side effects, such as severe headaches, depression, or fatigue. Athletes must be closely aware of their own symptoms and stay in contact with the treating physician.

SUMMARY

The athletic trainer must remember that not all abdominal distress is caused by gastrointestinal disease and must remain alert to possible cardiac, pulmonary, and reproductive system causes of symptoms in the abdomen.[20] Other than appendicitis, most gastrointestinal problems in athletes are not true emergencies. The symptoms can be safely managed with over-the-counter medications initially by the athletic trainer with referral to the physician only if the over-the-counter medications do not elicit a response. Severe gastrointestinal symptoms with accompanying high fever, however, need to be assessed by a physician.

Gastrointestinal problems may or may not interfere with performance, and return to participation is generally based on the severity of the symptoms. In addition, many gastrointestinal disorders are chronic and intermittent in nature. The athletic trainer can help the athlete in managing these symptoms as needed.

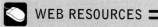

WEB RESOURCES

A Practical Guide to Clinical Medicine.

University of California San Diego School of Medicine
http://medicine.ucsd.edu/clinicalmed/links.html
A comprehensive physical examination and clinical education site for medical students and other health care professionals; offers medical examination information for the major systems of the body; has many links to pictures and videos

International Foundation for Functional Gastrointestinal Disorders
http://www.iffgd.org/GIDisorders/
http://www.GERD.org
http://www.IBS.org
A nonprofit education and research organization; websites address issues about gastrointestinal functional and motility disorders; general patient information as well as medical practitioner information available

Crohn's & Colitis Foundation (CCFA)
http://www.ccfa.org/
Sponsors basic and clinical research pertaining to Crohn's disease and colitis; also provides a support foundation for people affected by the diseases; site provides basic information on the diseases for patients and health professionals

The UNC Center for Functional GI & Motility Disorders
http://www.med.unc.edu/medicine/fgidc/
Offers up-to-date information on functional gastrointestinal and motility disorders for both the professional and the patient and provides information on the center and its research, training, patient education, and clinical treatment

The Merck Manual—Gastrointestinal Disorders
http://www.merck.com/mrkshared/mmanual/section3/sec3.jsp
Provides information about numerous medical conditions; this section specifically addresses gastrointestinal disorders, including gastroenteritis, diarrhea, irritable bowel syndrome, and inflammatory bowel diseases

REFERENCES

1. Seidel HM, Ball JW, Dains JE, Benedict GW: *Mosby's guide to physical examination*, ed 5, St Louis, 2003, Mosby.
2. Bergman RT: Assessing acute abdominal pain: a team physician's challenge, *Physician and Sportsmedicine* 24(4), 1996.
3. Patton RM: Thoracic and abdominal problems, In Mellion MB, et al, editors: *Sports medicine secrets*, ed 2, Philadelphia, 1999, Hanley & Belfus, Inc.
4. Gore JI, Surawicz C: Severe acute diarrhea, *Gastroenterology Clinics of North America* 32(4):1249-1267, 2003.
5. Noble J, editor: *Textbook of primary care medicine*, ed 3, St Louis, 2001, Mosby.

6. Griffith HW, Dambro MR: *Griffith's 5-minute clinical consult,* ed 11, Philadelphia, 2003, Lippincott Williams & Wilkins.

7. Juckett G: Prevention and treatment of traveler's diarrhea, *American Family Physician* 60:119-136, 1999.

8. Dambro M: *Griffith's 5-minute clinical consult,* ed 10, Philadelphia, 2002, Lippincott Williams & Wilkins.

9. Olden KW, Drossman DA: Psychologic and psychiatric aspects of gastrointestinal disease, *Medical Clinics of North America* 84:1313-1327, 2000.

10. Arce DA, Ermocilla CA, Costa H: Evaluation of constipation, *American Family Physician* 65(65):2283-2290, 2293, 2295-2296, 2002.

11. Devault KR, Castell DO: Updated guidelines for the diagnosis and treatment of gastroesophageal reflux disease. The Practice Parameters Committee of the American College of Gastroenterology, *American Journal of Gastroenterology* 94:1434-1442, 1999.

12. Housner JA, Green G: Gastrointestinal problems in athletes. In Salis RE, Massimino F, editors: *Essentials of sports medicine,* St Louis, 1997, Mosby.

13. Meurer LN, Bower DJ: Management of *Helicobacter pylori* infection, *American Family Physician* 65:1327-1336, 1339, 2002.

14. American College of Gastroenterology Functional Gastrointestinal Disorders Task Force: Evidence-based position statement on the management of irritable bowel syndrome in North America, *American Journal of Gastroenterology* 97: S1-S5, 2002.

15. Heymann-Monnikes I, Arnold R, Florin I, et al: The combination of medical treatment plus multicomponent behavioral therapy is superior to medical treatment alone in the therapy of irritable bowel syndrome, *American Journal of Gastroenterology* 95:981-994, 2000.

16. Hardin DH: Acute appendicitis: review and update, *American Family Physician* 60:2027-2034, 1996.

17. Graffeo CS, Counselman FL: Appendicitis, *Emergency Medicine Clinics of North America* 14:653-671, 1996.

18. Liu DS, McFadden DW, editors: *Acute abdomen and appendix,* ed 2, Philadelphia, 1997, Lippincott-Raven.

19. Rakel RE: *Saunders manual of medical practice,* ed 2, Philadelphia, 2000, WB Saunders.

20. American College of Emergency Physicians (ACEP): Clinical policy: critical issues for the initial evaluation and management of patients presenting with a chief complaint of non-traumatic acute abdominal pain, *Annals of Emergency Medicine* 36(4):406-415, 2000.

CHAPTER 7

Genitourinary and Gynecological Disorders

Joseph M. Garry and
Craig Whaley

OBJECTIVES

At the completion of this chapter, the reader should be able to do the following:

1. Recognize common genitourinary and gynecological disorders that athletic personnel encounter in the care of the athlete.
2. Recognize conditions of the genitourinary and gynecological systems that warrant referral.
3. Describe the physiology of ovulation and menstruation.
4. Describe the physiological changes that occur in pregnancy.

INTRODUCTION

Whereas injury to the genitourinary and gynecological systems is rare in athletics, disorders of these systems are common in the athletic population. This chapter focuses on these systems and discusses how an athletic trainer might recognize and refer conditions to a physician. Although athletic trainers do not perform most of the evaluations in this chapter, they do have a relationship with their athletes whereby they may be able to gather enough symptomatic data to warrant referral to the team physician. In addition, knowledge of the types of diagnostic tests will better enable the athletic trainer to explain them to the affected athlete.

OVERVIEW OF ANATOMY AND PHYSIOLOGY

Anatomy of the Kidneys, Ureters, and Urinary Bladder

The kidneys act to remove excess water, salts, and products of metabolism from the blood in order to maintain proper acid-base status. The body's waste products are then conveyed in the urine to the urinary bladder by the ureters. Normally, an individual has two kidneys, two ureters, and a single urinary bladder (Figure 7-1). The kidneys lie posterior to the peritoneum in the retroperitoneal space on the posterior abdominal wall, alongside the spine and against the psoas major muscles. The kidneys are bean-shaped organs whose upper poles are protected by the lower bony thorax. Because of the large size of the right lobe of the liver, the right kidney lies at a slightly lower level than the left. In muscular individuals and those with well-developed abdominal musculature, the kidneys are generally not palpable on exam.

The surrounding anatomy of the two kidneys differs anteriorly (Figure 7-2). The right kidney is associated with the liver and separated from it by the hepatorenal recess. The left kidney is associated with the left adrenal gland, stomach, spleen, pancreas, a portion of the small bowel, and the descending colon. They lie well protected posteriorly by the costovertebral angle between

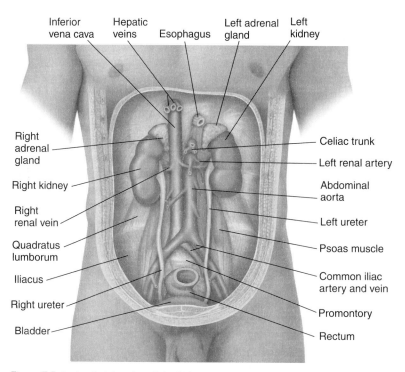

Figure 7-1 Anatomical location of the kidneys in the retroperitoneal aspect of the abdomen. (From Seidel HM, Ball JW, Dains JE, Benedict GW: *Mosby's guide to physical examination,* ed 5, St Louis, 2003, Mosby, p 527.)

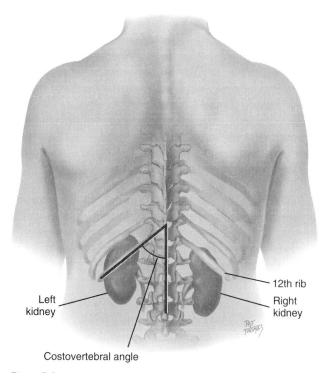

Figure 7-2 Posterior view of the kidneys protected within the costovertebral angle between the twelfth rib and the spine. (From Jarvis C: *Physical examination & health assessment,* ed 4, Philadelphia, 2004, WB Saunders, p 564.)

the twelfth rib and the vertebral spine. In addition, both kidneys are attached superiorly to the diaphragm and move slightly on respiration.

The kidneys are enclosed in a strong fibrous capsule that is surrounded by a layer of fat called **perirenal fat.** The unique characteristics of the density of the kidney itself and the perirenal fat allow for the kidneys to be visualized on abdominal radiographs. The kidney is a solid organ with a thick cortex under the fibrous capsule (Figure 7-3). The filtration system begins with the medulla moving interiorly to the calyx structures and ending in the collection area before the ureter.

The ureters are muscular ducts, or tubes, that carry urine from the kidneys to the urinary bladder. Urine passes from the kidneys through the ureters by peristaltic waves of muscular contractions. The ureters are approximately 25 cm long and retroperitoneal in location. Each descends almost vertically along the psoas major muscle just anterior to the tips of the transverse processes of the lumbar vertebrae (L2-L5). In the female, the ureters and uterine arteries are closely associated. The uterine artery crosses the ureter at the side of the cervix; therefore, during a surgical procedure to remove the uterus and cervix, the ureter may be inadvertently damaged.

The urinary bladder is a muscular sac or vesicle that functions to store urine. Its shape, size, position, and relation to other structures vary with the amount of urine it contains. It is composed chiefly of smooth muscle.

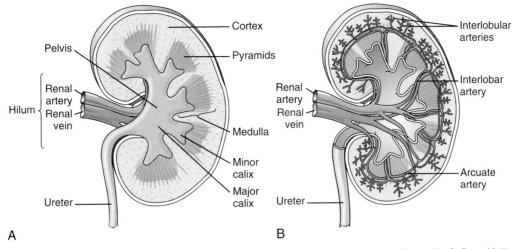

Figure 7-3 Cross section reveals two views of the internal structure of the kidney. (From Copstead LC, Banaski JL: *Pathophysiology: biological and behavioral perspectives,* ed 2, Philadelphia, 2000, WB Saunders, p 628.)

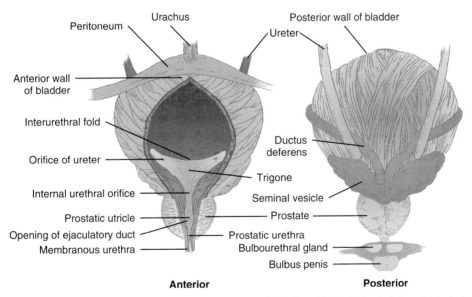

Figure 7-4 Anatomy of the urinary bladder. (From Copstead LC, Banaski JL: *Pathophysiology: biological and behavioral perspectives,* ed 2, Philadelphia, 2000, WB Saunders, p 710.)

In the adult, the empty urinary bladder lies posterior to the symphysis pubis within the pelvis (Figure 7-4). As it fills, it ascends into the lower abdomen. A full bladder may reach as high as the level of the umbilicus. The ureters enter at the superolateral aspect of each side of the bladder. The bladder is then drained by a single urethra that empties from the central inferior aspect.

The blood supply to the kidneys is provided by the right and left renal arteries, respectively. These branch off from the descending aorta at nearly right angles. Venous drainage is provided by the right and left renal veins that empty into the inferior vena cava. Blood supply to the ureters is more complex, but it is principally supplied by arterial branches from the renal,

aortic, common iliac, vesicular, or uterine arteries. The main arteries supplying the urinary bladder are branches of the internal iliac arteries. In the female, however, branches of the uterine and vaginal arteries also supply a portion of the blood supply to the bladder. Venous drainage occurs via the vesicular venous plexus that drains to the internal iliac vein (see Figure 7-1).

Lymphatic drainage from the kidneys and upper ureter empties into the aortic lymph nodes, whereas lymphatic drainage from the middle and lower ureter is directed to the common iliac lymph nodes. Drainage from the superior portion of the urinary bladder is directed to the external iliac lymph nodes, and the inferior portion of the bladder drains to the internal iliac lymph nodes.

The urinary bladder is supplied by parasympathetic motor fibers to the detrusor muscle of the bladder, and sensory fibers. The sensory fibers are stimulated by stretching of the bladder, causing a sensation of fullness and activating the micturition, or urination, reflex. Micturition is preceded by contraction of the diaphragm and abdominal wall. The neck of the bladder descends, the detrusor muscle contracts by reflex, and urine is voluntarily expelled from the bladder (see Figure 7-4).[1]

Anatomy of the Urethra

The urethra is a fibromuscular tube that conducts urine from the bladder (and semen from the ductus deferens in the male) to the exterior. The urethra originates at the central lower portion of the urinary bladder, traverses the pelvis, and terminates at the external urethral orifice.

The female urethra is approximately 4 cm long. It is closely associated, often fused, with the anterior vaginal wall. The urethral orifice is located between the clitoris (anteriorly) and the vagina (posteriorly).

The male urethra is considerably longer, averaging 20 cm in length. The male urethra consists of three parts: prostatic, membranous, and spongy. The proximal prostatic portion descends through the prostate gland. The membranous portion of the urethra descends from the lower portion of the prostate to the bulb of the penis. This portion of the urethra is surrounded by a sphincter (i.e., muscle). The lowermost portion of the membranous urethra is most susceptible to rupture or penetration by a catheter. The spongy portion of the urethra lies in the corpus spongiosum and traverses the bulb, shaft, and glans of the penis, terminating at the external urethral orifice or meatus.[1]

Male Genital Anatomy

The male genital organs comprise the penis, ejaculatory duct, prostate gland, bulbourethral gland, and paired testes, each with an epididymis, ductus or vas deferens, and seminal vesicle (Figure 7-5). Spermatozoa, formed in the testes and stored in the epididymides, are contained in the semen, which is secreted by the testes and epididymides, seminal vesicles, prostate, and bulbourethral glands. The sperm, on leaving the epididymides, pass through the ductus deferens and ejaculatory ducts to reach the urethra and pass through the external urethral orifice.

The testes are paired ovoid glands located in the scrotum and responsible for production of spermatozoa and steroid hormones. They reside away from the core of the body to maintain a slightly lower temperature of approximately 1° to 2° F below that of the body proper. The left testicle often lies slightly lower than the right testicle in the scrotum. The epididymis is associated with the posterior portion of each testicle. The testes and epididymides are covered by a dual-layered tunica vaginalis testis, which is derived prenatally from the processus vaginalis of the peritoneum (Figure 7-6). The potential cavity between these two layers or some part of the processus vaginalis may become distended with fluid, forming a hydrocele.

The testes and epididymides receive their blood supply from the testicular artery, and venous drainage occurs via the pampiniform plexus, which forms the bulk of the spermatic cord. The veins of the pampiniform plexus can become varicose, leading to the formation of a varicocele. Lymphatic drainage from the testes empties into the lower aortic lymph nodes.

The scrotum is a cutaneous pouch that houses the testicles and epididymides. A median raphe indicates the subdivision of the scrotum by a septum into right and left compartments. Smooth muscle, known as the dartos muscle, is firmly attached to the overlying skin. The dartos muscle contracts in response to cold, exercise, and sexual stimulation. Loose connective tissue underlying the dartos allows free movement and is the site for the accumulation of edema.

The prostate gland is a fibromuscular pelvic organ surrounding the male urethra and containing glands that contribute to the semen. It is located behind the symphysis pubis and directly in front of the rectum, which is where it can be palpated by a digital rectal exam. Venous drainage and lymphatic drainage of the prostate are important because these contribute to the distinct areas for the spread of prostate cancer. Venous drainage occurs via the prostatic venous plexus that drains into the internal iliac vein and communicates with the vertebral plexus, thereby allowing metastatic spread of prostate cancer to the vertebrae. Lymphatic drainage terminates in the internal and external iliac lymph nodes.[1]

Female Genital Anatomy

The female genital organs comprise the ovaries, fallopian tubes, uterus, vagina, and external genitalia, specifically the mons pubis, labia majora and minora, vestibule of the vagina, bulb of the vestibule, vestibular glands, and clitoris (Figure 7-7, A).

The ovaries are paired organs that produce oocytes (i.e., eggs) and secrete steroid hormones. The ovaries are situated on the lateral wall of the pelvis where they can be palpated bimanually. The paired fallopian tubes act to transmit the oocyte from the ovaries and spermatozoa from the uterus.

The fallopian tube is the usual site of fertilization because it conveys the early embryo to the uterus.

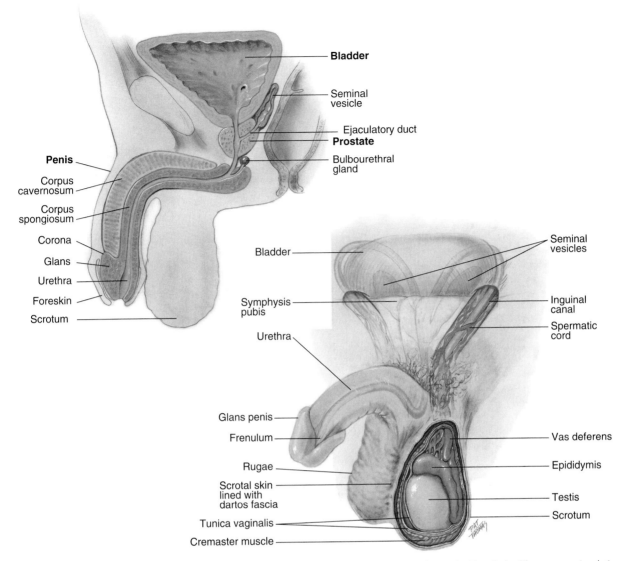

Figure 7-5 Anatomy of the male genitourinary system. (Adapted from Jarvis C: *Physical examination & health assessment,* ed 4, Philadelphia, 2004, WB Saunders, pp 722-723.)

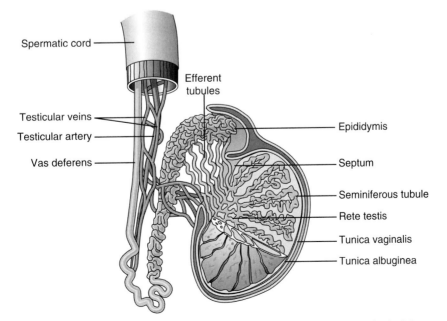

Figure 7-6 Anatomy of the testis and epididymis. (From Copstead LC, Banaski JL: *Pathophysiology: biological and behavioral perspectives,* ed 2, Philadelphia, 2000, WB Saunders, p 712.)

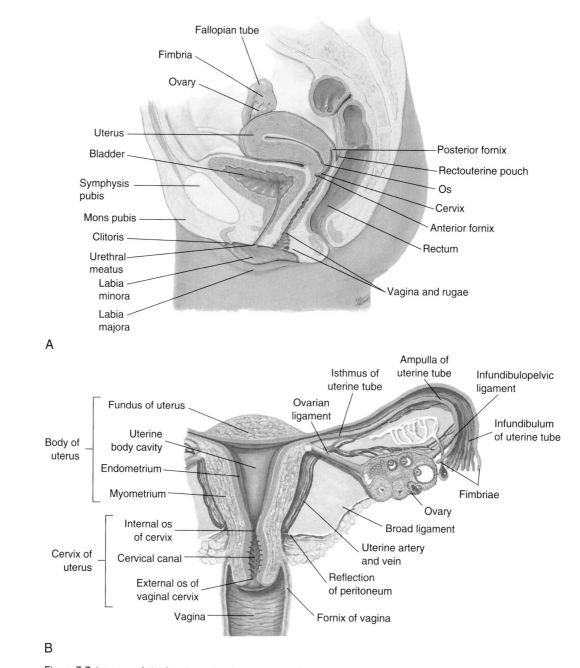

Figure 7-7 Anatomy of the female genitourinary system. (**A** from Jarvis C: *Physical examination & health assessment,* ed 4, Philadelphia, 2004, WB Saunders, p 767; **B** from Seidel HM, Ball JW, Dains JE, Benedict GW: *Mosby's guide to physical examination,* ed 5, St Louis, 2003, Mosby, p 587.)

As such, the fallopian tubes are the site of a tubal pregnancy and are susceptible to scarring associated with ascending infections (e.g., pelvic inflammatory disease [PID]), which can ultimately lead to an inability of the tube to transmit either oocytes or spermatozoa resulting in infertility.

The uterus is a muscular organ that lies within the pelvis (Figure 7-7, *B*). The uterus functions to accept the fertilized egg and allow for implantation and development of the fetus. The upper uterine segment receives the fallopian tubes. The lower uterine segment terminates in the cervix, which opens to the vagina.

The uterus has three distinct layers: a mucosa or endometrium, a muscular coat or myometrium, and a serosa or perimetrium.

The vagina lies posterior to the urinary bladder and anterior to the rectum. It serves as a receptacle for the penis, as the lower end of the birth canal, and as the excretory duct for the products of menstruation. The anterior and posterior walls of the vagina are approximately 7.5 and 9 cm long, respectively. The opening of the vagina into the vestibule may be partially closed by a membrane called the hymen. The opening is located posterior to the urethral orifice and anterior to the anus.

The vagina and cervix can be inspected through a speculum placed in the vagina. A Papanicolaou (Pap) smear is taken from the cervix to aid in the detection of cervical cancer.

Blood supply to the ovaries (i.e., ovarian arteries arising from the lower abdominal aorta), fallopian tubes (i.e., ovarian and uterine arteries), and uterus (i.e., uterine artery) is provided by their respective arteries and forms a complex anastomosis. The vagina and cervix are supplied by branches from the internal iliac arteries. Venous drainage for the ovaries is distinct for each side. The right ovarian vein drains to the inferior vena cava, whereas the left ovarian vein empties into the left renal vein. The veins of the fallopian tubes drain into the ovarian and uterine veins. The uterine veins form a uterine venous plexus on each side of the cervix and drain to the internal iliac veins. The uterine venous plexus connects with the superior rectal vein, forming a portal-systemic anastomosis. The vaginal veins form the vaginal venous plexuses and lie along the sides of the vagina, draining into the internal iliac veins. Lymphatic drainage, again, is related to the metastatic spread of cancer. The ovaries drain to the lumbar lymph nodes. The fallopian tubes have their lymphatic drainage directed to the lower lumbar lymph nodes with the ovaries and uterus. The uterus drains to the lower aortic and external iliac lymph nodes. The superior and middle portions of the vagina drain into the external and iliac lymph nodes, and the lower portion of the vagina (vestibule) drains into the superficial inguinal lymph nodes. The cervix drains to the external and internal iliac nodes and sacral lymph nodes.[1]

Physiology of Ovulation and Menstruation

Normal menstrual cycles depend on an intact hypothalamic-pituitary axis, functioning ovaries, and a normal outflow tract. The menstrual cycle, which averages 28 days, requires a well-coordinated series of events (Figure 7-8). The normal menstrual cycle is divided into two parts: a proliferative, or follicular, phase and a secretory, or luteal, phase. During the follicular phase, estrogen and luteinizing hormone (LH) levels increase as follicle-stimulating hormone (FSH) levels decrease. The endometrium thickens during this phase. Before ovulation, estrogen sharply declines, followed by a surge in LH and a steady rise in progesterone. It is shortly after this that ovulation occurs, followed by a slight increase in core body temperature. The remnant of the follicle (i.e., corpus luteum) supplies the progesterone for the second half of the cycle. During this time, the endometrium prepares itself for implantation. If fertilization and implantation do not occur, the corpus luteum involutes and progesterone levels decline, prompting menses.

Physiological Changes of Pregnancy

Noteworthy physiological changes occur in pregnancy.[2] Cardiac output (CO), defined as stroke volume (SV) × heart rate (HR), increases during pregnancy as a result of increases in both SV and HR. Plasma volume also increases with pregnancy. The high flow of blood exiting the heart can often create a benign heart murmur. Blood pressure, defined as CO × systemic vascular resistance (SVR), actually decreases because of a decrease in SVR.

Respiratory changes also occur in pregnancy and result in increased tidal volume, which translates into increased minute ventilation at rest despite a normal respiratory rate. Of note, FEV_1 (forced expiratory volume in 1 second) does not change, which is important with regard to asthmatic athletes since peak flow meter values would not need to be altered. Overall airway resistance is also decreased in pregnancy.

Physiological responses to exercise are somewhat different in pregnancy than in the nonpregnant female.[3] Respiratory rates increase with mild exercise in pregnancy compared with nonpregnant women, whereas maximal oxygen consumption (Vo_2 max) is less in pregnant women compared with nonpregnant women. The respiratory quotient (Vco_2/Vo_2) is also increased in exercising pregnant women suggesting that there may be a greater dependence on carbohydrates as the preferred fuel source. This may also explain the fact that hypoglycemia can develop more rapidly during prolonged strenuous exercise in pregnant athletes. In addition, the core temperature of a pregnant woman is higher than that of a nonpregnant athlete, which requires caution in the exercising expectant mother, especially in hotter climates.

Anatomical considerations because of the enlarging uterus result in common changes in pregnancy. Urinary frequency increases during pregnancy as a result of pressure of the uterus on the urinary bladder. Low back pain is another common complaint and is again the result of the enlarging uterus. In this scenario, however, changes in biomechanics lead to increased lumbar lordosis that is more commonly the cause of the low back discomfort. Lower extremity edema may also develop and is more common later in pregnancy.

PATHOLOGICAL CONDITIONS OF THE GENITOURINARY SYSTEM

Kidney Stones

Kidney stones, also known as renal calculi, arise in the kidney when urine becomes supersaturated with a salt that is capable of forming solid crystals. More than 5%

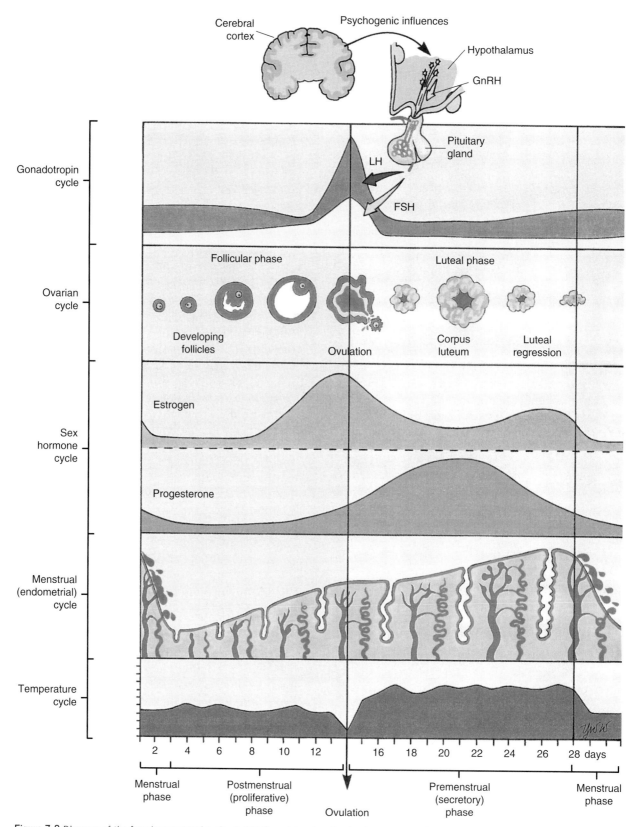

Figure 7-8 Diagram of the female menstrual cycle. *GnRH,* Gonadotropin-releasing hormone; *LH,* luteinizing hormone; *FSH,* follicle-stimulating hormone. (From Seidel HM, Ball JW, Dains JE, Benedict GW: *Mosby's guide to physical examination,* ed 5, St Louis, 2003, Mosby, p 589.)

Box 7-1   Types of Kidney Stones

Each of the following five commonly identified types of kidney stones, has its own causes:

1. Calcium stones are composed of calcium oxide, calcium phosphate, and calcium urate. Common causes of calcium stones include hyperparathyroidism, increased gut absorption of calcium, a renal phosphate leak, hyperuricosuria, hyperoxaluria, hypocitraturia, and hypomagnesemia.
2. Struvite stones are composed of magnesium ammonium phosphate. These stones are associated with chronic urinary tract infections secondary to gram-negative rods.
3. Uric acid stones are associated with high purine intake (diet rich in organ meats, legumes, fish, meat extracts, or gravies), gout, and malignancy.
4. Cystine stones are caused by an intrinsic metabolic defect resulting in failure of renal tubular reabsorption of cystine, ornithine, lysine, and arginine.
5. Indinavir stones typically appear in individuals with human immunodeficiency virus (HIV) infection who are treated with the protease inhibitor indinavir (Crixivan). These stones are composed entirely of the protease inhibitor.

of adults have had kidney stones.[4] Commonly renal calculi are composed of calcium (75%), struvite (15%), uric acid (6%), and cystine (2%) (Box 7-1). Recurrence rates after an initial kidney stone are 14% (1 year), 35% (5 years), and 52% (10 years). Males are affected approximately three times more commonly than females, and Caucasian males are affected more commonly than African-American males, although African-American males have a higher incidence of associated infection with renal calculi whereas females of all races have been noted to have a higher incidence of infected **hydronephrosis.** The age of onset of symptomatic renal calculi is generally in the third or fourth decades.

Approximately 80% to 85% of stones pass spontaneously, and 20% of individuals affected require hospitalization for unremitting pain, dehydration, associated urinary tract infection, or inability to pass the stone.

Signs and Symptoms

Most kidney stones originate within the kidney and proceed distally, creating varying degrees of urinary obstruction as they become lodged in the narrow canal areas. Acute passage of a kidney stone from the kidney through the ureter gives rise to pain so excruciating that it has been likened to that of childbirth. The location and quality of pain are related to the position of the stone within the urinary tract. Severity of pain is related to the degree of obstruction, presence of ureteral spasm, and presence of any associated infection. Pain is typically described as unilateral flank pain that radiates to the groin. The individual is often writhing in pain, moving about and unable to lie still. Nausea and vomiting are common. Examination demonstrates flank

tenderness, costovertebral angle tenderness, and occasionally testicular pain notably in the absence of any testicular tenderness. The abdominal examination is often normal although bowel sounds may be hypoactive because of a mild ileus (see Chapter 6). The presence of a fever raises the possibility of an infectious complication and warrants immediate referral.

Once a kidney stone passes to the urinary bladder it is often asymptomatic and can be passed during urination. During passage of the stone the athlete will usually note burning and some blood-tinged urine depending on the size of the stone.

Referral and Diagnostic Tests

An athlete with symptoms suggestive of a kidney stone should be referred immediately to the team physician if this is the first episode. Any athlete with new or recurrent presentation and an associated fever needs to be referred immediately for physician evaluation and a urology consultation. Also, an athlete with recurrent symptoms who is unable to tolerate oral fluids and has unrelenting pain with a history of renal failure or a single kidney should be referred for immediate physician evaluation and possible observation or hospitalization.

The mainstay of diagnostic testing for kidney stones is a urinalysis. Blood is often present in the urine and may be detectable in more than 90% of symptomatic individuals using both a urine dipstick and microscopy. Urine pH can also be helpful since a urine pH greater than 7 suggests the presence of urea-splitting organisms and struvite stones. Alternatively, a urine pH less than 5 suggests the presence of uric acid stones. The presence of **pyuria** (>5 white blood cells per high-power field) in a centrifuged urine specimen should prompt a careful search for an associated infection. (Normal urine values are listed in Table 2-4.) In these cases a complete blood count and differential, serum creatinine, and urine culture are in order.

Imaging studies may also be performed and are often done to confirm the initial diagnosis. The current imaging study most often used is the noncontrast helical computerized tomography (CT) scan.[5] This is a rapid test with sensitivity in the range of 95% to 100%. The principal disadvantage of CT is that indinavir stones are not well visualized by this method. Radiographs may also be obtained and may demonstrate a radiopaque stone. Radiographs are occasionally used to monitor the passage of a stone under certain circumstances. An **intravenous pyelogram (IVP)** may be used in the diagnosis of kidney stones but has essentially been replaced by CT. Last, ultrasound can also be used to identify stones. Although the sensitivity and specificity are poorer than other imaging techniques, there is no exposure to radiation, so this is an ideal imaging tool for pregnant women.

Differential Diagnosis

The differential diagnosis for kidney stones is long and often depends on what side of the body is involved, as well as the gender and age of the individual. The list includes urinary tract infection, **pyelonephritis,** urinary obstruction, testicular torsion, pelvic inflammatory disease, bowel obstruction, appendicitis, cholecystitis, **biliary colic,** and constipation. Among athletes older than 60 years of age, an **abdominal aortic aneurysm** may also be included as a differential diagnosis.[6]

Treatment

The crux of treatment for the uncomplicated passage of a kidney stone is pain management and maintenance of adequate hydration. Pain management is often obtained with narcotic analgesics or nonsteroidal anti-inflammatory agents, such as ketorolac.[7] An antiemetic medication also may be added when nausea is present and deters the use of oral analgesics or hydration. The forcing of oral or intravenous fluids has not been shown to alter outcome or improve the passage of the stone; therefore the focus should remain on maintenance of hydration. A strainer is useful to filter the urine during the passage of the stone in order to collect the stone for analysis. Antibiotics are necessary in the presence of an associated infection.

Prognosis and Return to Participation

The overall prognosis for kidney stones is very good. Approximately 80% to 85% of individuals will pass the stone in the outpatient setting, and 15% to 20% will require hospitalization for pain management or an associated complication. Recurrence rates escalate with time, but based on the type of stone present, treatment options to reduce the risk of recurrence are available. Return to sport can be achieved after passage of the kidney stone and adequate hydration. However, even after the diagnosis of a kidney stone, any athlete who develops fever, increasing pain, or emesis should be referred for immediate physician evaluation.

Prevention

Individuals with recurrent kidney stones may benefit from maintaining adequate hydration and avoiding dehydration. This may decrease the chance of urinary saturation with stone-forming salts. Daily consumption of coffee, tea, beer, or wine may decrease the risk of stone formation, whereas daily apple or grapefruit juice may increase the risk of stone formation.

Special Concerns in the Mature Athlete

Athletes 60 years and older with an initial presentation of a kidney stone actually may have an abdominal aortic aneurysm (AAA). In a series of 134 patients with a symptomatic AAA presenting to the emergency department, 18% had an initial misdiagnosis of a kidney stone.[6]

Sports Hematuria

Sports hematuria is the benign, self-limiting presence of three or more red blood cells per high-power field in a centrifuged urine specimen and is directly associated with exercise or activity. Sports hematuria is asymptomatic and has been documented to occur in both contact and noncontact sports. The degree of hematuria is believed to be related to the intensity and duration of the exercise. In most circumstances the hematuria will resolve within 72 hours of onset in athletes without any coexisting urinary tract pathology.[8]

The incidence of sports hematuria is estimated to be as high as 80% in swimming, lacrosse, and track and field; 55% in football and rowing; and 20% in marathon runners. These incidence levels have led to the development of several possible causes of sports hematuria (e.g., increased permeability of the glomerulus, direct or indirect trauma to the kidneys, renal ischemia, dehydration, release of a hemolyzing factor), all of which appear to be related to exercise duration and exercise intensity.[9]

Signs and Symptoms

By definition sports hematuria is asymptomatic. The finding of hematuria may occur during a routine urinalysis, such as those that may be performed during a physical examination or preparticipation exam. Occasionally individuals will present with gross hematuria (i.e., visible presence of blood in the urine) after a prolonged and strenuous workout. In these situations, the general rule is that the hematuria will resolve within 72 hours without any further intervention than rest.

Referral and Diagnostic Tests

The finding of asymptomatic hematuria in an athlete during some form of routine testing needs to be reviewed by the team physician. As a general rule, these athletes are retested at 24 to 72 hours to document resolution. Any athlete with symptomatic hematuria or systemic symptoms is referred to a physician for immediate evaluation.

Although sports hematuria is a benign condition, not all hematuria is benign so the evaluation must include some basic tests. A urinalysis or dipstick test will demonstrate the presence of blood in the urine. Because drugs, dyes, and myoglobin can mimic hematuria by causing a false-positive result on the urine dipstick, a microscopic examination of a spun urine specimen will confirm the presence of red blood cells. If symptoms of **dysuria** (i.e., painful urination) are present, a urine culture may be performed. If hypertension, renal disease, repeated urinary tract infections, or pyelonephritis is found in the athlete's history, an initial serum creatinine can be performed. A repeat urine dipstick and microscopic urine examination are performed at 24 to 72 hours after rest to document resolution. As a general rule, if hematuria persists beyond 72 hours, further evaluation is warranted. Additional tests include a renal ultrasound, CT, and possible **cystoscopy.**

Differential Diagnosis

The differential diagnosis includes causes of true hematuria (i.e., red blood cells in urine) and causes of a false-positive urine blood dipstick. True hematuria may result from a urinary tract infection, urethritis, interstitial nephritis, renal papillary necrosis, nephrolithiasis (i.e., renal stone), polycystic kidney disease, kidney laceration, a neoplasm arising from any structure in the urinary tract, coagulopathy, and prostatitis in males.[10] Causes of a false-positive urine dipstick exam for blood include drugs (i.e., phenazopyridine, rifampin, nitrofurantoin, phenytoin), food dyes, menses, and myoglobin in the urine.

Treatment, Prognosis, and Return to Participation

The treatment of sports hematuria is simply rest for 24 to 72 hours. Resolution is the rule and should be documented with a repeat urinalysis after rest. The prognosis is excellent because sports hematuria is a benign and self-limiting condition.

Urinary Tract Infection

Urinary tract infection (UTI) occurs in either the upper or lower urinary tract. These infections most commonly involve the urinary bladder, but they can also involve the urethra, ureters, and kidneys (i.e., pyelonephritis). UTIs are a leading cause of morbidity and health care expenditures in persons of all ages.

As many as 90% of uncomplicated UTIs are caused by *Escherichia coli*, 10% to 20% can be caused by coagulase-negative *Staphylococcus saprophyticus,* and up to 5% may be caused by Enterobacteriaceae species or *Enterococcus.*

Anyone can develop a UTI; however, sexually active young women are at highest risk. Several factors have been attributed to this higher risk: a short urethra, sexual activity, delays in micturition particularly after intercourse, and the use of diaphragms and spermicides.[11] Fortunately, the risk of a complicated UTI in this population is very low, yet up to 20% of young women with a UTI will develop recurrent UTIs.

UTIs in men are less common than in women but can occur. Overall, most UTIs in men are accounted for by older men: this is attributed to risk factors such as prostatic disease that can cause some degree of urinary obstruction and urinary tract instrumentation. In younger men, UTIs may occur in men who participate in anal sex, who are not circumcised, or whose sexual partner is colonized with an uropathogen.[12] Catheter-associated UTIs are also known to occur.

Signs and Symptoms

In most individuals a UTI is signaled by a constellation of symptoms, including dysuria, increased frequency of urination, and voiding small amounts of urine relative to their normal pattern. Occasionally lower pelvic discomfort or cramping may also be present. The presence of gross hematuria, abnormal vaginal bleeding, or fever warrants prompt physician attention.

Referral and Diagnostic Tests

Because of the relative discomfort associated with a UTI and the possibility of developing an ascending infection, symptomatic athletes need to be referred to a physician for evaluation and treatment. The presence of gross hematuria, fever, abdominal pain, nausea, or vomiting warrants immediate referral.

The diagnosis of an uncomplicated UTI is often made by the history, physical exam, and examination of a urine specimen. The urine specimen is examined specifically for the presence of leukocyte esterase, nitrite (i.e., a surrogate marker for bacteria), and the finding of leukocytes on microscopic examination. The use of a urine Gram stain can also aid in the identification of bacteria. The finding of a single bacterial organism, under high-power oil immersion, on an unspun urine specimen correlates with a count of more than 100,000 colony-forming units on urine culture. Because of the limited added value in determining treatment for most uncomplicated UTIs, a urine culture may not be performed in the initial evaluation. The evaluation of a recurrent, complicated, or catheter-associated UTI often necessitates obtaining a urine culture.

Urine culture results must be viewead in light of certain threshold values that have been shown to correlate with significant **bacteriuria.** In young women, a urine culture producing more than 100,000 colony-forming units of bacteria per 1 ml of urine is considered a positive culture because of its high specificity for the diagnosis of a true infection. In men, a urine culture yielding more than 1000 colony-forming units of bacteria is considered a positive culture, and in catheterized individuals this value falls to more than 100 colony-forming units of bacteria.

The use of additional urological testing for anatomical abnormalities is generally unrewarding. However, a urological evaluation should still be performed in an adolescent male with his first UTI and in men with pyelonephritis or recurrent UTI.[13]

Differential Diagnosis

Differential diagnoses for UTIs include urethritis, noninfectious cystitis, pyelonephritis, vulvovaginitis, sexually transmitted diseases (STDs), dehydration, mittelschmerz, endometriosis, and **balanitis.**

Treatment

UTIs are treated with antibiotics. An uncomplicated UTI can be treated with antibiotics such as trimethoprim-sulfamethoxazole, ciprofloxacin, or ofloxacin for a 3-day course (see Chapter 3). Recurrent UTIs in women or UTIs in men should be treated with a 7- to 10-day course of antibiotics with antibiotic choice based on the results of the urine culture. If a woman experiences more than three UTIs in a given year, prophylactic antibiotics may be used to prevent recurrence. Prophylactic antibiotics may be given after coitus, continuously at a lower dose than treatment dose, or as directed by the physician. Complicated UTIs require a longer course of treatment and should be treated for 10 to 14 days.

Prognosis and Return to Participation

The prognosis for an uncomplicated UTI is excellent and generally will not preclude participation in athletics. For the few individuals developing a complicated UTI, return-to-play decisions need to be based on the athlete's unique complication. Athletes with fever or poor fluid intake as a result of nausea or vomiting should be observed and return to play after symptoms resolve with treatment.

Prevention

Common sense will help prevent recurrent UTIs. Modification of risk factors associated with UTI includes urination after intercourse, avoidance of delays in urination, and limited use of either diaphragms or spermicides. Wearing breathable (cotton) underwear also reduces the chances of contracting a UTI.

Urethritis

Urethritis is an inflammation of the urethra caused by an infection and is typically reserved to describe a syndrome of sexually transmitted diseases (STDs), namely gonococcal urethritis (GU) and nongonococcal urethritis (NGU). Urethritis, in a more general definition, may also be a posttraumatic irritation and inflammation of the urethra.

Infectious causes of urethritis are typically sexually transmitted and may be caused by *Neisseria gonorrhoeae* (GU) or nongonococcal organisms such as *Chlamydia trachomatis, Ureaplasma urealyticum, Mycoplasma hominis,* or *Trichomonas vaginalis* (NGU).[14] Less common infectious causes of urethritis include **lymphogranuloma venereum,** herpes genitalis, or syphilis and may be associated with infectious conditions such as epididymitis, **orchitis,** prostatitis, or UTIs. The incidence of GU is in decline. Conversely, the incidence of NGU is rising and is notably higher during the summer months. Urethritis affects males and females equally although up to 50% of females may be asymptomatic and homosexual males are more commonly infected than heterosexuals or homosexual females. Infectious urethritis may occur in any sexually active person, but the incidence is highest among people ages 20 to 24 years.

Signs and Symptoms

Despite the infectious causes of urethritis, up to 25% of those with NGU will be asymptomatic. Symptom onset typically occurs between 4 and 14 days after contact with an infected partner. Urethral discharge may be present and may be yellow, green, brown, or blood tinged. Dysuria is usually localized to the urethral orifice and worst with a first-morning void. Urethral itching may be present. Males may report heaviness or aching in the testicles although associated tenderness should suggest orchitis or epididymitis. Females may report a worsening of symptoms with their menses. The presence of fever, chills, sweats, or nausea suggests a more systemic infection and warrants immediate referral to a physician.

Referral and Diagnostic Tests

Athletes suspected of having urethritis are referred to a physician for diagnosis and treatment. In the interim, the athlete should be counseled to refrain from sexual intercourse until seeing the physician so as to avoid infecting any other people.

The diagnosis of urethritis is most often based on history and examination. A urinalysis is not particularly helpful in establishing the diagnosis but may be helpful in the exclusion of cystitis or pyelonephritis. More than 30% of individuals with NGU do not have leukocytes in their urine. A urethral culture may be performed to examine for the presence of gonococcus or chlamydia. In cases of confirmed GU or NGU, testing for syphilis, hepatitis B, and human immunodeficiency virus (HIV) is encouraged. Women of child-bearing age who have experienced unprotected intercourse need a pregnancy test before treatment.

Differential Diagnosis

The differential diagnosis for urethritis is best considered by gender. Differential diagnoses to be considered in both men and women include STDs such as **chancroid,** chlamydia, gonorrhea, herpes, mycoplasma, syphilis, or trichomoniasis, dermatological diseases involving the urethral orifice (e.g., contact dermatitis secondary to spermicides), **molluscum contagiosum,** urethral stricture, urethral trauma, urethral warts, urethral diverticulum, and urethral cancer. Differential diagnoses affecting females are **oophoritis,** pelvic inflammatory disease, **salpingitis,** vaginitis, and vulvovaginitis. Differential diagnoses exclusive to males are epididymitis and prostatitis.

Treatment

Antibiotics are the mainstay of treatment for urethritis. Symptoms will resolve in all individuals with urethritis over time regardless of treatment. The use of antibiotics in the treatment of infectious urethritis is to prevent morbidity and reduce transmission to others. The antibiotic choice or choices are based on the likelihood of whether it is GU or NGU. Current recommendations are to treat individuals for both GU and NGU. Azithromycin in a single 2 g dose treats both GU and NGU, is the treatment of choice for urethritis, and is well tolerated. Ceftriaxone (intramuscularly), cefixime (oral), ciprofloxacin (oral), or ofloxacin (oral) can be used in single doses to treat GU only. Doxycycline can be taken for 7 days to treat NGU only. In the case of recurrent NGU, a prolonged course of erythromycin for 14 to 28 days is recommended. Antibiotic treatment is recommended for sexual partners of those with culture-positive urethritis, including *Trichomonas.*

Prognosis and Return to Participation

The overall prognosis for urethritis is excellent. The use of antibiotics helps to decrease any associated morbidity and prevent further transmission. Any individual with urethritis is counseled to abstain from sexual intercourse until all partners have been treated and is further encouraged to use barrier devices (condoms) when engaging in sexual intercourse with multiple partners. Uncomplicated urethritis should not interfere with an athlete's ability to train or compete.

Prevention

Prevention of urethritis equates to education. Sexually active athletes are encouraged to use barrier methods during intercourse. Education regarding STD risk factors can be beneficial. Risk factors include intercourse at a young age, unprotected intercourse, multiple sexual partners, intercourse with partners known to have infections, and drug abuse. The early diagnosis and treatment of individuals with urethritis help to limit the transmission, as does the identification and treatment of all partners.

Testicular Torsion

The testicle is covered by the tunica vaginalis, which attaches to the posterolateral surface of the testicle and allows for limited mobility. In the event that the testicle is able to twist or freely rotate (i.e., torsion), venous occlusion can occur, which subsequently leads to arterial ischemia causing infarction of the testicle (Figure 7-9).

The incidence of testicular torsion in males younger than 25 years is approximately 1 per 4000. The highest incidence is among males 12 to 18 years of age with a peak incidence at age 14 years.[15] Torsion predominantly affects the left testicle. A subgroup of individuals has a higher frequency of testicular torsion because of an inappropriately high attachment of the tunica vaginalis (i.e., **bell clapper deformity**).[15]

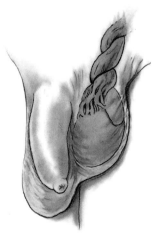

Figure 7-9 Testicular torsion. (From Jarvis C: *Physical examination & health assessment,* ed 4, Philadelphia, 2004, WB Saunders, p 744.)

A higher attachment allows the testicle to rotate freely on the spermatic cord. This congenital abnormality is found in as many as 12% of males.[16] Testicular torsion can also occur following exercise, sexual activity, or trauma, or it may develop at rest.

Signs and Symptoms

The history of testicular torsion includes the sudden onset of severe unilateral scrotal pain. The most common symptoms include scrotal swelling, abdominal pain, nausea, and vomiting. Less frequently a fever or urinary frequency may be documented. Examination of the scrotum reveals a tender and painful testicle that is often elevated in relationship to the contralateral testicle. The involved testicle often is in a horizontal position rather than its usual vertical orientation. The testicle may be enlarged with scrotal swelling and erythema.[15] Generally elevation of the involved testicle provides no relief of pain as compared with epididymitis, in which pain relief is notable with elevation of the involved testicle.

Referral and Diagnostic Tests

Testicular torsion is a urological emergency (Red Flags—Testicular Torsion).

> ### ⚐ Red Flags for Testicular Torsion
>
> Testicular torsion is a urological emergency requiring emergent medical attention. It presents as follows:
> - Scrotal swelling
> - Abdominal pain
> - Nausea and vomiting
> - Tender testicle
> - Elevated testicle compared with uninvolved one
> - Possible horizontal rather than vertical orientation

The consideration of a diagnosis requires immediate and emergent evaluation by the team physician or immediate referral to an emergency department. Diagnosis and treatment within 6 hours of the onset of pain result in an 80% to 100% salvage rate for the affected testicle. Beyond this time frame, the salvage rate steadily decreases and approaches 0% at 12 hours.[17]

Initial laboratory tests often include a urinalysis and complete blood count. The urinalysis is most often normal but may demonstrate leukocytes in up to 30% of cases. The serum leukocyte count is elevated in just 60% of individuals with testicular torsion.[15]

Imaging studies can provide useful information, but since testicular torsion is a clinical diagnosis, treatment should not be delayed for imaging if the diagnosis is clear. For those cases in which the diagnosis is less clear, color Doppler ultrasonography can be performed.[18] A color Doppler is used to assess arterial blood flow to the testicle. A radionuclide scan can also be performed to assess arterial blood flow, with decreased uptake indicating a lack of blood flow to the testicle.

Differential Diagnosis

Because testicular torsion is a urological emergency there is little room for error in diagnosis. The differential diagnosis, however, should include epididymitis, orchitis, hydrocele, varicocele, a hernia, and acute appendicitis.

Treatment

Early diagnosis and referral are the keys to successful treatment. Once testicular torsion is diagnosed, a manual reduction can be attempted by the physician. Because most testicular torsion involves a "turning in" toward the midline, the process of detorsion involves rotating the affected testicle 180 degrees from medial to lateral. This rotation may need to be repeated two or three times for a complete detorsion. Success is determined by a marked decrease in pain. Detorsion can be accomplished manually in 30% to 70% of affected individuals.[15] If manual detorsion is not successful, surgery is indicated for definitive treatment and involves detorsion and orchiopexy.

Prognosis and Return to Participation

The prognosis for testicular torsion depends on rapid referral and diagnosis. If detorsion is obtained within 6 hours of onset of symptoms, nearly 100% of torsive testicles can be salvaged. A delay in treatment up to 12 hours results in decreasing rates of salvage, and beyond 12 hours virtually all torsive testicles must be removed.[17] Return to participation is based on the result of the torsion and physician clearance.

Prevention

Other than early identification of the bell clapper deformity, no preventive measures can prevent a testicular torsion. Wearing an athletic supporter may lower the risk of torsion.

Hydrocele

Hydroceles are fluid collections within the tunica vaginalis of the scrotum or along the spermatic cord. Most hydroceles are developmental in origin because of persistence of a patent processus vaginalis. However, for unknown reasons hydroceles can also develop as a result of an imbalance between scrotal fluid production and absorption. It is estimated that approximately 6% of adult males have a clinically apparent hydrocele.

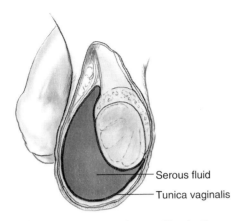

Figure 7-10 Hydrocele is a painless swelling in the scrotum. (From Jarvis C: *Physical examination & health assessment,* ed 4, Philadelphia, 2004, WB Saunders, p 746.)

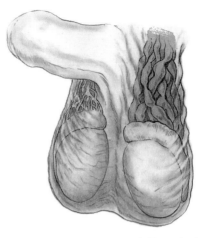

Figure 7-11 Varicocele in the spermatic cord. (From Jarvis C: *Physical examination & health assessment,* ed 4, Philadelphia, 2004, WB Saunders, p 745.)

Signs and Symptoms

Hydroceles are usually asymptomatic. Increased fluid collections, however, can cause a scrotal aching. A hydrocele typically manifests itself as a nontender fullness in the hemiscrotum and is palpable just anterior to the testicle. Inability to clearly delineate or palpate the testicular structures or the presence of tenderness raises the possibility of an alternate diagnosis (Figure 7-10).

Referral and Diagnostic Tests

Athletic trainers should immediately refer any male with painful scrotal swelling to a physician. Although a hydrocele is not an emergency, nontender scrotal swelling that is consistent with a hydrocele needs to be examined by a physician to document its presence. An experienced physician can confirm the diagnosis of a hydrocele. An ultrasound may be performed to confirm the diagnosis in some cases.

Differential Diagnosis

Differential diagnoses for hydrocele include varicocele, epididymitis, orchitis, inguinal hernia, testicular tumor, cancer, and testicular torsion.

Treatment

Asymptomatic adults with an isolated hydrocele can be observed indefinitely or until they become symptomatic. Surgical intervention is warranted for the following indications: inability to distinguish hydrocele from an inguinal hernia, failure to resolve spontaneously after an appropriate interval of observation, inability to clearly examine the testes, or association of hydroceles with suggestive pathology, such as testicular torsion or tumor. Return to sport may take 2 to 6 weeks following a simple hydrocele repair.

Box 7-2	Staging of Varicoceles

Varicoceles are staged according to size:
- Large: those easily identified by inspection alone
- Moderate: those identified by palpation without Valsalva's maneuver
- Small: those identified by palpation using Valsalva's maneuver to increase intraabdominal pressure, which will impede venous drainage and increase varicocele size

Prognosis and Return to Participation

The presence of a hydrocele does not preclude participation in athletics. If the hydrocele is symptomatic or has been surgically repaired, the treating physician will need to make a decision regarding return to play.

Varicocele

A **varicocele** is a dilation of the pampiniform venous plexus and the internal spermatic vein within the scrotum (Figure 7-11). The etiology of a varicocele is unclear. Varicoceles occur in approximately 20% of the adult male population; however, about 40% of infertile men may have a varicocele.[19]

Signs and Symptoms

Approximately 80% to 90% of varicoceles occur on the left side of the scrotum because of anatomical vascular differences.[19] Men are generally asymptomatic but will occasionally report an aching pain or heaviness in the scrotum. Physical examination demonstrates a soft thickening just above the testicle and has been described as feeling like a "bag of worms." Varicoceles are staged according to size (Box 7-2).

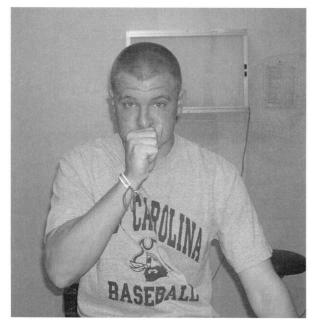

Figure 7-12 In Valsalva's maneuver the athlete is asked to exhale against a closed epiglottis (bearing down).

Referral and Diagnostic Tests

The development of a new varicocele or sudden onset of testicular swelling or pain requires immediate physician evaluation. Any male athlete with a known varicocele who develops increasing testicular pain also warrants physician evaluation. Referral to an urologist for a surgical opinion is indicated when there is significant testicular pain, impairment of testicular function as evidenced by decreased semen quality, or testicular atrophy (volume <20 ml or length <4 cm).

The diagnosis of a varicocele is typically clear by physical examination; Valsalva's maneuver may aid diagnosis (Figure 7-12). If the physical exam is equivocal a Doppler ultrasonogram may be performed to demonstrate the varicocele. Individuals who have a new or sudden-onset varicocele or a nonreducible varicocele in the recumbent position may warrant abdominal CT to evaluate for renal or vascular pathology as a cause of spermatic vein compression.

Differential Diagnosis

The differential diagnosis for a varicocele includes hydrocele, testicular torsion, epididymitis, orchitis, testicular cancer, and spermatic vein compression caused by a renal or vascular tumor.

Treatment

There is no medical treatment per se for an asymptomatic varicocele. Surgical treatment involves the ligation

of the involved veins in order to prevent continued abnormal blood flow.

Prognosis and Return to Participation

The presence of a varicocele poses no known risks to the athlete involved in individual or team sports. Following surgical correction of a varicocele, return to play is generally within 2 to 6 weeks but will depend on the specific circumstances for the athlete and the recommendations of the surgeon. Use of a protective cup is recommended for involvement in contact or collision sports if early return is allowed.[19]

Testicular Cancer

Testicular cancer is an abnormal growth of cells in the testicles. It accounts for 1% to 2% of all cancers in men and typically affects a single testicle. Because of the high cure rate if diagnosed early, nearly 100% of men with this cancer are cured.

Testicular cancer typically affects men between the ages of 18 to 44 years. Conditions that are associated with an increased risk of testicular cancer include **cryptorchidism** (i.e., failure of one or both testicles to descend into the scrotum during development), maternal exposure to **diethylstilbestrol** (DES) while pregnant, testicular atrophy, and some possible environmental and drug exposures.[20]

Signs and Symptoms

Any new or unexpected change in the testicles should prompt an evaluation by a physician. The most common findings noted by the athlete or during the self-testicular exam include a painless swelling (58%), a growth (27%), or pain (33%) in the testicle (Red Flags—Testicular Cancer). Less commonly, a sense of

---

> ► **Red Flags for Testicular Cancer** ═══
> Warning signs for testicular cancer include the following:
> - Painless testicular swelling
> - Testicular growth
> - Painful testicle

---

heaviness or prolonged aching in the testicles may be noted. Rarely, breast tenderness (3%) may occur as the initial sign and is the result of hormonal changes caused by the cancer.

Referral and Diagnostic Tests

Any male with an abnormal testicular exam, a new painless testicular growth, swelling, or testicular pain should be referred to the team physician for further evaluation. Physical examination of the testicles by the athlete or a physician can determine if a palpable mass or swelling is present. An ultrasound of the scrotum and testicles is then performed to document the presence or absence of an abnormality. Confirmatory testing is by tissue diagnosis that is most commonly obtained by radical **orchiectomy** (i.e., surgical removal of the testicle and spermatic cord). In the presence of testicular cancer, a chest radiograph and CT of the abdomen and pelvis are performed to evaluate for metastatic spread of the disease.

Differential Diagnosis

The differential diagnoses for testicular cancer include orchitis, epididymitis, hydrocele, and varicocele.

Treatment

The initial treatment for testicular cancer is a radical orchiectomy involving the testicle and spermatic cord. Therapy is then based on tumor type (i.e., **seminoma,** nonseminoma, or other), microscopic appearance, location and extension of the tumor, and both physician and patient preference. Treatment options include chemotherapy, radiation therapy, and surgical resection of lymph nodes.[20] Overall treatment success is high for testicular cancer. Follow-up care is essential, is based on tumor type, and involves periodic chest radiographs, CT scans, and blood tests for tumor markers.

Individuals undergoing orchiectomy are often counseled to consider sperm banking since return of testicular function following radiotherapy or chemotherapy can be prolonged.

Prognosis and Return to Participation

Cure rates for testicular cancer are high, ranging from greater than 80% for more disseminated cancers to nearly 100% for cancers localized to the testicle. During treatment, individual participation in athletics may be limited because of pain or discomfort afforded by the treatment. Specific decisions about the degree of involvement that can be undertaken in athletics will need to be determined by the treating physician in conjunction with the athlete. Following successful treatment of testicular cancer, there are no contraindications to participation in athletics, although use of a support cup is recommended in contact or collision sports to protect the remaining testicle.

Prevention

There is no known way to prevent testicular cancer. Recommendations are for men (particularly those ages 16 to 44 years) to perform monthly testicular self-exams (Box 7-3). This act can help in the early recognition and diagnosis of testicular cancer thereby improving overall survival.

Prostate Cancer

As discussed at the beginning of the chapter, the prostate gland is responsible for contributing to the seminal fluid and is located directly anterior to the rectum (see Figure 7-5). Prostate cancer is an abnormal growth of cells within the prostate gland. It is the second leading cause of cancer deaths for men in the United States, and African-American men have a higher death rate from this cancer than those in all other ethnic groups.[21] The incidence of prostate cancer increases with age with an estimate that 1 in 10 men will develop prostate cancer in his lifetime. Risk factors for the development of prostate cancer include advancing age, a family history of prostate cancer, tobacco use, ethnicity, and diets high in the consumption of animal fats or chromium.[22-24]

Signs and Symptoms

No reliable signs or symptoms suggest the early presence of prostate cancer. Advanced or metastatic prostate cancer may result in fatigue associated with anemia,

---

Box 7-3   Testicular Self-Exam

Men should perform testicular self-exam (TSE) monthly. It consists of examining and palpating the scrotum for lumps or swelling and bringing any abnormality to a physician's attention:

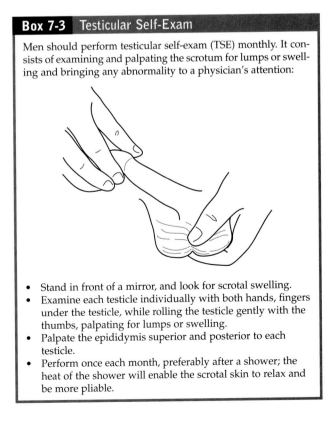

- Stand in front of a mirror, and look for scrotal swelling.
- Examine each testicle individually with both hands, fingers under the testicle, while rolling the testicle gently with the thumbs, palpating for lumps or swelling.
- Palpate the epididymis superior and posterior to each testicle.
- Perform once each month, preferably after a shower; the heat of the shower will enable the scrotal skin to relax and be more pliable.

weight loss, hematuria, urinary retention (caused by obstruction), urinary incontinence, back pain, pathological fractures, or spinal cord compression.

Referral and Diagnostic Tests

Any male athlete suspected of having prostate cancer should be referred to his physician, and any male athlete over the age of 40 years is encouraged to obtain a yearly digital rectal exam.

The early diagnosis of prostate cancer is based on a medical history, physical examination that includes a digital rectal exam in order to palpate the prostate, and a **prostate-specific antigen (PSA)** test. It is worth noting that the upper limit of a normal PSA is related to age, and elevated PSA levels may not always be present in relatively higher-grade prostate cancers.[25] When cancer is suspected, an ultrasound examination with a transrectal needle biopsy can often provide a definitive tissue diagnosis. Once prostate cancer is diagnosed, further testing and imaging for staging of the cancer are performed. These tests generally include complete blood count, serum chemistries, liver function tests, PSA, free PSA/total PSA ratio, alkaline phosphatase, and urinalysis. Imaging studies can include chest radiographs, CT or magnetic resonance imaging (MRI) of the abdomen and pelvis, Prostascint scan (i.e., immunoscintigraphy used to detect extraprostatic spread), and bone scan.

Differential Diagnosis

Conditions that involve the prostate gland include benign prostatic hypertrophy, both acute and chronic prostatitis, **prostatic calculi,** prostate cysts, and **prostatic tuberculosis.** Other cancers that can mimic prostate cancer include lymphomas. Occasionally **Paget's disease,** a bone disease, can mimic bony metastatic lesions of prostate cancer.

Treatment

The treatment strategies for prostate cancer are changing with new advances. At the present time, general recommendations favor early versus delayed treatment and radiation or hormone therapy for locally advanced prostate cancer. The management of metastatic prostate cancer involves the addition of palliative radiation therapy to sites of painful metastases. Specific treatment regimens will be outlined with the athlete and his physicians.

Prognosis and Return to Participation

Mortality rates from prostate cancer are declining in the United States. Early diagnosis of prostate cancer can lead to the detection of prostate cancer confined to the prostate gland and subsequently improved survival. The overall prognosis in terms of survival is related to the tumor size, lymph node involvement, and presence or absence of metastases. For small cancers, localized within the prostate gland itself, overall survival is excellent and a cure may be expected. In contrast, the 10-year survival rate for men with aggressive cancers that have metastasized is 25%.

Athletes may return to their sport during treatment for prostate cancer if they feel well and have no significant side effects to their treatment regimen.

Prevention

Prostate cancer prevention involves risk factor modification and regular prostate screening. Men at risk for the development of prostate cancer should consider diets low in animal fats and chromium, regular exercise, and digital rectal exams every year starting at age 40 years.

PATHOLOGICAL CONDITIONS OF THE GYNECOLOGICAL SYSTEM

Vaginitis

Vaginitis is an inflammation, usually derived from infection, of the vagina. In the sexually active athlete, bacterial vaginosis (BV), trichomoniasis, and candidiasis are three common conditions that may account for 90% of all cases of vaginitis.[26]

The normal vaginal environment is relatively stable. Bacteria are an important component of this environment and help to maintain an acidic pH. An abnormality or disruption in this system can create an environment that allows for the growth of pathogens and subsequent infection. Examples may include frequent douching, antibiotics or certain other medications, intercourse, foreign objects in the vagina, STDs, and pregnancy. Chemicals or foreign objects can also cause inflammation of the vagina. In addition, wearing certain undergarments (i.e., thongs) can transport bacteria from the anus, thereby introducing foreign bacteria to the vagina.

Bacterial vaginosis occurs when the normal balance of bacteria in the vagina is disrupted. A shift in the dominance or overgrowth of certain bacteria causes symptoms. This is not an STD but may be more common in sexually experienced individuals and occur secondary to sexual intercourse, which can change the vaginal environment.

Candidiasis also is not an STD, but it is more common than BV in the sexually naïve individual. Candidiasis is often called a yeast infection; individuals with diabetes or who are immunocompromised are at greater risk. Other risk factors may include pregnancy, obesity, and wearing nonbreathable or close-fitting underwear.

Signs and Symptoms

Vaginal discharge is a common symptom in vaginitis. However, the description of the discharge differs depending on the cause. BV discharge is typically thin, white or gray in color, and malodorous. The athlete may also experience vaginal itching.

An athlete with a *Trichomonas* infection may not have any symptoms, but a discharge described as thick, frothy, and green or yellow is not uncommon. The athlete may experience vaginal itching or discomfort with voiding, although this does not occur in the majority of cases.

Last, athletes with candidiasis may experience a thick, white discharge resembling cottage cheese that is associated with itching or burning. This may also involve the vulva and surrounding skin and is thus termed vulvovaginitis.

Referral and Diagnostic Tests

Any athlete with vaginitis benefits from referral to a physician because diagnosis requires a pelvic exam and treatment typically involves prescription medication.

Initially, a sexually active athlete with vaginal discharge is evaluated for STDs in general. The diagnosis of the common causes for vaginitis involves sampling the discharge or vaginal fluid, measuring pH of the secretions, and performing microscopic examination of the vaginal fluid. Trichomonads can be seen microscopically and are described as "swimming" on the slide. Microscopic findings for BV include "clue cells," which are vacuolated epithelial cells. Demonstration of pseudohyphae and budding yeast on a potassium hydroxide (KOH) preparation suggests candidiasis.

Another diagnostic tool, in which KOH is added to the sample, is called the whiff test. If the discharge is due to BV, a particular fishy odor may be noted. Measurement of the vaginal pH is also helpful with diagnosis. BV and trichomoniasis tend to occur when the pH is less acidic (>4.5). Other more sophisticated tests are available but not necessarily needed for the diagnosis.

Differential Diagnosis

The differential diagnosis for an athlete with vaginal discharge includes STDs. Other causes for vaginal inflammation include contact dermatitis, where the skin reacts to some chemical or object that has come in contact with it; a retained foreign object, such as toilet tissue, tampon, or condom; chemical irritants; and much less commonly a neoplasm, such as cervical or vaginal cancer.

Treatment

Metronidazole is used to treat both BV and trichomoniasis. The athlete must abstain from alcohol while taking the medication because the combination can cause nausea and vomiting. Treatment for vulvovaginal candidiasis includes the use of antifungal agents, either oral or topical, many of which are available over the counter (see Chapter 3). Occasionally, vaginitis of fungal origin is resistant to initial therapy and further evaluation and treatment are required. Including yogurt with active cultures in the diet can help with certain cases of vaginitis, such as those related to an athlete taking antibiotics, because yogurt helps promote stabilization of the normal bacterial flora. Partners of those found to have a *Trichomonas* infection also need to receive treatment to prevent further spread.

Prognosis and Return to Participation

The prognosis is good for common causes of vaginitis, and interference with athletic activity is not typical; therefore return to play is not usually delayed. Problems related to BV and trichomoniasis, however, can occur during pregnancy and may include the risk for premature labor and premature rupture of membranes. In addition, athletes with frequently recurring vulvovaginitis may have an underlying disorder, such as diabetes or a compromised immune system, although other systemic symptoms or complaints would likely be present in these cases.

Prevention

For **trichomoniasis,** an STD, prevention consists of abstinence from sexual intercourse or protection with a condom. The prevention of vaginitis caused by BV or *Candida* is aided by the promotion of a normal vaginal environment, which is facilitated by avoidance of douching, wearing breathable cotton underwear, and the use of condoms during intercourse.

Special Concerns

None of these causes of vaginitis are reportable to a public agency; however, a partner of an athlete with trichomoniasis must be treated for the disease in order to prevent its spread or recurrence.

It is especially important to treat vaginitis caused by BV or trichomoniasis in the pregnant female because it may place her at risk for complications (e.g., premature rupture of membranes or premature labor).

Such complications can be prevented with prompt diagnosis and treatment. The athletic trainer needs to encourage any athlete with recurrent or chronic vaginitis despite treatment to be carefully evaluated for underlying causes to ensure proper treatment.

Pelvic Inflammatory Disease

In generally accepted terms, primary pelvic inflammatory disease (PID) is defined as a bacterial infection of the upper genital tract that originates in and ascends from the lower genital tract (Figure 7-13). Sites of infection include the endometrium, parametrium, fallopian tubes, ovaries, and pelvic peritoneum. These infections usually are a result of sexually transmitted organisms, such as *Chlamydia trachomatis* and *Neisseria gonorrhoeae*.

Signs and Symptoms

The signs and symptoms of PID vary over a large spectrum, from mild or relatively few symptoms to severe symptoms. Diagnosing even the mildest cases is important, however, because sequelae from this disease can be problematic. Typically, symptoms begin within the first couple of weeks following menses, and subtle findings can include abnormal vaginal bleeding or **dyspareunia** (i.e., painful intercourse). Because no exam finding or laboratory test is optimal in diagnosing PID, the Centers for Disease Control and Prevention (CDC) list the minimum criteria: lower abdominal tenderness, **adnexal** tenderness, and cervix motion tenderness without evidence of a different, obvious source.

To further clarify diagnosis, the CDC also includes the following: fever above 38.3° C (101° F); elevated erythrocyte sedimentation rate (ESR); elevated C-reactive protein (CRP); the presence of leukocytes on a saline preparation of vaginal secretions; abnormal cervical or vaginal discharge particularly mucopurulent discharge, and documented cervical infection with *Neisseria gonorrhoeae* or *Chlamydia trachomatis* (Red Flags—Pelvic Inflammatory Disease). More definitive

> ### ▶ Red Flags for Pelvic Inflammatory Disease
> Female athletes with any of the following signs or symptoms should be referred to a physician:
> - Abnormal vaginal bleeding
> - Lower abdominal tenderness
> - Fever
> - Abnormal vaginal discharge
> - Amenorrhea (3 months or more)

answers can include surgical sampling of tissue, which is not without its own risks and can lead to false-negative results.

Referral and Diagnostic Tests

Symptoms or a health history that raises suspicion for PID warrants urgent referral to a physician. If appendicitis or other emergent surgical problems are suspected, immediate referral to a physician or emergency department is warranted.

Every female athlete of reproductive age presenting with pelvic complaints or symptoms requires a pregnancy test to evaluate the possibility of pregnancy. Because of the varying presence of signs and symptoms, it is prudent to obtain a urinalysis to evaluate for urinary tract problems. Other specific tests include a cervical or vaginal smear to be evaluated for the presence of leukocytes, overwhelming bacterial load, or trichomonads and possibly a Gram stain to identify specific organisms. A cervical culture for gonorrhea and chlamydia is performed. Blood tests with a CBC and differential, ESR, and CRP also are performed. If the diagnosis is unclear, a pelvic ultrasound may be performed to evaluate for other abnormalities.

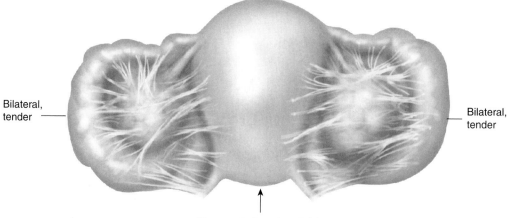

Bilateral, tender

Bilateral, tender

Movement of cervix painful

Figure 7-13 Pelvic inflammatory disease. (From Seidel HM, Ball JW, Dains JE, Benedict GW: *Mosby's guide to physical examination,* ed 5, St Louis, 2003, Mosby, p 644.)

Differential Diagnosis

The differential diagnosis of a female athlete suspected to have PID may include inflammation or infection that has occurred in close proximity to the upper genital tract. Appendicitis, classically described as periumbilical pain that radiates to the right lower quadrant, is another process that is typically diagnosed clinically and may be entertained as a possible cause of symptoms. This, however, would have no particular relationship to menses, and such a diagnosis would be more suspicious in someone with anorexia, nausea, and vomiting without symptoms of PID. Other possibilities include, but are not limited to, tubal pregnancy, corpus luteal cyst, endometriosis, mittelschmerz (typically described as a dull pain of short duration at midcycle), gastroenteritis, and lymphadenitis of intestinal lymph nodes. A careful history of symptoms, including fever, genitourinary complaints, and onset of pain especially with relation to the menstrual cycle, and an evaluation for risk factors can provide useful information in the diagnosis of PID.

Treatment

Treatment of PID in an inpatient versus outpatient setting is controversial; however, it is generally accepted that certain individuals need to be treated in a hospital setting (Box 7-4).[27] Medical treatment for PID includes antibacterials. Chapter 3 lists outpatient and inpatient medications geared toward treating the most common bacterial organisms.

Prognosis and Return to Participation

The prompt diagnosis and treatment of PID are crucial because of the sequelae, which include infertility, increased risk of ectopic pregnancy, recurrent infections, and chronic pelvic pain. The risk of infertility is relatively high, increases with subsequent infections, and depends on the severity of the infection and therefore the time between infection and initiation of treatment.

Before return to sports participation by the affected athlete, adequate antibiotic therapy is instituted, fever is resolved, nausea and vomiting are rectified to ensure adequate hydration status, and pelvic or abdominal pain is minimal. If a surgical procedure was performed, the surgeon will determine when return to activity will be allowed.

Prevention

Early diagnosis is important but is not nearly as crucial as prevention. It is important that athletes, both male and female, understand the problems associated with PID and the importance of preventing the transmission of STDs, especially in light of the fact that many who have *Neisseria gonorrhoeae* or *Chlamydia trachomatis* may be asymptomatic. The only proven prevention for transmission of many STDs, besides abstinence, is a correctly used condom. It should also be noted that intrauterine devices and douching may actually increase an individual's risk for disease.

Special Concerns

An athlete who is diagnosed with PID should be tested for other STDs, notably HIV and syphilis, and advised to receive hepatitis B vaccinations if she has not been previously immunized. A Pap smear also is performed to look for pathological changes caused by human papillomavirus (HPV). In addition, the athlete's sexual partner or partners need to be evaluated for gonorrhea and chlamydia infection and treated if there was sexual contact within 60 days of the patient's symptoms. The athlete should abstain from sexual activity until fully treated. Follow-up testing in 4 to 6 weeks for gonorrhea and chlamydia may be warranted and recommended by the physician. Last, information on STDs and their prevention needs to be made available to all athletes and prevention encouraged.

Dysmenorrhea

Dysmenorrhea is described as severe cramps and pain associated with menstruation or painful menstruation and is categorized as either primary or secondary. Essentially, primary dysmenorrhea is not associated with gross pathology but rather involves a type of prostaglandin that acts to constrict blood vessels within the uterus, causing ischemia and subsequently painful uterine contractions during menstruation.

Secondary dysmenorrhea, by contrast, is caused by a gross pathological process involving the uterus. This can include endometriosis in which endometrial tissue is found outside the uterus, PID, uterine fibroids or polyps, pelvic tumors, ectopic pregnancy, and spontaneous abortion. In these cases, the painful uterine contractions are a result of the associated condition.

Box 7-4   Hospitalization for Patients with Pelvic Inflammatory Disease

Patients with PID who require hospitalization for treatment include the following:
- Patients who require surgical intervention for an ectopic pregnancy or abscess that requires drainage
- Pregnant patients
- Patients not responding to outpatient therapy
- Patients noncompliant with therapy or follow-up within 48 to 72 hours
- Patients who are immunocompromised

Signs and Symptoms

Primary dysmenorrhea may be more common in the first few years after menarche and in those whose gravity and parity status is low. The athlete may also have a significant family history for this condition. In addition, smoking, early menarche, and a history of heavy flow and long menstrual periods may be risk factors associated with more severe dysmenorrhea.[28] Symptoms may include not only cramping of the lower abdomen or back, with occasional radiating pain to the thighs, but also nausea, vomiting, diarrhea, headaches, and other systemic problems. The pain and associated symptoms typically begin just before or at the onset of menses and last through the first day or two of menstruation. Physical examination yields no obvious pathology.

Secondary dysmenorrhea may not be as closely tied to the onset of menses, and symptoms last for a longer time but may still have some relation to the menstrual cycle. Physical exam may or may not provide an etiology, and symptoms may vary depending on the underlying pathology. If an athlete has been diagnosed with primary dysmenorrhea and treatment such as nonsteroidal antiinflammatory agents or oral contraceptives has failed, then a pathological cause must be considered and the athlete should be reevaluated.

Referral and Diagnostic Tests

Athletes who experience severe menstrual pain, who have pertinent systemic complaints as mentioned previously, or who have abnormal menstruation need to be routinely referred to a physician for evaluation.

As always, a thorough history and physical exam are warranted with a presentation of dysmenorrhea. A careful health history of the athlete's menstruation including age of onset, length, frequency, flow, and regularity of cycling; sexual activity history; family history; and type and severity of associated symptoms are all helpful. Any female athlete being evaluated for dysmenorrhea warrants a pregnancy test, regardless of sexual history. Depending on the athlete's history and the physical exam, other diagnostic tests may be necessary. Options include pelvic ultrasound; **laparoscopy,** which is a direct visualization of the pelvic organs via a surgical procedure; **hysteroscopy,** which views the inside of the cervix and uterus using an endoscope; and radiological procedures. In some cases tissue sampling or endometrial biopsy may be required for review by a pathologist.

Differential Diagnosis

Differential diagnoses for dysmenorrhea include endometriosis, PID, uterine fibroids or polyps, pelvic tumors, ectopic pregnancy, or spontaneous abortion.

Treatment

The management of dysmenorrhea varies according to its etiology. For primary dysmenorrhea, nonsteroidal antiinflammatory drugs (NSAIDs) as well as oral contraceptives have been the mainstay of treatment. NSAIDs should be taken just before the onset of menses and continued through the first few days of the menses. They function to decrease levels of the inciting prostaglandins. Oral contraceptives alone or in combination with NSAIDs can be beneficial.

Treatment for secondary dysmenorrhea depends on the pathological etiology as previously discussed. Secondary dysmenorrhea should be considered in someone with primary dysmenorrhea who does not respond well to treatment.

Prognosis and Return to Participation

Dysmenorrhea can certainly be disabling to those affected; however, several treatment options exist for the varying etiologies, and prognosis generally is good. Sports participation may be limited only by the athlete's symptoms, unless the athlete is being treated for a certain pathological condition that may, as directed by the physician, exclude her from strenuous physical activity.

Prevention

There is no primary prevention for primary dysmenorrhea. Secondary prevention for primary dysmenorrhea stems from its treatment. Starting NSAIDs before menses, when pain would typically develop, or taking oral contraceptives lends itself toward this secondary prevention. For secondary dysmenorrhea, only certain causes, such as PID and STDs, are preventable by employing safe-sex practices.

Special Concerns

Older female athletes with dysmenorrhea are more likely to have a secondary or pathological cause for their discomfort and warrant close evaluation.

Amenorrhea

Amenorrhea is typically categorized as primary or secondary. Primary amenorrhea is classically defined as the absence of menarche (i.e., onset of menses) before the age of 16 years. Secondary amenorrhea is less well defined but alludes to the fact that a female's menstruation has stopped after having been previously normal. Depending on the source, secondary amenorrhea may be defined as either (1) the absence of menses for 3, 4, 6, or 12 months in a previously menstruating female or (2) fewer than three menstrual cycles per year.[29] To add further confusion, **oligomenorrhea** is used to describe menstrual cycles whose intervals are greater than 36 days but less than 90 days. Since the cause for oligomenorrhea is often the same as for amenorrhea, this section will mainly focus on amenorrhea but with the knowledge that this may apply to many cases of missed menstrual periods in general.

The cause for amenorrhea, both primary and secondary, is highly variable. To understand the various etiologies, a basic understanding of ovulation is necessary. The ovulatory pathway consists of the hypothalamic-pituitary axis, the ovaries, a feedback loop, the uterus, and a subsequent outflow tract. The hypothalamus secretes gonadotropin-releasing hormone (GnRH) that stimulates the pituitary gland to secrete follicle-stimulating hormone (FSH) and luteinizing hormone (LH). These hormones then stimulate the ovaries to produce estrogen and progesterone, which each directly affect the menstrual process (see Figure 7-8). Low circulating levels of these hormones, in turn, have a direct feedback to the hypothalamus to produce more GnRH. One can therefore imagine both hormonal and anatomical problems that can interfere with normal ovulation.

The source of amenorrhea depends on the cause. In general terms, anatomical defects can occur that are congenital, genetic, or acquired. Ovarian failure can occur prematurely. Chronic anovulation or the absence of ovulation in the presence of estrogen, such as **polycystic ovarian disease** or certain tumors, can occur. Chronic anovulation also can occur in the absence of estrogen or in hypogonadotropic **hypogonadism,** such as occurs with athletic amenorrhea, stress, anorexia nervosa, and pituitary tumors.[29]

Signs and Symptoms

Signs and symptoms of amenorrhea vary greatly and depend on the etiology of the amenorrhea. For primary amenorrhea, genetic disorders and anatomical abnormalities of the reproductive system must be considered. A classic example of a genetic defect is **Turner's syndrome** (45X), which would have physical findings such as short stature, webbed neck, shield chest, increased carrying angle of the elbows, as well as other possible findings (Figure 7-14).

Problems with the outflow tract can also cause amenorrhea. If there is no exit path for the sloughed endometrial lining, then the athlete perceives there is no menses but may have severe cramping and pain from retained tissue and blood with each menstrual period. Obstruction can be congenital, such as imperforate hymen or labial **agglutination,** or can occur secondarily, such as with **uterine synechiae** or scarring as seen in **Asherman's syndrome** following a surgical procedure.

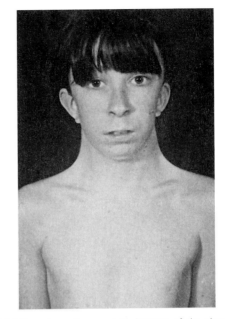

Figure 7-14 Turner's syndrome results because of the absence of one X chromosome. (From Epstein O, Perkin GD, Cookson J, de Bono DP: *Clinical examination,* ed 3, Philadelphia, 2003, Mosby, p 22.)

Proceeding further up the ovulatory chain, ovarian failure from various causes can lead to amenorrhea. It can be related to genetic defects, autoimmune disorders, or prior chemotherapy and can be associated with various symptoms. Not uncommonly, an individual may have symptoms similar to menopausal women, namely, hot flashes, vaginal dryness, and mood changes to name a few. The athlete may also have systemic symptoms common to particular autoimmune or endocrine disorders. For example, an athlete with hypothyroidism may exhibit fatigue, weight gain, constipation, or cold intolerance.

Problems with the hypothalamic-pituitary axis are varied as well. Deficient, absent, or inappropriate secretion of GnRH from the hypothalamus is common in female athletes, which in turn results in amenorrhea. Not all female athletes are affected, and some are at greater risk than others. The athlete's diet, her particular sport and level of activity, as well as genetic composition are among possible factors involved with athletic amenorrhea. Diagnosis of athletic amenorrhea is important since a hypoestrogenemia state, such as occurs with athletic amenorrhea and ovarian failure, can adversely affect bone mineral density, leading to fractures.[30] The athletic trainer needs to look for signs or symptoms of disordered eating in the evaluation of the athlete because this remains a common and well-described entity (see Chapter 15).[29]

Another potential cause for amenorrhea that involves the hypothalamic-pituitary axis is inhibition of gonadotropin-releasing hormone (GnRH) by increased prolactin levels, which can occur as a result of a pituitary tumor that could have neurological manifestations such as headaches and visual disturbances as well as a complaint of galactorrhea. Polycystic ovary syndrome is a common entity that is manifested by findings such as **hyperandrogenism** (with associated acne and **hirsutism**), obesity, and hyperinsulinemia.

Referral and Diagnostic Tests

Athletes with primary amenorrhea are referred to a physician for a complete evaluation. An athlete who has had normal menstrual cycles but who misses three consecutive periods or who is oligomenorrheic needs to be evaluated by a physician. However, missing just one or two menses is not always benign and one must not allow the number of missed menses to define the line between passiveness and concern.

The work-up for amenorrhea involves assessment of the neuroendocrine system, genetics, anatomy of the athlete, and a pregnancy test. A complete medical history, including exercise, nutrition, menstrual history, and physical examination, should be performed. Laboratory evaluation may include a urine pregnancy test and blood tests for thyroid-stimulating hormone (TSH), FSH, estradiol, and prolactin. Testing for levels of LH, dehydroepiandrosterone (DHEA), and testosterone may be indicated depending on the history and physical examination. In addition, the physician may elect to perform a progestin challenge to see if the endometrium has been primed by estrogen and if there is a patent outflow tract. With proper estrogen priming of the endometrium, its lining should slough after withdrawal of progesterone, as it would with normal menstruation.

Other laboratory evaluations may include karyotyping to check for any chromosomal abnormalities. This will also provide evidence for presence or absence of a Y chromosome. Depending on the history, laboratory, and exam findings, neuroimaging may be helpful to look for an intracranial mass, specifically involving the pituitary. Other imaging may include evaluation of the reproductive tract and the gonads.

A bone density assessment should be considered in all female athletes with a prolonged history of oligomenorrhea or more than 6 months of amenorrhea, particularly in those with a history of disordered eating.[29]

Treatment

The treatment of amenorrhea depends on its etiology and the sequelae one is trying to eliminate or prevent. One such problem is low bone mineral density or other effects of a hypoestrogenemia state. Treatment may consist of dietary changes to improve overall energy balance, hormone replacement therapy, and a decrease in the athlete's activity level. In some causes

of amenorrhea, surgery could be required, such as for an athlete with a pituitary tumor or with an outflow tract abnormality. Treatment for polycystic ovarian disease may include oral birth control pills and medications to control the **hyperinsulinemia.** Knowing the underlying cause for amenorrhea is the key in determining treatment.

In the case of athletic amenorrhea, treatment involves both pharmacological and nonpharmacological measures. Oral contraceptives are the mainstay of pharmacological treatment for athletic amenorrhea and should be strongly considered if nonpharmacological measures fail. In the presence of either osteopenia or osteoporosis, nasal calcitonin should be considered. Neither bisphosphonates nor selective estrogen receptor modulators (SERMs) have been well studied in young premenopausal women. Nonpharmacological measures include dietary changes and adjustments in physical activity in order to promote an overall positive energy balance, daily calcium and vitamin D supplements, nutrition counseling, and screening or treatment for disordered eating.

Prognosis and Return to Participation

As with treatment, prognosis relies on the etiology of amenorrhea. The concern for female athletes with amenorrhea caused by low gonadotropin stimulation is the increased risk for low bone mineral density and its sequelae, such as stress fractures. Correcting the underlying conditions, or providing hormone replacement when correcting the cause for hypoestrogenemia is not possible, is important in trying to prevent adverse outcomes for the athlete.

Because the etiology of amenorrhea is broad, return-to-play recommendations for each type are not presented here. Rather, for female athletes with athletic amenorrhea, although multiple factors may contribute to the overall etiology, an intense exercise routine can play a major role. Simply reducing the athlete's level of activity and ensuring an adequate and well-balanced diet may help the athlete to return to a regular menstrual pattern. Therefore returning to play is not prohibited but may be limited, at least initially. Such decisions and treatment plans require the involvement and communication of the athlete, athletic trainer, physician, registered dietitian, coach, and perhaps a mental health provider.

Prevention

Many causes for amenorrhea are not preventable. An important goal for athletes, however, is ensuring that their nutritional intake is adequate and meets the needs placed on them by their activity.

Special Considerations

As discussed previously, special care must be taken when evaluating an athlete for amenorrhea because of its possible complications. In addition to medical intervention, alterations in exercise routine may be required. Nutritional evaluation is also important, especially with athletic amenorrhea or in the presence of an eating disorder. Essentially, the approach may involve a multidisciplinary effort, depending on the cause. Sports participation and age are only relevant depending on the cause and required treatment.

Mittelschmerz

Mittelschmerz is pain secondary to ovulation and hence tends to occur at mid-cycle. The pain associated with ovulation is thought to be due to fluid that is released from the ovary, along with the ovum, during ovulation. This fluid can be irritating to intraabdominal tissue and can cause pain for the female athlete.

Signs and Symptoms

Pain can vary from one individual to another. However, the pain tends to be located in the lower abdomen and usually occurs on one side. This is probably secondary to the unilateral release of the ovum. The affected side may change from one month to the next. Typically, the pain will last minutes to hours and, occasionally, a day or two. Since mittelschmerz is related to ovulation, there will be a history of pain that occurs between menstrual periods.

Referral and Diagnostic Tests

A female athlete who presents with new-onset lower abdominal pain or pelvic pain needs to be referred to a physician for evaluation. If the athlete's pain is associated with nausea, vomiting, or fever, she should be immediately referred to a physician. She should also be referred if the pain is prolonged (i.e., lasts more than 2 days), if the pain is severe or unrelieved by over-the-counter medications, or if there is a suspicion of pregnancy or an STD.

There is no diagnostic test for mittelschmerz; rather, it is a diagnosis of exclusion. A good health history, including menstrual history, is very helpful. Depending on the history and type of pain, a pelvic exam may be warranted to exclude other etiologies. Occasionally imaging, such as ultrasound, can be helpful in looking at anatomy and ruling out certain structural causes. In addition, one should always have a low threshold for ordering a urine pregnancy test.

Differential Diagnosis

Lower abdominal pain in a female athlete can pose a diagnostic dilemma. However, as previously mentioned, a good history can be extremely useful. Certain signs or symptoms are considered serious. periumbilical or right lower quadrant pain associated with nausea, vomiting, or fever should always raise concern for appendicitis. A history (including sexual and menstrual data) along with a physical exam and possibly imaging and laboratory studies can help in diagnosing PID (see Pelvic Inflammatory Disease). Ectopic pregnancy may also be associated with lower abdominal pain and needs to be included in the differential diagnosis, especially if there is a history of PID or prior ectopic pregnancies. Endometriosis, UTI, kidney stones, constipation, and gastroenteritis should also be considered depending on history, onset, and symptoms.

Treatment

The standard treatment for mittelschmerz includes over-the-counter pain medications, including NSAIDs and acetaminophen (Tylenol). Heating packs can alleviate some of the discomfort. In addition, oral contraceptives prevent pain by preventing ovulation.

Prognosis and Return to Participation

The prognosis for mittelschmerz is generally good, and athletic activity is not contraindicated. Although the pain is generally tolerable, it can be significant for some. Again, pain unrelieved by standard medications as aforementioned may warrant referral to a physician.

Prevention

Mittelschmerz pain can be prevented by preventing ovulation through the use of oral contraceptives.

Special Concerns for the Mature Athlete

Ovulation must be occurring for a diagnosis of mittelschmerz; therefore it is not a diagnosis in an athlete who is no longer menstruating.

Ovarian and Cervical Cancer

Ovarian cancer is a malignant cell growth originating from an ovary and is the leading cause of death from a gynecological malignancy in women. Cervical cancer is a malignancy originating from the cervix and has significant morbidity and mortality as well.

Ovarian cancer is typically seen in the older female adult with symptoms usually presenting late in its course. Risk appears to be proportional to the number of times a woman ovulates. For example, women who have never had children are at increased risk. Oral contraceptives that prevent ovulation may decrease a woman's risk. Age is another factor and is related to the greater number of ovulatory cycles experienced. Other risks include family history, personal history of breast or colon cancer, and history of prolonged hormone replacement. Genetic predisposition is an important risk factor, especially with the *BRCA1* gene mutation.

Human papillomavirus (HPV) plays a large role in the development of cervical cancer.[31] Several HPV genotypes exist, but only a few are associated with cervical cancer. This may be why sexual activity plays an important role in the development of this malignancy. Risk factors include sexual activity beginning at a young age, a higher number of sexual partners, a history of other STDs, and smoking.

Signs and Symptoms

Signs and symptoms are not usually present with either ovarian or cervical cancer in the early stages, since symptoms may occur only after the tumor has grown large enough to have some mass effect. Unfortunately, by this time the tumor has likely metastasized to other sites. Symptoms may vary and depend on the size and location of the tumor and sites of metastasis. Gastrointestinal disturbances such as constipation or diarrhea may occur with either malignancy. An individual may also experience early satiety or unexplained weight changes. Vaginal bleeding and discomfort may occur with cervical cancer, as well as urinary complaints. Extension of cervical cancer may obstruct lymphatic and venous drainage causing lower extremity edema, perhaps unilaterally. Symptoms involving other organs depend on metastatic spread. Symptoms for either cancer can be nonspecific and of little diagnostic value.

Referral and Diagnostic Tests

Any suspicion for malignancy requires referral to a physician for evaluation. An athlete with a past history of or family history of malignancy and with unexplained symptoms as previously described needs to be referred. In addition, a female athlete should be encouraged to have routine pelvic exams and Pap smears as outlined by her physician.

Diagnosing ovarian cancer may prove somewhat difficult. Finding an adnexal or pelvic mass on examination is of concern, especially in an older female or a woman with other risk factors for ovarian cancer.

Unfortunately, no good screening test is available. Serum tumor markers are used in the initial evaluation of ovarian cancer but are not appropriate for use as screening tests at this time. Pelvic ultrasound may demonstrate an ovarian mass if suspected or symptoms warrant this examination. Laparoscopy plays an important role in diagnosis and staging of ovarian cancer, since no one laboratory test or imaging technique is sufficient.

The incidence of cervical cancer has decreased in recent years, largely because of screening examinations with the use of the Pap smear. Cells from the cervix are taken and evaluated for atypical or abnormal appearance, with further evaluation and treatment depending on the results. The U.S. Preventive Services Task Force currently recommends every woman be screened by Pap smear at least every 3 years (barring any previous abnormal results) beginning no longer than 3 years after first sexual activity or by age 21 years, whichever comes first. Certain individuals may not require routine screening, such as women over the age of 65 years who have had normal screenings in the past or individuals who have had total hysterectomies but without a history of malignancy or a questionable malignancy. These cases, however, must be individualized and the decision made by the individual woman in consultation with her physician.

Differential Diagnosis

Because the symptoms of ovarian or cervical cancer can be vague or nonspecific, the differential diagnosis can be broad. For both ovarian and cervical cancer, a definitive diagnosis is based on tissue biopsy. For ovarian cancer, a benign ovarian mass or complex cystic ovarian disease is considered in the differential diagnosis as well as localized spread of cancer from surrounding tissues. The differential diagnosis for cervical cancer includes severe cervical dysplasia, vaginal dysplasia or cancer, and uterine cancer with localized spread to the cervix.

Treatment

The treatment of ovarian cancer largely depends on the stage of disease, which is obtained by surgical exploration. There are four stages (I, II, III, IV), with stage IV being the least favorable. The degree of tumor extension plays a large role with regard to staging. Therapies include surgical removal of involved tissue and chemotherapy. Invasive cervical cancer therapies include surgery, radiation therapy, and chemotherapy. Here again, the choice depends on the stage of malignancy.

Several treatments are available for cervical dysplasia (i.e., precancerous lesions) discovered by Pap smear.

Treatment may be as simple as frequent follow-up and repeat Pap smears or may include colposcopy with biopsy or removal of the abnormal tissue.

Prognosis

Morbidity and mortality related to ovarian and cervical cancer are high because of the nature of the disease process and its lack of symptoms early in the course of the disease process. Screening for cervical cancer using the Pap smear has allowed great strides in the prevention of invasive disease. More progress will be made in the detection of HPV and possible prevention of infection, both of which will further aid in cervical cancer prevention.

Athletic participation for women undergoing treatment for ovarian or cervical cancer is limited by the toll of treatment, which can include nausea, vomiting, fatigue, and diarrhea. Treatment requires a multidisciplinary approach, and good communication among all involved is important for the athlete's well-being.

Prevention

Many risk factors for ovarian cancer are difficult to avoid. Probably the best form of prevention is routine medical examinations with special attention placed on those persons with risk factors, such as family history and prior medical history of gynecological malignancy.

As mentioned earlier, cervical cancer has risk factors associated with sexual activity. Therefore alteration in sexual behavior or practices as previously described may decrease an athlete's risk. Routine exams, including screening for cervical lesions, cannot be overemphasized. As previously discussed, current research involves detecting and even preventing infection with HPV genotypes linked to cervical cancer.

Breast Cancer

The breast consists of glands, blood and lymph tissue, fat, and fibrous or connective tissue (Figure 7-15). Underlying the breast is muscle. The lymph tissue drains to nodes in the axillae. To facilitate milk delivery, the breast has numerous milk glands, which open to lobules. Several lobules make up a lobe, and these lobes empty into ducts that deliver the milk to the nipple. The lymphatic system is also an important aspect of the breast (Figure 7-16) and can act as a conduit for cancer to metastasize to other regional or nonregional areas.

A neoplasm arising from the breast tissue is a breast cancer. The majority of breast cancers (~80%) originate in the ducts of the breast with another significant portion (~10% to 15%) originating within the lobules. These cells can escape the breast or metastasize and affect other areas of the body. With the exception of skin cancer, breast cancer is the most commonly

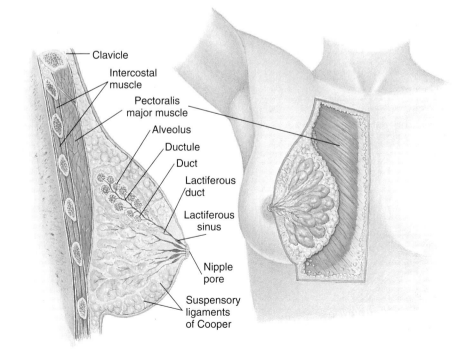

Clavicle
Intercostal muscle
Pectoralis major muscle
Alveolus
Ductule
Duct
Lactiferous duct
Lactiferous sinus
Nipple pore
Suspensory ligaments of Cooper

Figure 7-15 Anatomy of the female breast. (From Seidel HM, Ball JW, Dains JE, Benedict GW: *Mosby's guide to physical examination,* ed 5, St Louis, 2003, Mosby, p 497.)

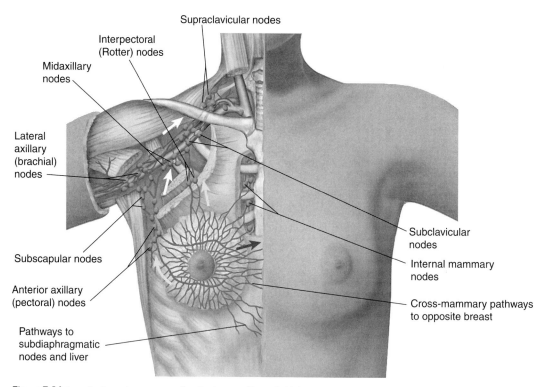

Supraclavicular nodes

Interpectoral
(Rotter) nodes

Midaxillary
nodes

Lateral
axillary
(brachial)
nodes

Subscapular nodes

Anterior axillary
(pectoral) nodes

Pathways to
subdiaphragmatic
nodes and liver

Subclavicular
nodes

Internal mammary
nodes

Cross-mammary pathways
to opposite breast

Figure 7-16 Lymphatic system surrounding the breast. (From Seidel HM, Ball JW, Dains JE, Benedict GW: *Mosby's guide to physical examination,* ed 5, St Louis, 2003, Mosby, p 498.)

diagnosed cancer among American women. In 2004, an estimated 40,580 women will die from breast cancer, and 75% of those diagnosed will be older than 50 years.[32]

Risk factors associated with breast cancer include a person's gender, age, prior history of breast cancer, family history of breast cancer, and genetics. An individual's overall exposure to estrogen, either physiological or by replacement, may increase the risk for breast cancer. Therefore women who have taken hormone replacement for several years, women who began menstruation at an early age, women who experienced menopause at a late age, and women who never had children or began childbearing at a later age may all be at increased risk.

The three major types of breast cancer are described on the basis of their location of origin and histology: infiltrating ductal carcinoma or ductal carcinoma in situ if localized, infiltrating lobular carcinoma or lobular carcinoma in situ if localized, and inflammatory breast carcinoma.

Signs and Symptoms

Early stages of breast cancer usually are silent. The initial tumor is typically painless, and the first sign may be a lump or abnormality noted on a mammogram. Certain findings may occur that should raise suspicion, however, such as a lump in the breast or axilla.

Many of these lumps are benign and associated with fibrocystic change, which may be manifested by breast tenderness just before menstruation. The lump in this case is a fluid-filled cyst rather than a solid, fixed nodule. Other warning signs include nipple discharge, change in size or shape of the breast, change in appearance of the skin overlying the breast, and inversion of the nipple (Box 7-5).

Although breast cancer in men is rare, it does occur. Concerns about breast cancer expressed by the male athlete should not be taken lightly.

Referral and Diagnostic Tests

Although many breast lumps are benign and can have characteristic findings, the importance of a medical evaluation of a lump cannot be underestimated. An athlete with any signs or symptoms of a breast mass or breast changes needs to be referred to a physician. As listed in Box 7-5, these signs include a breast or axillary lump or mass not previously evaluated, nipple discharge, changes in size or shape of the breast, changes in appearance of the skin of the breast, and a newly inverted nipple.

The diagnosis of breast cancer starts with a thorough medical history and physical examination, including breast palpation by a trained medical provider. In the presence of a suspicious palpable breast mass, imaging of the breasts with mammography or ultrasound

Clinical signs of breast cancer include the following:

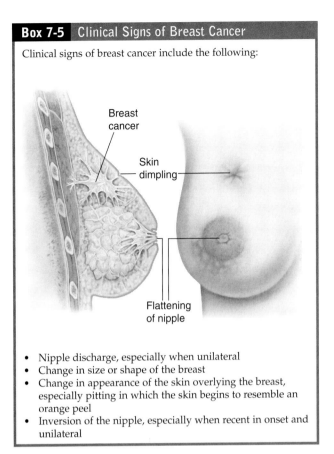

- Nipple discharge, especially when unilateral
- Change in size or shape of the breast
- Change in appearance of the skin overlying the breast, especially pitting in which the skin begins to resemble an orange peel
- Inversion of the nipple, especially when recent in onset and unilateral

may help further clarify the malignant potential of the mass. A potential difficulty in younger female athletes involves their relatively dense breast tissue that may make clear imaging of a mass more difficult.

Other diagnostic tools are more invasive and involve sampling or removing tissue for pathological examination. These tools include fine needle aspiration in which a needle is introduced into the lump and cells are aspirated for cytological examination; core needle biopsy, which introduces a large needle to obtain tissue for pathological review; and surgical biopsy, which involves surgical removal of a portion of the mass or the entire lump and surrounding tissue. These procedures provide a tissue sample to determine a definitive diagnosis.

Differential Diagnosis

The finding of a breast mass can be frightening. Not all masses are cancerous and in fact most are probably benign. In the very young athlete (i.e., before puberty), a lump may appear around the nipple that is followed by a similar occurrence on the other side with both remaining unchanged until some time during puberty. A **fibroadenoma,** which is a firm but painless mass, is typically a benign lesion that tends to occur in the young athlete during the late teens to early thirties.

It is typically well circumscribed and mobile on exam. These lumps tend to persist and sometimes calcify. Fibrocystic change is a common benign breast lesion that consists of fluid-filled cysts within the breast tissue. These cysts or lumps are typically tender, especially just before menses, and may be fluctuant on exam.

Treatment

Treatment for breast cancer largely depends on its progression, which is measured using a staging system. This system uses the tumor's size, lymph node involvement, and location of any metastatic spread in order to stage the cancer. For instance, stage 0 is noninvasive cancer such as **ductal carcinoma in situ** or **lobular carcinoma in situ.** This type of cancer is localized but has the potential for spreading. Stage IV represents the other end of the spectrum where the cancer has metastasized beyond the breast and its lymph nodes. In addition to staging, other factors are extremely important when treating breast cancer. These include the patient's age and general state of health, previous medical history, gender, pregnancy status, menopausal status, as well as the specifics of the tumor itself, such as the presence of certain receptors on the tumor cell.

Multiple therapies exist, including surgery, chemotherapy, radiation therapy, hormone therapy, and biological therapy. Surgery ranges from the common removal of the mass and surrounding tissue, including a sampling of the axillary lymph nodes, to the uncommon removal of the entire breast and its lymph nodes. Often some other form of therapy is used in addition to surgery, especially if only a portion of the breast is removed. This may include radiation, chemotherapy, or hormone therapy, which are also used before surgery for certain larger cancers that may require shrinkage preoperatively.

Prognosis and Return to Participation

The prognosis varies from individual to individual, but overall it is related to the stage of the cancer. Stage IV obviously offers the worst prognosis or 5-year survival. Other factors involved include those used for determining particular treatments, such as the individual's overall health, age, and tumor receptor status. The time to return to sport can range from days to weeks or months and is determined by the overall tumor burden, including metastases, side effects from the particular treatment, and the athlete's medical condition.

Prevention

Because many risk factors associated with breast cancer are not controllable, screening is very important.

Box 7-6   Monthly Breast Self-Exam

It is important for people to be familiar with the usual appearance of their breasts in order to be aware of any changes that occur quickly or over time and that might be warning signs for breast cancer. A monthly breast self-exam is performed by first palpating for lumps or abnormalities.

- Perform the exam 7 to 10 days following the first day of the menstrual cycle.
- Stand and visually inspect breast in a mirror in three positions.

Standing with arms at side

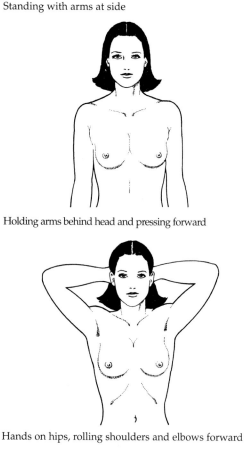

Holding arms behind head and pressing forward

Hands on hips, rolling shoulders and elbows forward

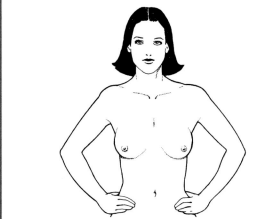

- In the shower, raise one arm, and using at least three or four soapy fingers, palpate the other breast in circles, covering the whole breast, moving in toward the nipple. Repeat with opposite breast.

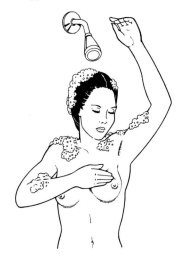

- Palpate the axillary area, since it is rich with lymph nodes and should not contain unusual lumps or masses. Repeat with other breast.
- Squeeze the nipple, and look for any discharge. Perform this bilaterally.

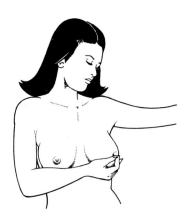

- Repeat the above three steps lying supine.

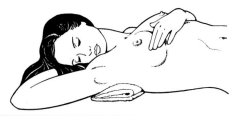

Illustrations from Seidel HM, Ball JW, Dains JE, Benedict GW: *Mosby's guide to physical examination*, ed 5, St Louis, 2003, Mosby, p 502.

Screening includes monthly breast exams performed by the individual athlete (Box 7-6) and exams performed by a medical professional every 2 to 3 years between the ages of 20 and 40 years and yearly thereafter.

Mammography is another screening tool and is recommended every 1 to 2 years after the age of 40 years. Recommendations for breast exams and mammography may need to be altered if the athlete has a past medical history or family history of breast cancer. It would be important for that athlete to seek the advice of a physician regarding screening in such instances.

Prevention for other risk factors may seem extreme but is not uncommon. Preemptive breast removal is occasionally performed for someone without cancer or a lump. For example, an individual with a strong family history for breast cancer or who is known to carry a gene associated with breast cancer (*BRCA1* or *BRCA2*) may elect to have breast removal to preempt the cancer.

Special Concerns

Breast cancer is more common in the mature athlete and in the young athlete who has a strong family history of breast cancer, especially at young ages. It is important that athletes perform regular self-exams and receive screening mammography as recommended.

PREGNANCY

Normal pregnancy consists of a series of remarkable changes that occur within the female body. Multiple organ systems are affected in order to support a growing fetus in addition to maintaining the health of the mother. A few of these important normal changes are highlighted here and a single pathological condition, ectopic pregnancy,v is discussed.

Before becoming pregnant, a woman should maintain proper nutrition, start the use of prenatal vitamins, and discontinue using or avoid potential harmful substances such as tobacco, alcohol, and illicit drugs. Folic acid is present in most prenatal vitamins and is important in helping to prevent neural tube defects in the fetus. It should be taken by all pregnant women.

The initial signs and symptoms of pregnancy include a missed menstrual period and breast swelling or tenderness. Nausea and vomiting, known as morning sickness, may also be present early in the pregnancy and if severe, may compromise hydration, nutrition, and weight gain. Severe cases of nausea and vomiting can lead to hospitalization for fluid replacement, electrolyte correction, and control of emesis. In general, however, symptoms are not this severe and typically subside. In fact, the pregnant woman's fluid status increases during pregnancy. Blood volume increases, as well as intracellular and extracellular fluid. Fluid tends to accumulate more during the day, and dependent swelling is very common.

Physiological changes also occur in pregnancy. As mentioned previously, plasma volume and cardiac output increase as a result of increases in stroke volume and heart rate. In addition, blood pressure decreases in the normal pregnancy because of an overall decrease in systemic vascular resistance. Respiratory changes include an increased tidal volume, increased minute ventilation, and decreased overall airway resistance. Despite these changes, the woman's FEV_1 and respiratory rate usually remain unchanged at rest.

Gastroesophageal reflux is another common symptom occurring among pregnant women and is due to both anatomical and physiological changes. An athlete may note that certain foods aggravate reflux, and avoidance of these foods is prudent. If avoidance of the offending foods does not help, pharmacological therapy may be necessary. This therapy can consist of calcium-containing antacids, histamine (H_2) antagonists, or proton-pump inhibitors as prescribed.

Low back pain is a common complaint as well and is largely due to the woman's altered center of gravity secondary to the enlarging fetus, uterus, and breast tissue. Low back pain is generally more of a problem during the latter stages of pregnancy. Interestingly, although the woman's bones may adjust to the various stresses placed on them, they appear to suffer no ill effects from the high calcium demands of the fetus.

Throughout the course of pregnancy, a woman's breasts enlarge and may become tender. It is also possible for a pregnant woman to notice that she is expressing fluid from her breasts before the birth of her child. The fluid expressed is known as colostrum and is a normal change associated with pregnancy.

Exercise and physical activity for healthy women should be encouraged in pregnancy. Women who exercise regularly in pregnancy have the benefits of improved cardiac function, limited weight gain, improved mental health, and decreased time in labor.[33] Little scientific data address the participation in vigorous and competitive sport by the pregnant athlete, but a few cautious recommendations are noteworthy. Pregnant athletes should avoid exercise in the supine position as much as possible, particularly after the first trimester. Scuba diving and the use of hot tubs, steam baths, and saunas place the fetus at potential risk and are discouraged during pregnancy. In addition, pregnant athletes are generally discouraged from participation in contact or collision sports after the fourteenth week of pregnancy, although this is based on indirect evidence. Further, a pregnant athlete who participates in competitive endurance sports should consider participation at the noncompetitive level for the duration of the pregnancy.

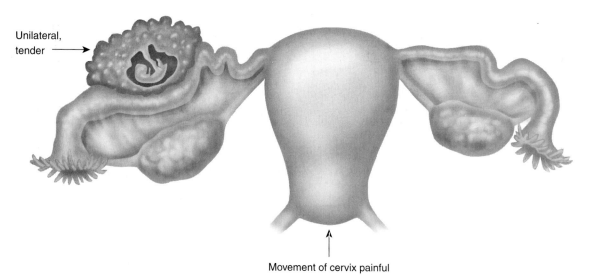

Unilateral, tender

Movement of cervix painful

Figure 7-17 Ectopic pregnancy. (From Seidel HM, Ball JW, Dains JE, Benedict GW: *Mosby's guide to physical examination,* ed 5, St Louis, 2003, Mosby, p 643.)

Box 7-7   NCAA Recommendations and Cautions on Exercise During Pregnancy

The pregnant athlete should do the following:
- Avoid supine exercise after the first trimester
- Be discouraged from heavy weight lifting
- Be discouraged from activities that require Valsalva's maneuver
- Avoid activities associated with a high risk of falling
- Consider noncompetitive activity for those athletes involved in endurance sports
- Avoid contact sports after the fourteenth week of pregnancy even though there are no data regarding contact sports and pregnancy
- Avoid any physical activity pending evaluation by her obstetrician when she has a previously diagnosed medical condition that may affect normal pregnancy, such as uncontrolled diabetes, hypertension, or cervical defects

Modified from Klossner D, editor: *2004-2005 NCAA sports medicine handbook,* Indianapolis, 2004-2005, National Collegiate Athletic Association.

Whereas exercise during pregnancy is safe in most cases, in some situations, exercise needs to be discontinued pending a complete evaluation by a physician. Contraindications to exercise in pregnancy include vaginal bleeding, pregnancy-induced hypertension, an incompetent cervix, preterm labor, premature rupture of membranes, and intrauterine growth restriction.[34] Warning signs that suggest the immediate cessation of exercise include back, pubic, or abdominal pain; dizziness; nausea; uterine contractions; excessive fatigue; and decreased fetal movements.[34] When in doubt, the athlete should discuss these issues with her physician. Box 7-7 gives National Collegiate Athletic Association (NCAA) recommendations.[35]

Ectopic Pregnancy

An infrequent yet important complication of pregnancy is an ectopic pregnancy. Ectopic pregnancy occurs when the fertilized egg implants outside the normal endometrial lining of the uterus (Figure 7-17). This is lethal for the fetus and can be for the mother as well. Appropriate diagnosis is therefore extremely important. The implantation can occur in numerous locations, but most occur in the ampulla of the fallopian tube. Symptoms may include amenorrhea, vaginal bleeding, and pain. An athlete may have hemodynamic compromise in severe cases when rupture and hemorrhage have occurred.

Common causes of ectopic pregnancy include anatomical abnormalities, such as scarring or obstruction of a portion of the egg's path that hinders the normal migration of the fertilized egg to its proper implantation site in the uterus. Some risk factors include a prior ectopic pregnancy, a history of PID, use of an intrauterine device, a history of tubal ligation, an abnormally formed uterus, and cigarette smoking. Diagnosis of an ectopic pregnancy involves serial measurement of serum beta-HCG (human chorionic gonadotropin) levels and pelvic or abdominal imaging with ultrasound.

Treatment most commonly involves aborting the fetus through the use of either methotrexate or surgical intervention. Methotrexate can be considered, under favorable circumstances, in order to avoid the risks and trauma of surgery. Each method of treatment carries its own risks, however, and is generally prescribed by the obstetrician in conjunction with the woman's personal wishes.

WEB RESOURCES

National Kidney and Urologic Diseases Information Clearing house (sponsored by the National Institute of Health)
> http://kidney.niddk.nih.gov/a-z.asp
> Information on kidney and urological diseases, such as urinary tract infections (UTIs) and kidney stones

The Testicular Cancer Resource Center
> http://tcrc.acor.org/index.html
> Information on testicular cancer, self-exams, varicocele, and hydrocele

National Cancer Institute
> http://www.meb.uni-bonn.de/cancer.gov/
>   CR0000257530.html
> Anatomy and information on testicular cancer

American Cancer Society
> http://www.cancer.org
> Information on all cancers, including testicular, prostate, ovarian, and breast cancers

National Cancer Institute (affiliated with National Institutes of Health)
> http://www.nci.nih.gov/
> Information on all cancers, including testicular, prostate, ovarian, and breast cancers

The prognosis for recovery from an ectopic pregnancy is generally very good as long as the pregnancy is identified early in its course and before rupture. In the event of either a delayed diagnosis or rupture of the fallopian tube, the prognosis is considered guarded. Ectopic pregnancy can easily become fatal if diagnosis is delayed and rupture occurs, resulting in hemorrhage and hemodynamic collapse. Following the successful treatment of an ectopic pregnancy, subsequent infertility may occur.

SUMMARY

Athletes are unique individuals by nature of their high-intensity exercise and the physical demands placed on their bodies; but, like all other people, they too have the potential to develop any number of genitourinary or gynecological problems. Some of these conditions are unique to athletes, such as sports **hematuria** and pregnancy in the athlete, and others are common to athletes and nonathletes alike.

The team of professionals caring for athletes must all be aware of the common medical problems that can occur in this group of individuals so that prompt attention and diagnosis can be obtained. Because of the sensitive nature of these systems and the unique relationship of the athletic trainer to the athlete, familiarity with the signs and symptoms is especially critical to assessing these disorders. Understanding the medical conditions affecting the genitourinary and gynecological systems can lead to prompt referral and diagnosis and the subsequent early return of the athlete to sport.

REFERENCES

1. O'Rahilly R: *Basic human anatomy*, Philadelphia, 1983, WB Saunders.
2. Hytten FE: *Clinical physiology in obstetrics*, Oxford, England, 1980, Blackwell.
3. Artal R: *Pulmonary response to exercise in pregnancy*, ed 2, Baltimore, 1991, Williams & Wilkins.
4. Stamatelou K, Francis M, Jones C, et al: Time trends in reported prevalence of kidney stones in the United States: 1974-1994, *Kidney International* 63:1817-1823, 2003.
5. Boulay I, Holtz P, Foley W, et al: Ureteral calculi: diagnostic efficacy of helical CT and implications for the treatment of patients, *American Journal of Roentgenology* 172(6):1485-1490, 1999.
6. Borrero E, Queral LA: Symptomatic abdominal aortic aneurysm misdiagnosed as nephroureterolithiasis, *Annals of Vascular Surgery* 2(2):145-149, 1988.
7. Larkin G, Peacock W, Pearl S, et al: Efficacy of ketorolac tromethamine versus meperidine in the ED treatment of acute renal colic, *American Journal of Emergency Medicine* 17(1):6-10, 1999.
8. Abarbanel J, Benet A, Lask D, Kimche D: Sports hematuria, *Journal of Urology* 143(5):887-890, 1990.
9. Jones G, Newhouse I: Sport-related hematuria: a review, *Clinical Journal of Sports Medicine* 7(2):119-125, 1997.
10. Gambrell R, Blount B: Exercise-induced hematuria, *American Family Physician* 53(3):905-911, 1996.
11. Sobel J: Pathogenesis of urinary tract infection. Role of host defenses, *Infectious Disease Clinics of North America* 11:531-549, 1997.
12. Foxman B, Ahang L, Tallman P, et al: Transmission of uropathogens between sex partners, *Journal of Infectious Diseases* 175:989-992, 1997.
13. Khan A, Schaeffer H, Evans H: Urinary tract infection in adolescent boys, *Journal of the National Medical Association* 65:1589-1596, 1996.
14. Bremnor J, Sadovsky R: Evaluation of dysuria in adults, *American Family Physician* 65:1589-1596, 2002.
15. Rupp T, Zwanger M, Rupp T: Testicular torsion, *Emedicine*. Available at http://www.emedicine.com/med/. Accessed October 2004.
16. Caesar R, Kaplan G: Incidence of the bell-clapper deformity in an autopsy series, *Urology* 44(1):114-116, 1994.
17. Cattolica E, Karol J, Rankin K, Klein R: High testicular salvage rate in torsion of the spermatic cord, *Journal of Urology* 128:66-68, 1982.
18. Baker LA, Sigman D, Mathews RI, et al: An analysis of clinical outcomes using color Doppler testicular ultrasound for testicular torsion, *Pediatrics* 105:604-607, 2000.
19. Kim E: Varicocele, *Emedicine*. Available at http://www.emedicine.com/med/topic 2757.htm. Accessed October 2004.
20. Kincade S: Testicular cancer, *American Family Physician* 59(9):2539-2544, 1999.
21. Centers for Disease Control: Prostate cancer: the public health perspective, Centers for Disease Control. Available at http://www.cdc.gov/cancer/prostate/prostate.htm#facts. Accessed November 2004.
22. Giovannucci E, Rimm E, Ascherio A, et al: Smoking and risk of total and fatal prostate cancer in United States heath professionals, *Cancer Epidemiology, Biomarkers and Prevention* 8:277-282, 1999.

23. Biarati I, Meyer F, Fradet Y, Moore L: Dietary fat and advanced prostate cancer, *Journal of Urology* 159(4): 1271-1275, 1998.
24. Key T, Silocks P, Davey G, et al: A case control study of diet and prostate cancer, *British Journal of Cancer* 76(5): 678-687, 1997.
25. Fowler J, Sanders J, Bigler S, et al: Percent free prostate specific antigen and cancer detection in black and white men with total prostate specific antigen 2.5 to 9.9 ng/mL, *Journal of Urology* 163(5):1467-1470, 2000.
26. Egan M, Lipsky M: Diagnosis of vaginitis, *American Family Physician* 62:1095-1104, 2000.
27. Committee on Infectious Diseases, American Academy of Pediatrics: *Red book: 2003 report of the committee on infectious diseases*, ed 26, Elk Grove Village, Ill, 2003, AAP.
28. Harlow S, Park M: A longitudinal study of risk factors for the occurrence, duration and severity of menstrual cramps in a cohort of college women, *British Journal of Obstetrics and Gynaecology* 103(11):1134-1142, 1996.
29. Fulton K, Nattiy A: A menstrual dysfunction. In Puffer J, editor: *20 common problems in sports medicine*, New York, 2002, McGraw-Hill.
30. Nattiy A, Agostini R, Drinkwater B, et al: The female athlete triad: the interrelatedness of disordered eating, amenorrhea and osteoporosis, *Clinics in Sports Medicine* 13:405, 1994.
31. Arends M, Wyllie A, Bird C: Papillomaviruses and human cancer, *Human Pathology* 21(17):686-698, 1990.
32. Centers for Disease Control: The national breast and cervical cancer early detection program: saving lives through screening, Centers for Disease Control. Available at http://www.cdc.gov/cancer/nbccedp/about 2004.htm. Accessed October 2004.
33. Clapp J: Exercise during pregnancy, a clinical update, *Clinics in Sports Medicine* 19(2):273-286, 2000.
34. Lively M: Sports participation and pregnancy, *Athletic Therapy Today* 7(1):11-15, 2002.
35. Klossner D, editor: *2004-2005 NCAA sports medicine handbook*, Indianapolis, 2004-2005, National Collegiate Athletic Association.

CHAPTER 8

Neurological Disorders

Rose Snyder and
Sara McDade

OBJECTIVES

At the completion of this chapter, the reader should be able to do the following:

1. Understand the anatomy and function of the nervous system.
2. Identify conditions that make an athlete susceptible to encephalitis or meningitis.
3. Recognize and refer an athlete with signs or symptoms of a life-threatening neurological condition.
4. Appreciate the symptoms of reflex sympathetic dystrophy/complex regional pain syndrome (RSD/CRPS).
5. Describe chronic neurological conditions and their effect on athletic participation.
6. Know when to refer an athlete to a physician for further neurological evaluation.

INTRODUCTION

Neurological disorders in athletes are generally placed in two categories: life-threatening conditions such as encephalitis, meningitis, or stroke; and those with chronic implications, which may include Guillain-Barré, multiple sclerosis, migraines, reflex sympathetic dystrophy (RSD), or epilepsy. Because of the age range and close living quarters shared by many college athletes, they are more susceptible to certain neurological diseases, such as meningitis. In addition, outdoor practices in the late afternoon warm weather are favorable to mosquitoes, the carrier of certain types of encephalitis.

The athletic trainer who appreciates these conditions will be better able to recognize and possibly prevent contact and spread of these deadly disorders.

Although chronic neurological conditions are less common, they produce symptoms that can interfere with normal daily function as well as prevent vigorous activity for periods of time. Most have no clear or distinguishable signs, and only the athlete's particular symptoms can guide the clinician to a correct impression. These conditions can also cause emergent situations that require immediate medical referral.

Many symptoms associated with neurological conditions are vague and fleeting and are sometimes passed off as a result of overtraining or fatigue, both of which are common to the athlete. This chapter reviews the pertinent neurological anatomy and highlights signs and symptoms associated with specific neurological conditions. A strong knowledge base will enable the athletic trainer to recognize important symptoms and properly refer the athlete to a physician.

NEUROANATOMY

Skull

The human skull is made up of two main components: the cerebral cranium that protects the brain and brainstem, and the anterior facial bony structure. The cerebral cranium consists of eight bones that include the frontal, two temporal, two parietal, occipital, sphenoid, and ethmoid bones. The facial skeleton is made up of

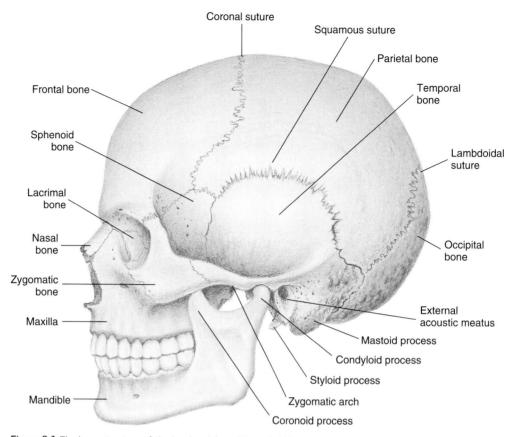

Figure 8-1 The bony structure of the head and face. (From Seidel HM, Ball JW, Dains JE, Benedict GW: *Mosby's guide to physical examination*, ed 5, St Louis, 2003, Mosby, p 252.)

the mandible, two zygomatic, two maxillary, and two nasal bones (Figure 8-1).

Meninges

The meninges lie just under the skull and provide three protective layers: the outermost dura mater, the arachnoid membrane, and the pia mater. The dura mater is a thick, tough, fibrous membrane functionally composed of two layers with the periosteum against the skull and the inner dura supporting structures of the brain. The real and potential spaces formed between these membranes allow for arteriovenous connections that can be disrupted by **hematomas** (i.e., accumulations of blood between the spaces) caused by trauma.

Blood supply to the meninges comes from vessels that follow grooves in the skull. Although the periosteum adheres directly to the skull bones, a potential epidural space exists and ruptured vessels or infection can cause an actual space to form as seen when a hemorrhage causes an epidural hematoma. In the spine, a true epidural space separates the dura from the periosteum of the vertebral bones that contains fat and epidural veins.

The inner lining of the dura mater forms folds in the cerebral hemispheres. The membranous plate known as falx cerebri divides the hemispheres into right and left halves as seen in Figure 8-2. Another plate formed by the dura, the tentorium cerebelli, separates the cerebral hemispheres from the cerebellum and brainstem.

Large sinuses or cavities that lie within the dura mater allow for the venous return from cerebral veins located between the two layers. The walls of these sinuses are made up primarily of dura. The function of the superior sagittal sinus is to collect venous blood, as well as excess cerebrospinal fluid (CSF), which drains through its arachnoid villi. The blood flows into the transverse sinuses, which also receive blood from other veins of the brain. Together with the sigmoid sinuses, these major venous pathways leaving the brain become the internal jugular vein.

The cavernous sinuses are smaller and receive venous blood from the hypothalamus. They are of clinical importance because the internal carotid artery and several nerves pass through them after entering the cranium at the base of the skull.

The arachnoid membrane is named for its delicate, spiderweb-like consistency. The arachnoid membrane and dura mater are separated by the subdural space,

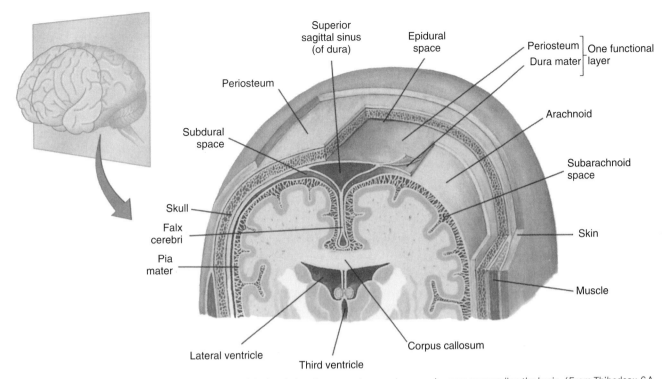

Figure 8-2 A frontal section of the superior portion of the head show bony covering, meninges, and spaces surrounding the brain. (From Thibodeau GA, Patton KT: *Anatomy and physiology*, ed 5, St Louis, 2003, Mosby.)

which is a potential space that contains only a few drops of CSF and numerous small veins. If the membrane is disrupted, it can become distended with blood, pus, or other fluids during pathological conditions. The subarachnoid space separates the arachnoid from the pia mater and is filled with fibrous connecting trabeculae, the major arteries, and CSF. Because the trabecular connections are subtle, the arachnoid and pia layers are sometimes called the **leptomeninges.**

The pia mater is the innermost meninges and is very thin, adhering directly to the surface of the brain and spinal cord. It follows every fold and enters every crevice, making it difficult to distinguish this membrane from the surface to which it adheres. No potential or actual spaces exist between the pia mater and neural tissue.

Meninges also provide a protective covering to the brainstem and spinal cord.

Cerebrum

The two cerebral hemispheres are composed of neural tissue. These hemispheres are divided into four principal lobes: frontal, temporal, parietal, and occipital (Figure 8-3, *A*). The lobes have been extensively researched in attempts to isolate the locations of specific brain physiological functions and pathological processes. The most commonly used classification is Brodmann's classification system, which identifies specific functional cortices of each lobe by numbers (see Figure 8-3, *B*).

The frontal lobe contains the primary motor area (area 4), the premotor area (area 6), the frontal eye field (area 8), Broca's speech area (areas 44 and 45), and the frontal association area (areas 9, 10, 11). The primary motor cortex is highly organized in a somatotopic fashion with the lips, tongue, face, and hands on the lowest part, moving upward to trunk, arm, and hips, and ultimately to the foot, lower legs, and genitalia that hang over the edge into the interhemispheric fissure. This cortical area is responsible for voluntary movement of skeletal muscle of the contralateral side of the body. The frontal eye fields coordinate contralateral deviation of the head and eyes.

Clinically, seizure activity within this cortex results in convulsions of the parts of the body represented in the area of electrical disruption. Damage to this cortex can lead to contralateral **flaccid** paresis or paralysis, and spasticity is usually present if there is concomitant injury to the premotor area. The left hemisphere usually influences and correlates with right hand dominance. Broca's area is located in the dominant hemisphere only, and, when this area is damaged, **Broca's aphasia** is the resulting disorder. Also known as expressive aphasia, Broca's aphasia presents with intact comprehension and impaired expression of speech.

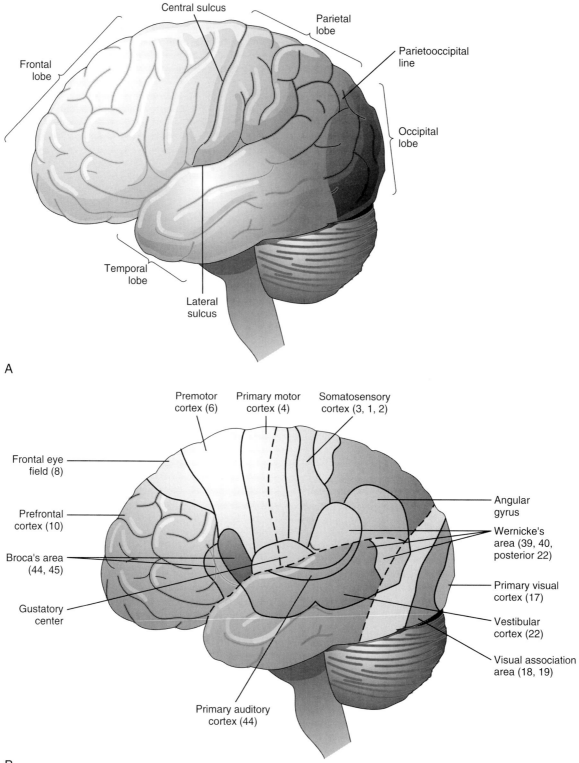

Figure 8-3 A, The four principal lobes of the cerebral cortex. **B,** A partial Brodmann's map of cortical areas of the brain. (From Copstead LEC, Banasik JL: *Pathophysiology: biological and behavioral perspectives,* ed 2, Philadelphia, 2000, WB Saunders, p 973.)

The parietal lobe contains the primary sensory cortex (areas 1, 2, and 3), the sensory association areas (areas 5 and 7), and the cortical taste area embedded in the facial sensory area (areas 1, 2, and 3). The primary sensory cortex, like the motor cortex, is also organized in a somatotopic way. This cortex receives sensory information from the skin and mucosa of the body and face. The types of sensory information processed here include pain, temperature, touch, and proprioception. Pathological injuries to this cortex, such as occur with cerebrovascular accidents (CVAs), lead to paresthesias, impaired sensation, and, rarely, complete anesthesia of the representative body areas on the contralateral side of the body.

The occipital lobe contains the primary visual cortex (area 17) and the visual association areas (areas 18 and 19). The visual cortex receives information from the ipsilateral half of each retina. Therefore, the right visual cortex receives information from the right half of each retina, which correlates clinically with the left visual field. Irritative lesions to this area, such as seizures or migraines, can lead to visual hallucinations; whereas cortical damage, such as in CVAs (strokes), results in contralateral homonymous visual field defects. Pathology of the visual association areas can lead to impairments of spatial orientation and visual disorganization in the same visual field.

The temporal lobe contains the primary auditory cortex (area 41), auditory association area (area 42), temporal association area (represented here by anterior area 22), and Wernicke's speech comprehension area (posterior area 22). The primary auditory cortex receives auditory input from the cochlea of both ears. Irritation of this area can cause buzzing or roaring sounds, and damage can cause hearing deficits ranging from mild caused by a unilateral lesion to severe loss or deafness caused by bilateral lesions. Wernicke's area, like Broca's area, is located in the dominant hemisphere only and is involved in higher auditory processing and in speech comprehension. Injury to this particular area can lead to word deafness, or **Wernicke's aphasia.**

It is important to realize that although specific areas of the brain may be critical to particular function, other areas also are involved in that function, which can adapt to play a more dominant role when necessary because of neural loss resulting from trauma or disease.

Brainstem

The brainstem acts as the main conduit for information between the brain and the spinal cord by way of three large bundles of fibers called the **cerebellar peduncles.** These bundles contain the ascending and descending tracts carrying motor and sensory information, descending tracts of the autonomic nervous system, and pathways of the monoaminergic system. In addition, the brainstem contains almost all the cranial nerve nuclei and houses the center that controls respiration, cardiovascular system functions, level of consciousness, sleep, and alertness.

The brainstem comprises the medulla oblongata, the pons, and the midbrain. Each of these areas is associated with neural fibers related to specific body function. The medulla oblongata contains the ascending and descending tracts; the nuclei of cranial nerves (CN) IX, X, and XII; and the inferior cerebellar peduncles. The pons consists of longitudinal neural tracts; the raphe nucleus, which is important in the modulation of pain as well as in controlling the level of arousal during the sleep-wake cycle; the nuclei of CN VI, VII, and V; auditory pathways; and the middle cerebellar peduncles. The midbrain contains ascending and descending longitudinal neural tracts; the nuclei of CN III and IV; the substantia nigra, which connects with the basal nuclei; superior and inferior colliculi, which are involved in the visual and auditory pathways; pathways of the monoaminergic system, which interact with the raphe nucleus and its functions; periaqueductal gray matter, which contains autonomic pathways and endorphin-producing cells that modulate pain; and the superior cerebellar peduncles.

Autonomic Nervous System

The autonomic nervous system innervates glands, smooth muscle, and cardiac muscle. It is divided into the parasympathetic and the sympathetic divisions. The parasympathetic division is also referred to as craniosacral because of its origins in the brainstem and the sacral levels of the spinal cord. The cranial division consists of parasympathetic fibers in four of the cranial nerves (III, VII, IX, X) that innervate the head and the thoracic and abdominal viscera. The sacral division comprises parasympathetic fibers from segments S2 to S4 and innervates the bladder, genitalia, descending colon, and rectum. The sympathetic nervous system is also referred to as thoracolumbar because it arises from the thoracic and lumbar areas of the spinal cord. These sympathetic fibers usually travel with the peripheral nerves or along the wall of a blood vessel to its target vessels in skeletal muscle.

Box 8-1 lists the major functions of the parasympathetic and sympathetic nervous systems, which are generally antagonistic. The sympathetic nervous system is responsible for the fight-or-flight response and is catabolic in nature, expending energy as it prepares the body for danger. Conversely, the parasympathetic nervous system dominates during times of rest.

Disruption of the sympathetic system can lead to several clinical conditions. **Horner's syndrome** is a

---

Box 8-1 | Major Functions of the Sympathetic and Parasympathetic Nervous Systems

Sympathetic Nervous System
- Increases heart rate and breathing
- Dilates blood vessels in skeletal and cardiac muscles and constricts them in the gastrointestinal tract
- Dilates the bronchial passages
- Dilates the pupils
- Erects the hairs for protection and display
- Increases sweat secretion
- Mobilizes glucose

Parasympathetic Nervous System
- Constricts the pupils
- Decreases the heart rate
- Increases gastrointestinal peristalsis and secretion
- Expels wastes

---

neurological condition manifested by facial flushing of the affected side, ipsilateral miosis, and moderate ptosis of an eye. It is caused by a lesion or tumor at the level of the carotid plexus, cervical sympathetic chain, upper thoracic cord, or brainstem. Sympathetic pathway disruption at the level of the peripheral vascular system can lead to the severe vasoconstrictive episodes characteristic of **Raynaud's disease** (see Chapter 11). **Reflex sympathetic dystrophy** and **causalgia** also involve abnormalities at the level of the peripheral blood vessels leading to sympathetic overactivity.

Cerebellum

The cerebellum is located dorsal to the pons and medulla oblongata and consists of two hemispheres connected by the vermis. The cerebellar peduncles connect the cerebellum to the brainstem and contain communicating neural pathways. The cerebellum controls function in the higher-level coordination of voluntary movements and in the maintenance of balance, equilibrium, and muscle tone. Therefore injuries to this structure generally result in the loss of muscle tone (i.e., **hypotonia**) and the loss of muscle coordination (i.e, **ataxia**). Other clinical signs of cerebellar disease include **nystagmus,** dysmetria, intention tremor, and **dysdiadochokinesia.**

Spinal Cord

The spinal cord is the body's communication system, transmitting nerve impulses to the brain from the spinal nerves that innervate sensory organs and muscles. The cord is divided into white and gray matter. The gray matter consists of neurons or nerve cells. The anterior, or ventral, gray matter contains nerve cells for axons in the ventral roots carrying motor output. The intermediolateral gray matter contains nerve cells

carrying autonomic nerve fibers. The posterior, or dorsal, gray matter comprises sensory fibers conveying pain, temperature, proprioception, and touch input. These nerve cells are further mapped out into laminae on the basis of the types of information being carried. The white matter surrounds the gray matter and consists of the ventral, lateral, and dorsal columns, which contain myelinated and unmyelinated nerve fibers.

The dorsal columns comprise the ascending sensory tracts called the fasciculus gracilis and the fasciculus cuneatus. Together they relay information on touch, proprioception, and two-point discrimination. The lateral columns contain the spinothalamic tracts, dorsal and ventral spinocerebellar tracts, and the spinoreticular pathway. The crossing-over, or decussation, that occurs between the axons of the dorsal columns and the spinothalamic tracts in the spinal cord is clinically important. Brain injuries involving these areas lead to contralateral deficits, whereas injuries within the spinal cord result in ipsilateral touch and proprioception deficits and contralateral pain perception deficits.

Injuries to the motor tracts result in two different clinical conditions based on the level of injury. Injuries at or peripheral to the anterior horn cell within the spinal cord gray matter present as lower motor neuron syndromes, whereas injuries in the lateral white column or above are associated with upper motor neuron syndrome (Key Points—Upper and Lower Motor Neurons).

KEY POINTS
Upper and Lower Motor Neurons

- Upper motor neurons pertain to the brain or spinal cord. Damage to these structures present as weakness, paralysis, increased muscle tone, spasticity, hyperactive deep tendon reflexes, and the presence of Babinski's reflex. Typically, damaged or destroyed upper motor neurons do not regenerate.
- Lower motor neurons relate to nerve cell bodies or axons or both and are located in the anterior horn of the spinal cord and peripheral nerves. Damage to these nerves causes decreased muscle tone, flaccidity, diminished or absent deep tendon reflexes, muscular twitching, and progressive atrophy of the affected muscles.

Spinal Nerves

The 31 paired spinal nerves in the body arise from the spinal cord as ventral or dorsal roots. The dorsal roots contain sensory fibers of pain and temperature from the muscles and also contain axons from muscle spindles and skin and joint mechanoreceptors. The ventral roots are primarily composed of motor neuron fibers from skeletal muscle, as well as muscle spindle fibers, autonomic axons, and axons carrying thoracic and abdominal visceral sensory information.

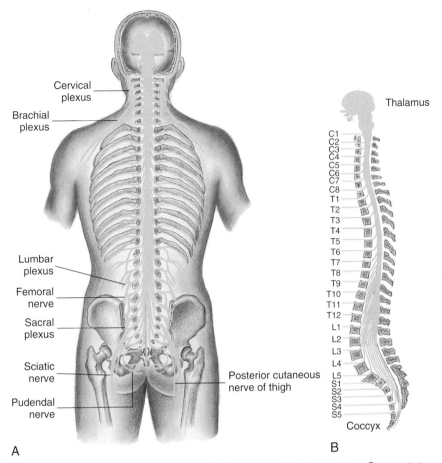

Cervical plexus
Brachial plexus
Lumbar plexus
Femoral nerve
Sacral plexus
Sciatic nerve
Pudendal nerve

Thalamus

C1
C2
C3
C4
C5
C6
C7
C8
T1
T2
T3
T4
T5
T6
T7
T8
T9
T10
T11
T12
L1
L2
L3
L4
L5
S1
S2
S3
S4
S5
Coccyx

Posterior cutaneous nerve of thigh

A   B

Figure 8-4 A, Posterior view of the location of spinal nerves exiting the vertebrae. **B,** Lateral view of the spine and spinal cord. (From Rudy EB: *Advanced neurological and neurosurgical nursing,* St Louis, 1984, Mosby.)

The spinal nerves combine to form the cervical, brachial, lumbar, and sacral plexuses and then innervate the limbs via peripheral nerves (Figure 8-4). Therefore peripheral nerves generally contain fibers from several different spinal nerves. Dermatomes represent the area of skin supplied by a specific spinal nerve and are clinically significant in diagnosing the sensory area of nerve injury (Box 8-2). Nerve injury needs to be distinguished from the cutaneous innervation of the peripheral nerves. A myotome is a muscle or group of muscles supplied by one ventral (motor) nerve. Motor deficits may be attributed to damage in specific myotomes.

Myelination is a process in which a nerve is enveloped in a myelin sheath. In the peripheral nervous system, this is accomplished by the encircling of a nerve axon by Schwann cells. Gaps between the Schwann cells are called the **nodes of Ranvier** (Figure 8-5) and expose unmyelinated axons. The significance of this is that nerve conduction in these myelinated nerves is saltatory, jumping from node to node, which increases the conduction velocity.[1] This type of myelination ceases just before the interface of the dorsal or ventral nerve root with the spinal cord. At this juncture between the peripheral nervous system (PNS) and the central nervous system (CNS), known as the **Obersteiner-Redlich zone,** astrocytes and oligodendrocytes form the myelin covering.

Demyelinating conditions such as multiple sclerosis, which affects the CNS, and Guillain-Barré syndrome, which affects both the PNS and CNS, can lead to varying degrees of sensory and motor loss. Remyelination often takes place in the PNS; however, it occurs sluggishly, if at all, in the CNS.

ASSESSMENT OF THE NEUROLOGICAL SYSTEM

Warning Signs of Neurological Diseases

Assessment of the neurological system begins with the athlete's clinical history, coupled with listening carefully to the complaints and terms the athlete uses to describe the condition. In general, neurological diseases can present with positive or negative signs or manifestations.

Box 8-2 Dermatomes

Nerves exit the spinal cord in an orderly manner similar to a ladder. A dermatome is an area of skin supplied mainly by one spinal cord segment through a particular spinal nerve. Fortunately, dermatomes overlap so if one nerve is severed, sensations can be transmitted by the nerve above or below. Following this generalized map of the spinal cord and spinal nerves and their related dermatomes it is easy to find useful landmarks that aid in assessment.

- The thumb, middle finger, and fifth finger are each in the dermatomes of C6, C7, and C8
- The head and neck are at the level of C2 and C3
- The chest is at the levels of C5 through T7
- The groin is in the region of L1

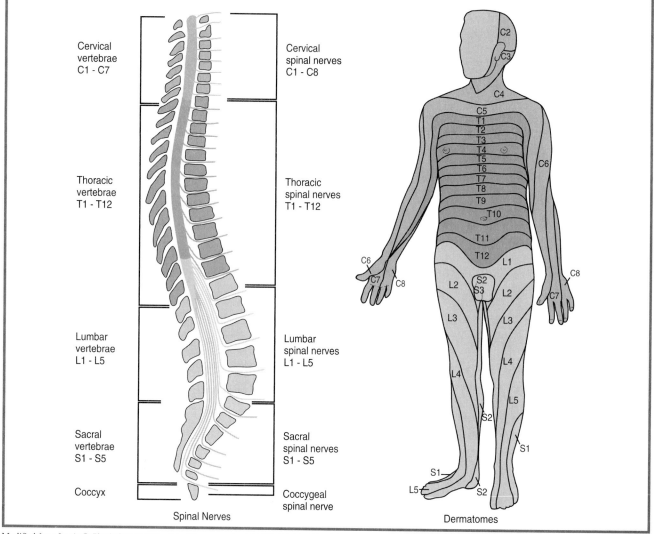

Modified from Jarvis C: *Physical examination & health assessment*, ed 4, Philadelphia, 2004, WB Saunders, p 668.

Positive manifestations represent inappropriate excitation of the nervous system. These include hypersensitivity; seizures; movement disorders that include tremor, spasm, and tics; and upper motor neuron signs, such as spasticity, hypertonicity, and hyperreflexia. Some descriptions given by the athlete to indicate positive symptoms include the following: heaviness, weakness, cramps, slow reacting, tired, tremors, visual disturbances, incoordination, deadened, numb, tingling, or pins and needles. Negative signs or manifestations represent a loss of function. These include paresis; paralysis; hyposensitivity; dementia; **aphasia** including receptive-sensory, expressive-motor, and

anomic; syncope; neck stiffness; gait dysfunction; movement disorders; incoordination; sensory ataxia or proprioception loss; and lower motor neuron signs including hypotonicity-flaccidity, hyporeflexia, and atrophy.

The physical examination of the athlete begins with a visual inspection of the spinal column, assessing for deviations, muscular imbalance, or surgical scars. The athlete's musculature, although typically stronger on the dominant side, should not be particularly unilaterally hypertrophic. The athletic trainer assesses bilaterally for tremors, atrophy, and muscular tone. The dermatomes are bilaterally assessed for

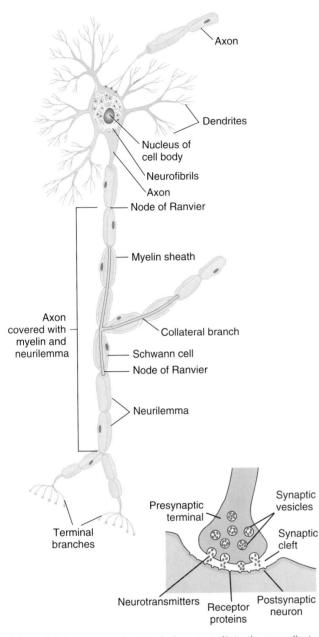

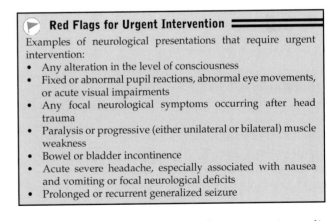

Figure 8-5 A neuron and a chemical synapse. Note the unmyelinated areas in the nodes of Ranvier. (From Black JM, Hawks JH: *Medical-surgical nursing: clinical management for positive outcomes*, ed 7, St Louis, 2005, WB Saunders, p 2008.)

sensation as described in Chapter 2, followed by bilateral comparison of the reflexes. Evaluation of the cranial nerves (described in the next section) and muscular strength tests follow. Muscular strength tests include both range of motion and break tests for the brachial plexus as well as heel and toe walking for the lower extremity. The athletic trainer notes any weakness or differences and refers the athlete to a physician when a discrepancy occurs in either. Functional knowledge of the myotomes and dermatomes is instrumental in assessment of any neurological issue.

Clinical neurological signs can assist in differentiating muscle weakness. The pattern of muscle weakness varies depending on the area of injury within the motor unit from nerve cell to muscle: upper motor neuron, lower motor neuron, neuromuscular junction, muscle itself, or manifestation as functional weakness. Upper and lower motor neurons have been previously discussed. Neuromuscular junction disorders are characterized by signs of injury that include fatigable weakness, normal or decreased muscle tone, and normal deep tendon reflexes. Decreased or absent reflexes present with injury at the muscle level (i.e., myopathy). Functional weakness, in contrast to actual weakness, is associated with decreased power in the presence of normal tone, reflexes, and muscle girth.

Understanding the basic anatomy and physiology of the neurological system also helps in identification of injury to higher neurological systems. Cerebral injuries may present with aphasias, **apraxias,** paresis, paralysis, sensory deficits, and visual and auditory dysfunction. Cerebellar damage leads to varying degrees of ataxia and incoordination, as well as **dysmetria** and tremors. Neurological injury to the brainstem may manifest with cranial nerve palsies (CN III to CN XII). In addition to these symptoms, many other common signs associated with neurological disease have special terminology (Box 8-3).

Neurological presentations can range from emergent, to urgent, to routine in severity and in their need for medical evaluation and management. The box entitled Red Flags—Urgent Intervention provides a framework

---

▶ Red Flags for Urgent Intervention

Examples of neurological presentations that require urgent intervention:
- Any alteration in the level of consciousness
- Fixed or abnormal pupil reactions, abnormal eye movements, or acute visual impairments
- Any focal neurological symptoms occurring after head trauma
- Paralysis or progressive (either unilateral or bilateral) muscle weakness
- Bowel or bladder incontinence
- Acute severe headache, especially associated with nausea and vomiting or focal neurological deficits
- Prolonged or recurrent generalized seizure

---

of warning signs and symptoms that warrant immediate referral to a physician or an emergency department. Indications for referral of specific disorders will be addressed under Pathological Conditions.

Cranial Nerves and Cranial Nerve Testing

The cranial nerves emerge from the cranium, as opposed to spinal nerves, which emerge from the spinal cord (Figure 8-6). The cranial nerves provide sensory and

Box 8-3   Terminology Associated with Neurological Diseases

Agnosia—Inability to recognize and interpret sensory stimuli (CVA)

Agraphia—Inability to express thoughts in writing (CVA)

Allodynia—Sensitivity or pain to nonpainful stimuli (RSD/CRPS)

Anisocoria—Pupil size inequality of 0.5-2.0 mm (neurological disease)

Aphasia—Impaired comprehension or expression of written or spoken language (CVA, encephalitis, dysphasia, head trauma)

Apraxia—Inability to perform purposeful movements in the absence of weakness, sensory loss, poor coordination, or lack of comprehension (CVA)

Ataxia—Incoordination of voluntary movement (CVA, head trauma, GBS, MS)

Aura—Sensory or motor phenomenon that indicates the start of a seizure or an impending classical migraine (migraine, seizure)

Babinski's reflex—Abnormal extension of the great toe and extension of the toes with plantar foot stimulation (CVA, head trauma, MS, meningitis)

Brudzinski's sign—Flexion of the hips and knees in response to passive flexion of the neck (meningitis, trauma, SAH)

Decerebrate rigidity—Abnormal extensor responses in the upper and lower limbs (cerebral trauma)

Decorticate rigidity—Abnormal flexor response in the upper extremity and extensor response in the lower extremity (CVA, head trauma)

Deep tendon reflexes—Abnormally brisk muscle contraction with tapping; hyperactive on the muscle tendon (CVA, MS); abnormally slow muscle contraction with tapping; hypoactive on the muscle tendon (GBS)

Diplopia—Double vision (CVA, encephalitis, MS, head trauma, migraine)

Drooling—Loss of saliva from the mouth (CVA, GBS, seizure)

Dysarthria—Impaired articulation (CVA, MS)

Dysdiadochokinesia—Difficulty performing rapidly alternating movements (CVA- cerebellar)

Fasciculations—Irregular contractions of groups of muscle fibers (GBS)

Footdrop—Plantar flexion of the foot caused by impaired ability to dorsiflex the foot (CVA, MS, GBS)

Gait, spastic—Abnormal gait with extended stiff legs causing dragging of the foot (MS, CVA)

Gait, steppage with footdrop—Abnormal gait with exaggerated hip and knee flexion to clear the dragging toes (GBS, MS)

Headache—Pain in the head, retroorbital, and cervical areas

Hemianopia—Loss of vision in one half of the visual field (CVA)

Hyperesthesia—Increased sensitivity to touch, pain, and temperature (CVA, RSD)

Incontinence—Involuntary loss of urine or feces (CVA, MS, head trauma)

Kernig's sign—With a patient in the supine position and leg flexion, there is resistance and pain with leg extension (meningitis, SAH)

Level of consciousness—Reduced alertness ranging from lethargy to stupor (CVA, encephalitis, head decreased trauma—bleeds, seizure, meningitis)

Light flashes—Bright stars, streaks, or spots in the visual field (migraine, head trauma)

Miosis—Unilateral constriction of a pupil (cluster headache)

Muscle atrophy—Wasting of muscle size (CVA, MS)

Muscle flaccidity—Profound weakness with lack of active muscle movement and resistance (CVA, GBS, seizures)

Muscle spasticity—Increased resistance to movement (CVA, MS, head trauma)

Muscle weakness—Reduced muscle strength (CVA, MS, head trauma GBS, seizure)

Myoclonus—Spasms of a muscle or group of muscles (viral encephalitis)

Nuchal rigidity—Profound stiffness of the neck with flexion (meningitis, encephalitis, head trauma—bleeds)

Nystagmus—Involuntary oscillations of one or both eyes (CVA, MS, encephalitis, head trauma)

Ocular deviation—Abnormal movement of one or both eyes (CVA, MS, encephalitis, head trauma, meningitis)

Paralysis—Complete loss of voluntary movement (CVA, encephalitis, MS, migraine, seizure, head trauma—bleeds)

Paresthesia—Abnormal sensations in the distribution of peripheral nerves (CVA, GBS, migraine, MS, head trauma, seizure)

Photophobia—Increased sensitivity to light (meningitis, migraine)

Ptosis—Drooping of the upper eyelid (migraine)

Pupils, nonreactive—Absence of constrictive response of the pupil to light (encephalitis)

Pupils, sluggish—Abnormally slow constrictive response of the pupils to light (encephalitis, MS)

Rhinorrhea—Loss of thin mucus from the nasal passages (cluster headache)

Romberg's sign—Impaired balance with eyes closed and feet together (MS)

Scotoma—Focal area of darkness or blindness in the visual field (migraine)

Seizure—Abnormal cerebral electrical activity presenting disturbances (CVA, MS, head trauma, with motor, sensory, autonomic, or psychic encephalitis)

Signorelli's sign—Pain with pressure anterior to the mastoid process (meningitis)

Tremors—Rhythmical shaking of an extremity from involuntary contraction and relaxation of opposing muscles (MS)

Vision, blurred—Impaired visual acuity (CVA, MS, migraine, concussion)

Vision, lost—Inability to sense visual stimuli (concussion)

CVA, Cerebrovascular accident; *RSD,* reflex sympathetic dystrophy; *CRPS,* complex regional pain syndrome; *GBS,* Guillain-Barré syndrome; *MS,* multiple sclerosis; *SAH,* subarachnoid hemorrhage.

motor innervation to the head and neck, including voluntary as well as involuntary muscle function, and sensation (see Table 2-7, Cranial Nerve Function). Testing these nerves is essential to ascertaining their integrity as well as noting discrepancies that may indicate a medical condition.

The olfactory nerve (CN I) can be tested by placing different-smelling substances underneath a single nostril with the other nostril occluded. Both nares are tested since injuries to this nerve are usually unilateral. The clinical spectrum of pathology can range from normal function, to **anosmia** in which the patient can only discern ammonia, to organic dysfunction in which the patient cannot recognize any smells.

The optic nerve (CN II) carries visual information within the complex visual system. The fibers of the optic nerve carrying information from the right half of the retina cross over and join with those same fibers of the contralateral optic nerve. Together, these fibers form the optic tract. The optic tract then forms optic radiations that eventually synapse on the primary visual cortex. Different clinical visual defects will occur

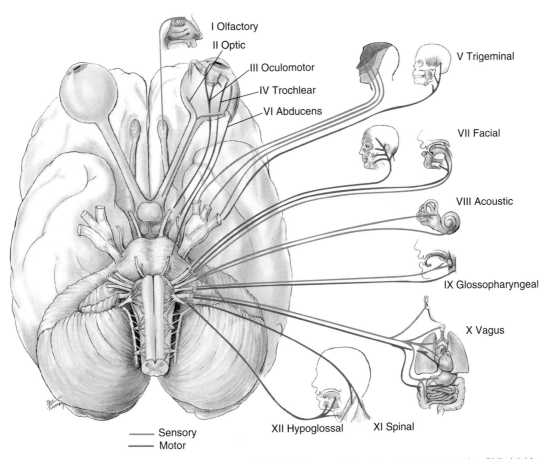

Figure 8-6 The cranial nerves of the brain. (From Jarvis C: *Physical examination & health assessment*, ed 4, Philadelphia, 2004, WB Saunders, p 667.)

depending on the area of lesion within the optic pathway.[1] Complete assessment of the optic nerve requires testing the visual fields, acuity, and pupillary light reflex.

To test the visual fields, the athletic trainer faces the athlete, who is looking straight ahead. The athletic trainer moves fingers of one hand within the athlete's peripheral vision and monitors the athlete's response about which finger is moving. Next the athletic trainer focuses on individual eye deficits by repeating this test while the athlete closes one eye. The Snellen eye chart, which is described in Chapter 9, is used to test visual acuity. Alternatively, the athlete may be asked to read something.

The oculomotor nerve (CN III) controls direct pupillary light reflex. The constriction of the pupil is normal when a light shone into the athlete's eye. Then the light is shone in the other eye, and that pupil should constrict as well, demonstrating consensual pupillary light reflex. Any deviation from this is abnormal. This nerve is also responsible for eye adduction (toward the midline) and downward movement.

The trochlear (CN IV), and abducens (CN VI) nerves can also be tested by monitoring the movements of the extraocular muscles. The athlete is asked to visually follow a pen as it is slowly moved within the visual field. Then the athletic trainer passes the pen across the midline space toward the athlete's nose, watching for movement of both eyes in toward the midline and testing for convergence. **Saccadic eye movements** are tested by having the athlete look in each direction and watching the coordination and quality of movement. Specifically, the trochlear nerve (CN IV) is responsible for upward eye movement and the abducens nerve (CN VI) coordinates eye movement laterally away from the nose (Figure 8-7).

The athletic trainer tests response of the trigeminal nerve (CN V) and the facial nerve (CN VII) by observing for symmetry when the athlete bares teeth, whistles, looks up at the ceiling, and clenches eyes closed (Figure 8-8). Sensory testing of the trigeminal nerve is performed with light touch and pinprick in the divisions of the trigeminal nerve on both sides. If any abnormalities are found, further tests are warranted. When testing the motor function of the trigeminal nerve, the athletic trainer has the athlete clench teeth while placing a hand under the athlete's chin to resist jaw opening. Any noticeable muscle atrophy or elicited muscle weakness indicates an abnormal test.

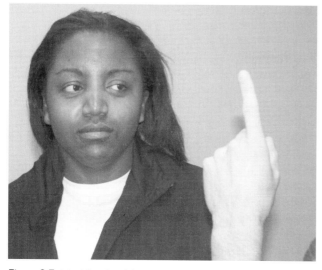

Figure 8-7 A test for the abducens nerve (CN VI) is to have the athlete move the eyes laterally, following the finger of the examiner.

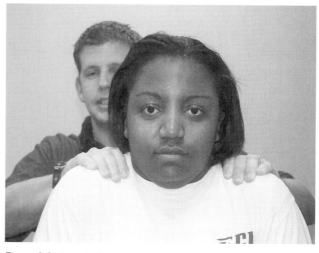

Figure 8-9 The spinal accessory nerve (CN XI) is tested by a resisted shrug, which determines the bilateral integrity of the trapezius muscle.

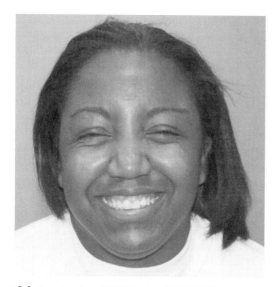

Figure 8-8 The trigeminal (CN V) and facial (CN VII) nerves are tested by clenching the teeth and facial expressions, respectively.

Sensory testing of CN VII as well as CN IX (glossopharyngeal) appraises the athlete's ability to distinguish taste. For example, the athlete might be asked to tell the difference between sweet and sour.

Testing of the vestibulocochlear nerve (CN VIII) involves auditory testing of hearing and equilibrium. Auditory testing is performed using the Rinne test and the Weber test (see Box 10-2). In both tests a vibrating tuning fork is placed at various points on the patient's head and the patient is asked to identify which placement is louder. Conductive deafness occurs when conduction of sound is impaired, as opposed to sensorineural deafness in which there is neurological disruption. Auditory testing may also be conducted by creating a sound—such as snapping fingers—behind each of the athlete's ears and looking for a response.

Tests to the glossopharyngeal (CN IX), vagus (CN X), and hypoglossal (CN XII) motor nerves involve observing the athlete's tongue and mouth anatomy and watching for deviations in tongue movement when the mouth is opened and the tongue stuck out. The athlete is asked to push tongue against cheek or a depressor to demonstrate strength. The athletic trainer watches the uvula for deviation from midline as the patient says "aah." The vagus nerve (CN X) controls the gag reflex, which is assessed by touching each side of the pharyngeal wall behind the tonsils and observing movement of the uvula. The vagus nerve is also responsible for movement of the larynx and pharynx, which can be tested together by observing the quality and coordination of movement while the athlete swallows water.

The athletic trainer tests the spinal accessory nerve (CN XI) by focused examination of the sternocleidomastoid and the trapezius muscles on both sides of the body. The strength of the trapezius muscle is assessed through a resisted shoulder shrug (Figure 8-9), and the sternocleidomastoid muscle is assessed by resisting both turning and lifting of the chin. The presence of atrophy or weakness during resisted muscle movement suggests nerve injury.

PATHOLOGICAL CONDITIONS

Encephalitis

Encephalitis literally translated means inflammation of the brain. Generally, encephalitis is caused by a viral infection, but it can also be a sequela of immunizations or vaccines. The same organisms responsible for aseptic meningitis are also responsible for encephalitis, although their relative frequencies differ.

Encephalitis takes two forms: primary and secondary with complications from a viral infection. Primary encephalitis is due to a direct viral invasion of the brain and spinal cord. The virus can be sporadic or epidemic. Sporadic infection arises from herpes simplex, varicella-zoster, mumps, and other viruses.[2] Epidemic encephalitis is typically caused by mosquito-borne arboviruses. **Arboviruses** are a large group of viruses recovered largely from bats, rodents, and arthropods (e.g., insects and crustaceans). Disease is typically transmitted through blood-feeding practices (e.g. by mosquitoes and ticks). These arboviruses are also known as distinct disorders: eastern and western equine encephalitis, both named after the horses that are attacked by the virus, and St. Louis, La Crosse, and West Nile viruses, which are named for the areas of the United States where they were first discovered.

Secondary encephalitis is typically a complication of a viral infection in another part of the body that then enters the brain. All forms of encephalitis have a similar presentation that may begin as a minor illness with headache and fever, followed by more serious symptoms. Whereas primary encephalitis is the most serious, the secondary form is more common. People often do not seek medical care because of the milder nature of secondary encephalitis; therefore physicians see more cases of primary encephalitis.

Although encephalitis is rare, it is the most common mosquito-borne disease in the United States. The mortality rate varies with the source of the virus. Insect-borne sources might cause low morbidity one year but severe mortality the next.[2] The five major types of mosquito-borne encephalitis that infect people in the United States are eastern equine encephalitis, western equine encephalitis, St. Louis encephalitis, La Crosse encephalitis, and more recently, West Nile encephalitis.

Birds are the conduit that spread the virus to mosquitoes through their food chain. A newly infected bird carries high levels of the virus in its blood stream before developing immunity. Mosquitoes who feed on these birds become lifelong carriers of the disease. The mosquito then easily passes the infection on to more birds, which in turn spread it to more mosquitoes.[3] Although most mosquitoes would choose birds over mammals for their primary food source, they do attack humans and other warm-blooded creatures (Box 8-4). The risk of this occurrence is highest during the warm

Box 8-4   Vector Transmission of Disease

Organisms that transmit disease from one animal host to another are called vectors.
Mosquitoes are vectors for the transmission of encephalitis from small creatures, usually birds and rodents, to humans.

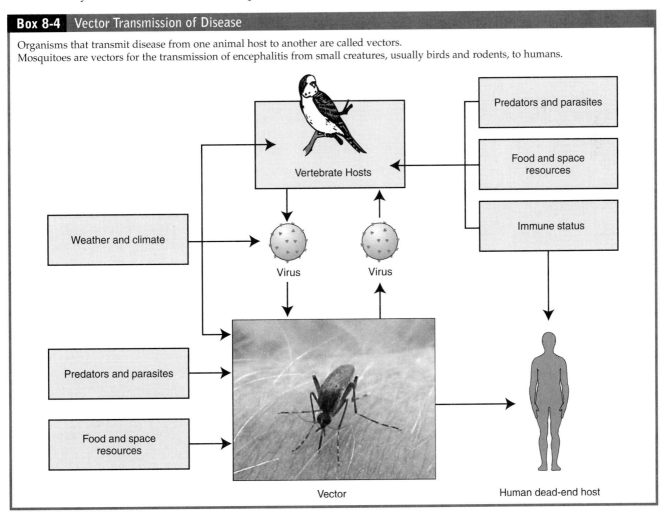

months when birds and mosquitoes reproduce.[2] Because athletes practice in the late afternoon and early evening during the warmer months their activity coincides with the highest mosquito activity; therefore their risk is highest.[4] In addition, mosquitoes congregate in bodies of water, however small. This would make puddles of water from a hydration station or a discarded water bottle a haven for these pests.

Eastern equine is the most serious viral encephalitis found in North America, primarily in the eastern United States. It affects horses, as its name infers, and humans. Western equine encephalitis also affects horses and humans and is prevalent in the central and western plains. It is a very serious variety of encephalitis but not as fatal as the eastern variety. Both are rare in the United States.[3]

Arboviruses also include St. Louis, La Crosse, and West Nile virus strains. The St. Louis variety was first discovered in the Midwest and is responsible for approximately 128 cases per year. La Crosse encephalitis is one of the few mosquito-borne viruses common in hardwood forests and is primarily found in the upper Midwest.[3] It is transmitted to mosquitoes via chipmunks and squirrels rather than birds. However, it is the West Nile virus, with activity in 40 states in 2004, that gathers the most media attention.[5] The *Culex* mosquito is the primary culprit for West Nile virus (see Box 8-4), which was first reported in Africa, Europe, and Asia and reached the United States in 1999.[6]

The West Nile virus has been transmitted through blood transfusions, through donated organs, by breastfeeding, and during pregnancy from mother to fetus.[6,7] First reported in New York, West Nile virus is now found coast to coast (Figure 8-10). It has been found in birds, horses, dogs, squirrels, and bats, as well as humans.[5] In 2000, the virus infected 19 people in the United States and resulted in two deaths, whereas in 2003, 264 fatalities resulted from more than 9862 cases.[8] Although symptoms of West Nile encephalitis are generally mild, the disease can become severe, especially in older people and those with weakened immune systems.[9]

Signs and Symptoms

Signs and symptoms of encephalitis generally appear within 5 to 15 days of being bitten by an infected mosquito. These include sudden fever, headache, vomiting, photophobia, stiff neck and back, confusion, drowsiness, clumsiness, unsteady gait, and irritability. A rash may also be an early indicator. Symptoms that require emergency treatment include loss of consciousness, seizures, poor responsiveness, muscle weakness, memory loss, sudden and severe dementia, impaired judgment, coma, and paralysis.[10,11]

Referral, Diagnostic Tests, and Differential Diagnosis

Encephalitis is potentially serious and life threatening. Early referral to a physician or hospital emergency department may be necessary. The cardinal symptoms for immediate referral include severe headache, stiff neck, photophobia, and mental disturbances.

The keystone diagnostic test is CSF examination and analysis. Neuroimaging studies, magnetic resonance imaging (MRI), computed tomography (CT) scan, and

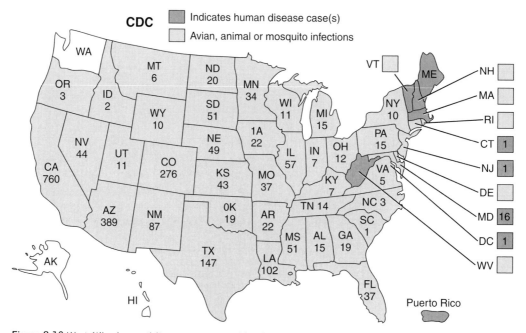

Figure 8-10 West Nile virus activity map as reported by the Centers for Disease Control in November 2004. (From www.cdc.gov/ncidod/westnile/surv&control104Maps_PrinterFriendly.htm.)

Table 8-1	Cerebrospinal Fluid (CSF) Values and Indicators	
	Normal Values	**Notes**
Pressure	50-80 mm H$_2$O	High: acute bacterial meningitis, cerebral hemorrhage, perhaps Lyme disease
Appearance	Clear	Cloudy: infection, meningococcal meningitis Red: cerebral hemorrhage, obstruction Orange: high protein, old bleeding
Protein	20-45 mg/dl	High: tumors, trauma, infection, inflammation, acute bacterial meningitis, Guillain-Barré syndrome
Glucose	40-70 mg/dl	Low: acute bacterial meningitis, hypoglycemia, infection, cancer High: hyperglycemia
Leukocytes	Up to 5 cells	500-10,000: acute bacterial meningitis 0-500: Lyme disease 0-100: Guillain-Barré syndrome Presence of red blood cells (RBCs): cerebral hemorrhage

Data from http://www.bbc.co.uk/health/talking/tests/samples_csf.shtml; Beers M, Berkow R, editors: *The Merck manual of diagnosis and therapy*, ed 17, Whitehouse Station, NJ, 1999, Merck Research Laboratories; Ferri F: *Ferri's clinical advisor instant diagnosis and treatment*, St Louis, 2004, Mosby; Tierney L, McPhee S, Papadakis M, editors: *Current medical diagnosis and treatment*, ed 43, New York, 2004, McGraw-Hill.

often an electroencephalogram (EEG) may be performed as well. An EEG is a graphic record of the electrical activity of the brain. Electrodes are placed on the patient's scalp to measure electrical waves, frequencies, and amplitudes. These tests help identify or exclude alternative diagnoses (Table 8-1). They also determine if the disease process is focal or diffuse.[10]

Differential diagnosis for encephalitis includes bacterial meningitis, brain abscess, parasitic diseases, metastatic tumors, and collagen diseases.

Treatment

Viruses are not responsive to antibiotics. Antiviral agents such as acyclovir are only used in the early stages for the herpes simplex virus. In general, treatment is geared toward symptom management and maintenance of body systems. This will include adequate nutrition, ventilation, and hydration. Control of seizures and increased cerebral edema with resultant pressure along with prevention of secondary infection may be necessary.

Prognosis and Return to Participation

The overall prognosis for recovery is good depending on the infecting agent and the speed with which treatment is begun. Some cases are mild, and the patient has a full recovery. In severe cases, however, permanent impairment or death is possible within 48 hours despite early treatment. The acute phase of the infection may last 1 to 2 weeks. Resolution of fever and neurological symptoms may be sudden or gradual. Neurological symptoms may require many months before full recovery, and rehabilitation with speech therapy is often required.

Public Health Implications

All cases of encephalitis caused by an arbovirus (e.g., eastern equine encephalitis, western equine encephalitis, St. Louis encephalitis, La Crosse encephalitis, West Nile virus) should be reported to the local public health authority. Each state authority is allowed to determine whether to report these diseases immediately, within 1 working day or within 1 week.

Prevention of many forms of secondary encephalitis caused by a viral infection in another part of the body, such as mumps, chickenpox, rubeola, or rubella, is best accomplished through immunization.

Public health measures that control mosquitoes can reduce the incidence of many types of viral encephalitis. Effective local mosquito control includes the use of appropriate pesticides and cleanup of containers with standing water that may offer breeding sites.[4] Common containers that may hold enough water to breed mosquitoes include discarded cups and water bottles, football sleds, flowerpots, tire swings, and birdbaths. Individual prevention measures include wearing a hat, wearing long pants with pant legs stuffed into socks, and liberal use of an insect repellent that contains DEET on the face, neck, ears, and arms (Figure 8-11).

Aseptic Meningitis

Aseptic or viral **meningitis** is the most common form of this infection and inflammation of the meninges and CSF surrounding the brain and spinal cord.

Even though viral meningitis is a benign, self-limiting illness, it is associated with approximately 36,000 hospitalizations each year in the United States.[12] It is generally less severe than bacterial meningitis and is rarely fatal in adults with normal immune systems. Care focuses on management of the symptoms, which typically last 7 to 10 days before complete recovery.

Many different viruses cause meningitis, including the enterovirus, arboviruses, mumps, varicella-zoster virus, and herpes simplex virus.[13-16] The most common causative agent is the enterovirus. However, a specific source cannot be identified in one third or more of cases of aseptic meningitis.[17] It is also interesting that

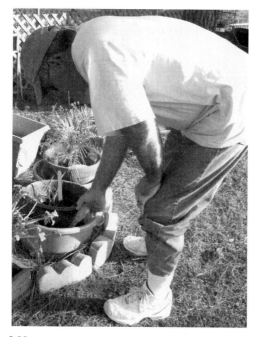

Figure 8-11 Prevention of mosquito bites entails wearing long pants; stuffing pant legs into socks; liberal use of DEET on the face, neck, ears, and arms; and wearing a hat. Note how using a common turkey baster to drain excess water in the container of a potted plant will eliminate a common breeding place for mosquitoes.

this disease has been associated with undiagnosed skull fractures.[18]

The organisms that cause viral meningitis are contagious. An **enterovirus** is most commonly spread through direct contact with respiratory secretions, such as the saliva, sputum, or nasal mucus of an infected person. Thus the typical pathway for infection occurs by shaking hands with an afflicted person or touching something that the person has handled before rubbing the nose, mouth, or eyes. Kissing an infected person on the mouth can also spread the disease.[19]

In temperate climates, most cases are seen in the summer and early fall. The incubation period for an enterovirus is generally between 3 and 7 days from the time of infection until symptoms develop. An infected person can spread the virus to someone else during a period of about 3 days after infection until approximately 10 days after symptoms develop.

Signs and Symptoms

Signs and symptoms of acute viral meningitis are common to all pathogens. Often the disease is accompanied or preceded by a nonspecific malaise or upper respiratory infection. Viral meningitis is similar in presentation to meningococcal infections because it appears with a sudden high fever, headache, and cervical rigidity (Box 8-5).

Box 8-5   Signs and Symptoms of Meningitis

- Headache increasing in severity is the first symptom, typically frontal or retroorbital
- Rapid onset
- Fever up to 104° F (40° C)
- Nausea and vomiting, especially in the early stages
- Confusion
- Drowsiness, progressive lethargy
- Convulsions or seizures: more common in children, especially with influenzal meningitis; rare in adults
- Cervical rigidity
- Positive Brudzinski's sign
- Positive Kernig's sign
- Skin rash, especially near the armpits or on the hands or feet
- Rapid progression of small petechiae under the skin
- Malaise
- Irritability
- Photophobia
- Muscle aches

Referral and Diagnostic Tests

The three indicators that occur abruptly and develop rapidly are a severe headache, high fever, and stiff neck; these indicators should alert the athletic trainer that immediate referral to a physician or hospital emergency department is necessary. Applying stress on the spinal cord through **Brudzinski's** (Figure 8-12) and **Kernig's** (Figure 8-13) **signs** can exacerbate pain in the meninges, but it is not as definitive an indicator of the disease as is a stiff neck (Red Flags—Meningitis).

Red Flags for Meningitis

Warning signs of meningitis that warrant immediate referral include the following:
- Severe headache
- High fever
- Stiff neck

In the early stages it is impossible to separate viral meningitis from acute bacterial or meningococcal meningitis without laboratory studies. It is necessary to examine the CSF to distinguish between the two infections as well as to rule out differential diagnoses. CSF is obtained through a spinal tap, which is also known as a lumbar puncture (Box 8-6).

With viral meningitis, the spinal fluid on gross inspection is usually clear to the naked eye, and no organisms are seen on microscopic examination nor can they be cultured. The glucose content also is normal.

Treatment

Once a diagnosis of viral meningitis is made, treatment is supportive. It consists of symptom management with bed rest, increased fluids, analgesics, and medications to prevent or relieve nausea and vomiting. Antibiotics are not helpful with a viral disease.

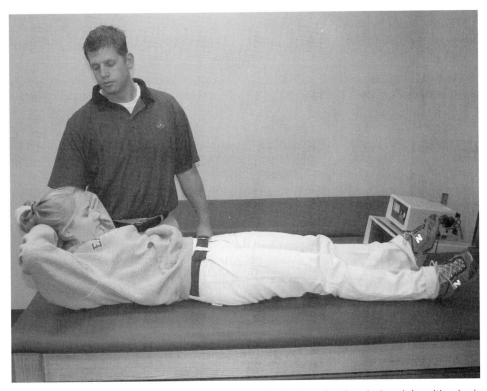

Figure 8-12 Brudzinski's sign involves active neck flexion, thereby elongating the spinal cord. A positive sign is increasing pain localized or radiating in the lower extremity, which indicates meningeal or nerve root irritation.

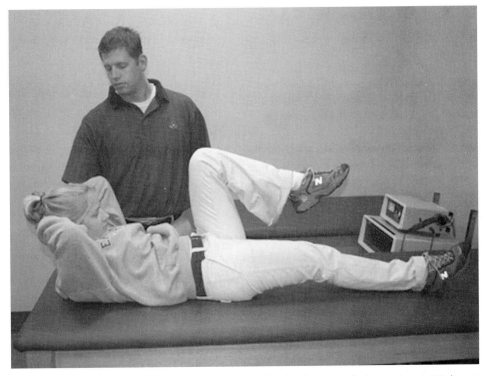

Figure 8-13 Kernig's sign can be a component of Brudzinski's sign. It involves flexing one knee to 90 degrees while actively maintaining cervical flexion. Increasing pain with this exercise can indicate the meningeal irritation associated with meningitis, or nerve root impingement.

Box 8-6 | Lumbar Puncture

Lumbar puncture is performed by having the patient in a side-lying position with knees pulled up to the chest and head fully flexed. This position helps to open the spaces between vertebrae in the lumbar column. Lumbar puncture is performed under strict sterile conditions. A sterile hollow needle is inserted between two lumbar vertebrae (typically L3 and L4) and enters the subarachnoid space to draw out cerebrospinal fluid (CSF) for assessment.

The CSF is assessed for pressure and color before being sent to the laboratory for evaluation of white blood cells (WBCs), glucose, and protein. The lumbar puncture is a good diagnostic tool for meningitis, Lyme disease, Guillain-Barré syndrome, multiple sclerosis, tumors, and other neurological disorders. A physician will sometimes use this procedure to inject drugs or anesthetic for other medical procedures. Following the puncture, the patient is typically kept prone for 4 to 6 hours to reduce the risk of headache.

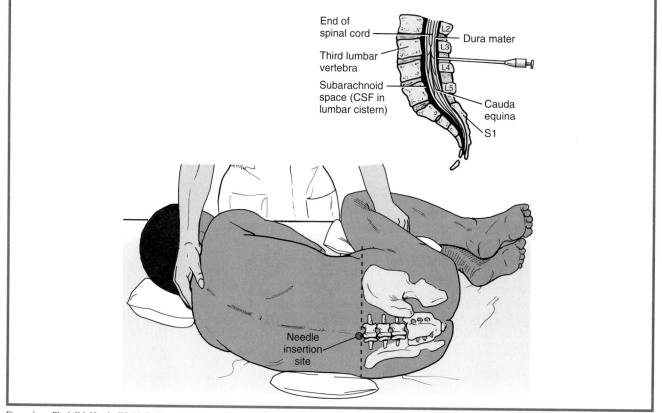

Figure from Black JM, Hawks JH: *Medical-surgical nursing: clinical management for positive outcomes*, ed 7, St Louis, 2005, WB Saunders, p 2044.

Public Health Implications and Prevention

Although aseptic or viral meningitis is the most common type of meningitis, the Centers for Disease Control and Prevention (CDC) in 1999 dropped it from a list of illnesses that need to be reported to the agency. It is still reportable to some state public health agencies. The time period within which to report a case or suspected case of aseptic meningitis varies from state to state but is usually within 1 week. A passive, voluntary database through the CDC and the National Enterovirus Surveillance System (NESS) is in place to gather information about enterovirus detection and outbreaks from state public health agencies and private laboratories as well as treating physicians.

The most effective method of prevention against enterovirus is adherence to good hygiene practices that include frequent and thorough hand washing and avoidance of shared utensils and drinking containers.

In institutional settings, washing objects and surfaces with a dilute bleach solution (as described in Chapter 1) can be a very effective way to destroy the virus.[20] Other preventive methods encompass the mosquito prevention techniques mentioned earlier.

Bacterial Meningitis

Unlike aseptic meningitis, bacterial meningitis is an acute, and potentially life-threatening infection of the meninges and the CSF. It is also called meningococcal meningitis. Three types of bacteria account for more than 80% of all cases: *Haemophilus (Haemophilus influenzae)*, *Pneumococcus (Streptococcus pneumoniae)*, and *Meningococcus (Neisseria meningitidis)*.[10]

The athletic trainer needs to fully appreciate meningococcal disease. This potentially life-threatening bacterial infection is the leading cause of bacterial meningitis in older children and young adults in the United States. The disease most commonly is expressed either as meningococcal meningitis, an inflammation of the membranes surrounding the brain and spinal cord, or as meningococcemia, a serious infection of the blood. Meningococcemia blood infections are caused by gram-negative *Neisseria meningitidis* but do not present with associated meningitis.[13] Most cases occur during the winter and spring.

It is estimated that 100 to 125 cases of meningococcal disease occur annually on college campuses and 5 to 15 students die as a result. The disease can result in permanent brain damage, hearing loss, learning disability, limb amputation, kidney failure, or death. When Harrison and colleagues[21] examined meningococcal outbreaks on college campuses in Maryland, the overall incidence of meningococcal infection in college students was similar to the incidence in the general population. It appeared, however, that college students living on campus were at a higher risk for meningococcal disease than students living off campus.

None of the bacteria that cause meningitis are as contagious as the common cold or the flu. Meningococcal disease is not spread by casual contact or by simply breathing the air where a person with meningitis has been. The bacteria are spread through the exchange of respiratory and throat secretions (i.e., coughing, kissing). Sometimes, however, bacteria have spread to other people who have had close or prolonged contact with a patient with meningitis caused by *N. meningitidis*. People in the same household, such as college students living in dormitories, or anyone with direct contact with a patient's oral secretions from coughing, sneezing, kissing, or oral contact with shared items such as cigarettes or drinking glasses would be considered at increased risk of acquiring the infection. People who qualify as close contacts of a person with meningitis caused by *N. meningitidis* should receive prophylactic antibiotics to prevent them from getting the disease. Many people carry the bacteria in their nose and throat without signs of illness; however, they can spread the disease to others.

Signs and Symptoms

As stated earlier, meningitis strikes suddenly; therefore early diagnosis and treatment are especially important. All forms of acute meningitis, bacterial or viral, have common symptoms that may also be mistaken for the flu. This disease has also been erroneously dismissed as torticollis because of its proclivity for stiff neck (see Box 8-5).[22] In addition, meningococcal meningitis presents with myalgia, tachycardia, tachypnea, and hypotension.[2,13]

Referral and Diagnostic Tests

Bacterial meningitis is a medical emergency. Ultimately a satisfactory outcome depends on the speed with which treatment is initiated. As with viral meningitis, the three indicators that occur abruptly and rapidly are a severe headache, high fever, and stiff neck. These warnings should alert the athletic trainer to immediately refer an athlete to a hospital emergency department.

Diagnosis is based on clinical history, physical examination, and specific diagnostic tests. The definitive diagnosis of bacterial spinal meningitis is made by examination of CSF (see Table 8-1) obtained through a lumbar puncture; opening pressure of the CSF will be elevated (>180 mm H_2O). On visual inspection the CSF appears cloudy or purulent. Further evaluation of the CSF includes culture, protein, glucose, and white blood cell count.[10] Other key laboratory tests include blood cultures, chest radiograph, and electrolyte and glucose measurement.[23] CT or MRI brain scanning may also be desirable.

Differential Diagnosis

A diagnosis of bacterial meningitis is not difficult to make when careful attention is paid to the patient's clinical history and physical examination that note sudden onset of severe headache accompanied by high fever and lethargy or confusion. Until results of the CSF analysis are known, however, several other processes need to be considered. These include herpes simplex virus (HSV) encephalitis, aseptic meningitis, encephalitis caused by arthropod-borne viruses, brain abscess, torticollis, skull fracture, and subarachnoid hemorrhage.[10,18,22]

Treatment

Bacterial meningitis can be treated effectively with a number of antibiotics. Treatment is two pronged. First, because of the severity and emergent nature of the disease, antimicrobial treatment is started before results of the CSF cultures are known. Once the specific pathogen is identified, specific intravenous drug therapy is begun. Second, other associated complications, such as hearing loss, brain swelling, shock, convulsions, and dehydration, must be addressed with appropriate supportive treatment and drug therapy.[10]

Prognosis and Return to Participation

The prognosis for bacterial meningitis depends on several factors, including the type of infecting organism and the speed with which medical treatment is initiated. Untreated bacterial meningitis is fatal. The mortality rate for uncomplicated meningococcal meningitis and *H. influenzae* is about 5%. Meningococcal infections in adolescents and young adults from 15 to 24 years of age show much higher mortality rate (22.5%) than for younger patients (4.6%) and older adult patients (16.5%).[10] In general, early and effective treatment leads to recovery with no residual symptoms. Late or inadequate treatment may incur permanent damage. Common sequelae include memory impairment, decreased intellectual function, hearing loss and dizziness, seizures, and gait disturbances.[2,10]

Return to participation will depend on the complete resolution of symptoms and medical clearance from the treating physician or medical team.

Public Health Implications

At the national level, meningococcal meningitis is listed as a reportable disease. State and local public health agencies also set guidelines with respect to reportable diseases. Guidelines are typically in place in universities regarding proper reporting procedures. Notification to local, state, and national agencies is usually done through the hospital or treating physician. Meningococcal infections require immediate reporting to the public health department.[13]

A vaccine is available against four of the most common strains of *N. meningitidis* in the United States. The vaccine is 85% to 100% effective in preventing disease in older children and adults. Studies suggest that up to 80% of college cases are vaccine preventable.[21] The CDC, the American College Health Association (ACHA), and the American Academy of Pediatrics (AAP) recommend that parents and college students, particularly freshmen who plan to live in dormitories, learn about meningococcal disease and the potential benefits of vaccination. Other college undergraduates wishing to reduce their risk may also choose to be vaccinated.

Guillain-Barré Syndrome

Guillain-Barré syndrome (GBS) is an acute, diffuse demyelinating disorder of the spinal roots and peripheral nerves. Rarely, it also attacks the cranial nerves. This polyneuropathy is an autoimmune syndrome that is acute, frequently severe, and rapidly progressive.[17] Specific lymphocytes are thought to produce antibodies against components of the myelin sheath and may contribute to destruction of myelin. As noted previously, without myelin, nerve conduction is interrupted.

GBS occurs year-round at a rate of approximately 1 case per 1 million per month; there are approximately 3500 cases per year in North America. The condition may occur in either gender and at any age but is uncommon in early childhood. Race is not a factor.

The incidence increases with age, and over one half of GBS patients experience symptoms of viral respiratory or gastrointestinal infection 1 to 3 weeks before onset of neurological symptoms.[2] Other reported triggers include pregnancy, minor surgical procedures, or minor medical procedures such as vaccination or flu vaccine.[2,11] GBS is not contagious.

An athletic trainer needs to be able to recognize the symptoms of rapid onset of bilateral muscle weakness in the lower extremities with the absence of fever or other systemic symptoms and refer the athlete immediately to the appropriate medical facility, usually the hospital emergency department.

Signs and Symptoms

The major clinical symptom of GBS is distal muscle weakness and loss of deep tendon reflexes that occurs bilaterally. The pattern is typically an ascending paralysis initially noted in the legs. The weakness evolves quickly over several hours or days and may be accompanied by tingling and dyesthesias in all extremities. The trunk, intercostals, neck, and cranial muscles may be involved later. Weakness may progress to total motor paralysis with death from respiratory failure within a few days. Frequently, early symptoms will also include paresthesias and numbness. A varying degree of sensory loss occurs in the first days and in a few days is barely detectable. When sensory deficits are present, deep sensations such as touch, pressure, and vibration are likely to be more affected than superficial sensations to pain or temperature. Complaints of pain and an aching discomfort especially in muscles of the hips, thighs, and back occur in 50% or more of the patients.[17,24]

Referral, Diagnostic Tests, and Differential Diagnosis

An athlete who experiences bilateral, rapidly evolving muscle weakness with absence of fever or other systemic symptoms and has a history of a recent viral upper respiratory infection (URI) or gastrointestinal illness must be referred to a physician immediately. Recently immunized or vaccinated athletes with the aforementioned complaints should be referred as well. GBS in its most severe form is a medical emergency. Most patients require hospitalization, and almost 30% require breathing assistance at some time during the course of the illness.[25] Severe GBS may result in total paralysis and inability to breathe without the help of a ventilator (Red Flags— Guillain-Barré Syndrome).

Key diagnostic and laboratory tests include an electromyelogram (EMG) (Box 8-7) and CSF analysis. CSF findings are distinctive but only conclusive after the first week.[24] They include an elevated CSF protein level (100 to 1000 mg/dl) without an accompanying increase in cells. When symptoms have been present for less

---

⦿ Red Flags for Guillain-Barré Syndrome

Signs and symptoms of Guillain-Barré syndrome include the following:
- Progressive weakness beginning distal and moving proximal
- Areflexia
- Afebrile state
- Pain with slightest movement of affected area
- Nocturnal muscular cramps

Box 8-7   Electromyography

An electromyogram (EMG) records and measures the electrical activity produced by a specific skeletal muscle. The test is performed by applying surface electrodes or inserting small needle electrodes into a muscle.

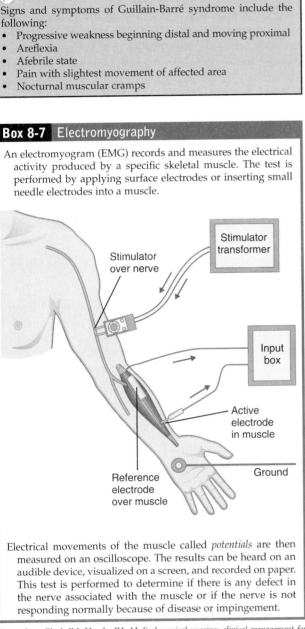

Electrical movements of the muscle called *potentials* are then measured on an oscilloscope. The results can be heard on an audible device, visualized on a screen, and recorded on paper. This test is performed to determine if there is any defect in the muscle or if the nerve associated with the muscle is not responding normally because of disease or impingement.

Figure from Black JM, Hawks JH: *Medical-surgical nursing: clinical management for positive outcomes,* ed 7, St Louis, 2005, WB Saunders, p 2047.

Box 8-8   Diagnostic Criteria for Guillain-Barré Syndrome

- Progressive weakness of two or more limbs because of neuropathy
- Areflexia
- Disease course <4 weeks
- Exclusion of other causes
  - Systemic lupus erythematosus
  - Toxins
  - Lead poisoning
  - Botulism
  - Diphtheria
  - Localized spinal cord trauma
  - Cauda equina syndrome
- Also consider the following:
  - Relatively symmetrical weakness
  - Mild sensory involvement
  - Facial nerve or other cranial nerve involvement
  - Afebrile state
  - Normal cerebrospinal fluid (CSF) readings
  - Electrophysiological evidence of demyelination

From Braunwald E, Fauci AS, Hauser SL, et al: *Harrison's principles of internal medicine,* ed 15, New York, 2001, McGraw-Hill.

---

the pattern of rapidly evolving signs of paralysis, diminished or absent reflexes, lack of fever or other systemic symptoms, and the results of laboratory tests, EMG, and CSF analysis. If the diagnosis is strongly suspected, treatment is initiated without waiting for the occurrence of characteristic EMG and CSF findings. Box 8-8 lists diagnostic criteria for GBS.

Differential diagnoses for GBS include metabolic myopathies, poliomyelitis, spinal cord compression, heavy metal intoxication, botulism, tick paralysis, and basilar artery occlusion.[2,11,25]

Treatment

Treatment is initiated as soon after diagnosis as possible. There is no cure for the syndrome, and although patients do get better, they rarely recover completely. Therapies are aimed at lessening the severity of the symptoms, accelerating the rate of recovery in most patients, and managing complications of the syndrome, such as fluctuations in blood pressure and heart rate, inability to breathe without respiratory assistance, and inability to chew and swallow. Some controversial studies[24,26] demonstrate that patients with GBS respond well to corticosteroids alone. In addition, plasmaphoresis and high-dose immunoglobulin therapy have been demonstrated to be effective.[17]

Rehabilitation involves being prudent with respect to possible thrombophlebitis, urine retention, and airway management for the sickest of patients. Skin conditions such as bedsores and contractures can occur. These can be circumvented with diligent skin care and inspection and range-of-motion exercises.

---

than 48 hours, the CSF is often normal. Nearly 75% of those diagnosed reach their lowest point of clinical function within 1 week, and the remainder reaches it within 1 month.[25]

Nerve conduction results are mild or absent in the early stages of GBS. The principal EMG findings are a reduction in the amplitudes of muscle action potentials, slowed conduction velocity, or conduction block in motor nerves.[17] GBS is described as a syndrome and not a disease because there is no specific disease-causing agent. Diagnosis is made by a physician carefully evaluating the athlete's symptoms and recognizing

Prognosis and Return to Participation

Most people reach the stage of greatest weakness within the first week after symptoms appear, and by the fourth week of the illness 98% of all patients are at their weakest.[25] The recovery period may be as short as a few weeks or as long as several years. Approximately 85% of patients with GBS recover completely or nearly completely with mild motor deficits in the feet or legs. About 30% of those with GBS still have residual weakness after 3 years. About 3% may suffer a relapse of muscle weakness and tingling sensations many years after the initial attack. The residual disability is pronounced in about 10% of the patients[26]: those with the most severe and rapidly progressing form of the disease when there has been evidence of widespread axonal damage as well as those who required early and prolonged mechanical ventilatory assistance. EMG findings are consistent predictors of residual weakness. The mortality rate is less than 5%.[17]

Return to participation will be determined by the level of symptom resolution and clearance of the medical team. It may take 1 year or more for symptoms to resolve.

Headaches

There are many different types of headaches, but 90% of them are classified as vascular, tension muscle contraction, or a combination of the two. The remaining 10% consist of headaches associated with intracranial, systemic, or psychological disorders. Vascular headaches include migraines, cluster headaches, toxic headaches, exertional headaches, and some types of posttraumatic headaches. A migraine is a type of vascular headache that may present with or without neurological symptoms. The neurological symptoms that occur depend on the location of the disturbance in the intracranial vascular system because they can be caused by either vasoconstriction or vasodilation.

Usually the onset for vascular headaches is during puberty or in the second to third decade of life between 10 to 40 years of age, with a familial occurrence of 50%. Vascular headaches, especially migraines, strike women more than men and may partially or completely remit after age 50 years. In many women, symptoms worsen during oral contraceptive or vasodilating medication use and improve, both in frequency and intensity, after menopause. Symptoms also appear to worsen during the spring months.

Pediatric and Adolescent Athletes

About 5% of children experience migraines during grade school years, with an increase to 20% of adolescents during high school.[27,28] A strong female predominance is also evident in this age group. When boys experience migraine, it usually occurs between 10 to 12 years of age. A study conducted with nearly 800 NCAA Division 1 basketball athletes concluded that although women have an increased prevalence of migraines, these athletes in general had lower incidence of migraines than did the general population.[28]

Some preventive strategies for younger athletes include eating regularly, avoiding skipping meals, getting adequate sleep by keeping a regular sleep schedule, and being aware of things that might trigger an attack such as particular foods. Other contributing factors are excessive exercise or physical activity, specific exercise regimens, physical or emotional stress, and maintaining a regular schedule of recreational exercise or organized sport.

Signs and Symptoms

Vascular headaches usually have a rapid onset and present with unilateral throbbing pain in the frontal or temporal area. The headaches may occur in an episodic pattern and often last for hours as opposed to days. Specifically, migraines tend to start in the morning, peak about 2 hours later, and resolve after 1 day although they can recur on a daily basis. As with most vascular headaches, migraines consist of a vasoconstriction phase of painless sensory phenomena before a headache and a vasodilation phase of a throbbing headache.

A migraine diagnosis is based largely on presenting symptoms. The classical migraine is the typical vascular headache that begins with an aura. The aura may consist of visual disturbances, usually unilateral, such as **scotomas** (i.e., darkness), flashes of light, and bright-colored or white objects. These phenomena commonly last for 20 minutes and usually resolve before any pain or throbbing begins. In contrast to the classical migraine, common migraines may be unilateral or bilateral and do not begin with an aura. These headaches generally last for days as opposed to hours, with associated symptoms including nausea, vomiting, diarrhea, weight gain, dizziness, and a prodromal period of endocrine dysfunction resulting in fluid retention. In addition, photophobia often accompanies these headaches. Cigarette smoking, sleep deprivation, stress, chocolate, and tyramine-containing cheeses are precipitating factors in the development of both the classical and common forms of migraines (Box 8-9).

Other types of migraines are associated with neurological deficits, such as the basilar artery migraine and the hemiplegic or ophthalmoplegic migraine. The basilar artery migraine is common in young women, occurring before their menstrual period; symptoms, which last for minutes to hours, may include facial or

Box 8-9   Precipitating Factors for Migraine

- Endocrine changes
  - Premenstrual
  - Menstrual
  - Oral contraceptive pills
  - Pregnancy
  - Puberty
  - Menopause
  - Hyperthyroidism
- Metabolic changes
  - Fever
  - Anemia
- Rhinitis
- Change in temperature or altitude
- Change in activity
- Alcohol, especially red wine
- Foods
  - Chocolates
  - Cheese
  - Nuts
  - Hot dogs
- Drugs
  - Nitroglycerin
  - Nitrates
  - Indomethacin
- Blood pressure changes
- Sleep, too much or too little

finger paresthesias, vertigo, ataxia, **dysarthria,** and tinnitus. The hemiplegic or ophthalmoplegic migraine is more common in young adults and can present in two ways. One condition involves extraocular muscle palsies (CN III) and ptosis, which may become permanent in recurrent cases. The other involves hemiplegia and hemiparesis that can persist even after the headache resolves.

Referral and Diagnostic Tests

A detailed and thorough clinical history helps to differentiate migraines from other types of headaches. Merely recognizing the key presenting symptoms of vascular headaches can help to exclude tension headaches.

Physical examination assesses commonly affected cranial nerves by testing visual acuity and visual fields, pupil reaction, extraocular muscle movements, and facial symmetry. A physician may also order a complete blood count (CBC), biochemistry profile, skull and cervical spine radiographs, CT or MRI of the brain, EEG, or lumbar puncture. In addition, treatment responses can help pinpoint the diagnosis. For instance, tension headaches caused by muscle contraction tend to respond positively to traditional nonsteroidal antiinflammatory drugs (NSAIDs), whereas migraines, generally, do not.

It is important to distinguish whether an athlete's headache is associated with exercise. These types of headaches include exercise-induced migraine, benign exertional headache also referred to as weight lifters' cephalgia, and vascular headache resulting from prolonged exercise. All three of these headaches are classified as vascular but have definite distinguishing factors.

An effort or exercise-induced migraine is a unilateral retroorbital headache that presents with a visual aura and is more prominent at the end of activity. The symptoms are more likely in hot weather and accompanying dehydration. In benign exertional headache, the symptoms are bilateral, have rapid onset and short duration, and occur at the beginning of activity. They are often associated with the increased intrathecal pressure associated with lifting weight with a closed glottis (Figure 8-14). Exertional headaches generally decrease in frequency over time. It is critically important that a physician evaluate athletes with this type of headache because 10% will have associated intracranial pathology such as arteriovenous malformation, **Arnold-Chiari malformation,** subdural hematoma, brain tumor, aneurysm, or basilar impression. The vascular headache with prolonged activity presents true to its name and may last for up to 24 hours after exercise. It may also have associated transient or persistent neurological deficits depending on the presence and severity of cerebral ischemia.

The athletic trainer also needs to recognize the features of headaches associated with intracranial hemorrhage and head trauma for on-the-field evaluation of the athlete. Headaches associated with intracranial hemorrhage usually present with more severe neurological signs, especially involving altered levels of consciousness, than those associated with head trauma.

After head trauma, two headaches of special concern include posttraumatic migraines and **dysautonomic cephalgia.** Posttraumatic migraines are common in soccer players secondary to heading a ball. This headache presents as a classical migraine with prominent visual symptoms and usually has an associated neck headache component. Dysautonomic cephalgia occurs with trauma to the anterior triangle of the neck and causes injury to the sympathetic nerve fibers near the carotid artery. Sympathetic nerve injury results in autonomic dysfunction presenting as Horner's syndrome often with ptosis, **hyperhidrosis,** and a unilateral headache.

In addition, athletes with headache should always be referred for medical evaluation if there is a history of head trauma or loss of consciousness, signs of a postconcussion syndrome, or an exertional headache. Box 8-10 lists general headache symptoms that warrant further evaluation by a physician.

Differential Diagnosis

Differential diagnoses include headaches associated with a head injury; facial pain such as temporomandibular joint (TMJ) pain, sinus headache, cluster

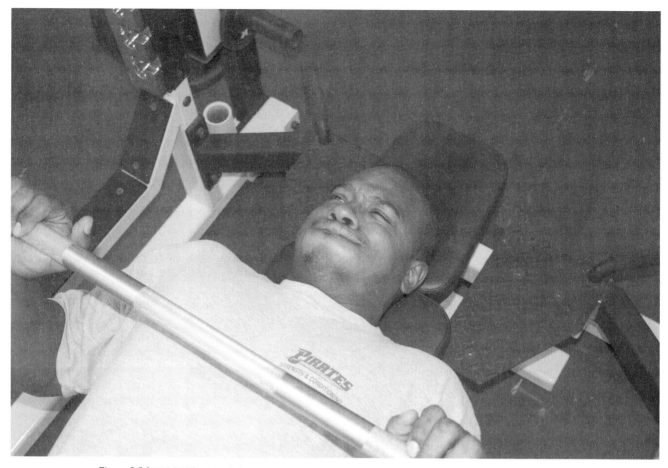

Figure 8-14 Weight lifter's cephalgia can occur when athletes attempt to lift weight while holding their breath.

| Box 8-10 | Headaches That Warrant Medical Evaluation |

- New or unusual headache
- Sudden onset of severe headache
- Change in the pattern of a headache
- Chronic headache with localized pain
- Headache that interrupts sleep during the night or in the early morning
- Headache that worsens over days
- Headache with severe nausea and vomiting leading to dehydration
- Visual disturbances
- Numbness, paralysis, or weakness of one side of the face or body
- Headache with associated
  - stiff neck or meningeal signs
  - systemic symptoms, such as fever or weight loss
  - neurological symptoms
  - local extracranial symptoms

headache, or **trigeminal neuralgia;** systemic conditions that include hypertension or infection whether viral, sinus, or influenza; side effects from medications such as mood-altering medications, antidepressants, analgesics, antibiotics, antihypertensives, caffeine, steroids, or nicotine; and environmental factors including high altitude, hypercapnia, and hyperthermia. Headaches associated with hunger are also possible in the athlete who comes to practice without adequate caloric intake.

Treatment, Prognosis, and Return to Participation

Treatment for migraines includes identifying the cause and appropriately treating the mechanism. Athletic trainers need to help the athlete learn the precursors of an episode and how to avoid them.

Persons with migraines may be discouraged from specific athletic activities, such as scuba diving where the diving environment itself can induce migraines that are often of increased severity. Typical stresses experienced in the diving environment include anxiety, associated sinus barotrauma, cold exposure, and possible saltwater aspiration (Figure 8-15).

Prevention

The key to prevention is identifying and avoiding precipitating factors such as stress, smoking, sleep deprivation, red wine, chocolate, and tyramine-containing cheeses. In addition, good control of blood pressure and monitoring medication side effects are important. Supportive psychotherapy can also assist in headache

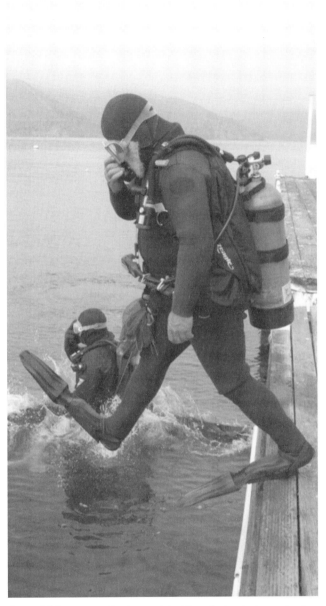

Figure 8-15 Scuba activity is not advised in patients who have migraines because the diving environment is contraindicated for migraines. (Courtesy Bill Dent.)

prevention by teaching techniques to reduce and relieve stress and tension.

Two preventive treatment protocols are specific to exercise-related headaches. Exercise-induced migraines brought on because of effort may be prevented by a graded warm-up period before exercise, which primes the sympathetic system. In addition, avoiding training in hot weather and ensuring adequate hydration may also reduce the occurrence of these migraines. Rarely, in cases of severe unrelenting headache, the offending activity needs to be significantly reduced or discontinued. Benign exertional headache is generally successfully treated with NSAIDs, neck massage, and

hydration, and it may be prevented by administration of acetaminophen or ibuprofen prior to exercise.

Simple treatment options for migraines include placing the athlete in a quiet dark room and encouraging sleep, which will often neutralize the headache. Pharmacological treatment is often necessary. Medical therapy for migraines consists of two classes of drugs: abortive and preventive medications.

Stroke

A stroke, also called a **cerebrovascular accident** (CVA), is a condition caused by lack of oxygen to the brain that may lead to reversible or irreversible paralysis and other neurological damage. Such damage to a group of nerve cells in the brain is often caused by interrupted blood flow from a blood clot or aneurysm in which the blood vessel bursts. Depending on the area of the brain that is damaged, a stroke can cause coma, paralysis, speech problems, or dementia.

Although the causes of stroke in adolescents and younger adults (15 to 45 years) are quite different from those in middle-aged and older adults, stroke is not uncommon in the younger age group. This group accounts for an estimated 3% of CVAs.[17,29] Rohr and colleagues[30] identify cardiac embolism, hematological stroke, and lacunar stroke as the most common causes in young adults. Nearly one third of first and recurrent strokes had no identifiable cause.[30] In athletes, a primary cause of stroke may be head injury. Head injury frequently causes intracranial bleeding, with common sites including intracerebral areas, especially inferior frontal and temporal lobes, and the subarachnoid, subdural, and epidural spaces (see Figure 8-2).[10] Another cause of stroke associated with intracerebral hemorrhage in young adults is drug abuse, specifically the "designer drugs" amphetamine, cocaine, and ecstasy.[29] In such cases, evaluation may be hindered when a cause is not readily apparent. A careful clinical history from the athlete or especially close friends and acquaintances is vital.

Signs and Symptoms

The athletic trainer needs to appreciate the signs and symptoms of a possible stroke (Red Flags—Stroke).

> **Red Flags for Stroke**
>
> Signs and symptoms of a possible stroke include sudden occurrence of the following:
> - Numbness or weakness of the face, arm, or leg, especially on one side of the body
> - Confusion, trouble speaking or understanding
> - Vision difficulties in one or both eyes
> - Problem with speaking, slurred speech
> - Trouble walking, dizziness, loss of balance or coordination
> - Severe headache with no known cause

Knowledge of the cranial nerves and their functions also are helpful in determining the extent of neurological involvement. Awareness of Brodmann's areas of the brain is very helpful in diagnosing where a possible problem may lie (see Figure 8-3).

Referral and Diagnostic Tests

A stroke is a medical emergency. Emergency treatment is crucial because every minute lost from onset of symptoms to the time of emergency contact limits the window of opportunity for intervention. Many patients do not go to the emergency department until 24 hours or more after the onset of symptoms. The longer the delay, the greater damage and loss of potential for recovery related to the stroke.

Diagnosis requires a complete medical history, physical and neurological examination, CBC including electrolyte levels, and a battery of specific diagnostic tests. The tests fall into three categories: imaging tests including CT scan and MRI; EEG and evoked potentials test to record electrical activity and sensory response patterns; and Doppler blood flow studies to reveal the patency of the arteries at the base of the skull or in the neck and arteriography injecting dye into the vessels combined with radiograph to reveal blood flow through the vessels in the brain and the size and location of any blockages.[10]

Differential Diagnosis

In the athletic setting, differential diagnoses for a stroke may include epileptic seizure with postictal **Todd's paresis,** a focal weakness following generalized or focal motor seizures that is uncommon in persistence for more than a few hours; tumor; migraine; metabolic encephalopathy caused by fever or infection; hyperglycemia; or hypercalcemia.[10] In addition, drug interactions, overdose, or abuse should not be overlooked.

Treatment

Acute treatment is designed to reverse or lessen the amount of tissue death. This involves medical support to optimize tissue perfusion and prevent complications such as infection, deep vein thrombosis (DVT), and pulmonary embolism (PE). Administration of pharmaceutical agents through intravenous or intraarterial lines may be combined with anticoagulant and antiplatelet agents, heparin or aspirin, and possibly hypothermia to mitigate cell destruction secondary to ischemia.[17]

Poststroke rehabilitation starts in the hospital as soon as possible after the stroke. Stable patients can begin rehabilitation 2 days after the stroke has occurred and continue as necessary after release from

| Box 8-11 | Rehabilitation Options After Stroke |

The choice of rehabilitation options after stroke depends on tissue damage and severity and includes the following:
- Rehabilitation unit in the hospital
- Subacute care unit
- Rehabilitation hospital
- Home therapy
- Home with outpatient therapy

the hospital (Box 8-11). Other therapy includes occupational and speech-language therapy.

The goal of rehabilitation is to improve function so that the stroke survivor can continue an independent lifestyle. Such training must be accomplished in a way that preserves dignity and motivates the patient to relearn basic skills for the activities of daily life that may have been lost, including communicating, eating, dressing, and walking.

Prognosis and Return to Participation

It is not fully understood how the brain compensates for the damage caused by stroke. A slight interruption in the flow of oxygenated blood may damage a few brain cells temporarily that later resume functioning. In some cases because different areas of the brain overlap in function, the brain can reorganize with one area taking over for the area damaged by the stroke. Because of this organ fluidity, stroke survivors sometimes experience remarkable and unanticipated recoveries.

Return to full athletic participation following a stroke depends primarily on the level of recovery and residual impairment as well as the type of sport (i.e., contact or collision sports versus noncontact sports). Certainly an athlete who has incurred a stroke as a result of a head injury may be ruled medically ineligible to participate even when recovery has been complete. Any athlete who has sustained a stroke related to a medical issue that could be exacerbated by activity should refrain from dangerous activity in the future. Further, the risk of additional injury may be too great to continue participation in sports such as hockey, football, or lacrosse.

In regard to participation in physical activity and exercise, studies have well documented the positive effects of physical training on the recovery and rehabilitation process following a stroke.[31,32] In addition to the obvious physical benefits of a training and reconditioning program, a return to physical activity may also assist the athlete with psychological recovery.[32] Elements of activity choice, intensity, duration, and volume are best chosen with the guidance of the medical team and athletic trainer supervising the athlete's recovery. Recovery is generally slow and tedious and may take many months.

Prevention

Prevention of stroke encompasses two distinct components for the athlete: lifestyle risk factors and trauma prevention factors. Lifestyle risk factors such as obesity, diabetes, hypertension, alcohol, and smoking may not be implicated during the robust years of collegiate and professional participation, but athletes need to be well aware of their significance to cerebrovascular disease later in life. Death from stroke is the third leading cause of fatalities in the United States.

In addition, hypertension in the athlete cannot be underestimated for the risk of stroke. Athletes who are hypertensive on the preparticipation examination should have serial blood pressures taken before and after exercise for several weeks to see if the high readings continue. If blood pressures continue to be hypertensive, the athlete needs to be referred to a physician for further evaluation and possible medications.

Trauma protection is key in the prevention of stroke for an athlete involved in contact sports and may include proper helmet fitting and the use of a correctly fitted mouth guard. Although no direct links have been established between stroke and helmet or mouth guard fit and use, both have been well documented for preventing or minimizing head injury.[33] Stroke caused by intracranial hemorrhage from head trauma is considered one of the most severe sequelae.

Multiple Sclerosis

Multiple sclerosis (MS) is a neurodegenerative, lifelong chronic disease diagnosed primarily in young adults. It is characterized by the gradual accumulation of focal plaques of demyelination in the brain. Peripheral nerves are not affected. The pathophysiology of MS involves myelin cells being destroyed and replaced by hard sclerotic tissue. The result may be permanent disability in the affected nerves. In Western societies, MS is second only to trauma as a cause of neurological disability arising in early to middle adulthood.[34]

Current evidence indicates that MS is an autoimmune disease. The precise cause of MS remains unknown, but a number of epidemiological facts have been clearly established. MS develops in genetically susceptible individuals who reside in certain permissive environments. It affects approximately 400,000 Americans and 1.1 million individuals worldwide and is approximately twice as common in females as in males. In both genders, the incidence rises steadily from adolescence to age 35 years and declines gradually thereafter. About two thirds of cases have an onset between 20 and 40 years of age.[34] Manifestations of MS vary from a benign illness to a rapidly evolving and incapacitating disease requiring profound adjustments in lifestyle and goals for patients and their families. Complications from MS affect multiple body systems.[2,10,17]

Signs and Symptoms

Symptoms of MS may be mild or severe, may be of long or short duration, and appear in various combinations. Most frequently, the disease is a relapsing-remitting disorder with symptoms that may come and go over time.[35] Weakness or numbness in one or more extremities is the initial symptom in approximately one half of the patients. The initial presentation in about 25% of all MS patients is an episode of optic neuritis.[2] **Optic neuritis** is a syndrome in which partial or total loss of vision, usually in one eye, evolves rapidly over several hours to days. Some patients may experience pain within the orbit that may be made worse with eye movement or palpation of the globe 1 or 2 days before visual loss. Other visual symptoms may include blurred or double vision or red-green color distortion. About one third of patients with optic neuritis recover completely, and others generally improve significantly even in cases in which the initial visual loss was profound.

Systemic fatigue is also a common complaint associated with MS. Sixty percent of people with MS judge fatigue the worst symptom of their disease.[36] This symptom makes diagnosis challenging in active college-aged athletes in whom fatigue is common.

MS patients who experience muscle weakness in their extremities will have difficulty with coordination and balance. Most people with MS exhibit paresthesias, transitory abnormal sensory feelings such as numbness or "pins and needles." Some may also experience pain or loss of feeling. About one half of people with MS experience cognitive impairments such as difficulties with concentration, attention, memory, and judgment. Such impairments are usually mild and rarely disabling, and intellectual and language abilities are generally spared.[1,37]

Heat is a culprit for the worsening of many MS symptoms, and athletes with this disorder should be monitored carefully during warmer days.[13]

Referral, Diagnostic Tests, and Differential Diagnosis

The symptoms of MS are often vague, insidious, and nonspecific. However, any athlete who experiences fatigue; numbness and tingling in the arms, legs, or elsewhere in the body; or vision irregularities must be referred to the team physician. These are among the early indications of MS. Often the symptoms will be unilateral and occur without trauma. Static tremors may be present, and a physician will determine whether a neurological condition such as MS may be the cause.

Physicians use a neurological examination and take a medical history when they suspect MS. Imaging technologies include MRI, which provides an anatomical picture of lesions, and magnetic resonance spectroscopy (MRS), which yields information about the biochemistry of the brain. Other tests include a spinal tap to obtain a sample CSF to study the immunoglobulin G antibody, an EEG, sensory evoked potential (EP) studies, and an EMG. No single test unequivocally detects MS. Other tests performed to diagnose MS include testing deep tendon reflexes, which are generally increased in the disease.

A number of other diseases produce symptoms similar to those seen in MS. The possibility of an alternate diagnosis must be considered and eventually ruled out. Initially MS may mimic stroke, lupus, a progressive myelopathy, migraine, spinal cord tumor, arteriovenous disorders, Lyme disease, arthritis, Guillain-Barré syndrome, and syphilis, among other conditions.[2,10]

Treatment

There is no cure for MS. Approximately 85% of people with MS have the relapsing-remitting form of the disease in which they experience acute exacerbations or relapses with or without complete recovery.[35] Treatment is divided into two categories: treatments designed to modify the course of the disease, and symptom management. Several disease-modifying medications are available for relapsing-remitting MS: interferon beta-1a (Avonex, Rebif), interferon beta-1b (Betaseron), and glatiramer (Copaxone). All require daily or weekly self-injection of the medication, which in turn reduces the number of exacerbations.[38]

MS may also be progressive. Medications to relieve symptoms in progressive MS include corticosteroids, muscle relaxants, and medications to reduce fatigue. Many medications are used for the muscle stiffness, depression, pain, and bladder control problems often associated with MS. Drugs for arthritis and medications that suppress the immune system may slow MS in some cases.

In addition to medications, other treatments may relieve MS symptoms. These include physical and occupational therapy with the goal of preserving independence by performing flexibility, strengthening, and proprioceptive exercises and using assistive devices to ease daily tasks.

Counseling for individuals or in group therapy sessions may help both the athlete and family cope with MS and relieve emotional stress.[38] Exercise is an excellent treatment for MS patients when performed in moderation (Box 8-12). Exercise may also have some

---

| **Box 8-12** | **Benefits of Mild to Moderate Exercise for Individuals with Multiple Sclerosis** |

- Decreases fatigue
- Allows more independent functioning
- Helps overcome depression
- Improves
  - stamina
  - strength
  - muscle tone
  - balance
  - coordination
  - overall mood
  - sense of well-being

---

adverse effects, particularly if prolonged or practiced in heated environments; these bad effects include increased fatigue, weakness, pain, and spasticity. MS or medications used to control some symptoms can alter the body's ability to dissipate heat. Overheating will increase MS symptoms. In addition, muscle weakness around joints can leave individuals with MS unstable and vulnerable to injury, which causes pain that makes spasticity worse and promotes more weakness.

Prognosis and Return to Participation

Because the exact cause of MS remains unknown, the clinical course and prognosis are as variable as the symptoms. Whereas one patient may present with the disease and have a virtually benign course, another may rapidly progress to dependency on wheelchairs and catheters for voiding.

The majority of people with MS have a normal life expectancy. The remission-exacerbation components of the disease make it challenging to predict future disability. In general, patients who experience minimal neurological impairment 5 years after the initial symptoms are least likely to be severely disabled 10 to 15 years later.[11,13] Those who experience a disease course that is progressive from the start are more likely to experience progression of disability. In the worst cases, MS can render a person unable to write, speak, or walk.

A young athlete who develops this chronic, debilitating disease can be particularly devastated. One of the first questions may be, "Can I continue to exercise or train?" The answer is "yes, but ..." Research has shown that although exercise does not change the impairment, physical exercise does result in an improvement in disability and has a positive impact on the mental aspect of health-related quality of life perception.[39-42]

Because MS strikes people in different ways, some athletes who have completely or almost completely recovered from an exacerbation may be able to run 5 or 10 miles or bicycle 75 miles per day. Others may be severely disabled and need to use a powered wheelchair. Finding the optimal exercise management program requires a team effort among the physician, athletic trainer, physical therapist, and athlete. The best program combines elements of cardiovascular training, strength, flexibility, balance, coordination, and appropriate functional exercises and is designed with independence and quality of life in mind.

Reflex Sympathetic Dystrophy and Complex Regional Pain Syndrome

Reflex sympathetic dystrophy (RSD) is a condition involving overactivity of the sympathetic nervous system after minor injury or, more commonly, a condition of unknown etiology. Historically, it has been referred to by other names, such as sympathetically mediated pain, shoulder-hand syndrome, **Sudeck's atrophy,** and posttraumatic edema, which are all synonymous with the same constellation of symptoms. On the other hand, causalgia has been mistakenly used interchangeably with RSD. Although both conditions present with sympathetic nervous system overactivity, the underlying etiology in causalgia is nerve injury.

RSD and causalgia have recently been incorporated into a newly reorganized syndrome called **complex regional pain syndrome** (CRPS). Table 8-2 lists the new definitions, but despite new terminology, definitions, and classification systems, the old term of RSD is familiar and still commonly in use. Therefore this chapter refers to this condition as RSD/CRPS.

RSD/CRPS presents with the hallmark symptom of pain out of proportion to the degree or severity of injury. It generally presents posttraumatically with underlying ligament, bone, or nerve injury, although more than 30% of all cases occur without any identifiable associated trauma.[43] Although rare, RSD/CRPS can occur in children, but it is more common in adolescents. The presentation in children is quite different from in adults. For example, RSD/CRPS in adults has a higher incidence of upper extremity involvement, especially the shoulder, compared with a predominance of lower extremity involvement in children and adolescents, where ankle or foot sprains are the likely trigger. The prognosis and actual outcomes of RSD/CRPS treatment are generally better in children as well.

Signs and Symptoms

Athletes with RSD/CRPS usually experience intense unrelenting pain at a joint. The pain is generally worse with any weight bearing or loading of the affected extremity and relieved by rest and joint immobilization in severe cases. This pain is accompanied by varying degrees of autonomic dysfunction, including vasomotor disturbances or dystrophic changes. In addition, the affected area may exhibit edema, sweating, nerve hypersensitivity (e.g., **allodynia** in 90% of cases), and **dermatographia.** The vasomotor disturbances encompass vasodilation responses of warmth and erythema and vasoconstrictive responses of coolness, cyanosis, and mottling. RSD/CRPS may progress through three distinct phases of deteriorating function: acute within less than 3 months, dystrophic over 3 to 6 months, and atrophic after more than 6 months.[43]

Often, the most notable findings for the clinician are reduced joint range of motion, complaints of acute pain with movement of the affected limb, and delayed injury recovery. Of interest is the high incidence of associated anxiety and depression with RSD/CRPS, which is probably a function of and proportional to the chronic nature of the pain.

Referral and Diagnostic Tests

Often the best diagnostic tool for identifying and confirming RSD/CRPS is the clinical response to a coordinated comprehensive rehabilitation program. Therefore it is not at all uncommon for the athlete to initially be referred by the therapeutic clinician to the physician for further evaluation. As the rehabilitation course progresses, delayed recovery from that expected is one of the first clues that RSD/CRPS may be developing. This finding alone may warrant referral back to the physician for assessment as to whether other underlying or associated injuries that were not initially identified or early RSD/CRPS changes are present. Delayed recovery in the presence of pain disproportionate to the degree of injury, reduced joint motion, or hypersensitivity to touch and movement (Red Flags—RSD/CRPS) require prompt referral back to the physician for further evaluation for definite RSD/CRPS.

Table 8-2	Complex Regional Pain Syndrome	
New Terminology	**Old Terminology**	**Definition**
CRPS I	RSD	Chronic nerve disorder causing pain after a major or minor injury
CRPS II	Causalgia	Chronic nerve disorder causing pain specifically after nerve injury

CRPS, Complex regional pain syndrome; *RSD,* reflex sympathetic dystrophy.

> ### ▶ Red Flags for RSD/CRPS
> Signs and symptoms of a patient with RSD/CRPS include the following:
> - Severe burning pain
> - Hyperanhidrosis
> - Pain beyond what would be expected for the injury
> - Local edema
> - Pathological changes in skin
> - Radiographic changes in bone
> - Extreme sensitivity to pressure or touch

RSD/CRPS, Reflex sympathetic dystrophy/complex regional pain syndrome.

RSD/CRPS is primarily a clinical diagnosis arrived at after performing a thorough medical history and examination and excluding other more common conditions that prompt a high level of suspicion. Physical examination, in particular, can be very helpful in accurate identification of RSD/CRPS and may even assist in determining its severity and chronic prognosis. Findings may reveal a warm, swollen joint with reduced and painful range of motion. There may be tenderness over the third metacarpophalangeal joint with palpation in upper extremity syndromes. The overlying skin may be sweaty and erythematous with dense hair growth and accelerated nail growth. These findings may change depending on the stage of RSD/CRPS at the time of presentation.[2] Over time, fat atrophy leads to thin, waxy, pale skin, muscle atrophy is prominent, nails become brittle and fractured, muscle spasms ensue, and extremity pain and stiffness progress. At the end stages of RSD/CRPS, irreversible changes to the extremity have resulted in a nonfunctional atrophic extremity with joint contractures, lost mobility, and severe pain.

Diagnostic tests are generally nonspecific. Radiographs taken early may be negative; however, within 2 to 3 months, patchy **juxtaarticular** demineralization or osteoporosis may develop. Nuclear bone scans, although not very helpful, can also show changes of increased uptake in the juxtaarticular areas of bones, often involving the joints distal to the actual site of injury. Yet, again, the expected results will vary depending on the stage of the disorder, with these variations being much more common in children and adolescents.[11]

Another diagnostic approach tests the function of the sympathetic nervous system compared with the uninvolved side by skin wheal assessment, **thermography,** and sympathetic nerve blocks. Dermatographia is abnormally prolonged wheal and erythematous response that can develop in RSD/CRPS after writing on the skin of both extremities. An abnormal test suggests sympathetic nervous system dysfunction. Thermography is often used in pain centers to assist in the diagnosis of RSD/CRPS. Because it also depends on the stage and severity of the condition, thermography is often inconsistent, nonspecific, and overall inconclusive.

One procedure that can be therapeutic as well as diagnostic is a sympathetic anesthetic block. This block may be performed at the cervical level of C6 for upper extremity conditions, at the celiac plexus for upper abdominal area conditions, or at the lumbar level of L2 for lower extremity conditions.

Differential Diagnosis

As stated earlier, in some respects RSD/CRPS is a diagnosis of exclusion. It is vital to rule out other conditions that have a similar clinical presentation as well as underlying conditions that could actually be the cause of the presenting RSD/CRPS. In the latter case, if these conditions are not identified and treated, the RSD/CRPS may never resolve or improve. Diagnoses to exclude include Raynaud's phenomenon, systemic lupus erythematosus, **polymyositis,** gout, myofascial pain syndrome, heterotopic ossification (i.e., myositis ossificans), and thrombophlebitis. Demonstrated underlying causes of RSD/CRPS are peripheral nerve entrapment such as carpal tunnel syndrome and tarsal tunnel syndrome, nerve injury caused by laceration or neuroma, ligament sprain or tear, and fracture.

Treatment

The mainstay in the treatment of RSD/CRPS is early motion and pain control. Prompt initiation of a physical rehabilitation program is critical. The goals of rehabilitation for RSD/CRPS are to do the following:

- Desensitize the extremity
- Increase joint and extremity range of motion
- Reduce pain
- Effect control of the extremity
- Restore strength and function

Desensitization techniques for hypersensitivity consist of challenging the area with increasingly abrasive textured materials and stress loading the affected extremity. Range-of-motion activities are the central focus of rehabilitation, and they may be facilitated by the concomitant use of ultrasound, transcutaneous electrical nerve stimulation (TENS), muscle stimulation (Figure 8-16), or hydrotherapy. Contrast baths and range-of-motion exercises (Figure 8-17) may both assist in reducing the edema of the extremity. In addition, biofeedback may allow the patient to gain some control over the autonomic nervous system functions of sweating, skin temperature variations, and blood flow. Often, supportive psychotherapy provides these patients with various skills to assist in the acceptance, coping, and treatment of pain. Some of these skills are relaxation training, biofeedback, and distraction techniques.

Pharmacological treatment is available in the pain management with RSD/CRPS. Traditional treatment with NSAIDs may be used but often brings incomplete and ineffective relief. Narcotic medications may also be given but should be prescribed judiciously because of an increased risk of addiction in patients with RSD/CRPS and other chronic pain conditions. NSAIDs and narcotic medications may successfully reduce the pain's intensity, but the actual course of RSD/CRPS is not changed. Other medications available for treatment of RSD/CRPS include tricyclic antidepressants such as amitriptyline and the anticonvulsants gabapentin (Neurontin), phenytoin, and phenobarbital.[43] In addition, either oral methylprednisolone or injected steroid

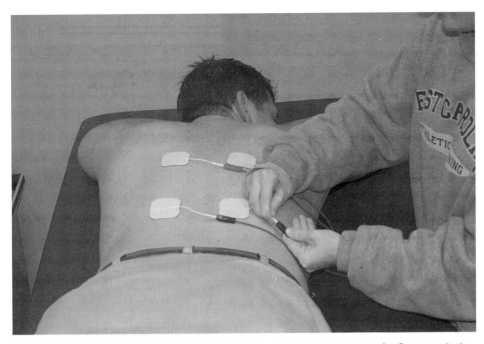

Figure 8-16 Muscle stimulation has been shown to be beneficial in the treatment of reflex sympathetic dystrophy/complex regional pain syndrome (RSD/CRPS).

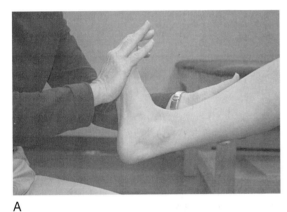

A

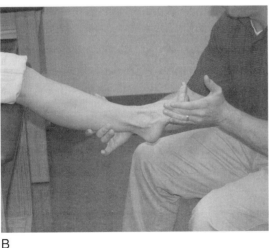

B

Figure 8-17 A, Maintaining range of motion shown here as passive dorsi-flexion and, B, light resistance training shown as eversion following an injury is a treatment for reflex sympathetic dystrophy/complex regional pain syndrome (RSD/CRPS) from occurring.

preparations may give pain relief in some cases. More than 50% of children and adolescents with RSD/CRPS achieve satisfactory results with the noninvasive treatments discussed, and their recovery is generally quicker than seen in adults.

Chemical blockade, as mentioned earlier, consists of sympathetic anesthetic blocks to the cervical, celiac, or lumbar ganglia and may be the most effective form of treatment. If a therapeutic response is obtained with this technique, three to six blocks may be performed during a 2- to 3-month period. The blocks are almost always successful in relieving the pain. In fact, if a person does not respond to a block, the diagnosis of RSD/CRPS is questioned.[2]

It is important to note that a program of range-of-motion activities and stress-loading exercises to the affected joint or extremity amplifies the potential for good treatment response. Exercise provides a means for the individual to continue desensitizing the affected extremity. For example, in RSD/CRPS of the hand, a stress-loading protocol may consist of household chores that include scrubbing a 3 foot–square area of floor for 20 minutes three times daily or lifting and carrying books several times each day. In some cases, the pain recurs during rehabilitation so intensely that a somatic block such as an epidural block or brachial plexus block may be necessary to calm down the noxious stimuli coming from the muscles and joints in the affected extremity.

At the far end of the spectrum of treatment options, permanent interruption of the sympathetic pathways either by a sympathetic neurolytic blockade or by surgical sympathectomy exists. It is important that the patient realize that the goal of surgical blockade is to treat the pain and that surgical blockade has less benefit in restoring impaired function, especially in more severe conditions. In addition to the potential for unsatisfactory functional outcomes from surgery, there is often incomplete pain relief. Although surgical procedures are a viable treatment option in the face of other treatment failures, they are to be avoided if at all possible because, in some cases, the procedure itself can reactivate the RSD/CRPS. Further, the changes in vascular flow that occur after sympathectomy could affect bone and limb growth in children and should be performed only after due deliberation and with extreme caution.

Adolescent Athletes

A high level of suspicion for RSD/CRPS in adolescent athletes is always wise because they will often hide or downplay the severity of their symptoms in order to return to play sooner or to avoid missing any activity at all. Precautions also need to be taken in prescribing medications to this age group. The physician and athletic trainer must persist in encouraging compliance with therapy and maintenance programs in young athletes to ensure recovery and prevent chronic limitations, deformities, or disabilities.

Mature Athletes

The major concern with mature athletes is the tendency for stiffness to develop faster and to a greater degree than in younger people. Therefore prompt initiation of joint and extremity mobilization in these athletes is critical.

Prognosis, Return to Participation, and Prevention

Prognosis in RSD/CRPS depends on the degree of severity and the progression of the condition. Most changes associated with RSD/CRPS are reversible in the early stages of the disease within the first 4 to 6 months but can become irreversible with time, often after 8 to 9 months. In most athletes, the condition is usually identified and treated early in its course because of the overt limitations that it places on the athlete's activity and performance. Generally, an athlete will not wait or stay quiet long when unable to perform in sport. This propensity for early recognition and initiation of treatment in athletes is beneficial to both the athlete's recovery potential and return to participation.

Given that recovery will vary depending on RSD/CRPS severity, the nature of the underlying injury, the extremity affected, and the athlete's sport, only general guidelines can be given for return-to-participation schedules (Box 8-13).

Functionally, the athlete must be able to perform challenging agility tasks that simulate sport activity

---

Box 8-13   Criteria for Return to Participation with RSD/CRPS

An athlete with RSD/CRPS can return to participation in sports when the following occur:
- Affected extremity and joint have full and pain-free range of motion.
- Flexibility is symmetrical to the unaffected extremity.
- Strength is at least 80% of the unaffected limb.
- Coordinated firing patterns of the supporting muscles and muscular groups have been reestablished.

RSD/CRPS, Reflex sympathetic dystrophy/complex regional pain syndrome.

---

with sound biomechanics and appropriate skill. The return to participation can be expedited if the affected extremity is not critical in the performance of the sport. In these cases, modification of the athletic activity may assist in the athlete's return given adequate protection of the affected extremity.

In essence, the mainstay in the prevention of RSD/CRPS is early rehabilitative intervention for traumatic injuries. The athlete must progress through a complete rehabilitation course focused on restoring mobility, attaining strength, and regaining function.

Epilepsy

Although an estimated 10% to 30% of individuals will have a seizure at some time, **epilepsy** is a chronic condition consisting of unprovoked, randomly recurring seizures that occur in approximately 1% to 2% of the population.[2] Epilepsy is diagnosed before the age of 21 years in 75% of these cases and shows a prevalence of 0.5% in children less than 9 years of age.[11] It is important to know that the diagnosis of epilepsy is based on the occurrence of more than two seizures; therefore single-seizure episodes during a person's lifetime, including infantile febrile seizures, do not meet the clinical definition.

A seizure is abnormal electrical activity in the brain that causes systemic convulsions depending on the area of brain involvement. There are many underlying causes of seizures although more than one half of the cases are idiopathic. In fact, more than 75% of seizures in young adults and a smaller percentage in children under the age of 3 years have no identifiable cause. The etiology is presumed to be some form of inherited neuronal abnormality. In general, most idiopathic seizures develop between the ages of 2 and 14 years of age. Other seizures occurring in children younger than 2 years are usually related to developmental defects, birth trauma, or metabolic diseases of the brain. In people older than 25 years, the etiology is usually identified.[38] Some identifiable causes of seizures include recent or old brain injury, brain tumor, stroke, infection, metabolic disturbances, inherited disorders, alcohol or drug ingestion or withdrawal, sleep deprivation, heat stroke, and extreme emotional and physical stress.

Exercise-induced seizures occur very infrequently and present during or immediately after exercise. In sports of prolonged activity, such as marathons and triathlons, the underlying cause may be metabolic imbalance as opposed to the exercise itself. Other reasons for convulsions during activity include head trauma and heat illness. The best diagnostic approach for these seizures, outside of the history and physical examination, is an EEG performed during exercise.

Signs and Symptoms

Seizures result in systemic activity that can affect the level of consciousness and manifest as motor activity, sensory phenomena, psychic disturbances, or inappropriate behavior. With this in mind, the classification of seizures is based on the clinical manifestations of the abnormal electrical activity, which assist in making an accurate diagnosis and initiating appropriate treatment depending on that diagnosis. Seizures are divided into two major categories: generalized seizures and partial or focal seizures.

Generalized seizures involve electrical activity in both cerebral hemispheres. These types of seizures may have bilateral cerebral hemisphere involvement from onset or evolve from a partial seizure to involving both cerebral hemispheres. Generalized seizures are further classified as **tonic-clonic seizures** such as seen in intermittent or status epilepticus, absence seizures, or a various array of less common seizures. Intermittent tonic-clonic seizures are one of the most common types of seizures and are associated with an aura of smells or sounds that alert the person to impending seizure; tongue biting caused by uncontrolled muscle contraction; **incontinence;** and a postictal state of disorientation, confusion, exhaustion, or lethargy. These seizures are generally of short duration and self-limited, at times requiring no medication. Continuous tonic-clonic seizures are called **status epilepticus** and are medical emergencies. These are defined as continuous tonic-clonic convulsions lasting more than 30 minutes or recurrent tonic-clonic convulsions without regaining consciousness between attacks. These seizures require immediate intervention with monitoring and support of the airway, breathing, and circulation and prompt administration of medications to abort the continued pattern.

Absence seizures are another type of generalized seizure and are characterized by brief episodes of loss of attention or awareness lasting between 3 to 15 seconds without an aura or postictal state. Associated automatisms may include chewing, lip smacking, swallowing, or facial twitching. As many as 15 other types of generalized seizures occur, including myoclonic seizures and febrile seizures.

Partial seizures start with a focal presentation of a motor, sensory, autonomic, or psychic disturbance that manifests on the basis of the area of the origin in one cerebral hemisphere. Examples of these disturbances include involuntary motor activity of the face, limbs, or head; sensory symptoms of tingling, numbness, or pins and needles; special senses involvement of visual, auditory, olfactory, or **gustatory hallucinations;** autonomic dysfunction of **diaphoresis** (i.e., sweating) and flushing; and psychic phenomena such as **déjà vu, jamais vu,** paranoia, and fear. In simple partial seizures, consciousness is not impaired and the manifestations are usually restricted to one anatomical area on only one side of the body. In complex partial seizures, consciousness is impaired and may occur alone or in association with integrated purposeful movements or experiences such as automatisms or psychic disturbances. Automatisms may be simple, such as chewing, lip smacking, and swallowing, or complex, such as walking into a room or getting dressed. Both types of partial seizures can evolve into generalized seizures. There are also obvious partial seizures that cannot be further differentiated as simple or complex and account for approximately 7% of all seizures.[2]

Referral and Diagnostic Tests

Any athlete who experiences a seizure, whether of new or established onset, needs to be referred for neurological assessment to ensure appropriate diagnosis and management in new cases and to review medical management for effective control in established cases. Also, any athlete with a syncopal event needs to be referred for medical examination.

General evaluation of an athlete with a seizure disorder involves a detailed medical history including occurrences and precipitating factors and a physical examination thoroughly reviewing the neurological system. Laboratory tests include a CBC, chemistry panel, and urinalysis. Neurological testing may include an EEG, MRI or CT of the brain, lumbar puncture in cases of suspected infection, and possibly a positron emission tomography (PET) scan.

Differential Diagnosis

Convulsive activity caused by seizures must be differentiated from that prompted by other disorders, such as concussive convulsions and convulsive syncope. Concussive convulsions are brief periods of tonic posturing that are expressions of the concussion event, are benign, and require no specific treatment outside of that for the underlying concussion. Convulsive syncope involves generalized convulsive movements,

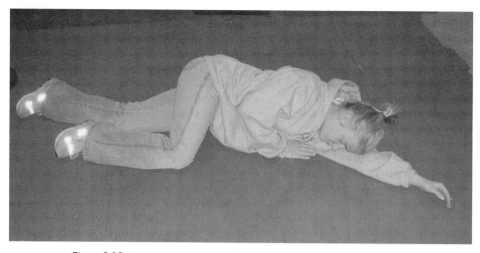

Figure 8-18 The correct recovery position for an individual following a seizure.

tongue biting, and incontinence during a syncopal or fainting event. Both entities involve convulsive movements related to reflex phenomena rather than abnormal cerebral electrical activity.

Treatment

Acute management of a seizure includes protecting the athlete from further harm by ensuring all dangerous objects are out of the way during a seizure. This includes moving desks, chairs, and anything the athlete may hit while seizing. It is neither necessary nor indicated to restrain someone undergoing a seizure. Following a seizure, the athlete is placed in the recovery position, on the left side with head resting on the left arm (Figure 8-18).

Medical management of epilepsy follows some general guidelines. Initially, a single medication is used to control the seizures with a second agent added when maximal dosage of the first is attained, side effects or toxicity limits further dosage increases, or adequate seizure control is not attained using a single agent. It is important to monitor the serum levels of the medications and the blood chemistry that may be affected by these medications.

The athletic trainer must also assess and treat underlying complications that can occur during seizures, such as fractures, dislocations, and head and neck injuries.

Prognosis and Return to Participation

Participation by an epileptic athlete in sports or physical activity depends on a number of issues that include the type of sport, risk of injury, and presence of preexisting neurological injury or dysfunction (Box 8-14).

In determining an athlete's ability to return to sport, the medical team considers the level of risk, which is

Box 8-14	Criteria for Return to Participation with Epilepsy

The following criteria must be carefully considered before an individual with epilepsy returns to participation:
- Sport type—collision, contact or noncontact
- Risk of severe injury or death if seizure occurs during the activity
- Preexisting brain injury and neurological dysfunction
- Risk of traumatic brain injury from athletic participation
- Seizure control—frequency, association with exercise, medications
- Effects of medications on performance—sedation and impaired judgment

lower when the athlete has been seizure free for 1 year on medications or seizure free for 2 years without medications. High-risk sports, including gymnastics, high diving, sky diving, rock climbing, and motor sports, should be avoided.[44] Noncontact sports that are still worrisome include archery, riflery, swimming, weightlifting events, and activities involving height.

Return-to-participation guidance is approached with caution and on an individual basis with the final determination made with respect to factors for sports participation, and consideration of high-risk sports. One factor to consider is the ability of the athlete to commute because individuals with epilepsy commonly need to prove stable management of their seizures before obtaining or reinstating their driver's license.

Public Health Implications

An individual with epilepsy must meet certain additional legal obligations when operating a motor vehicle. The athlete and, as appropriate, the parents are alerted to this requirement. The actual reporting of epilepsy to an appropriate governing authority varies from state

WEB RESOURCES

National Headache Foundation
http://www.headaches.org
Education about causes and treatment of headaches

American Council for Headache Education
http://www.achenet.org
Nonprofit organization of physicians and health providers studying headache causes and treatments

National Institute of Neurological Disorders and Stroke
http://www.ninds.nih.gov
Research and news on neurological disorders

Multiple Sclerosis Association of America
http://www.msaa.com
Information for the newly diagnosed; publications and programs for MS

Multiple Sclerosis Foundation
http://www.msfocus.org
Symptoms and treatment of MS; research and special events supporting research

National Multiple Sclerosis Society
http://www.nmss.org
Information for the newly diagnosed; research; special events

National Rehabilitation Information Center
http://www.naric.com
Information for anyone with a disability or brain rehabilitation issue

National Institute of Health
www.nih.gov
Reflex sympathetic dystrophy/complex regional pain syndrome (RSD/CRPS), epilepsy

Centers for Disease Control
http://www.cdc.gov/ncidod/dvbid/arbor/
Fact sheet about encephalitis: transmission, prevention, treatment, etc.

National Institute of Neurological Disorders and Stroke
http://www.ninds.nih.gov/health_and_medical/disorders/encmenin_doc.htm
Information on meningitis and encephalitis
http://www.ninds.nih.gov/disorders/gbs/gbs.htm
Guillain-Barré syndrome information

Epilepsy Foundation
www.epilepsyfoundation.org/answerplace/Social/driving
Epilepsy information

to state, and guidelines are available from the National Institutes of Health or Epilepsy Foundation websites as well as the local drivers-licensing facility. More stringent legal requirements exist for commercial licensing because the U.S. Department of Transportation has made it illegal to license anyone with a history of epilepsy for interstate trucking.

The main approach to prevention of an epileptic seizure is the avoidance of or prompt treatment of precipitating factors.

SUMMARY

Neurological disorders are alarming in the athletic population because they may be overlooked as a symptom of a benign condition. Without trauma, headaches are not typically a cause for concern in the healthy person. This chapter demonstrates conditions ranging from encephalitis to meningitis, including chronic disabling diseases, RSD/CRPS, epilepsy, and stroke that can begin with a simple headache.

Identifying conditions that expose an athlete to encephalitis or meningitis as well as understanding that strokes do occur in apparently healthy people are two of the critical aspects involved in recognition of neurological disorders. Rehabilitation of seemingly minute injuries that present with exaggerated pain prompts the athletic trainer to consider RSD/CRPS. Having the knowledge to consider atypical neurological conditions in otherwise healthy individuals is critical to the future health of athletes.

REFERENCES

1. Waxman S, deGroot J: *Correlative neuroanatomy,* ed 22, Norwalk, Conn, 1995, Appleton & Lange.
2. Beers M, Berkow R, editors: *The Merck manual of diagnosis and therapy,* ed 17, Whitehouse Station, NJ, 1999, Merck Research Laboratories.
3. Centers for Disease Control and Prevention: Arboviral encephalitides. Available at: http://www.cdc.gov/ncidod/dvbid/arbor/index.htm. Accessed March 2005.
4. Anderson, A: Arthropod pests and the diseases they carry: prevention in community and athletic settings, *Athletic Therapy Today* 9(3):16-21, 2004.
5. Centers for Disease Control and Prevention: West Nile virus activity—United States, October 13-19, 2004, *Morbidity & Mortality Weekly Report* 53(41):971-972, 2004.
6. Huhn GD, Sejvar JJ, Montgomery SP, Dworkin MS: West Nile virus in the United States: an update on an emerging infectious disease, *American Family Physician* 68(4):653-660, 2003.
7. Centers for Disease Control and Prevention, editor: *West Nile virus: what you need to know,* Atlanta, 2004, CDCP.
8. Centers for Disease Control: 2003 West Nile Virus Activity in the United States. Available at: http://www.cdc.gov/ncidod/dvbid/westnile/surv&controlCaseCount03_detailed.htm. Accessed March 2005.
9. Petersen L, Marfin A: West Nile virus: a primer for the clinician, *Annals of Internal Medicine* 137(3):173-179, 2002.
10. Braunwald E, Fauci AS, Hauser SL, et al: *Harrison's principles of internal medicine,* ed 15, New York, 2001, McGraw-Hill.
11. Ferri F: *Ferri's clinical advisor instant diagnosis and treatment,* St Louis, 2004, Mosby.
12. Khetsuriani N, Quiroz ES, Holman RC, Anderson LJ: Viral meningitis-associated hospitalizations in the United States, 1988-1999, *Neuroepidemiology* 22:345-352, 2003.

13. *Professional guide to diseases*, ed 7, Springhouse, PA, 2001,Springhouse.

14. Jhaveri R, Sankar R, Yazdani S, Cherry JD: Varicella-zoster virus: an overlooked cause of aseptic meningitis, *Pediatric Infectious Disease Journal* 22(1):96-97, 2003.

15. Makela A, Nuorti J, Peltola H: Neurologic disorders after measles-mumps-rubella vaccination, *Pediatrics* 110(5): 957-963, 2002.

16. Dylewski J, Bekhor S: Mollaret's meningitis caused by herpes simplex virus type 2: case report and literature review, *European Journal of Clinical Microbiology & Infectious Diseases* 23(7):560-562, 2004.

17. Victor M, Ropper A, editors: *Adam's and Victor's principles of neurology*, ed 7, Philadelphia, 2001, McGraw-Hill.

18. Emby D: Recurrent meningitis due to unrecognized skull fracture, *South African Medical Journal* 93(3):160-161, 2003.

19. Chin J, editor: *Control of communicable diseases manual*, ed 17, Washington, DC, 2000, American Public Health.

20. Centers for Disease Control and Prevention, editor: *Viral meningitis*, Atlanta, 2004, CDCP.

21. Harrison LH, Dwyer DM, Maples CT, Billmann L: Risk of meningococcal infection in college students, *JAMA* 281(20):1906-1910, 1999.

22. Mukherjee S, Sharief N: Bacterial meningitis presenting as acute torticollis, *Acta Paediatrica* 93(7):1005-1006, 2004.

23. Ellner P, Neu H: *Understanding infectious disease*, Boston, 1992, Mosby.

24. Goldman L, Ausiello D, editors: *Cecil textbook of medicine*, ed 22, vol 2, Philadelphia, 2004, WB Saunders.

25. Newswanger D, Warren C: Guillain-Barré syndrome, *American Family Physician* 69(10):2405-2410, 2004.

26. National Institute of Neurological Disorders and Stroke: *Guillain-Barré syndrome*, Available at http://www.ninds.nih.gov/disorders/gbs/detail_gbs_pr.htm. Accessed November 2004.

27. Lewis DW: Headaches in children and adolescents. *American Family Physician* 65(4):625-632, 635-636, 2002.

28. Kinart C, Cuppett M, Berg K: Prevalence of migraines in NCAA Division I male and female basketball players. National Collegiate Athletic Association. *Headache* 42(7): 620-629, 2002.

29. McCrory P: Headache and exercise, *Sports Medicine* 30(3): 221-229, 2000.

30. Rohr J, Kittner S, Feeser B, et al: Traditional risk factors and ischemic stroke in young adults: the Baltimore-Washington cooperative young stroke study, *Archives of Neurology* 53(7):603-607, 1996.

31. Albright A: Head injury. In Sherry E, Wilson SF: *Oxford handbook of sports medicine*, Oxford, UK, 1997, Oxford University Press.

32. Asthagiri A, Dumont A, Sheehan J: Head and neck injuries in sports medicine, *Clinics in Sports Medicine* 22(3): 559-576, 2003.

33. Guskiewicz K: Cumulative effects associated with recurrent concussion in collegiate football players, *JAMA* 290:2549-2555, 2003.

34. National Multiple Sclerosis Society, editor: *Just the facts 2004-2005*. Available at www.nationalmssociety.org. Accessed November 2004.

35. Tierney L, McPhee S, Papadakis M, editors: *Current medical diagnosis and treatment*, ed 43, New York, 2004, McGraw-Hill.

36. Zifko U: Management of fatigue in patients with multiple sclerosis, *Drugs* 64(12):1295-1304, 2004.

37. Finlayson M, Van Denend T, Hudson E: Aging with multiple sclerosis, *Journal of Neuroscience Nursing* 36(5): 245-251, 259, 2004.

38. University of Washington, Woodley M, Whelan A, editors: *The Washington manual: manual of medical therapeutics*, Boston, 1992, Brown & Co.

39. Petajan J, White A: Recommendations for physical activity in patients with multiple sclerosis, *Sports Medicine* 27(3): 179-191, 1999.

40. Sutherland G, Anderson MB: Exercise and multiple sclerosis: Physiological, psychological, and quality of life issues. *Journal of Sports Medicine and Physical Fitness* 41(4): 421-432, 2001.

41. Solari A, Filippin G, Gasco P, et al: Physical rehabilitation has a positive effect on disability in multiple sclerosis patients, *Neurology* 52(1):57-62, 1999.

42. Freeman J, Allison R: Group exercise classes in people with multiple sclerosis: a pilot study, *Physiotherapy Research International* 9(2):104-107, 2004.

43. Kirkpatrick A: *Clinical practice guidelines*, Milford, Conn, 2000, Reflex Sympathetic Dystrophy Syndrome Association.

44. Boyajian-O'Neill L, Cardone D, Dexter W, et al: Determining clearance during the preparticipation evaluation, *Physician and Sportsmedicine* 32(11):29-41, 2004.

CHAPTER 9

Disorders of the Eye

David Eichenbaum and
Charles B. Slonim

OBJECTIVES

At the completion of this chapter, the reader should be able to do the following:

1. Describe the basic anatomy and physiology of the eye.
2. Perform a basic eye exam.
3. Describe appropriate initial management of common conditions and injuries of the eye.
4. Recognize conditions of the eye that require referral.
5. Recognize conditions of the eye that may preclude the athlete from participation.

INTRODUCTION

Acute vision is vital to the success of the competitive athlete, and even "minor" eye disorders will sideline most athletes. An athletic trainer must understand the basic anatomy and physiology of the eye, be able to perform a basic eye examination, and know the common sport-related eye conditions and injuries for which referral to an eye care specialist is appropriate. This chapter discusses the structures of the eye, examination techniques for both healthy and injured eyes, and the pathological eye conditions that the athletic trainer might encounter.

OVERVIEW OF ANATOMY AND PHYSIOLOGY OF THE EYE

The anatomy of the eye consists of external and internal structures. The external eye includes the eyelids, the conjunctivae, and the lacrimal glands (Figure 9-1).

These structures serve to protect the eye from foreign objects and to distribute tears evenly across the eye. The eye socket (Figure 9-2), anatomically known as the bony orbit, comprises four walls made up of seven different facial bones of the skull, connective tissue, fat, blood vessels, and nerves.

Anteriorly, the orbit rim is created by the frontal, zygomatic, and maxillary bones (see Figure 8-1). The sphenoid, lacrimal, ethmoid, and maxillary bones form the posterior and medial aspect of the orbit. The palatine, zygomatic, and maxillary bones create the floor of the orbit, and the zygomatic and sphenoid bones form the lateral aspect. The orbit provides protection for the eyeball (globe) and contains the lacrimal gland that produces the tears that lubricate and rinse the surface of the eye. The bony orbit also provides anchorage for the six small extraocular muscles that move the eye. The optic nerve passes through the posterior aspect of the orbit. The visual cortex is located in the occipital lobe of the brain.

The eyelids provide protection for the external surface of the eye. They help lubricate the ocular surface with their blinking action. The eyelid skin is the thinnest skin of the body. Within each eyelid is a relatively rigid tarsal plate containing meibomian glands, which secrete the oily component of the three-layered tear film. The conjunctiva is a thin, essentially transparent, highly vascular mucous membrane that covers the anterior sclera and the posterior surfaces of both the upper and lower eyelids.

The eye consists of the sclera, cornea, iris, lens, retina, choroid, optic disc, and macula (Figure 9-3). The sclera is the dense white connective tissue that makes up more than 90% of the outer layer of the globe and provides structure for the contents of the eyeball. The cornea serves as the barrier between the environment

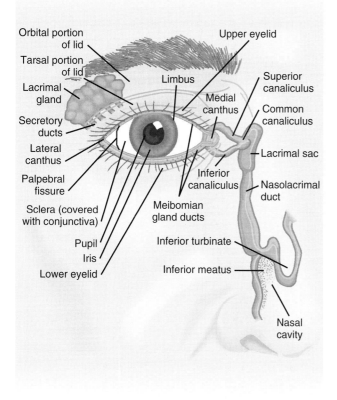

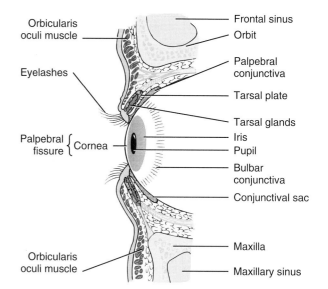

Figure 9-1 The external eye showing the eyelids, the conjunctiva, and the lacrimal glands. (From Black JM, Hawks JH: *Medical-surgical nursing: clinical management for positive outcomes,* ed 7, St Louis, 2005, Mosby, p 1911.)

Figure 9-2 A side view of the eye socket, anatomically known as the bony orbit of the eye. (From Black JM, Hawks JH: *Medical-surgical nursing: clinical management for positive outcomes,* ed 7, St Louis, 2005, Mosby, p 1911.)

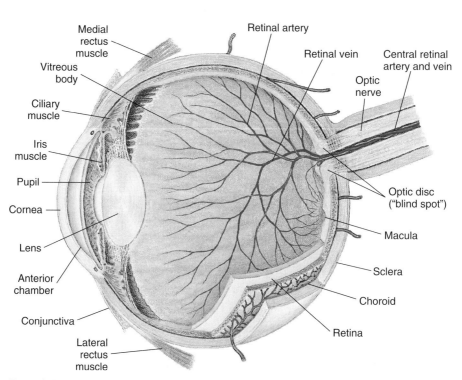

Figure 9-3 The internal eye. (From Seidel HM, Ball JW, Dains JE, Benedict GW: *Mosby's guide to physical examination,* ed 5, St Louis, 2003, Mosby, p 279.)

and the aqueous humor. The cornea is made up of several layers and is the clear window of the eye through which light passes. The iris creates the color of the eye. The pupil is the round, central opening in the iris that creates a pathway for light to reach the retina. This aperture dilates or constricts to regulate the amount of light that enters the eye. Between the cornea and the iris is the anterior chamber. This space is filled with a clear fluid known as aqueous humor.

The crystalline lens is a round, transparent tissue located directly behind the iris. Tiny filaments called zonules that are attached to the ciliary body suspend it and control the thickness of the lens by contracting or relaxing it, allowing the image to be focused onto the retina. The ciliary body is responsible for the production of the aqueous humor that fills the anterior chamber of the eye. The large space behind the lens is filled with the transparent gelatinous fluid of the eye known as the vitreous humor.[1]

The retina is the thin, transparent membrane lining the back of the eye that receives light and sends the initial visual signal through the optic nerve to the brain, where it is processed and interpreted. Between the retina and the sclera is the vascular tissue called **choriocapillaris.** The choriocapillaris supplies blood and nourishment to the outer layers of the retina. The reflection of light that occurs during a camera flash through a dilated pupil and against the choriocapillaris gives the red reflex or red eye seen in a photograph. As the nerve fibers from the retina exit the eye through the optic nerve, they bunch together at the origin of the optic nerve to form the optic disc. The optic disc is the visible portion of the optic nerve that can be seen when examining the eye. The other structure that can be seen during examination with an ophthalmoscope is the macula, or fovea, which is considered the site of central vision and color perception of the eye. The majority of color receptors called cones are found in the macula (Figure 9-4).[2]

BASIC EXAMINATION TECHNIQUES

Testing Visual Acuity

The most important part of an eye exam is the testing of visual acuity. The ability of the eye to focus clearly on distant or near objects is directly related to the structural integrity of all its parts. It is crucial to know an athlete's visual acuity before any injury (i.e., preparticipation vision screening) and to assess visual acuity immediately after an injury.[3] The visual acuity is assessed while athletes wear their spectacles or contact lenses for distance vision. It is recorded as a fraction comparing the athlete's performance with the standard or normal person's performance. This fractional notation is known as the Snellen visual acuity, based on the Snellen letter chart that is placed 20 feet away from the athlete (Figure 9-5, *A*).

The first number, or numerator, represents the athlete's distance from the eye chart, which should be 20 feet, and the second number, or denominator, represents the distance at which a "normal" person could read the same-size letter or letters on the same line of the chart. For example, reading the 20/40 line (from 20 feet away) indicates that the athlete can see a specific-sized letter at 20 feet.[4] A person with normal visual acuity can see the same-size letter from 40 feet away (Key Points—Visual Acuity), revealing that the athlete has suboptimal acuity.[1,5] Each eye is tested

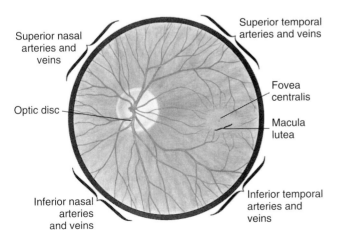

Figure 9-4 The retinal structures of the eye. (From Seidel HM, Ball JW, Dains JE, Benedict GW: *Mosby's guide to physical examination*, ed 5, St Louis, 2003, Mosby, p 294.)

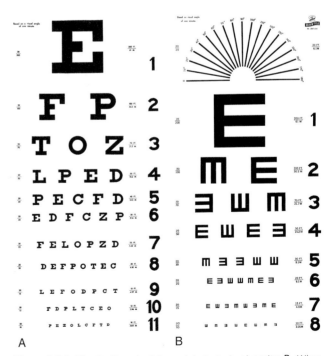

Figure 9-5 A, The Snellen chart is used to test visual acuity. B, When examining young children or those who do not read, an illiterate E or C or picture chart may be used to test visual acuity. (From Seidel HM, Ball JW, Dains JE, Benedict GW: *Mosby's guide to physical examination*, ed 5, St Louis, 2003, Mosby, p 72.)

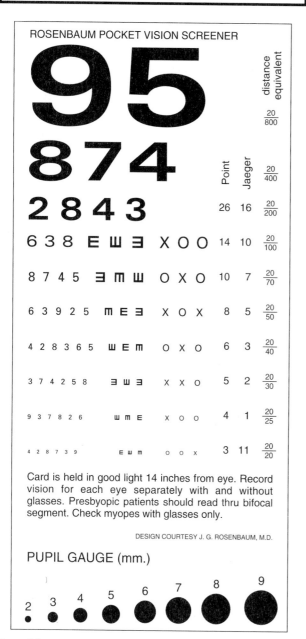

Figure 9-6 The Rosenbaum chart for testing near vision. (From Seidel HM, Ball JW, Dains JE, Benedict GW: *Mosby's guide to physical examination,* ed 5, St Louis, 2003, Mosby, p 73.)

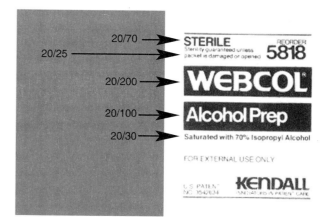

Figure 9-7 A common alcohol prep pad may be used in lieu of a near vision card or Snellen eye chart when held at 14 inches.

These small cards can be easily added to a standard first-aid kit. If near vision is tested, then athletes should wear their reading glasses or bifocals if they typically require corrective lenses to read with. In lieu of a vision card or a Snellen chart, a common alcohol prep pad may be used to test visual acuity (Figure 9-7).

When an athlete cannot see the largest letters of an eye chart, the athletic trainer can hold up some of the fingers of one hand and ask the athlete to count them at progressively closer distances to the eye. This is documented as "count fingers vision at, for example, 2 feet." If the athlete cannot count fingers, the examiner can wave a hand in front of the eye and ask if the athlete can detect the motion. This is documented as "hand motion vision." If the athlete cannot detect hand motion, any bright light source (e.g., a penlight) can be used to detect ability to detect light. This is documented as "light perception vision."

Reduction of visual acuity in an injured eye is a serious ocular emergency. Immediate referral to an eye care specialist is warranted.

Testing Pupillary Responses

The ability of the pupil to react to light is a basic feature of a normal functioning ocular system. A brisk pupil constriction to a bright light also suggests the presence of vision in the absence of any standard eye chart. While the athlete is looking into the distance, a light is moved in toward the eye from the side and shined directly into the pupil (Figure 9-8). The speed (briskness) of the pupillary constriction is noted. Each eye is examined separately and should have similar findings.

After examining each eye for its light reactivity and responsiveness, the athletic trainer performs a swinging light test by swinging a light from the normal eye to the injured one. This test is based on the fact that the

independently, with the other eye occluded by the palm of one's hand or an opaque object. When testing acuity in children or nonreaders, an illiterate E or C or picture chart is used (Figure 9-5, *B*).

If a standard eye chart is not available, a near-vision card can be used to assess visual acuity (Figure 9-6).

same quantity of light (i.e., from the same light source) should constrict each pupil by the same amount. When internal ocular damage or optic nerve damage occurs in one eye, the pupil of the injured eye will appear to dilate when the light is moved from the normal eye to the injured eye, indicating that the same amount of light is not being transmitted through the optic nerve in the injured eye. This is known as an **afferent pupillary defect** and represents a potentially severe ocular emergency. Immediate referral to an eye care specialist is warranted.

A pupil that is larger in the injured eye or does not react to light (i.e., traumatic mydriasis) or a pupil that is no longer round (e.g., peaked or oval) may represent significant intraocular trauma (e.g., **traumatic iritis**).

Immediate referral to an eye care specialist is warranted. It is important for the athletic trainer to know if the athlete has a previously existing or congenitally larger pupil on one side, or **anisocoria,** because this may confuse the findings of the examination.

Testing Extraocular Muscle Motility

Part of the basic assessment of an athlete's eye is the examination of ocular motility. The inability of one or both eyes to move into the cardinal fields of gaze (Figure 9-9), especially after an eye injury, indicates a severe eye injury with possible eye socket pathology or entrapment of the extraocular muscles (Figure 9-10).[6]

The athletic trainer asks the athlete to follow an object or a fingertip up, down, left, and right with both eyes together. The examiner assesses the athlete for smooth, uninterrupted movements of both eyes in all fields of gaze. There should be no restriction of gaze in either eye; movements of the two eyes should be harmonious and parallel. When the eyes do not move in synchrony, the athlete will commonly complain of double vision, or diplopia. This is the result of each eye being focused in a different place because of their misalignment. Diplopia after an injury may also represent a variety of neurological conditions and requires immediate medical attention.[7]

Testing Peripheral Vision

Although arguably not as crucial as central visual acuity, peripheral vision allows athletes to view the entire field of sport around them and see where their teammates or competitors might be while they focus

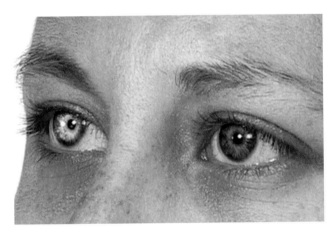

Figure 9-8 To test pupillary response, the athlete looks into the distance while a light is moved in toward the eye from the side and shined directly into the pupil. The speed of the pupillary constriction is compared with the opposite eye.

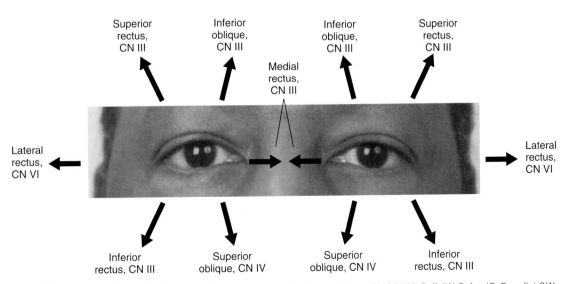

Superior rectus, CN III

Inferior oblique, CN III

Medial rectus, CN III

Inferior oblique, CN III

Superior rectus, CN III

Lateral rectus, CN VI

Lateral rectus, CN VI

Inferior rectus, CN III

Superior oblique, CN IV

Superior oblique, CN IV

Inferior rectus, CN III

Figure 9-9 Test eye motility in all six cardinal fields of gaze. *CN,* Cranial nerve. (From Seidel HM, Ball JW, Dains JE, Benedict GW: *Mosby's guide to physical examination,* ed 5, St Louis, 2003, Mosby, p 291.)

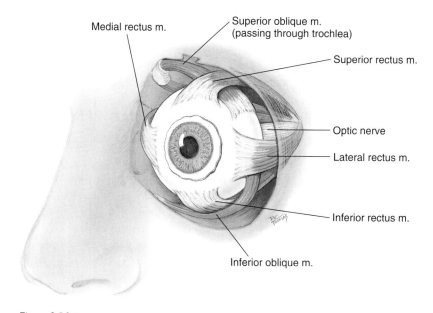

Figure 9-10 Extraocular muscles of the eye. *m*, Muscle. (From Jarvis C: *Physical examination & health assessment*, ed 4, Philadelphia, 2004, WB Saunders, p 299.)

their vision centrally. It is important that the range of an athlete's peripheral vision be known before any injury (i.e., preparticipation peripheral vision testing).

The athletic trainer tests the athlete's peripheral vision one eye at a time. To test the right eye, the examiner sits approximately 3 feet directly in front of the athlete. The athlete, left hand over left eye, focuses only on the examiner's left eye. Conversely, the examiner's right eye is closed. This allows the examiner to watch his or her own open hands during the examination while fixating on the athlete's right eye.

The examiner holds up one, two, or three fingers on each hand equidistant between the examiner and the athlete and equidistant on either side of the direct line of sight between the athlete's right eye and the examiner's left eye. Examiners must be able to see their own fingers during this kind of examination. The athlete is asked to add the total number of fingers seen while fixating only on the examiner's left eye and without looking at the examiner's fingers. The examiner will be able to detect if the athlete looked away from the examiner's left eye. It is best not to hold up the same number of fingers on each hand at the same time. This will allow the examiner to know exactly which field of vision was defective. Next, the other eye is examined in a similar fashion. All the cardinal fields of vision—right, left, above, below, above and to the right, above and to the left, below and to the right, and below and to the left—need to be tested. Any finding of the athlete's inability to see in a particular field of vision should be referred to an eye care specialist before participation.

Examining the Anatomical Structures of the Injured Eye

A good assessment of the eye can usually be made by simply having athletes open their eyes and examining them directly. Occasionally, the eyelids may have to be held apart by either the athlete or the examiner. Eyelid swelling is a common consequence of direct trauma to the eye. Therefore the eye must be examined as soon as possible before the swelling of the eyelids makes direct assessment impossible.

The athletic trainer can use room lighting or a directed source of light (e.g., flashlight or penlight) to assess the anterior portion of the ocular anatomy (Figure 9-11). Inspection of the lids and palpation of the bony orbital rim can reveal serious trauma after a blunt injury. If there is any suspicion that the trauma was severe enough to penetrate or rupture the eyeball then no external pressure should ever be placed on the eye or surrounding structures (i.e., eyelids).

A light is directed toward the eye with the lids retracted while the athlete is asked to look up while the examiner retracts the lower lid (Figure 9-12, *A*) or look down while the examiner retracts the upper lid (Figure 9-12, *B*). This facilitates examination of the entire anterior aspect of the globe including the conjunctiva, sclera, and cornea. Foreign bodies are commonly found in the conjunctival fornices. The **fornices** are the most posterior portions of the upper and lower conjunctivae where the conjunctiva overlying the sclera (**bulbar conjunctiva**) and the conjunctiva lining the eyelids (**palpebral conjunctiva**) join together.

Obscuration of the structures behind the cornea (e.g., iris or lens) because of a cloudy anterior chamber is an ominous sign of potential blood in the anterior chamber (i.e., hyphema). This can frequently be detected with a penlight and indicates a very serious eye injury. If the eye is anatomically distorted or bleeding, it is prudent to discontinue any further palpation or examination and to seek emergency medical attention and urgent ophthalmological referral.

Examining the Eye with the Ophthalmoscope

To examine an athlete's eye with the ophthalmoscope, the athletic trainer turns on the ophthalmoscope and selects the large aperture (see Chapter 2). This should project a large round light on the examiner's hand or the wall. Next the room is darkened. The examiner holds the handle of the ophthalmoscope in the right hand (to examine the athlete's right eye) with the index or middle finger on the lens selector wheel. To examine the left eye, the left hand is used. The ophthalmoscope is held firmly against the bony orbit of the examiner's eye (right eye for examining the athlete's right eye and left eye for the athlete's left eye) with the handle tilted laterally. This will prevent the athletic trainer and the athlete from bumping noses during the examination.

The athlete is instructed to look up over the shoulder of the athletic trainer. The examiner should start about 15 inches away from the athlete, shining the light into the eye to visualize the reddish orange "glow" (red reflex) of the eye. The athletic trainer should approach the athlete from the lateral side (at about a 15-degree angle). Shining the light directly into the athlete's eye must be avoided because it will cause the pupil to constrict, making it more difficult to visualize the internal eye through an undilated pupil. While keeping the light focused on the red reflex, the athletic trainer moves in close to the eye, almost touching the athlete's eyelashes. Absence of a red reflex is often the result of an improperly positioned ophthalmoscope.

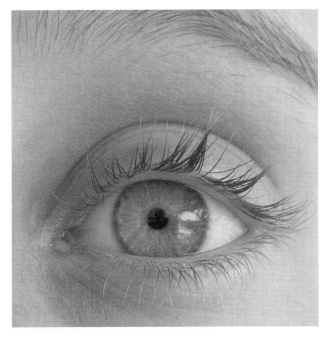

Figure 9-11 The normal eye.

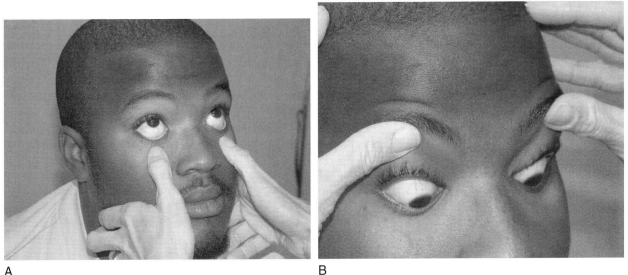

A   B

Figure 9-12 A, Examining the anterior aspect of the globe with the lower lid retracted. B, Examining the anterior aspect of the globe with the upper lid retracted.

Box 9-1   Using the Ophthalmoscope

During examination of the internal structures of the eye with an ophthalmoscope, the lens selector wheel is used and adjusted so that the examiner can focus on the retina. Depending on whether the patient's, or the examiner's, eye is myopic or hyperopic, the dial on the lens selector wheel is turned to either the red or black numbers. Each number represents the strength of each lens in the wheel, measured in diopters. The red numbers indicate concave lenses used to neutralize myopia, and the black numbers indicate convex lenses used to neutralize hyperopia.

Normal Eye

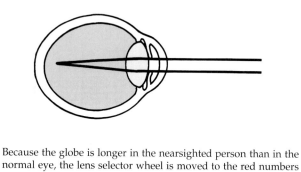

0 Diopter

The diopter is set at zero (clear glass) when both the patient's and the examiner's eyes are normal.

Myopia (Nearsighted)

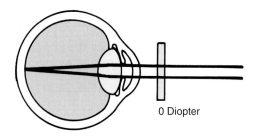

Because the globe is longer in the nearsighted person than in the normal eye, the lens selector wheel is moved to the red numbers

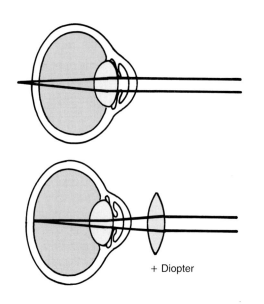

− Diopter

(concave lens) to adjust for myopia in either the patient or the examiner.

Hyperopia (Farsighted)

+ Diopter

The globe in a hyperopic eye is shorter than normal. The black numbers (convex lens) on the ophthalmoscope lens selector wheel are used so the focal point is on the retina.

Modified from Jarvis C: *Physical examination & health assessment*, ed 4, Philadelphia, 2004, WB Saunders, p 317.

To view the internal structures of the eye, such as the optic disc, arteries, veins, and retina, the athletic trainer may need to turn the lens selector wheel to focus on various structures. If the athlete is myopic, a minus (red) lens will be used (Box 9-1). The fundus or retina will appear as a yellow or pink background with blood vessels branching away from the optic disc (see Figure 9-4). It is often easier to find the blood vessels and follow them back to the optic disc than to try to locate the optic disc by itself. The arterioles are smaller than the venules and reflect brighter light (Key Points—Retinal Vessels). The vessels should be followed as far as possible in each of the four quadrants of the eye (i.e., superior, inferior, nasal, temporal) as they go away from the optic disc. When the optic disc is visualized, it should appear yellow to creamy pink but may be darker in dark-skinned individuals. The borders of the disc should be sharp and well defined. Moving in

KEY POINTS
Retinal Vessels

The eye is the only place in the body where the blood vessels may be viewed directly through the use of an ophthalmoscope. Many systemic diseases that affect the vascular system may show signs in the retinal vessels.

a temporal direction from the optic disc, the macula (fovea centralis) may be able to be visualized.[4] To bring the fovea into the field of vision, the examiner asks the athlete to look directly at the light of the ophthalmoscope. It will appear as a yellow dot surrounded by a deep pink periphery and will not have any blood vessels running through it.[2] Considerable practice is needed to visualize the macula, and it may be impossible to view without the pupil being dilated.

PATHOLOGICAL CONDITIONS

Refractive Error

Signs and Symptoms

For clear vision, both near and distant images must be sharply focused onto the retina, which lines the back of the eyeball. The ability of the eye to focus these images is directly related to the length of the eye, the curvature of the cornea, the clarity of the ocular media, and the flexibility of the crystalline lens. The first two parameters, length of eye and curvature of cornea, determine the refractive error of an eye. **Myopia,** or nearsightedness, is a longer than normal eye. A distant object is focused in front of the retina instead of on it (Figure 9-13, *A*). **Hyperopia,** or farsightedness, is a shorter than normal eye (Figure 9-13, *B*). A distant object is out of focus when it reaches the retina and, theoretically, focuses behind the retina.[8] The shape of the cornea is typically spherical (just like a tennis ball) on its anterior curvature. When this curvature is not spherical and has multiple curvatures (such as an egg or football), the eye is considered astigmatic[8] (i.e., astigmatism, Figure 9-13, *C*). After the age of 40 years, the crystalline lens inside the eye loses its flexibility and the ability to focus on near objects. This is known as **presbyopia.** Presbyopic athletes require reading glasses for near vision. Mild degrees of refractive errors can remain undetected for years until very clear distance vision is needed, such as when an adolescent first begins an athletic season.

Referral and Diagnostic Tests

Athletes who complain of poor vision, either at a distance or close up, need to be referred to an eye care practitioner who will perform a refraction along with other ocular tests. The refraction determines the refractive error of an eye. The refractive error will change over time as the shape and length of the eye change up to the ages of 23 to 25 years. After that the refractive error tends to stabilize.

Treatment

The refractive error can be corrected with spectacles or contact lenses. Refractive surgery, such as laser-assisted in situ keratomileusis (LASIK), is also an option for treatment, but it should not be performed until the refraction has been stable for at least 2 years, especially in the adolescent or young adult.

Prognosis, Return to Participation, and Prevention

The prognosis for the vast majority of refractive errors is excellent. Return to participation can be immediate after the athlete has received correction for the refractive error. A refractive error is an anatomical feature of the shape of the eye and cannot be prevented (Box 9-2).

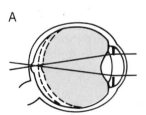
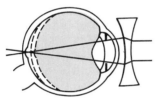

Myopia (nearsightedness)   Corrected with biconcave lens

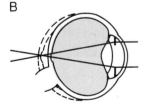
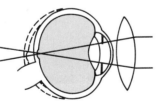

Hyperopia (farsightedness)   Corrected with biconvex lens

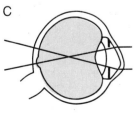

Astigmatism   Corrected with astigmatic lens

Figure 9-13 A comparison of the common refractive disorders with their corrections. **A,** Myopia or nearsightedness. **B,** Hyperopia or farsightedness. **C,** Astigmatism. The dashed lines in **A** and **B** show the contours of a normal eye. (From Black JM, Hawks JH: *Medical-surgical nursing: clinical management for positive outcomes,* ed 7, St Louis, 2005, Mosby, p 1964.)

Box 9-2   Common Misconceptions About Vision and the Eyes

The following statements are often passed along as advice, but *all* are *false:*
- Reading in the dark is harmful to the eyes.
- Children will outgrow crossed eyes.
- A cataract is a film growing over the surface of the eye.
- One should avoid reading to save eyesight when vision is failing.
- Children must be cautioned not to sit too close to the television.
- Wearing someone else's glasses may damage your eyes.
- Misuse of the eyes in childhood results in the need for glasses later in life.
- Emotional stress increases intraocular pressure.

From Black JM, Hawks JH: *Medical-surgical nursing: clinical management for positive outcomes,* ed 7, St Louis, 2005, Elsevier, p 1920.

Conjunctivitis

Conjunctivitis is a general term for an inflammation of the conjunctiva, the transparent, vascular tissue covering the anterior sclera and the posterior surface of the eyelids. It is commonly caused by bacteria, viruses, allergies, or dry eye or as a response to a corneal injury or irritation.

Signs and Symptoms

The symptoms of conjunctivitis are not specific to the causative agent and can include all or some of the following: redness, burning, itching, tearing, irritation, and foreign body sensation (Box 9-3). Allergic conjunctivitis is classically characterized by itching. The most obvious signs of conjunctivitis are redness or vascular engorgement (Figure 9-14). There may be a discharge, ranging from watery to mucoid to frank purulence (pus). Viral conjunctivitis is often associated with recent cold or flu symptoms or recent contact with someone with a red eye.[9,10] Redness of the conjunctiva in the space between the eyelids associated with a burning sensation is common after exposure to sun, wind, or dusty conditions, which are all common to outdoor athletics.

Referral, Diagnostic Tests, and Differential Diagnosis

Viral conjunctivitis is highly contagious, and therefore referral to an eye care practitioner for diagnosis is important in most cases of conjunctivitis.

Without the benefit of a slit lamp biomicroscope used by the ophthalmologist or optometrist, an absolute diagnosis may be difficult (Box 9-4). A few basic features can help differentiate bacterial, viral, and allergic conjunctivitis. A watery or mucous discharge can be seen in both allergic and viral conjunctivitis. Typically, the discharge in bacterial conjunctivitis is purulent (Figure 9-15). Allergic conjunctivitis itches. Viral conjunctivitis frequently involves the cornea, which is difficult to visualize without high magnification. Viral conjunctivitis frequently presents with **preauricular lymphadenopathy** (i.e., a small tender lymph node located just in front of the tragus of the ear).

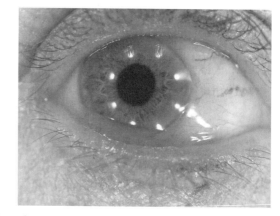

Figure 9-14 This photograph of allergic conjunctivitis shows the redundant conjunctiva rising over the edge of the lower lid margin in addition to redness and vascular engorgement of the sclera.

Box 9-3　Evaluation of Red Eye

Follow these steps to assess the need for referral of an athlete with red eye:
1. Check the athlete's visual acuity.
2. Inspect for a pattern of redness. A diffuse "pink" color is quite different from a deep localized redness.
3. Observe for the presence of discharge.
4. Use a fluorescein stain and blue cobalt light to observe for corneal defects if an abrasion is suspected.
5. Use an ophthalmoscope to observe the inner structures of the eye for irregularities.

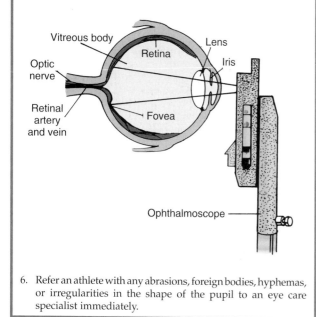

6. Refer an athlete with any abrasions, foreign bodies, hyphemas, or irregularities in the shape of the pupil to an eye care specialist immediately.

Modified from Black JM, Hawks JH: *Medical-surgical nursing: clinical management for positive outcomes*, ed 7, St Louis, 2005, Elsevier, p 1920.

Box 9-4　The Cause of Red Eye

Athletic trainers often encounter athletes whose chief complaint is a "red eye." An engorgement of the conjunctival vessels causes the eye to be red. It may be associated with a subconjunctival hemorrhage that requires no treatment, or it may be a manifestation of a serious eye disorder that requires immediate attention. Common disorders involving red eye include the following:
　Conjunctivitis: bacterial, viral, allergic, and irritative
　Herpes simplex keratitis: inflammation of the cornea
　Scleritis: inflammation of the sclera
　Subconjunctival hemorrhage: accumulation of blood in the potential space between the conjunctiva and the sclera
　Abrasions and foreign bodies: hyperemic response

Modified from Black JM, Hawks JH: *Medical-surgical nursing: clinical management for positive outcomes*, ed 7, St Louis, 2005, Elsevier, p 1920.

Treatment

Standard treatment for mild acute bacterial conjunctivitis includes topical antibiotic eye drops or ointments. Viral conjunctivitis usually resolves spontaneously within 2 weeks and cannot be treated effectively with topical antibiotics. Typically the third to the fifth day produces the worst signs and symptoms. Because antiviral therapies are not effective in treating viral conjunctivitis, treatment is directed at symptomatic relief (e.g., redness, burning). This may involve the use of over-the-counter vasoconstrictors (i.e., whiteners), topical antiallergy drops, or simply artificial tears to lubricate the ocular surface. Allergic conjunctivitis is frequently self-treated using a variety of over-the-counter topical ophthalmic antihistamine or decongestant products. There are also prescription antiallergy ophthalmic products that can be prescribed by the eye care practitioner. These include topical ophthalmic antihistamines, mast cell stabilizers, mast cell stabilizer/antihistamine combinations, nonsteroidal antiinflammatories, and steroids.

Prognosis and Return to Participation

Viral conjunctivitis is highly contagious. Therefore any athlete with acute watery conjunctivitis should not be in close contact with others until the condition is resolved. A persistent or worsening conjunctivitis may be secondary to more aggressive bacteria or a moderately severe allergy. Ophthalmic assessment should be ascertained with such progression of signs and symptoms. After 2 or 3 days, the athlete can return to participation. Some extremely virulent strains of viral conjunctivitis can cause corneal clouding that can persist for weeks to months. This can adversely affect the athlete's visual performance. Bacterial conjunctivitis, although contagious, is not as easily spread from one individual to another as is viral conjunctivitis.[7] After 1 or 2 days of topical antibiotic therapy, the athlete can return to participation.

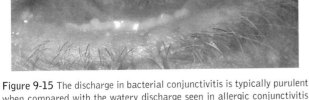

Figure 9-15 The discharge in bacterial conjunctivitis is typically purulent when compared with the watery discharge seen in allergic conjunctivitis in Figure 9-14.

Prevention

Appropriate hygiene and hand washing as well as isolating the athlete who has a red eye until it is properly diagnosed can prevent the spread of a viral conjunctivitis. Team members are advised not to share cosmetics or other products used around their eyes.

Hyphema

Blood in the anterior chamber of the eye is known as a hyphema, and it is a common complication of blunt trauma to the eyeball, often associated with other types of orbital or ocular damage, such as corneal abrasions, orbital fractures, eyelid contusions, and open globe injuries (Figure 9-16). The blood often comes from a damaged blood vessel in the iris or ciliary body. Spontaneous hyphemas in the absence of trauma are rare and are associated with a variety of rare ocular syndromes.

Signs and Symptoms

The two main symptoms of a hyphema are pain and blurred vision. The pain is associated with both the initial trauma and the inflammatory effect that the blood has on the anterior structures of the eye (e.g., the iris). The blurred vision is associated with the interruption of the clear aqueous humor in the anterior chamber by the opaque blood. The blood can frequently be seen by close examination with an external

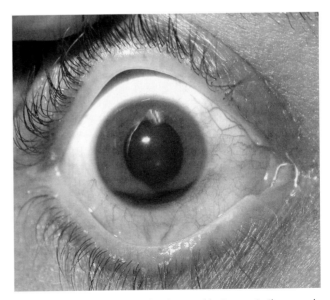

Figure 9-16 A hyphema most often is caused by trauma to the eye as in this racquetball player's injury. This injury points out why it is important to always wear eye protection. The appearance of blood in the anterior chamber of the eye begins as a crescent shape inferiorly and may progress such that the entire anterior chamber is filled with blood.

light source. With a vertical head position, the blood will form a layer in the anterior chamber with the heavier blood settling to the bottom and the lighter aqueous humor rising to the top. Occasionally, the blood creates a very thin, microscopic layer at the bottom of the anterior chamber. This may be imperceptible to the naked eye of the examiner.

Referral and Diagnostic Tests

A hyphema represents a serious, sight-threatening condition that requires immediate referral to an eye care specialist. During transport, the athlete should keep the head elevated in order to allow the blood to settle to the bottom of the anterior chamber. This will give the eye care specialist a better opportunity to visualize the rest of the ocular structures.

Differential Diagnosis

In the presence of trauma, blood in the anterior chamber can only represent a hyphema. Occasionally, the source of the bleeding can be visualized. Hyphemas are associated with a number of other sight-threatening conditions and complications. The differential diagnosis is aimed at looking for other potential ocular damage that may have occurred in association with the hyphema. These conditions include a ruptured globe, corneal abrasion, dislocated lens, traumatic **cataract,** bleeding in the vitreous cavity (i.e., vitreous hemorrhage), increased intraocular pressure (e.g., secondary glaucoma), and retinal tear or detachment. The presence of a hyphema may make it difficult to examine the more posterior structures of the eye (e.g., the retina).

Treatment

An uncomplicated hyphema is typically managed with bed rest and the administration of topical steroids, pupil-dilating drops known as **mydriatics,** and, if required, eye pressure–lowering (i.e., antiglaucoma) agents.[11] The athlete should sleep with the head of the bed slightly elevated. One of the greatest risks of hyphema is a rebleed that typically occurs between the third and the fifth day after the initial injury that can result in a complete filling of the anterior chamber with blood called an 8-ball hyphema. This can produce an elevated intraocular pressure as well as blood staining of the cornea, both of which are sight threatening. Occasionally, systemic medication may be required to control the bleeding and the high intraocular pressure. In cases of very high intraocular pressure or severe bleeding filling the front of the eye, the athlete may require hospitalization or surgical evacuation of the blood.

Prognosis, Return to Participation, and Prevention

The prognosis for an uncomplicated hyphema is excellent. Depending on the size of the hyphema and the intraocular pressure measurement, daily follow-up by an eye care specialist until the blood starts to resorb may be required. The athlete can return to participation 2 to 3 weeks after the blood has completely resolved. Less frequent examinations by the eye care specialist over the following months after the injury may be required to rule out late complications such as secondary glaucoma. Undetected high intraocular pressures can cause irreversible damage to the optic nerve. Blood staining of the cornea may require months to resolve.

Protective eyewear can prevent the vast majority of hyphemas caused by direct trauma to an eye. The athlete must wear protective eyewear after sustaining a hyphema to prevent a recurrence as a result of minimal ocular trauma.

Subconjunctival Hemorrhage

Bright red blood appearing acutely in a sector of the eye under the clear conjunctiva and in front of the white sclera is termed a **subconjunctival hemorrhage.** Although striking in appearance, this condition is benign. It represents a broken blood vessel under the conjunctiva and is analogous to a subcutaneous hematoma.

Signs and Symptoms

Subconjunctival hemorrhages can be caused by trauma, coughing or straining, high blood pressure, breath-holding or Valsalva's maneuvers, bleeding disorders, and ingestion of blood thinners (e.g., aspirin). They can occur spontaneously without a known cause and are usually without symptoms; however, other people observing the eye can easily detect the blood (Figure 9-17).

Referral, Diagnostic Tests, and Differential Diagnosis

Unless there has been blunt trauma, subconjunctival hemorrhage does not require ophthalmic evaluation as long as no other signs or symptoms are present and vision is unaffected. Rarely, more serious conditions such as conjunctival tumors can emulate a subconjunctival hemorrhage.

Treatment

For mild irritation, artificial tears can be given. A simple subconjunctival hemorrhage usually clears within

2 or 3 weeks; it may change color as the blood resolves, similar to a subcutaneous hematoma (e.g., a bruise).

Prognosis, Return to Participation, and Prevention

Prognosis is excellent. Athletic participation is not restricted because of subconjunctival hemorrhage.

If there are recurrent bleeding episodes, visual symptoms, pain, or persistence of blood, an ophthalmic referral should be sought.

Because of the nature of its pathophysiology, with the exception of direct trauma, there is no way to prevent a subconjunctival hemorrhage. Protective eyewear should prevent subconjunctival hemorrhages caused by direct trauma to the conjunctival surface.

Corneal Abrasions

A corneal abrasion results from a scratch to the surface of the cornea that causes a defect in the most superficial layer of cells called the epithelium.[12] The most common cause of a corneal abrasion is direct trauma with a foreign object.

Signs and Symptoms

The most common symptom of a corneal abrasion is the sensation of having something in the eye referred to as a foreign body sensation. Other symptoms are decreased vision, tearing, sensitivity to light, **blepharospasm** (i.e., squeezing eyelids), and reactive conjunctivitis.

Referral and Diagnostic Tests

Most corneal abrasions should be referred to an eye care specialist in order to rule out an injury that might be deeper into the cornea than just the epithelial surface. A corneal abrasion can be difficult to see with a penlight exam. It is best visualized with a special ophthalmic staining technique. This technique involves placing a water-soluble, orange dye, called fluorescein, on the ocular surface (Box 9-5). Fluorescein dye stains areas of abrasions on the cornea and conjunctiva that have lost their epithelial surface layer. The dye fluoresces as a bright yellowish green color when a cobalt blue light is shined on it (Figure 9-18). The fluorescein stain is best seen in a darkened environment.

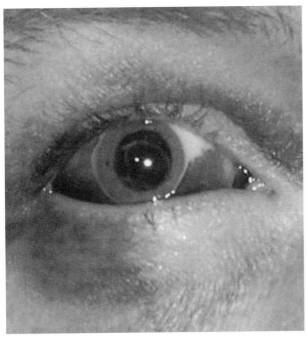

A

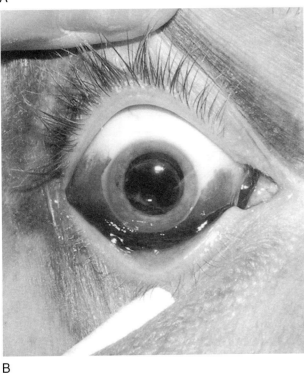

B

Figure 9-17 Eyelid contusion (**A**) with subconjunctival hemorrhage (**B**).

Box 9-5 Fluorescein Dye Test

Follow these steps:
1. Wet the tip of the fluorescein strip with sterile saline.
2. Touch the tip of the strip to the lower lid conjunctiva.
3. Do *not* place the strip directly on the globe of the eye.
4. Ask the athlete to blink in order to spread the dye.
5. Darken the room.
6. Use a cobalt blue light to illuminate the eye.
7. Observe the eye; the dye fluoresces as a bright yellowish green color under the cobalt blue light and pinpoints abrasions (see Figure 9-19).

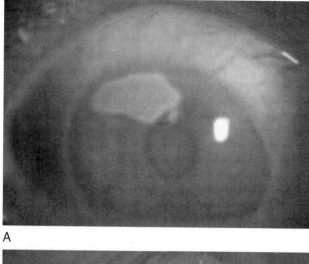

A

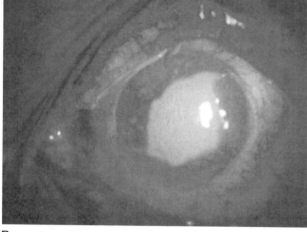

B

Figure 9-18 Two different corneal abrasions stained with fluorescein dye and "excited" with a cobalt blue filter.

Differential Diagnosis

Some corneal infections can have a similar presentation to a corneal abrasion, and it is important to make their distinction with staining and magnification. Frequently, a corneal abrasion is caused by an embedded foreign body that remains stuck to the ocular surface or possibly stuck onto the surface of the conjunctiva under the eyelids. Persistence of a foreign body sensation in the absence of an abrasion requires looking for a retained foreign body somewhere on the eye.

Treatment

The treatment of a simple corneal abrasion is lubrication with artificial tears and occasionally a topical antibiotic drop or ointment if the potential for a corneal infection exists. The antibiotic preparation should be administered as directed, and follow-up should be with the eye care practitioner as prescribed.

Corneal abrasions are frequently patched for 24 to 48 hours to prevent the eyelid from rubbing over the abrasion during blinking. Contact lenses should not be worn until the eye care specialist feels it is appropriate.

Prognosis, Return to Participation, and Prevention

Simple noninfected corneal abrasions usually resolve clinically within 24 to 72 hours.[13] After reepithelialization (i.e., healing) of the uncomplicated corneal abrasion, the area of the corneal abrasion is typically undetectable during future examinations and will not pose future problems for the athlete. The athlete can return to participation as soon as the foreign body sensation is gone. Larger abrasions may require more time for reepithelialization and resolution of symptoms. Protective eyewear can prevent corneal abrasions caused by direct trauma to the corneal surface.

Corneal Lacerations

One of the most serious traumatic eye injuries is a corneal or corneal-scleral laceration, also known as an open globe.[14] An open globe is an eyeball that has been ruptured following blunt or sharp trauma or injury with a projectile foreign body (Figure 9-19). Lacerations allow leakage of intraocular fluid or extrusion of intraocular tissues and contents. They also allow the introduction of infectious pathogens from the environment into the intraocular spaces.

Signs and Symptoms

The symptoms of an open globe are decreased vision and pain following trauma. The athlete often has a hyphema, dense subconjunctival hemorrhage, decreased eye movements, or bloody tears. An open globe should be considered after any ocular trauma.

Referral, Diagnostic Tests, and Differential Diagnosis

If a rupture is suspected, it is imperative that the eye not be touched and the athlete be immediately transported to the nearest emergency room.

Corneal lacerations can be penetrating, identified as open globe lacerations, or nonpenetrating. Some penetrating or perforating injuries may or may not have an extrusion of intraocular contents. The differential diagnosis is left to the eye care specialist.

Treatment

The treatment of a lacerated eye is prompt surgical repair, often followed by several days of intravenous and topical antibiotics. Infection of the eye after an open globe can be catastrophic and cause loss of vision or even loss of the eye.

Prognosis, Return to Participation, and Prevention

Visual rehabilitation of an eye with a corneal laceration is prolonged. Even after prompt diagnosis and appropriate treatments, the eye may still develop a cataract (i.e., clouding of the lens of the eye) or permanent scarring of the cornea. Scar tissue inside the eye often requires several eye surgeries to restore vision. Frequently, the pretrauma vision is not attainable even after the most heroic efforts at anatomical restoration of the normal eye structure.

Protective eyewear can prevent the vast majority of corneal lacerations caused by direct trauma to the eye.

Corneal and Conjunctival Foreign Bodies

Any object embedded in or adherent to the conjunctiva or cornea is defined as an ocular foreign body (Figure 9-20). The athlete may or may not recall getting something in the eye. The majority of ocular bodies are washed off the surface of the eye by the rinsing lubrication of the tear film or brushed off the surface by the blinking action of the eyelids. Those foreign bodies that remain on the eye can cause the athlete significant discomfort.

Signs and Symptoms

The symptoms of a foreign body are typically immediate. The athlete may complain of a sensation of "something in the eye" or of "scratchiness." There is

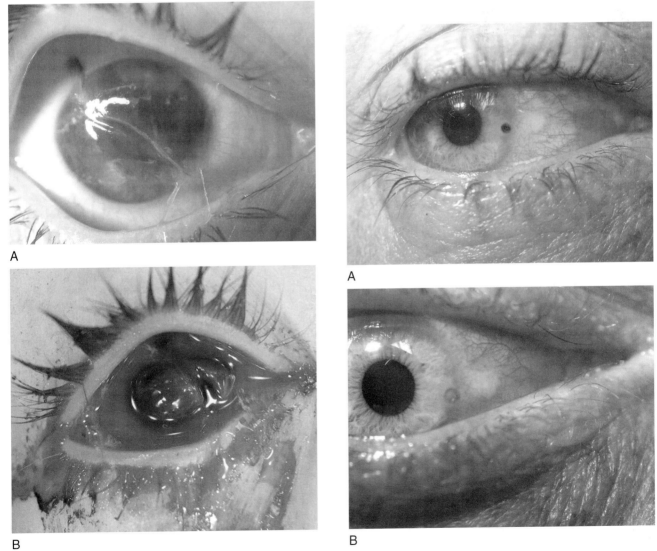

A

B

Figure 9-19 Two different corneal lacerations (i.e., open globe) caused by paintball injuries.

A

B

Figure 9-20 A, A metallic corneal foreign body in the eye. **B**, The same eye with a residual rust ring after the foreign body was removed.

frequently an associated "reflex" tearing as the eye reacts to the foreign body and tries to relieve the eye by lubricating it. The foreign body may not be visible to the examiner depending on its size, shape, and color.

Referral and Diagnostic Tests

Most foreign bodies lodged on the less sensitive conjunctival surface can be removed on site. Those on the extremely sensitive corneal surface may require referral to an eye care specialist if they cannot be removed with a few simple maneuvers.

Differential Diagnosis

A corneal or conjunctival abrasion without a foreign body can mimic the symptoms of a foreign body as the blinking eyelids continue to rub over the abraded surface. Frequently, the athlete will feel as if the foreign body is under the upper eyelid even if the foreign body or abrasion is in the middle or lower part of the eye.

Treatment

A loose foreign body on the ocular surface can frequently be rinsed off the eye with additional lubrication such as an eye rinse or just a few drops of an artificial tear supplement. The contact lens in the affected eye should be removed before treatment. It is appropriate to wash an eye with a foreign body at an eyewash station if available. If the foreign body sensation persists after irrigation, the upper eyelid can be gently pulled away from the eyeball by grasping the upper lid eyelashes and pulling the upper eyelid down over the lower eyelid lashes. The lower eyelid lashes will then act as a "brush" against the back (conjunctival) side of the upper lid and potentially dislodge a loose foreign body from under the upper eyelid.

If the foreign body sensation persists after the brushing maneuver, the upper lid can be everted to allow a direct inspection of its conjunctival surface.[15] The examiner can pull the upper lid away from the eye by gently grasping the upper lid lashes and having the athlete look down. When a small cotton-tipped applicator is placed against the upper eyelid crease (found approximately 0.5 inch above the margin of the eyelid), the eyelid can be rotated around the applicator (Figure 9-21, *A*). The examiner's finger can maintain the lid eversion by pressing the lashes against the brow. If the foreign body is located, the same applicator can be used to gently lift the foreign body off the surface of the conjunctiva (Figure 9-21, *B*).

The cornea should never be touched. No attempt to remove a foreign body from the cornea should be made because inadvertent pressure on a sharp corneal foreign body could potentially push the foreign body

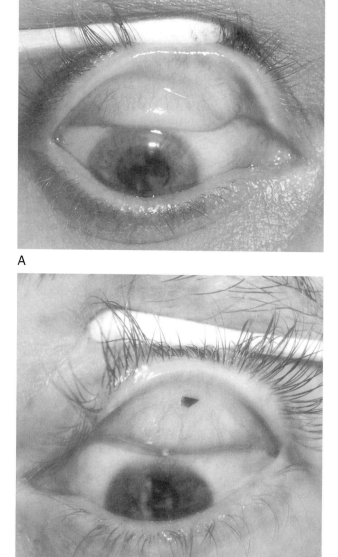

A

B

Figure 9-21 A, The upper eyelid is everted with a cotton-tipped applicator. **B,** A foreign body (plastic) on the upper eyelid. Foreign bodies that are not embedded may be removed from the lid with a cotton-tipped applicator. The cornea, however, must never be touched.

deeper or even perforate the thin cornea. If the foreign body cannot be removed and remains embedded on the conjunctival or corneal surface, the athlete needs to be referred to an eye care specialist.

Prognosis, Return to Participation, and Prevention

The prognosis for simple conjunctival foreign bodies is excellent. The athlete can typically return to participation immediately after the foreign body has been removed. Sometimes the maneuvers to remove the foreign body may create an additional ocular surface abrasion. Although the foreign body is gone, the foreign body sensation may remain for another 24 hours. The prognosis for removing corneal foreign bodies depends on their depth and size. The recovery time is usually a little longer and may require 24 to 48 hours for the symptoms to completely resolve.

Protective eyewear can prevent the vast majority of ocular surface foreign bodies caused by direct trauma to the eye.

Orbital Fracture

Among the seven bones that make up the walls of the bony orbit are some of the thinnest bones of the body. When there is a blunt injury to the eye, the forces against the orbit create a sudden increase in pressure within the orbit. The orbital contents including the eyeball are displaced posteriorly toward the back of the orbit. This pressure (i.e., force) can break the thin orbital walls, causing an orbital wall fracture frequently referred to as a *blow-out fracture*. Frequently, the nearby orbital contents (e.g., the extraocular muscles and orbital fat) can be forced through the fracture site and become incarcerated into the space behind the fractured wall. The two most common orbital walls that fracture during blunt trauma are the inferior wall (orbital floor) and the medial wall. The spaces behind these two walls are the maxillary and ethmoid sinuses, respectively.

Signs and Symptoms

Depending on the severity of the injury and fracture, the symptoms of an orbital fracture can include pain with attempted eye movement, double vision (i.e., **diplopia**) when orbital contents are trapped in the fracture site, and numbness, or hypesthesia, in the distribution of the infraorbital nerve, which gives sensation to the cheek, upper lip, and upper teeth. The double vision resolves when the athlete covers one eye. The athlete may show signs of restricted eye movements in up or down gaze, decreased sensation in the cheek or upper lip on the same side of the injury, misalignment of the orbital rim on palpation along with point tenderness, and sometimes a "crunchy" sensation under the skin of the orbit (Figure 9-22, *A*, *B*, and *D*). This **orbital emphysema** is a result of air from the sinus that has become trapped beneath the skin. Eyelid ecchymoses are often common.

Referral and Diagnostic Tests

An athlete with a suspected orbital fracture requires orbital imaging studies. The most important diagnostic test is a computerized tomography (CT) scan of the orbit with both coronal and axial views

(Figure 9-22, *C* and *E*). It is also important to examine the eye for potential intraocular injuries (e.g., retinal detachment, hyphema, open globe injury).

Differential Diagnosis

Blunt head trauma can cause damage to certain cranial nerves associated with extraocular movements (e.g., cranial nerves III, IV, and VI) that can present with diplopia. Localized swelling over the infraorbital nerve can cause temporary hypesthesia over its sensory distribution. Retrobulbar (i.e., behind the globe) hematomas can cause irreversible optic nerve damage.

Treatment

Not all orbital fractures require a surgical repair. Depending on the size, location, and whether there is tissue entrapment, an orbital fracture can be observed to see if the athlete's signs and symptoms spontaneously resolve with time. An orbital fracture technically represents an open fracture because the normally closed orbital space can allow sinus air to enter through the fracture site. For this reason, systemic antibiotics are administered. Iced compresses for the first 24 to 48 hours can help reduce the periorbital swelling. No compresses are used until the eyeball has been cleared of any injuries. Athletes with suspected orbital fractures are instructed not to blow their noses because this can force bacteria-laden air from the paranasal sinuses into the eyelids or orbit and cause a secondary infection. For large fractures or persistent diplopia in primary or down gaze, surgical repair of the fracture is often required. The athlete can be observed for up to 2 weeks before any surgical intervention to see if the signs and symptoms resolve spontaneously. Ophthalmologists, otolaryngologists, plastic surgeons, and maxillofacial surgeons perform this surgery.

Prognosis, Return to Participation, and Prevention

The prognosis for the complete resolution of the signs and symptoms of an orbital fracture depends on the spontaneous resolution of symptoms or the success of the surgical outcome. Persistent diplopia may require further extraocular muscle surgery. Shrinkage of the orbital fat after orbital trauma may cause delayed **enophthalmos** (i.e., movement of the eyeball deeper into the orbit). Infraorbital nerve hypesthesia may be transient or permanent depending on the extent of the injury to that nerve. Athletes may return to sport participation in approximately 2 to 4 weeks with facial and eyewear protection for approximately 4 to 6 months.

Protective eyewear can prevent the majority of orbital fractures caused by direct trauma to the orbit.

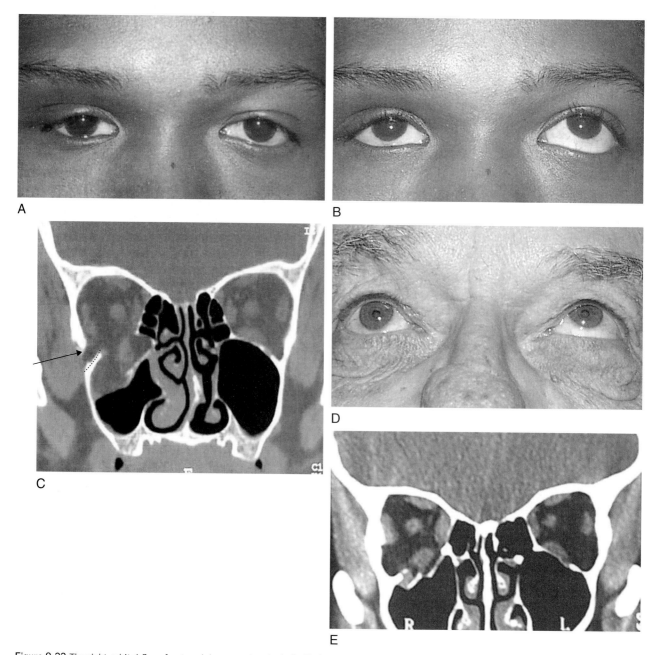

Figure 9-22 The right orbital floor fracture injury seen in a basketball player is assessed by, **A**, having the athlete look straight ahead and, **B**, noting the restricted upward gaze of the right eye, which is on the reader's left. **C**, A CT scan showing the floor in the maxillary sinus (*thick dotted oval*) The floor is supposed to be where the thin dotted line appears. A lateral wall fracture is shown by the *arrow* on the left. **D**, An injury in an older adult shows restriction in upward gaze on the right side, or reader's left. **E**, The CT scan shows a floor fracture.

Retinal Tear and Detachment

The retina is the delicate transparent tissue lining the back of the eye. Light-sensitive retinal fibers receive images projected through the lens and send them to the brain through the optic nerve for interpretation as a visualized image. When the retina is damaged, the transmission of the images is distorted or absent.

Retinal tears and retinal detachments may occur through illness, injury, or heredity or as the result of normal aging. These conditions are most typically found in people who are nearsighted, have undergone previous eye surgery, have experienced eye trauma, or have a family history of retinal detachments. Middle-aged and older individuals are at higher risk than the younger population. Retinal tears and detachments are also likely to recur in athletes with a history of a previous retinal tear or detachment. Retinal detachment typically begins with one or more small holes or tears in the retina. These holes are caused by the shrinkage (e.g., aging process) or sudden movement (e.g., in trauma) of the vitreous humor that is intimately attached to the retina. Once a tear has occurred, more liquid vitreous humor may flow through the hole or tear causing the retina to elevate and detach.

Signs and Symptoms

A retinal tear or detachment typically occurs in only one eye. The most common symptoms from a tear in the retina are brief flashes of light (**photopsia**) in the peripheral visual field or an abrupt increase in vitreous floaters. The most common symptoms of a retinal detachment are the same as a retinal tear plus a curtain or shadow moving over the field of vision. Sometimes central visual acuity may be lost. The signs of a retinal tear or detachment are essentially limited to the actual direct visualization of the elevated or torn retina by an eye care specialist.

Referral and Diagnostic Tests

Any athlete with a new onset of flashes and floaters, especially after trauma, needs to be immediately referred to an eye care professional. These athletes are frequently referred to retinal specialists. The proper examination requires pharmacological dilation of the pupil along with a detailed exam of the retinal periphery with specialized ophthalmic instrumentation (Figure 9-23).

Differential Diagnosis

As people age, the vitreous begins to liquefy. Eventually, it becomes so liquid that it collapses into itself and peels away from the retina. This phenomenon is

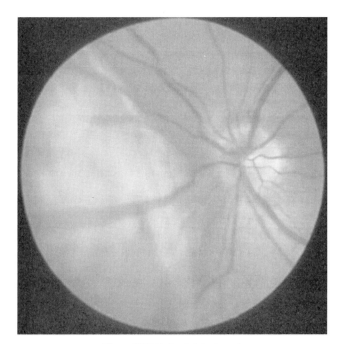

Figure 9-23 Retinal detachment.

called a **posterior vitreous detachment** (PVD) or posterior vitreous separation. Individuals who have had a PVD frequently notice floaters in their vision caused by small opacities in the vitreous that cast shadows on the retina. They may also experience a split-second flash of light (i.e., photopsia) in the corner of their vision. These symptoms are similar to those of a retinal tear.

Treatment

Retinal detachments caused by traumatic breaks or tears to the retina are treated surgically. Ophthalmologists use lasers or cryoprobes (i.e., freezing) to create adhesions between the detached retina and the back surface of the eye. Silicone oil, filtered air, or special gases are sometimes injected into the vitreous cavity to push the retina against the back of the eye during the healing process.

Prognosis and Return to Participation

The prognosis of a retinal tear or detachment is based on the number of tears or holes or the size and location of the detachment. Early diagnosis and treatment are critical factors in the successful surgical outcomes. If the central retina (macula) responsible for central 20/20 acuity is not detached, a successful surgery can preserve excellent central vision. However, complications of surgery, infection, redetachment, or a primary detachment of the central part of the retina can drastically decrease vision. Once an athlete has had retinal surgery, the eye requires several weeks to heal. The risk of a redetachment is higher in an athlete with a previous history of one. Return to participation depends on the extent of the retinal injury and the success of the repair. It also depends on the sport involved (e.g., contact versus noncontact). Lengthy discussions between the athlete and the retinal specialist are necessary in determining the athlete's safety and risks of future visual loss when returning to sports.

Prevention

Athletes with risk factors associated with retinal tears or detachments should avoid contact sports where head or eye trauma is possible. Protective eyewear can prevent direct trauma to the eye that can cause retinal tears or detachments; however, blunt head trauma without direct eye trauma can also cause these conditions.

Dislocated Contact Lens

More than 30 million Americans wear contact lenses as a substitute for glasses to correct refractive errors and improve their visual acuity. Contact lenses are categorized by the flexibility of the plastic material from which they are manufactured. Soft contact lenses are relatively large, soft, and pliable. They are designed to cover the entire corneal surface and extend approximately 1 to 2 mm beyond the cornea onto the conjunctiva and sclera. Rigid contact lenses, whether hard or gas permeable, are relatively small, hard, and less flexible. They are designed to fit only on the corneal surface. Contact lenses can be moved from their normal central location over the cornea when the eye is subjected to a shearing force, such as a tangential trauma from a ball or a hand.

Signs and Symptoms

The symptoms of a displaced contact lens are loss of visual acuity and the presence of a foreign body sensation. Most currently available contact lenses have a visible tint for easy handling. This makes it easier for the examiner to identify a dislocated lens against the background of the white sclera. Nontinted lenses may be more difficult to see. Soft lenses may become rolled up and lodged in the upper limits of the conjunctiva under the upper eyelid.

Referral and Diagnostic Tests

If the dislocated lens is located but cannot be removed by either the athlete or the athletic trainer, then a referral to an eye care specialist may be necessary. If no lens is found but a foreign body sensation remains, the athlete may need the services of an eye specialist to rule out a possible corneal or conjunctival abrasion and to further examine the eye for the dislocated lens. If an athlete feels that a contact lens has become dislocated, the athletic trainer should help locate the position of the lens. Frequently the athlete can manipulate the lens and reposition it.

Differential Diagnosis

Other acute conditions associated with contact lens wear can present with decreased acuity and a foreign body sensation, including corneal abrasions, corneal foreign bodies, some corneal infections, an inside-out contact lens, and hypersensitivity to a new or overused contact lens cleaning solution.

Treatment

Pulling the upper and lower lids away from the eye to inspect the conjunctiva will often locate the dislocated contact lens. Everting the upper eyelid will often reveal a displaced soft or rigid contact lens.

Before a displaced contact lens is removed, the eye should be lubricated with saline eyewash, an artificial tear solution, or contact lens rewetting solution. If the contact lens is dislodged under the upper lid, which is usually the case, the lid must be everted. Once the lens is located, the eyelid is allowed to assume its normal position by simply asking the athlete to look up. The lens can be moved to the lower portion of the eye by applying gentle, direct pressure through the eyelid. The athletic trainer must avoid excessive pressure on the contact lens. If the contact lens is dislodged under the lower lid, the conjunctiva is exposed by pulling the lower eyelid away from the eye. The lens can be repositioned with gentle finger pressure through the eyelid or removed from the eye. Applying a small contact lens suction cup, which should be included in the athletic trainer's kit, to a rigid lens can assist in lifting the lens out. The suction cup technique is not effective with soft contact lenses, and the suction cup should never be placed on the cornea.

Prognosis and Return to Participation

A rigid lens may be reinserted on the cornea, if necessary. A soft lens should not be reinserted until it has been disinfected. Once good acuity is achieved, either through contact lens replacement or spectacle correction, the athlete may return to sport participation.

Prevention

Protective eyewear can prevent shearing forces from displacing contact lenses. The use of prescription safety goggles eliminates the risks associated with contact lenses and simultaneously protects the eyes from other trauma.

Chemical Burns

Any chemical substance that comes into contact with the ocular surface has the potential to cause a serious chemical burn. Common chemicals that can produce serious, vision-threatening conditions and that are found in athletic training facilities include cleaning solutions or solvents, detergents, and aerosol hygiene products.

Signs and Symptoms

The symptoms of a chemical burn are the rapid onset of pain, a foreign body sensation, and frequently loss of vision following contact with a chemical substance. The signs of a chemical burn of the ocular surface range from defects on the corneal surface to corneal opacification with pronounced swelling and blanching of the cornea or conjunctiva (Figure 9-24). Burns of the surrounding skin of the face may also occur as the substance touches these surfaces.

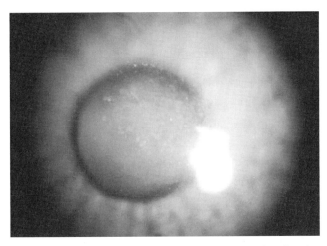

Figure 9-24 A chemical burn to the cornea; note the tiny white dots that are the irregularities on the corneal surface. Each dot represents a tiny corneal abrasion.

Referral and Diagnostic Tests

Any chemical burn of the eye should be evaluated by an eye care professional. Treatment must be initiated before transporting the athlete to the nearest emergency facility. Evaluation of the eye with a chemical burn requires a biomicroscopic (i.e., slit lamp) examination, occasional assessment of the pH of the eye with test strips, and fluorescein staining of the cornea.

Differential Diagnosis

A radiation burn (e.g., ultraviolet light) to the cornea can present with similar symptoms as a chemical burn to the ocular surface. The differential diagnosis is based on the presence or absence of a history of contact with a noxious substance.

Treatment

The most important treatment of a chemical burn to the ocular surface is the immediate irrigation of the eye with copious amounts of any available clean fluid or liquid (Key Points—Chemical Burns). These include

> **KEY POINTS**
> **Chemical Burns**
>
> Immediate irrigation of a chemical burn to the eye with copious amounts of clean water or saline solution is necessary. Irrigate from nasal side of the eye to temporal side of the eye whenever possible to avoid flushing the chemical into the nonaffected eye.

saline eyewash, sink or shower water, a very low-pressure water fountain or hose, or noncarbonated sports beverages. Irrigation should be performed from the nasal corner of the eye to the temporal (lateral) side of the eye whenever possible to avoid flushing the

chemical into the other eye. Irrigation should continue until the eye can be assessed at an emergency facility. A cooperative athlete should have the conjunctival pockets under the upper and lower eyelids swept with a moistened cotton swab and have the upper eyelid everted and irrigated. Irrigation is continued at the emergency facility until the pH of the eye has returned to normal. Associated complications, such as corneal damage or opacification and elevated intraocular pressure, may require further treatment.

Prognosis and Return to Participation

The prognosis for chemical burns of the eye has a broad range depending on the severity of the burn and the type of chemical causing the injury. Alkali burns tend to create more serious injuries than do acid burns. Most chemical burns create large corneal or conjunctival abrasions. A rapid resolution, with a similar rehabilitation course to that of a corneal abrasion, is common when irrigation is promptly initiated. However, if irrigation is delayed, vision-threatening ocular surface damage can result. Return to sport participation depends on the severity of the chemical burn.

Prevention

Chemical compounds typically found around an athletic facility should be well labeled and kept away from areas where accidental spills and splashes can occur. Protective eyewear can prevent some ocular damage as a result of splash injuries.

Periorbital Contusion

Direct trauma to periorbital structures (e.g., eyebrows, eyelids, cheeks) can result in localized swelling and subcutaneous hemorrhages. Periorbital contusion is commonly referred to as a "black eye." The dark purple, or "black and blue," appearance beneath the skin of the tissues around the eye is due to damaged blood vessels in the skin and muscles (ecchymoses) of the eyelids and face. These hemorrhages may extend to the subconjunctival space. The collection of blood and fluid produces the discoloration as well as the swelling within the surrounding ocular tissues.

Signs and Symptoms

Anyone who suffers a periorbital contusion can present with localized pain from the initial traumatic event. The swelling and hemorrhages can be so severe that the eyelids may be swollen shut and not allow access to the eyeball for an appropriate examination (Figure 9-25). The external signs of a periorbital

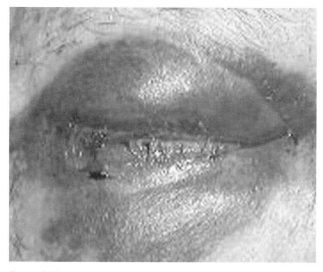

Figure 9-25 A severe periorbital contusion. An examiner would not be able to do an appropriate examination of the eye because the eyelids are swollen shut.

contusion with hemorrhage are usually obvious to the examiner. They include facial and eyelid ecchymoses with or without tissue edema and swelling. Extraocular muscle motility may be reduced as a result of severe periorbital swelling that prevents the eye from moving in all fields of gaze. Diplopia may occur. An increase in the pressure around the eye or inside the anterior orbit may give the appearance that the eyeball is being pushed forward (i.e., **proptosis**).

The typical appearance of a "black eye" with bruising and swelling often worsens within 1 to 2 days after blunt periorbital trauma. Prolonged increased pressure within the orbit can damage the optic nerve as well as damage the function of the extraocular muscles (Red Flags—Conditions for Immediate Referral).

> ### Red Flags for Conditions for Immediate Referral
>
> - Persistent blurred vision
> - Diplopia
> - Restricted eye movement
> - Hyphema
> - Distorted pupil
> - Unilateral pupil dilation or constriction
> - Foreign body protruding into the eye
> - Large lacerations of the eyelids
> - Lacerations that involve the margins of the eyelid
> - Persistent floaters

Referral and Diagnostic Tests

In the absence of any intraocular or visual damage, treatment of periorbital contusions can be performed without a referral to an eye care specialist. If there are any visual symptoms or evidence of intraocular injury (e.g., hyphema, difficulty moving the eye, or persistent or worsening pain) the athlete is referred to an eye care specialist for a complete ophthalmic examination.

Differential Diagnosis

All orbital and ocular injuries resulting from blunt trauma may present with mild to severe periorbital contusions. Therefore all potential orbital or ocular injuries (e.g., open globe, hyphema, orbital fracture) must be ruled out.

Treatment

In the absence of intraocular or visual damage, conservative therapy consisting of ice compresses for the first 48 hours followed by warm compresses until the ecchymoses have resolved will typically result in resolution within 1 to 2 weeks. Pain can usually be controlled with non–aspirin-containing analgesics.

Prognosis, Return to Participation, and Prevention

Most periorbital contusions resolve spontaneously and uneventfully. Most athletes without visual complaints or increasing or persistent pain can return to sport participation as long as the swelling of the periorbital tissue does not compromise their vision. Protective eyewear can prevent the many orbital contusions caused by direct trauma to an eye.

Traumatic Iritis

A traumatic iritis refers to an inflammation of the iris secondary to a blunt traumatic injury to the eye. The term is frequently used to refer to an inflammation within the anterior chamber of the eye. The many nontraumatic causes for iritis are related to various medical and ocular conditions.

Signs and Symptoms

Inflammation of the iris or anterior chamber of the eye is associated with a dull, deep aching pain when either the iris or pupil moves. The most common symptom of a traumatic iritis is **photophobia** or pain when light is shined into the eye. This is due to the constriction and movement of the pupil and iris when stimulated by a direct light source. A traumatic iritis can occur 1 to 7 days after the initial trauma. In addition to a mild to marked sensitivity to light, the athlete may also complain of decreased vision, different-sized pupils (i.e., **traumatic mydriasis**), or a red eye with the redness forming a ring just outside the edge of the cornea.

Referral and Diagnostic Tests

An eye care specialist must evaluate a suspected traumatic iritis. Only under the high magnification of a biomicroscope or slit lamp can the diagnosis of an iritis be made. Microscopic inflammatory white cells can be seen floating in the aqueous humor within the anterior chamber of the eye. These cells can plug up the outflow tract of aqueous causing the intraocular pressure to rise (e.g., secondary glaucoma).

Differential Diagnosis

In the presence of blunt ocular trauma, light sensitivity is a traumatic iritis until proven otherwise. Other ocular injuries associated with blunt trauma (e.g., corneal abrasion, hyphema, retinal detachment) need to be ruled out through a complete ophthalmic exam.

Treatment

The treatment of traumatic iritis is to prevent the iris from moving and to reduce the internal ocular inflammation. Dilation and temporary paralysis of the pupil with mydriatic (dilating) drops will typically alleviate the photophobia. Topical ophthalmic steroid drops are used to reduce the anterior chamber inflammation. Depending on the severity of the inflammation, the treatment may last 2 to 4 weeks. The topical steroid needs to be tapered to prevent a rebound of the inflammatory response. Occasionally, additional drops to treat a secondary glaucoma may be necessary.

Prognosis, Return to Participation, and Prevention

The prognosis for traumatic iritis is excellent. Improvement of symptoms begins as soon as the pupil is dilated. Reduction of the internal inflammation often occurs between 5 and 7 days. Eye drops are discontinued once the inflammation is resolved. It is important for the athlete to have a very thorough eye exam within 1 month after resolution of symptoms to check for other subtle signs of anatomical damage from the blunt trauma. Athletes can return to sport participation once the inflammation has subsided. Protective eyewear can prevent the majority of cases of traumatic iritis by preventing direct trauma to the eye.

Proptosis

Direct trauma to the orbit can result in deep orbital swelling and hemorrhages. Swelling that occurs behind the eye can push the eyeball forward, causing a bulging of the eye from between the eyelids (Figure 9-26). This is called **proptosis** or **exophthalmos.**[16,17] Swelling and hemorrhages behind the eyeball can cause direct damage to the optic nerve by compromising its blood supply. This same swelling can put pressure on the outside of the eyeball, which can subsequently increase the pressure inside the eye (secondary glaucoma).

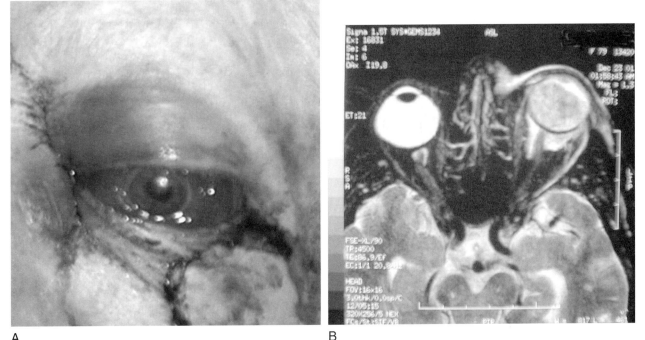

A   B

Figure 9-26 A, A retrobulbar hemorrhage with proptosis. **B,** Note the blood behind the eye on the CT scan.

The hemorrhages may extend to the subconjunctival space.

Signs and Symptoms

Athletes who suffer from traumatic proptosis will frequently present with a bulging eye. The extraocular movements may be significantly reduced or absent. The athlete may complain of diplopia. The eyelids may not close all the way (i.e., **lagophthalmos**), or there may be a severe **subconjunctival hemorrhage** that protrudes between the eyelids. Frequently the athlete will complain of pain and may be nauseous. Eyelid ecchymoses are not uncommon. These may not be evident for a day or two after the injury. Prolonged increased pressure within the orbit can damage the optic nerve as well as damage the function of the extraocular muscles.

Referral and Diagnostic Tests

Protrusion of the eye after blunt trauma must be referred immediately to an eye care specialist. An athlete with a suspected orbital hemorrhage requires orbital imaging studies. Either CT scans or magnetic resonance (MR) scans of the orbit with both coronal and axial views should be performed. It is also important to examine the eye for potential intraocular injuries (e.g., retinal detachment, hyphema, **open globe** injury).

Differential Diagnosis

In the presence of blunt trauma, proptosis may also be caused by significant orbital ecchymosis originating from a sinus as a result of an orbital fracture. All potential orbital or ocular injuries, including open globe, hyphema, and orbital fracture, must be ruled out.

Treatment

In the absence of any intraocular or visual damage, conservative therapy consisting of ice packs for the first 24 to 48 hours, ocular lubricants to protect the cornea from drying out, and careful observation may be all that is required. Pain can usually be controlled with non–aspirin-containing analgesics. In the presence of any intraocular or visual damage, orbital decompression surgery may be required to preserve vision.[11] Systemic and topical medications to reduce intraocular pressure may be necessary.

Prognosis, Return to Participation, and Prevention

Traumatic proptosis has a guarded prognosis depending on the severity of the proptosis and damage to the ocular structures. Many cases resolve spontaneously and uneventfully whereas others require surgical intervention.[17] Most athletes without visual complaints or increasing or persistent pain can return to sport participation after the proptosis has completely subsided. Protective eyewear can prevent traumatic proptosis caused by direct trauma to the eye.

Eyelid Lacerations

The eyelids and periorbital skin are very susceptible to both blunt and sharp trauma. The eyelid skin is the thinnest skin in the body. The thicker periorbital skin overlies a relatively solid orbital rim. These tissues are readily vulnerable to direct trauma (Figure 9-27).

Signs and Symptoms

In the presence of trauma, eyelid lacerations will present as an open wound of the eyelids or surrounding tissues.

Referral and Diagnostic Tests

Lacerations that are not amenable to adhesive strip bandages (e.g., Steri-strips) and require suturing need to be referred to the appropriate oculofacial surgeon or ophthalmologist. Complete examination of the eyeball remains the highest priority before closure of the wounds.

Differential Diagnosis

As with any tissue laceration, the presence of a foreign body needs to be ruled out. An examination for other evidence of ocular damage must be performed.

Treatment

Although the eyelids are not amenable to adhesive strips for closure of lacerations, for small wounds around the periorbital area (e.g., eyebrows) adhesive strips usually work well. Tissue adhesives (e.g., Dermabond) can be used to close small eyelid or periorbital wounds. Suturing the wound closed is the most effective way to close an eyelid wound. During wound cleaning and antisepsis, care must be taken to avoid getting nonophthalmic antiseptic solutions, rinses, and ointments in the eye.

Prognosis, Return to Participation, and Prevention

Most eyelid and periorbital lacerations heal nicely and uneventfully. Most athletes without visual complaints or increasing or persistent pain can return to sport participation as long as the swelling of the eyelid or

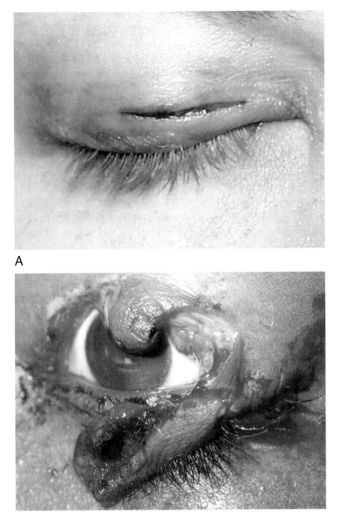

A

B

Figure 9-27 Two views of different lacerations to the eye. **A**, An eyelid laceration caused by being hit with a tennis racket. **B**, An eyelid laceration caused in a fall on a trampoline.

periorbital tissue does not compromise their vision. Protective eyewear can prevent eyelid and periorbital lacerations caused by direct trauma to the eye.

PROTECTIVE EYEWEAR

More than 100,000 sports-related eye injuries are reported each year, and the overwhelming majority of such injuries occur to athletes under 25 years of age. Baseball and basketball are the highest-risk sports for eye injuries, followed by water sports, racquet and court sports, and football.[18] Many eye injuries sustained in athletics are permanent and associated with serious vision loss.[19] Appropriate eye protection reduces the risk of eye injuries by at least 90% during any sport.[20] The American Academy of Ophthalmology recommends specific protective lenses for both low–eye-risk

and high–eye-risk sports, which are ANSI Standard No. Z87.1 with a strap fit, and sports goggles with polycarbonate lenses stronger than CR-39 plastic, respectively.[21] For athletes who are functionally monocular, such as those with a history of **amblyopia** (i.e., "lazy eye") or a history of a prior eye injury, wearing protective eyewear should be mandatory at all times during any sport participation (Box 9-6). Athletes with functional vision in only one eye should consider alternative sports rather than contact sports (e.g.,

Box 9-6   Tips for Choosing Protective Eye Guards

1. Fit an athlete who wears prescription glasses with prescription eye guards.
2. Purchase nonprescription eye guards at sports specialty stores or optical stores.
3. Only "lensed" protectors are recommended for sports use.
4. Fogging of lenses can be a problem for an active athlete. Some eye guards are available with antifog coating; others have side vents for additional ventilation.
5. Look for an indication on the eye guard's packaging that it has been tested and approved for the athlete's sport. Polycarbonate eye guards are the most impact resistant.
6. Make sure the eye guard is padded or cushioned along the brow and bridge of the nose. Padding will prevent the eye guard from cutting the athlete's skin during rugged sports activity.
7. Adjust the eye guard straps to be secure on the face but not too tight that the eye guard is uncomfortable.

WEB RESOURCES

American Academy of Ophthalmology
http://www.aao.org
The primary association of ophthalmologists; provides information on the latest news relevant to the eye for both the practitioner and the patient and includes case studies and self-assessments that may be of interest to the athletic trainer

National Library of Medicine
http://www.nlm.nih.gov/medlineplus/eyeinjuries.html
Offers definitions, basic explanation of eye conditions and injuries, as well as information on vision correction; includes anatomy of the eye and links to other resources and databases

American Optometric Association
http://www.aoa.org/eweb/startpage.aspx?site=aoastage
Provides information on eye conditions and vision with both preventive and clinical information for the patient and the practitioner

National Eye Institute
http://www.nei.nih.gov
A part of the National Institutes of Health (NIH) that conducts and supports research to prevent and treat vision disorders and diseases of the eye; site includes descriptions of common eye disorders as well as anatomy of the eye and resources for both the medical practitioner and the patient

Glaucoma Research Foundation
http://www.glaucoma.org
Dedicated to information and research about glaucoma

boxing, wrestling, martial arts) or sports involving high-velocity projectiles (e.g., ball sports, hockey).

Contact lenses offer no protection from eye injuries, and protective eyewear without a refractive correction should be worn over contact lenses.

SUMMARY

It is imperative that the athletic trainer recognize the eye conditions that require immediate attention and referral to an ophthalmologist. This chapter describes how to perform a basic examination of the eye including visual acuity and eye motility. If blurred vision is prolonged or eye motility is hindered, the athlete should be referred. The athlete who presents with an abnormally shaped pupil or diplopia also needs to be immediately referred. In addition, the athletic trainer should be skilled in the basic visualization of the internal structures of the eye and recognize abnormal conditions. The skilled use of an ophthalmoscope is necessary to visualize the internal structures of the eye. The reader is encouraged to use the accompanying DVD to watch a video of an eye examination and to complete the interactive exercises, including identification of the conditions discussed in this chapter.

REFERENCES

1. Jarvis C: *Physical examination & health assessment*, ed 4, Philadelphia, 2004, WB Saunders.
2. Seidel H, Ball J, Dains J, Benedict G: *Mosby's guide to physical examination*, ed 5, St Louis, 2003, Mosby.
3. Vaughan D, Asbury T, Riordan-Eva P: *General ophthalmology*, ed 15, Stamford, Conn, 1999, Appleton & Lange.
4. Curnyn KM, Kaufman LM: The eye examination in the pediatrician's office, *Pediatric Clinics of North America* 50(1):25-40, 2003.
5. Bradford CA: *Basic ophthalmology for medical students and primary care residents*, San Francisco, 1999, American Academy of Ophthalmology.
6. Starkey C, Ryan J: *Evaluation of orthopedic and athletic injuries*, ed 2, Philadelphia, 2002, FA Davis.
7. Beers MH, Berkow R, editors: *The Merck manual of diagnosis and therapy*, ed 17, Whitehouse Station, NJ, 1999, Merck Research Laboratories.
8. Fay A, Jakobiec FA: Diseases of the visual system. In Goldman L, Ausielllo D, editors: *Cecil textbook of medicine*, ed 22, Philadelphia, 2004, WB Saunders, pp 2406-2426.
9. Ferri F: *Ferri's clinical advisor instant diagnosis and treatment*, St Louis, 2004, Mosby.
10. Goldman L, Ausiello D, editors: *Cecil textbook of medicine*, ed 22, Philadelphia, 2004, WB Saunders.
11. Rhee DJ, Pyfer MF: *The Wills eye manual, office and emergency room diagnosis and treatment of eye disease*, ed 3, Philadelphia, 1999, Lippincott Williams & Wilkins.
12. Holmes HN, editor: *Professional guide to diseases*, ed 7, Springhouse, Pa, 2001, Springhouse.
13. Michael JF, Hug D, Dowd MD: Management of corneal abrasion in children: a randomized clinical trial, *Annals of Emergency Medicine* 40(1), 2002.
14. Rodriguez JO, Lavina AM, Agarwal A: Prevention and treatment of common eye injuries in sports, *American Family Physician* 67(7):1481-1488, 2003.
15. Bickley L: *Bates' guide to physical examination and history taking*, ed 8, New York, 2003, Lippincott.
16. Capao Filipe JA, Rocha-Sousa A, Falcao-Reis F, Castro-Correia J: Modern sports eye injuries, *British Journal of Ophthalmology* 87(11):1336-1339, 2003.
17. Giovinazzo VJ, Yannuzzi LA, Sorenson JA, et al: The ocular complications of boxing, *Ophthalmology* 94(6): 587-596, 1987.
18. Beckerman SA, Hitzeman S: The ocular and visual characteristics of an athletic population, *Optometry* (St Louis, Mo) 72(8):498-509, 2001.
19. Miller BA, Miller SJ: Visual fields with protective eyewear, *Journal of Orthopaedic and Sports Physical Therapy* 18(3): 470-472, 1993.
20. Livingston LA, Forbes SL: Eye injuries in women's lacrosse: strict rule enforcement and mandatory eyewear required, *Journal of Trauma, Injury, Infection, and Critical Care* 40(1):144-145, 1996.
21. American Academy of Pediatrics, Committee of Sports Medicine and Fitness: Protective eyewear for young athletes, *Ophthalmology* 111(3):600-603, 2004.

THE EYE

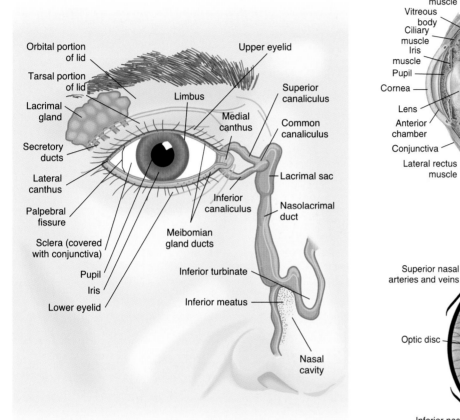

Figure 9-1. External eye

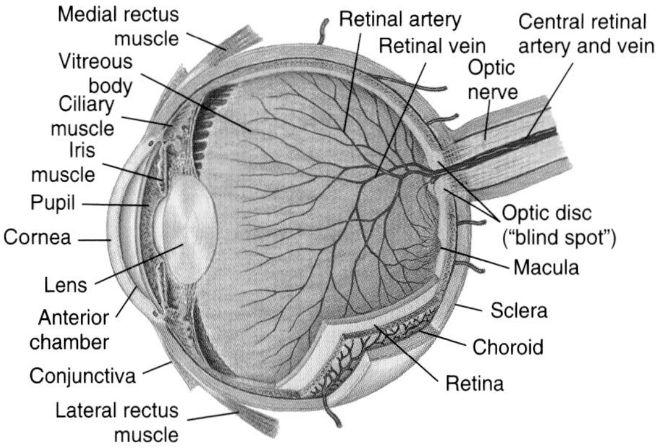

Figure 9-3. Internal eye

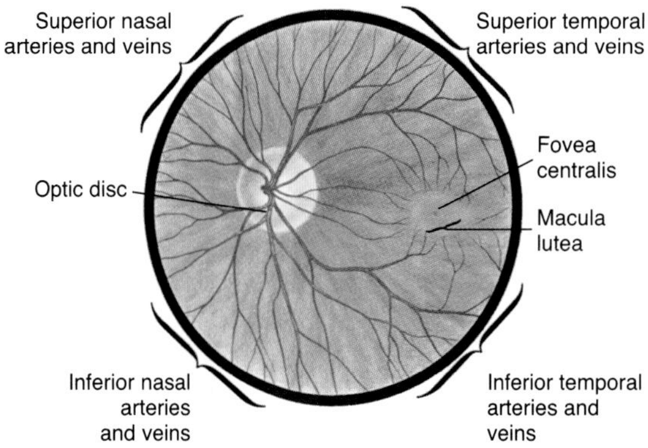

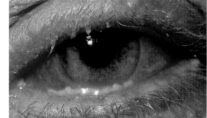

Figure 9-4. Retinal structures of the eye

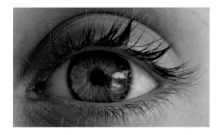

Figure 9-11. Normal eye

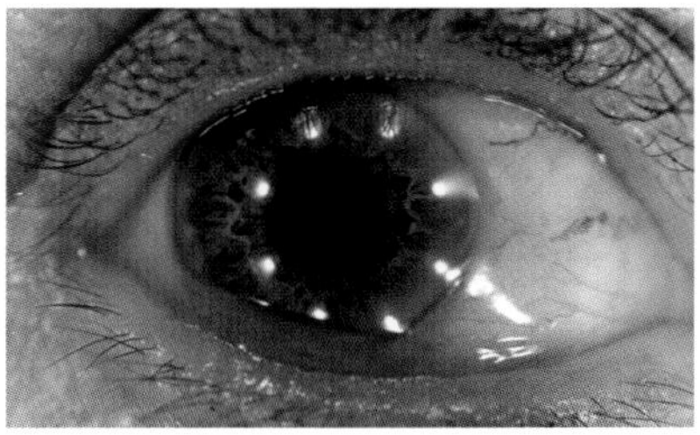

Figure 9-14. Allergic conjunctivitis

Figure 9-15. Bacterial conjunctivitis

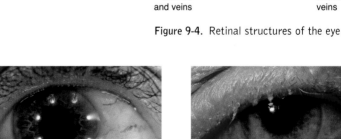
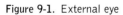

THE EYE

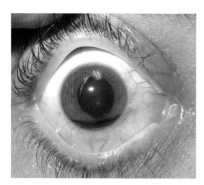

Figure 9-16. Hyphema

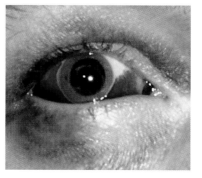

Figure 9-17, **A.** Subconjunctival hemorrhage

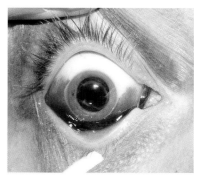

Figure 9-17, **B.** Subconjunctival hemorrhage

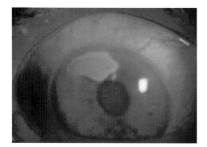

Figure 9-18, **A.** Corneal abrasion stained with fluorescein

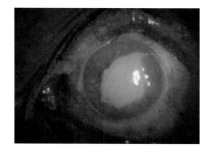

Figure 9-18, **B.** Corneal abrasion stained with fluorescein

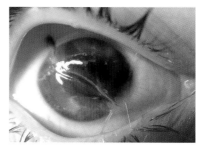

Figure 9-19, **A.** Corneal laceration (open globe)

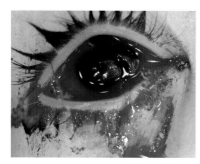

Figure 9-19, **B.** Corneal laceration (open globe)

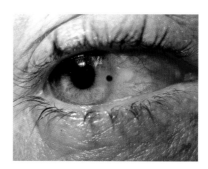

Figure 9-20, **A.** Metallic corneal foreign body

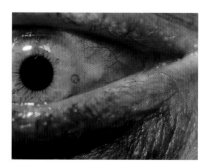

Figure 9-20, **B.** Residual rust ring from metallic corneal foreign

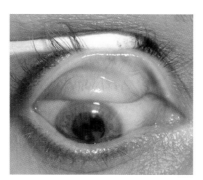

Figure 9-21, **A.** Everting upper eye lid

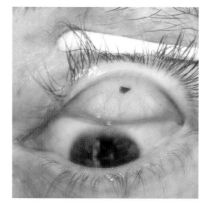

Figure 9-21, **B.** Plastic foreign body

THE EYE

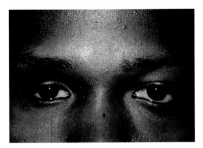

Figure 9-22, **A.** Right orbital floor fracture, athlete looks straight ahead

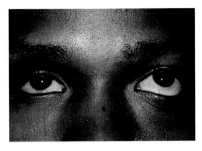

Figure 9-22, **B.** Right orbital floor fracture, restricted upward gaze

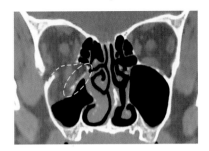

Figure 9-22, **C.** Right orbital floor fracture, CT scan

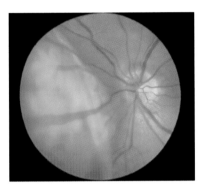

Figure 9-23. Retinal detachment

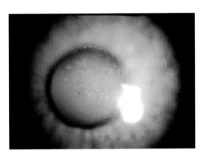

Figure 9-24. Chemical burn to cornea

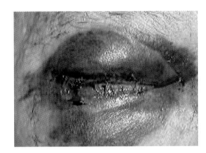

Figure 9-25. Severe periorbital contusion, assault

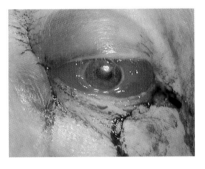

Figure 9-26, **A.** Retrobulbar hemorrhage with proptosis

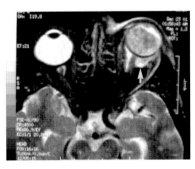

Figure 9-26, **B.** Retrobulbar hemorrhage with proptosis

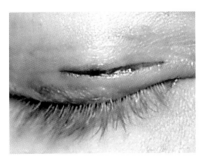

Figure 9-27, **A.** Eyelid laceration, tennis racket

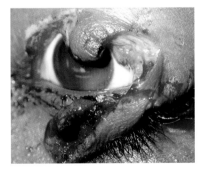

Figure 9-27, **B.** Eyelid laceration, trampoline

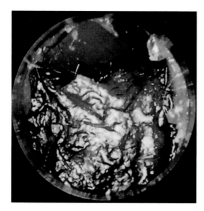

Figure 10-10. Impacted cerumen

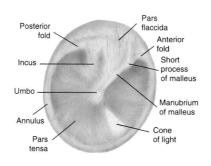

Figure 10-11, **A.** The tympanic membrane

Posterior fold
Pars flaccida
Anterior fold
Incus
Short process of malleus
Umbo
Annulus
Manubrium of malleus
Pars tensa
Cone of light

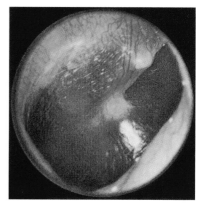

Figure 10-11, **B.** Normal tympanic membrane

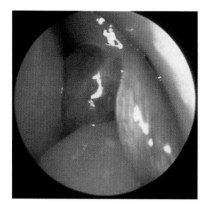

Figure 10-16, **A.** Nasal polyps

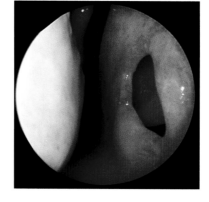

Figure 10-16, **B.** Perforated septum

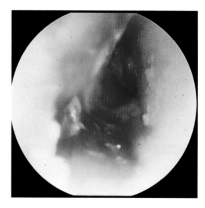

Figure 10-20. Otitis externa

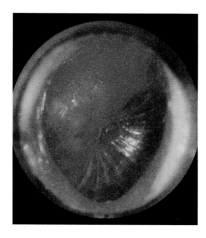

Figure 10-21. Otitis media

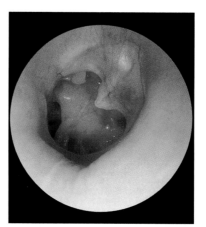

Figure 10-22. Large tympanic membrane perforation

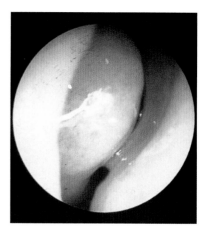

Figure 10-23. Allergic rhinitis

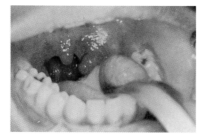

Figure 10-25, **B.** Acute viral pharyngitis

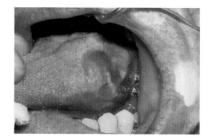

Figure 10-27, **B.** Carcinoma

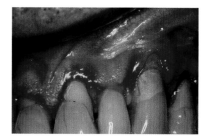

Figure 10-28. Gingivitis

CHAPTER 10

Disorders of the Ear, Nose, Throat and Mouth

Micki Cuppett

OBJECTIVES

At the completion of this chapter, the reader should be able to do the following:

1. Describe the basic anatomy of the ear, nose, mouth, and throat.
2. Perform a basic examination of the ear, nose, mouth, and throat, identifying normal and pathological conditions.
3. Properly use an otoscope to examine the ear and the nose.
4. Recognize common pathological conditions of the ear, nose, mouth, and throat, including signs and symptoms, differential assessment, and when to refer the athlete to a physician.
5. Appreciate the common diagnostic tests and standard medical treatment for conditions of the ear, nose, mouth, and throat.
6. Identify the implications for participation in athletics with various conditions of the ear, nose, mouth, and throat.

INTRODUCTION

This chapter covers nontraumatic conditions of the ear, nose, mouth, and throat. Many of these conditions are common occurrences in physically active individuals, and the athletic trainer may have ample opportunity to observe them. The athletic trainer needs to understand the anatomy and physiology discussed in this chapter and feel comfortable performing an examination of the athlete. Diagnosis of these conditions can usually be made on the basis of the athlete's history, signs and symptoms, and the caregiver's observations.

OVERVIEW OF ANATOMY AND PHYSIOLOGY

Ear

The ear serves two main functions: (1) to identify, locate, and interpret sound and (2) to maintain equilibrium. It consists of three distinct parts: the external, middle, and inner ears (Figure 10-1). The external ear consists of the pinna, or auricle; the external auditory canal; and the lateral surface of the tympanic membrane. The pinna has a cartilage framework that is covered in skin, whereas the ear lobe is fat covered in skin. The shape of the pinna is designed to gather or channel the sound into the canal. The approximately 2.5 cm long canal is lined with epithelial cells, hairs, sebaceous glands, and ceruminous glands.[1] The ceruminous glands function to produce cerumen, or ear wax, that lubricates the ear canal and tympanic membrane while serving as a protective barrier from foreign matter and bacteria. The outer third of the canal is flexible as it attaches to the pinna but is rigid for the last two thirds as it enters the skull.

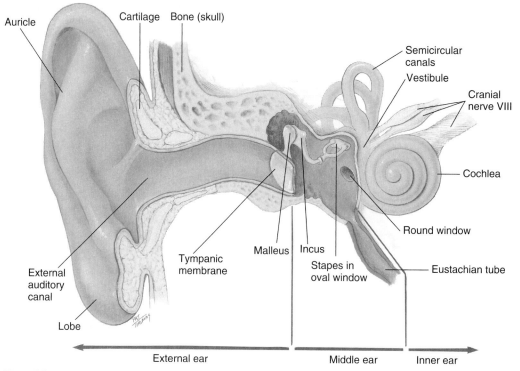

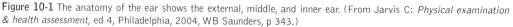

Figure 10-1 The anatomy of the ear shows the external, middle, and inner ear. (From Jarvis C: *Physical examination & health assessment,* ed 4, Philadelphia, 2004, WB Saunders, p 343.)

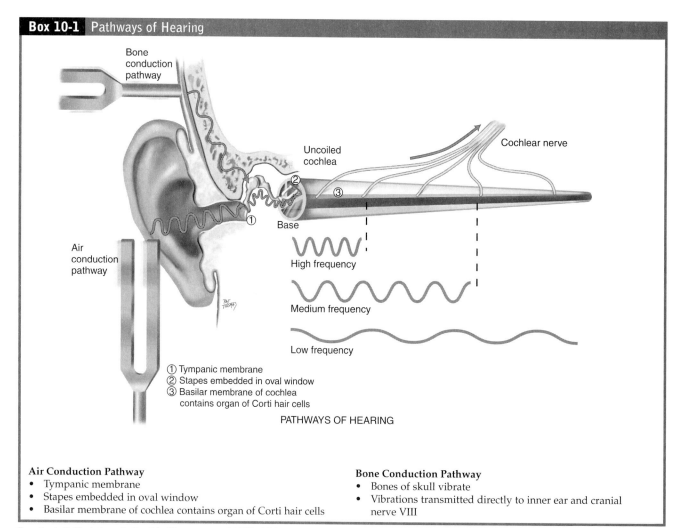

Box 10-1 Pathways of Hearing

① Tympanic membrane
② Stapes embedded in oval window
③ Basilar membrane of cochlea contains organ of Corti hair cells

PATHWAYS OF HEARING

Air Conduction Pathway
- Tympanic membrane
- Stapes embedded in oval window
- Basilar membrane of cochlea contains organ of Corti hair cells

Bone Conduction Pathway
- Bones of skull vibrate
- Vibrations transmitted directly to inner ear and cranial nerve VIII

From Jarvis C: *Physical examination & health assessment,* ed 4, Philadelphia, 2004, WB Saunders, p 344.

The external ear and the middle ear are separated by the tympanic membrane. The translucent tympanic membrane permits visualization of the middle ear, which is an air-filled cavity in the temporal bone that contains the ossicles: the malleus, incus, and stapes. These bones transmit vibrations from the tympanic membrane mechanically to the inner ear where the mechanical vibrations are changed to electrical signals. The middle ear is connected to the nasopharynx by the **eustachian tube.** This passage opens briefly to equalize pressure within the middle ear that occurs with changes in atmospheric pressure caused by swallowing, sneezing, or yawning.[2-4]

The inner ear consists of the vestibule, semicircular canals, and cochlea. The cochlea encodes the previous mechanical vibrations to electrical impulses that are then sent to the eighth cranial nerve (i.e., vestibulocochlear). The vestibule is directly responsible for balance as the fluid in the semicircular canals shifts with head movement. The feedback from this movement is provided to the brain, assisting to maintain upright posture and balance.[2]

Hearing is an interpretation of sound waves received via an air conduction path. The most efficient and normal hearing pathway is through air conduction; however bone also conducts sound whereby the vibrations of the skull are transmitted directly to the vestibulcochlear nerve. (Box 10-1).

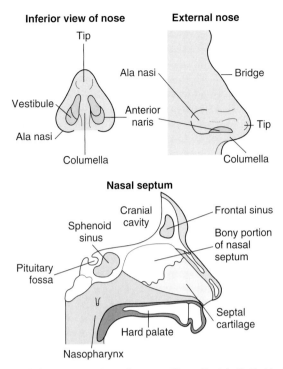

Figure 10-2 The nose and nasal septum. (From Epstein O, Perkin GD, Cookson J, de Bono DP: *Clinical examination,* ed 3, Philadelphia, 2003, Mosby, p 81.)

Nose and Nasopharynx

The external nose consists of bone in the proximal third of the nose and cartilage in the lower two thirds covered by skin. The nasal bones arise from extensions of the frontal and maxillary bones, forming the nasal bridge (Figure 10-2). The hard and soft palates form the floor of the nose, and the frontal and sphenoid bones form the roof. The external nose humidifies, filters, and warms inspired air and serves as a passageway for expired air.[1,4,5]

The internal nose is divided into two anterior cavities, or vestibules, by the septum. Air enters the nose through the nostrils and passes posteriorly to the **nasopharynx** through one of the **choanae,** separated by one of three turbinate bones. The **cribriform plate** that is part of the ethmoid bone on the roof of the nose houses the sensory endings of the olfactory nerve (i.e., CN I). A group of small fragile arteries and veins is located on the anterior superior portion of the septum. This group of arteries and veins is called **Kiesselbach's plexus** and is often responsible for epistaxis.[6,7] The **adenoids** lie on the posterior wall of the nasopharynx.

Three turbinate bones form the lateral walls of the nose. Covered by vascular mucous membrane, the turbinates separate the nose into a superior meatus, medial meatus, and inferior meatus (Figure 10-3). The turbinates help to increase the surface area for warming, filtering, and humidifying the air.

The paranasal sinuses are air-filled spaces within the cranium.[2,3] They are generally named for their location and drain into respective nasal cavities. The sinuses lighten the weight of the skull bones and serve as resonators for sound production. They also produce mucus from the membranes that line the cavities, which drains into the nasal cavity. Because the sinus openings are narrow and occlude easily, they are a common site for inflammation.

Mouth, Oropharynx, and Throat

The oral cavity consists of the lips, cheeks, tongue, teeth, and salivary glands (Figure 10-4). It functions in several capacities, including serving as a passage for food as well as the initiation of digestion by mastication and salivary secretion. The mouth and oropharynx also serve to emit air for vocalization and expiration.

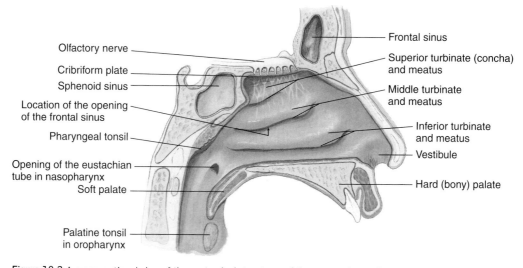

Figure 10-3 A cross-sectional view of the anatomical structures of the nose and nasopharynx including the turbinates. (From Jarvis C: *Physical examination & health assessment*, ed 4, Philadelphia, 2004, WB Saunders, p 373.)

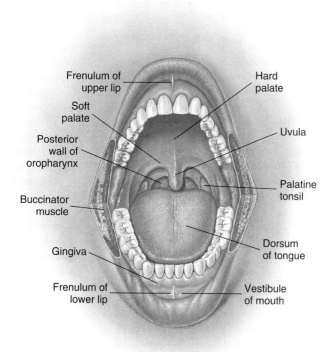

Figure 10-4 The anatomical structures of the oral cavity. (From Seidel HM, Ball JW, Dains JE, Benedict GW: *Mosby's guide to physical examination*, ed 5, St Louis, 2003, Mosby, p 320.)

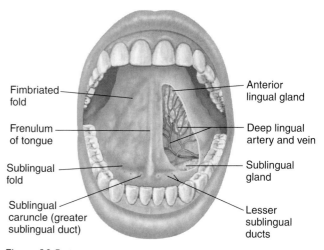

Figure 10-5 The ventral surface of the tongue showing anatomical landmarks. (From Seidel HM, Ball JW, Dains JE, Benedict GW: *Mosby's guide to physical examination*, ed 5, St Louis, 2003, Mosby, p 320.)

The oral cavity may be divided into the mouth and vestibule. The vestibule is the area between the buccal mucosa and the outer surface of the teeth and gums.[1] The roof of the mouth, which is formed by the hard and soft palates, separates the oral cavity from the nasal cavity. The soft palate is muscular tissue covered by mucous membrane that plays an active role in swallowing and vocal resonance. The soft palate, the tonsillar pillars, tonsils, base of the tongue, and posterior pharyngeal walls make up the oropharynx. The tongue is a skeletal muscle covered by mucous membrane, which helps to form the floor of the mouth and is anchored to the floor of the mouth by the **frenulum** (Figure 10-5).[1,4] Papillae cover the surface of the tongue to assist in movement of food. Taste buds are contained within the papillae that allow people to taste what they are eating.[4]

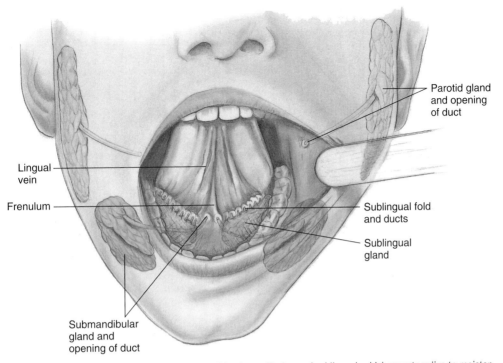

Figure 10-6 The salivary glands include the parotid, submandibular, and sublingual, which excrete saliva to moisten food and begin the digestive process. (From Jarvis C: *Physical examination & health assessment,* ed 4, Philadelphia, 2004, WB Saunders, p 375.)

Three pairs of salivary glands are located in the mouth. The parotid, submandibular, and sublingual glands secrete saliva to moisten and lubricate food and to begin the digestion process (Figure 10-6). The parotid gland lies within the cheeks just anterior to the ear with its duct, known as **Stensen's duct,** and extends to an opening on the buccal mucosa opposite the second molar.[3] The submandibular gland lies beneath the mandible at the angle of the jaw. Its duct runs to the floor of the mouth with the opening on either side of the frenulum. The sublingual gland is the smallest of the three glands and is located under the tongue.[3,4]

The teeth are embedded in the alveolar ridges and are protected by **gingivae** that cover the neck and roots of each tooth. Adults typically have 32 permanent teeth that are divided into upper and lower rows (Figure 10-7). Each tooth consists of the enamel, dentin, and pulp. The enamel is an extremely hard surface that covers the dentin. The periodontal ligament that surrounds the root of the tooth helps keep the tooth stable. The pulp chamber contains the pulp, nerves, and blood vessels (Figure 10-8).[1]

The pharynx consists of the combined upper parts of the respiratory and digestive tracts: the nasopharynx, oropharynx, and laryngopharynx (see Figure 4-1).[4]

The larynx functions in respiration, prevents food and saliva from entering the respiratory tract, and produces sound. It is protected anteriorly by the thyroid cartilage and inferiorly by the cricoid cartilage.

EVALUATION OF THE EAR, NOSE, MOUTH, AND THROAT

Examination of the Ear

When examining the ears, the athletic trainer begins with a general inspection of the auricle, or pinna (Key Points—Ear Exam), noting its general size, shape, and symmetry. The athletic trainer notes any deformities

KEY POINTS
Ear Exam

- Use the largest speculum that can comfortably fit in the ear.
- Pull the pinna up and back to straighten the canal.
- Do not insert the speculum too deep.
- Expect the normal ear canal to look pink without scaling or discharge.
- Expect the normal tympanic membrane to be "pearly gray" with no perforations, bulging, or redness.

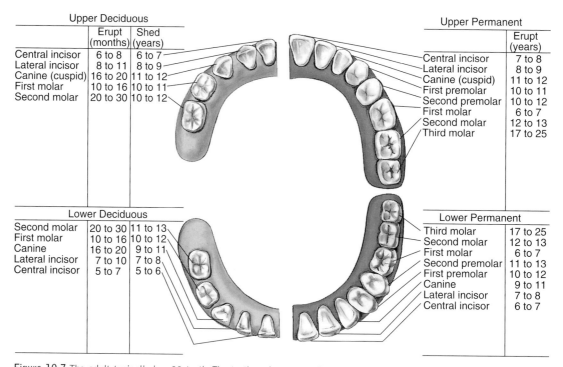

Upper Deciduous		
	Erupt (months)	Shed (years)
Central incisor	6 to 8	6 to 7
Lateral incisor	8 to 11	8 to 9
Canine (cuspid)	16 to 20	11 to 12
First molar	10 to 16	10 to 11
Second molar	20 to 30	10 to 12

Upper Permanent	
	Erupt (years)
Central incisor	7 to 8
Lateral incisor	8 to 9
Canine (cuspid)	11 to 12
First premolar	10 to 11
Second premolar	10 to 12
First molar	6 to 7
Second molar	12 to 13
Third molar	17 to 25

Lower Deciduous		
Second molar	20 to 30	11 to 13
First molar	10 to 16	10 to 12
Canine	16 to 20	9 to 11
Lateral incisor	7 to 10	7 to 8
Central incisor	5 to 7	5 to 6

Lower Permanent	
Third molar	17 to 25
Second molar	12 to 13
First molar	6 to 7
Second premolar	11 to 13
First premolar	10 to 12
Canine	9 to 11
Lateral incisor	7 to 8
Central incisor	6 to 7

Figure 10-7 The adult typically has 32 teeth. The teeth and gums are inspected during any evaluation of the mouth. (From Jarvis C: *Physical examination & health assessment,* ed 4, Philadelphia, 2004, WB Saunders, p 376.)

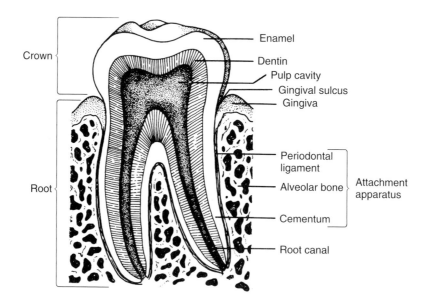

Figure 10-8 The anatomy of a tooth. (From Marx J, Hockberger R, Walls R: *Rosen's emergency medicine: concepts and clinical practice,* ed 5, St Louis, 2002, Mosby, p 892.)

or discoloration indicating trauma to the external ear. The athletic trainer also looks for lesions or nodules. Visual inspection of the external auditory canal for obvious discharge or odor is included in the ear examination. Straw-colored fluid draining from the ear following a head injury could be **cerebrospinal fluid** (CSF) indicative of a brain injury. The auricles and mastoid areas are palpated for point tenderness, swelling, and nonvisible nodules. The consistency of the auricle should be firm and mobile without nodules.

The athletic trainer conducts a gross determination of hearing when it is anticipated that the athlete's ability to hear has been lost. The athlete's response to questions or directions may give a good indication of gross hearing ability. To distinguish between sensorineural and conductive hearing loss, the Weber and Rinne tests may be used (Box 10-2).

An otoscope with a disposal speculum is used to inspect the ear canal. Specula come in different sizes to conform to different-sized ears.[5] The largest speculum

Box 10-2 Weber and Rinne Tests to Distinguish Between Sensorineural and Conductive Hearing Loss

When an athlete appears to have hearing loss, the Weber or Rinne test may be used to distinguish whether it is sensorineural or conductive in nature.

Weber Test for Lateralization of Sound
1. Hold the tuning fork at its base, and tap lightly against the palm of the hand to start its vibrations.
2. Place the tuning fork at the vertex of the athlete's head.
3. Ask the athlete if the sound is heard better in one ear or equally in both.

Results

Normal

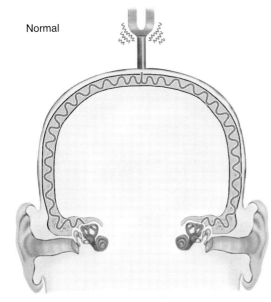

Normal finding: sound heard equally in both ears

Conductive loss

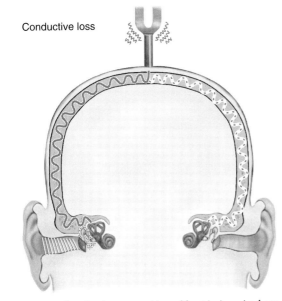

Conduction hearing loss: sound heard best in impaired ear

Sensorineural loss

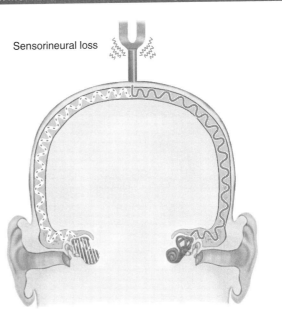

Unilateral sensorineural hearing loss: sound identified only in normal ear

Rinne Test
1. Hold the tuning fork at its base, and tap lightly against the palm of the hand to start its vibrations.
2. Place the stem of the tuning fork against the athlete's mastoid process.
3. Count the seconds when sound is no longer heard, and note the number of seconds.
4. Quickly, place the still-vibrating tines $\frac{1}{2}$ to 1 inch from the ear canal.
5. Ask the athlete to say when the sound is no longer heard. Count the seconds the sound is heard through air conduction.
6. Compare the number of seconds the sound is heard through the air and when in contact with the bone.

Results

Normal

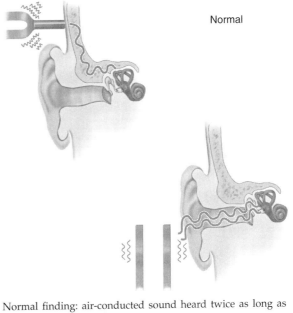

Normal finding: air-conducted sound heard twice as long as bone-conducted sound

Continued

Box 10-2 Weber and Rinne Tests to Distinguish Between Sensorineural and Conductive Hearing Loss—cont'd

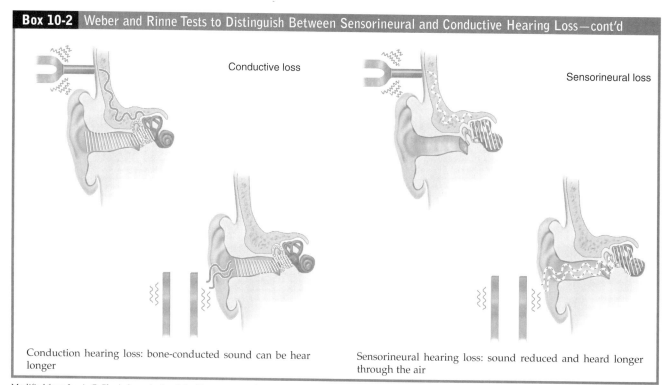

Conductive loss

Sensorineural loss

Conduction hearing loss: bone-conducted sound can be hear longer

Sensorineural hearing loss: sound reduced and heard longer through the air

Modified from Jarvis C: *Physical examination & health assessment*, ed 4, Philadelphia, 2004, WB Saunders, pp 368-369.

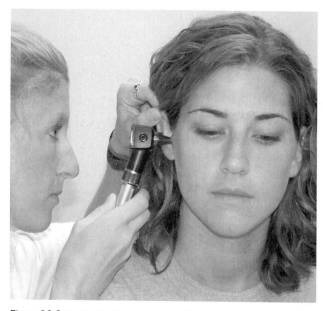

Figure 10-9 To view the inner structure of the ear with the otoscope, the ear canal must be straightened by pulling the pinna up and back.

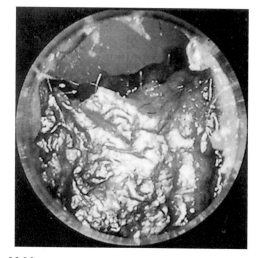

Figure 10-10 Impacted cerumen may be a cause of otalgia or hearing loss and will make examination of the tympanic membrane difficult. (From Seidel HM, Ball JW, Dains JE, Benedict GW: *Mosby's guide to physical examination*, ed 5, St Louis, 2003, Mosby, p 329.)

that can be comfortably fit into the ear is used to allow the best view of the canal and the tympanic membrane. The otoscope is turned on by rotating the dial on top of the handle. The athletic trainer asks the athlete to tip the head slightly toward the opposite shoulder and to avoid moving during the exam.

Because the canal slopes inferiorly and forward toward the eye the external auditory canal must be "straightened" from its S shape by pulling up and back on the pinna. Otitis externa is suspected if the athlete experiences pain while the athletic trainer is pulling on the pinna. The speculum is inserted gently and slightly down and forward approximately ½ inch into the ear canal. The athletic trainer places a finger or side of the hand against the cheek to guard against inserting the speculum too far into the ear (Figure 10-9).

The canal lining is lubricated with cerumen that is secreted by the **sebaceous glands** in the distal one third of the canal. Cerumen often builds up in the external canal and may impair the athlete's hearing

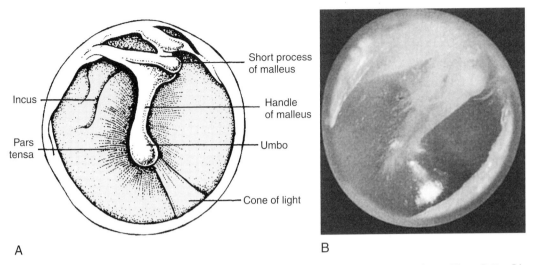

Figure 10-11 A, The anatomic landmarks of the typmanic membrane. B, Normal tympanic membrane. (From Potter PA, Weilitz PB: *Mosby's pocket guide to health assessment*, ed 5, St Louis, 2003, Mosby, p 225. Color plates from Jarvis C: *Physical examination and health assessment*, ed 4, Philadelphia, 2004, WB Saunders, pp 343, 351.)

and make examination more difficult (Figure 10-10). The skin in the external auditory canal is examined and should be smooth and somewhat pink or "fleshy" colored. The athletic trainer looks for and notes any scaling or increased redness in the canal as well as any discharge, lesions, or foreign bodies. A reddened canal with discharge signifies inflammation or infection.

To visualize the tympanic membrane the otoscope must be slowly moved in a circular direction as if looking at a large area through a small window. The tympanic membrane appears translucent and "pearly gray" in color. The translucent nature of a healthy tympanic membrane allows visualization of the middle ear cavity including the malleus. The tympanic membrane is concave as it is pulled in at the center, or umbo, by the malleus, allowing a light reflex to be visible when inspected by an otoscope (Figure 10-11). The tympanic membrane should be free from holes or breaks and should not be bulging or bloody. These signs may indicate a tympanic membrane puncture. Redness of and around the tympanic membrane indicates infection in the middle ear, whereas a white color may indicate pus behind the tympanic membrane (Table 10-1).

Examination of the Nose and Nasopharynx

Nasal disorders may present with local symptoms or may be a result of disorders from other structures, such as the paranasal sinuses (Key Points—Nose Exam). The major nontraumatic problems related to the nose are nasal obstruction, drainage, facial pain or headache, epistaxis, and change in smell or taste.[7] A thorough history of symptoms will help the athletic trainer determine the nature of the nasal disorder. The athletic trainer asks the athlete about the onset and duration

Table 10-1	Abnormal Findings of the Tympanic Membrane
Abnormal Finding	**Possible Indication**
Pink or red bulging	Inflammation of the tympanic membrane
Bluish or dark color	Blood behind the tympanic membrane
White color	Pus behind the tympanic membrane
Perforations or scarring	Current or previous tympanic membrane rupture

KEY POINTS
Nose Exam

- Use universal precautions when bleeding or discharge is present.
- Stop the epistaxis before performing an exam.
- Look for deformity of the external nose.
- Compare the sizes of the nares bilaterally.
- Determine the characteristics of any discharge.
- Determine the nature of any obstruction: unilateral or bilateral.
- Use short speculum for examination of septum and nasal cavity.

of the symptoms. In the case of nasal obstruction, it is important to determine if trauma was involved or whether the nasal obstruction or congestion onset was insidious. It is also important to determine if the obstruction is bilateral or unilateral and if it is constant or intermittent. Assessment of inspiratory and expiratory airflow is done by occluding one nostril at a time while the athlete inspires (Figure 10-12).

Unilateral obstruction may indicate an anatomical problem, such as a deviated septum or **polyp,** whereas bilateral obstruction could arise from a simple cold.[7] If drainage is present, it is helpful to determine its characteristics. Is it unilateral or bilateral? Is it clear or discolored? Clear drainage suggests **rhinitis,** either allergic or nonallergic, whereas yellow, green, or brown drainage suggests bacterial or viral infection (Table 10-2). Straw-colored drainage following a head injury could be cerebrospinal fluid (CSF) and an indicator of possible brain injury. If discharge is present, the examiner should wear gloves for the examination.

The athlete may also experience facial pain and headache. Many nasal or sinus disorders will present with headaches but should be differentiated from headache or face pain caused by migraine, tension headache, or temporomandibular joint (TMJ) pain. Dental disorders may also cause diffuse facial pain. When pain and swelling occur over the sinuses accompanied by **purulent** drainage, **sinusitis** may be suspected.

During or after the history, the athletic trainer visually examines the external nose, noting its shape, size, and color. The athlete is asked whether there are subtle changes in shape. Sometimes standing behind the athlete and looking down the nose while the athlete is sitting allows better visualization of whether the nose is straight. Next, the nares are examined

for discharge as well as any unilateral flaring or narrowing.

Palpation may reveal swelling, tenderness, or masses, as well as any displacement of bone or cartilage. The **patency** of the nares is evaluated by gently squeezing the nares together. Unilateral variations may indicate a deviated septum or polyp in the nose. One must remember that recent trauma may cause ecchymosis and edema of the nose and surrounding areas as well as localized tenderness.

The athletic trainer palpates the facial bones and the sinuses to determine any areas of tenderness, swelling, or deformity. The facial areas over the frontal sinus are palpated by the examiner positioning the thumb up and under the athlete's eyebrow (Figure 10-13, A). The maxillary sinus is palpated by pressing with thumbs up under the zygomatic process (Figure 10-13, B). Healthy sinuses are not generally tender to the touch, and pain with palpation of the facial bones over the sinuses often indicates inflammation from infection or allergy.

Transillumination

The sinuses also may be transilluminated. This skill is often performed by the physician; however, the athletic trainer may elect to try the technique. Transillumination is done in a darkened room using a penlight or an otoscope. The frontal sinus may be transilluminated by placing a light against the medial aspect of each supraorbital rim while looking for a slight red glow of light just above the eyebrow.[1,5] An absence of a glow in the sinus indicates that the sinus contains secretions. Likewise, the maxillary sinus may be illuminated by placing the light lateral to the athlete's nose beneath the medial aspect of the eye while asking the athlete to open the mouth. If the sinus is clear, the hard palate will be illuminated (Figure 10-14).

Speculum Exam

To view the septum and turbinates the athletic trainer tips the athlete's head slightly backward. The nares of the nose may be dilated and viewed by the use of a speculum and a light, or the speculum on an otoscope may be used. The speculum is held in one hand while the other guides the patient's head.

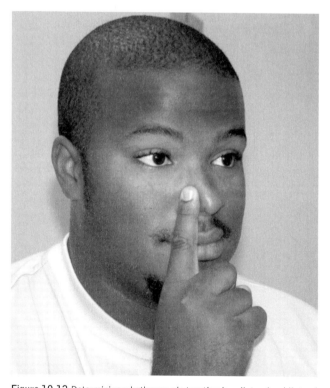

Figure 10-12 Determining whether an obstruction is unilateral or bilateral may be accomplished by occluding one nostril at a time during inspiration and expiration.

Table 10-2 Differential Diagnosis of Nasal Conditions with Drainage		
Nasal Drainage	**Other Symptoms**	**Most Likely Conditions**
Bilateral watery discharge	Usually associated with sneezing, watery eyes, and congestion	Allergic or nonallergic rhinitis
Bilateral purulent discharge	Associated with sinus or upper respiratory infection	Sinusitis (bacterial or viral)
Bloody discharge	Traumatic or dry nasal mucosa	Epistaxis

Modified from Potter PA, Weilitz PB: *Mosby's pocket guide to health assessment*, ed 5, St Louis, 2003, Mosby, p 247.

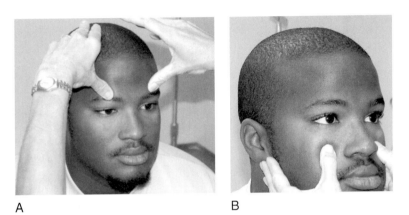

Figure 10-13 Palpation. A, Frontal sinuses. B, Maxillary sinuses.

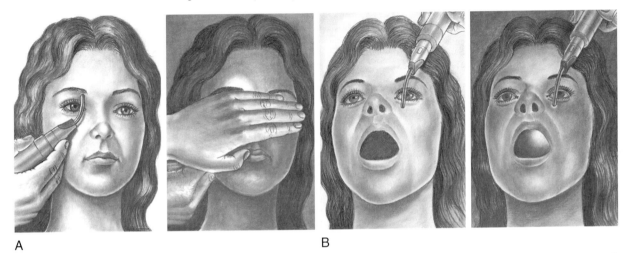

Figure 10-14 Transillumination. A, Frontal sinuses. B, Maxillary sinuses. (From Seidel HM, Ball JW, Dains JE, Benedict GW: *Mosby's guide to physical examination*, ed 5, St Louis, 2003, Mosby, p. 341.)

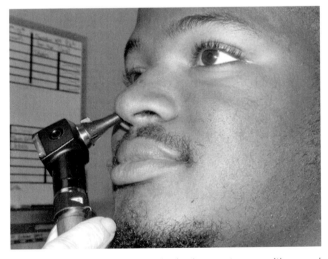

Figure 10-15 The septum is examined using an otoscope with a nasal speculum.

The septum may be visualized by tipping the speculum toward the midline (Figure 10-15). The septum is normally pink and glistening and should be thicker anteriorly. The athletic trainer checks for any discoloration, perforations, bleeding, or crusting (Figure 10-16, *A*) and notes differences such as polyps, holes, swelling, or abnormal coloring (Figure 10-16, *B*).[3,5] The septum should be straight and positioned close to the midline. To determine the position of the septum, it is best to compare sides bilaterally, ensuring that the space between the lateral wall of the nose and the septum is the same in both nostrils.

After determining the integrity of the septum, the vestibule and the turbinates can be visualized with the athlete's head fairly erect (Figure 10-17). The athletic trainer tilts the athlete's head backward to see the middle meatus and middle turbinates. The turbinates should be pink, moist, and free of any lesions or discoloration.

Examination of the Mouth and Throat

The assessment of the mouth and oropharynx starts with inspection of the face, head, and neck. The face, ears, and neck are observed, noting any asymmetry or changes on the skin. The lymph nodes are palpated bilaterally to detect enlargement. Examination continues with evaluation of the lips with the mouth both

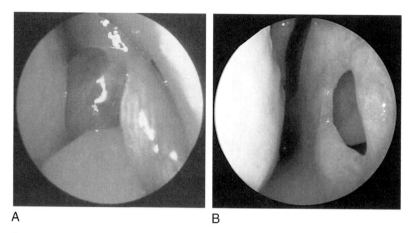

A   B

Figure 10-16 Abnormalities of the nose. **A**, Nasal polyps. **B**, Perforated septum. (From Jarvis C: *Physical examination & health assessment,* ed 4, Philadelphia, 2004, WB Saunders, pp 396, 397.)

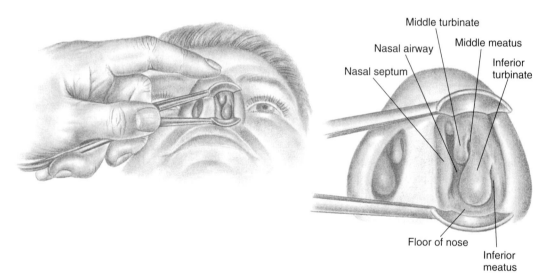

Figure 10-17 The athlete's head is tilted backward in order to view the nasal mucosa and middle turbinate through a nasal speculum. (From Seidel HM, Ball JW, Dains JE, Benedict GW: *Mosby's guide to physical examination,* ed 5, St Louis, 2003, Mosby, p 333.)

open and closed, noting the texture, color, and any surface abnormalities (Figure 10-18, *A*).

The athletic trainer asks the athlete to open the mouth to visually examine the labial mucosa as well as the maxillary and mandibular vestibules and notes the color and texture as well as any swelling of the mucosa or gingivae. The buccal mucosa is examined extending from the **labial commissure** back to the anterior tonsillar pillar. A tongue depressor or gloved finger may be used to pull the buccal mucosa away from the teeth (Figure 10-18, *B*). The athletic trainer notes pigmentation, color, texture, mobility, and other abnormalities of the mucosa (Key Points—Mouth and Throat Exam).

KEY POINTS
Mouth and Throat Exam

- Inspect the lips, noting color and lesions.
- Note any cracking of the lips that may indicate dehydration.
- Note the condition of the teeth and gums as an overall indicator of general health.
- Inspect the tongue and buccal mucosa for color, lesions, and presence of white plaque.
- Inspect the sides of the tongue for lesions.
- Use a tongue depressor to hold down the tongue to visualize the tonsils, uvula, and pharynx; redness, swelling, exudates, or spots indicate inflammation or infection.
- Palpate the mouth when indicated, being sure to wear gloves.
- Palpate the cervical lymph nodes for swelling.

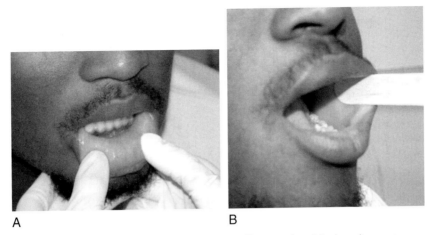

Figure 10-18 Inspection. **A,** Inner oral mucosa. **B,** Retraction of the buccal mucosa.

First, the athletic trainer examines the buccal and labial aspects of the gingivae and alveolar ridges (i.e., processes) by starting with the right maxillary posterior gingivae and alveolar ridge and then moving around the arch to the left posterior area.[1,5] The inspection continues with the left mandibular posterior gingivae and alveolar ridge and moves around the arch to the right posterior area. The athletic trainer looks for any abnormal lesions, especially white or dark pigmented areas. Stensen's duct, the opening of the parotid gland, will look like a small dimple opposite the upper second molar.

With the patient's tongue at rest and mouth partially open, the dorsum of the tongue is inspected for any swelling, ulceration, coating, or variation in size, color, or texture. The athletic trainer visualizes the papillae pattern on the surface of the tongue, asks the athlete to stick out the tongue, and notes any abnormality of mobility or positioning. Then the tip of the tongue is grasped with a piece of gauze to assist in its full protrusion and aid in examination of the more posterior aspects of the tongue's lateral borders (Figure 10-19). The ventral surface of the tongue is examined along with the floor of the mouth.

The examiner is looking for changes in color, texture, swelling, or other surface abnormalities. With the mouth wide open and the patient's head tilted back, the base of the tongue is gently depressed using a tongue blade. The hard palate is examined followed by the soft palate and oropharyngeal tissues. Movement of the soft palate may be evaluated by asking the athlete to say "ah." This also tests cranial nerves IX and X, the glossopharyngeal and vagus nerves.

Next, the oropharynx is inspected while keeping the tongue depressed with a tongue blade. The tonsillar pillars should be pink and blend in with the integrity of the retropharyngeal wall. Hypertrophied or reddened tonsils that may be covered in exudates indicate a viral or bacterial infection. The posterior

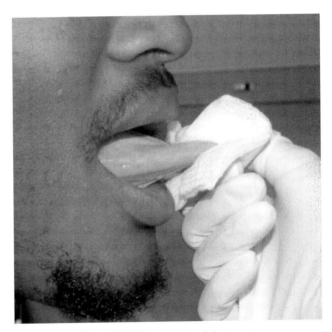

Figure 10-19 Examination of the tongue.

wall is normally pink and smooth, although some irregular spots of lymphatic tissue may be present. A yellowish film may indicate postnasal drip. The athletic trainer may elicit the gag reflex at this point in the examination, which also tests the glossopharyngeal and vagus nerves (i.e., CN IX and CN X, respectively).

PATHOLOGICAL CONDITIONS OF THE EAR

Hearing Loss

Hearing loss may include the inability to hear a specific pitch or the inability to detect any sound. It is estimated that 10% to 15% of the population has some degree of hearing impairment.[7] The inability to detect any sound is referred to as deafness. The most efficient and normal hearing pathway is through air conduction; however, bone also conducts sound (see Box 10-1). In bone conduction of sound, the vibrations of the skull are transmitted directly to the vestibulocochlear nerve (i.e., CN VIII).[1,3,8]

Hearing loss may be divided into conductive hearing loss and sensorineural hearing loss. In conductive hearing loss, the sound conduction pathway is blocked and sound does not pass through the external and middle ear to reach the inner ear, resulting in a loss of hearing. It is considered a mechanical dysfunction because the person is able to hear if the sound is amplified enough. A buildup of impacted wax, injury, foreign body, or infection in the external ear can cause conductive loss. Otitis media, sinus infections, small or blocked eustachian tubes, and allergies can also cause conductive loss.[8]

Sensorineural loss is more serious and involves the inner ear where sensory receptors convert sound waves into neural impulses that are transmitted to the brain for translation. Most people who are born deaf have this type of loss. Causes of this type of loss are generally idiopathic. Other identified causes include hereditary factors, **meningitis, measles,** scarlet fever, mumps, and **encephalitis.** Gradual nerve degeneration, known as **presbycusis,** often occurs with aging and may cause the person to be unable to understand words. Simple amplification of sound will not increase the ability to hear if sensorineural hearing loss is present.[3] Balance problems may also accompany this type of loss. A combination of both conductive and sensorineural hearing loss in the same ear is called a mixed hearing loss. If hearing impairment is suspected, the athlete should be referred as soon as possible for proper diagnosis and treatment. Treatment depends on the cause of the hearing loss.

Signs and Symptoms

The athlete experiences difficulty in hearing in either general or specific situations. Often the athlete will complain of hearing loss following bathing or swimming and may also note hearing loss associated with upper respiratory infection. It should be noted whether the athlete has any pain, dizziness, or tinnitus.

Referral and Diagnostic Tests

Quick tests for hearing may be performed during the patient history and include observing the responses to questions spoken at different intensities. Comparing the athlete's ability to hear sounds with whispering, normal conversational intensity, and shouting gives rough estimates of the amount of hearing loss.

Additional tests include the Rinne test and the Weber test to differentiate between conductive and sensorineural hearing loss[3-5] (see Box 10-2). **Audiometry** may be performed by an audiologist to determine the extent of the hearing deficit.

Prognosis and Return to Participation

The prognosis and ability of the athlete to return to sports after hearing loss are usually determined by the cause of the hearing deficit. Treatment of the condition responsible for the hearing loss may return the hearing to normal. Chapter 16 discusses concerns for athletes with permanent hearing loss.

Prevention

Prevention of hearing loss largely depends on preventing those things that may cause damage to the ear: sharp objects in the ear that may perforate the tympanic membrane, extremely loud noises, blows to the ear, and excessive buildup of cerumen. Since some hearing loss is congenital or occurs with age, there is no definitive method of prevention.

Otitis Externa

Otitis externa is an inflammation or infection of the external auditory canal and tympanic membrane (Figure 10-20). Subgroups include acute localized otitis externa or furunculosis, acute diffuse bacterial otitis externa or swimmer's ear, chronic otitis externa, eczematous otitis externa, fungal otitis externa or otomycosis, and rarely, invasive or necrotizing otitis externa.[9] Otitis externa occurs in 4 of every 1000

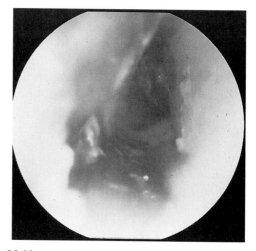

Figure 10-20 Otitis externa. (From Zitelli BJ, Davis HW: *Atlas of pediatric physical diagnosis*, ed 3, St Louis, 1997, Mosby.)

Americans each year, with the incidence being higher during the summer months. It is more prevalent in individuals who have narrow inner ear canals or in someone whose canals slope downward more than normal.[9] Because prolonged water exposure causes tissue swelling and oozing, otitis externa is a common malady seen in swimmers and others involved in water sports. Eczema, **seborrhea**, or **psoriasis** may also be present. Excessive cleaning of the external auditory canal may also contribute to otitis externa by removing the protective cerumen from the canal.[8,9] A normal acidic balance in the external canal maintains the level of *Pseudomonas aeruginosa* that is present in virtually all auditory canals. When the epidermal barrier is compromised, the pH protection is lost and the *Pseudomonas* organisms proliferate, causing serous exudates.[7,9]

Signs and Symptoms, Referral, and Diagnostic Tests

Signs and symptoms include pain, itching, or burning with possible drainage. The external auditory canal will be edematous and erythematous, perhaps causing narrowing of the canal. Scaling or crusting of the epithelial cells of the canal and an apparent absence of cerumen may be noted. Pulling on the pinna will increase pain in a person with otitis externa.[3,5] The athlete may present with inflammation outside the ear canal as well. This is typically cellulitis and not otitis externa. With otitis externa, the middle ear is generally not involved and the athlete will not have systemic symptoms, such as fever or chills.

A thorough history and physical examination are typically the primary diagnostic tests. Cultures are generally ordered only when the athlete is not responding to treatment.

Differential Diagnosis

Acute otitis externa should be distinguished from acute otitis media, impacted cerumen, cellulitis, and ruptured tympanic membrane. The telltale symptom of otitis externa that is not present with middle ear problems is pain the patient experiences when the pinna is pulled. Other conditions to consider are herpes zoster and foreign bodies in the ear.[10]

Treatment

Treatment typically includes the application of ear drops, three or four times daily, which may contain an acidifying agent such as aluminum acetate or vinegar and a drying agent that is often isopropyl alcohol. Many ear drops also contain broad-spectrum antibiotics or topical steroids. The efficacy of topical antibiotics and steroids in the treatment of otitis externa

has been debated; however, oral antibiotics may be appropriate for swimming athletes.[10-12] Treatment with ear drops will usually cure acute otitis externa in 1 or 2 days. Chronic conditions will take much longer, that is, weeks or even months. Oral analgesics may be used for pain. Some physicians advocate a hot pack applied to the side of the face for its soothing properties.

Prognosis and Return to Participation

Athletes other than those in water sports may participate as symptoms allow provided the head stays dry. Aquatic athletes with otitis externa are kept out of the pool until completing at least 24 hours of antibiotics. Persistent or recurrent otitis externa may require that the swimming athlete discontinue in-pool training for longer. When the athlete is restricted from the pool, on-land exercises such as weight training or conditioning may be continued. Mild infections may be treated with rubbing alcohol or a mixture of alcohol and vinegar. Creating a more acidic atmosphere will prevent the growth of bacteria.[13]

Prevention

Although recurrent otitis externa is not completely preventable, several measures may help reduce its occurrence. Swimming in potentially contaminated waters, such as lakes or rivers, increases the incidence of otitis externa over swimming in a chlorinated pool.[14] The ear canals should be emptied of water and dried carefully after swimming or bathing. Self-inflicted trauma to the ears, such as using cotton swabs or inserting objects into the canal, should be avoided. Frequent washing of the ears with soap may leave an alkaline residue in the ear canal, thereby reducing the normally acidic pH of the ear canal. Using an acidifying ear drop after swimming to assist in drying and acidifying the ear is helpful in the athlete who is susceptible to recurrent otitis externa.[8,14]

Otitis Media

Otitis media is the presence of fluid in the middle ear accompanied by signs and symptoms of infection (Figure 10-21). The peak incidence is between 6 and 36 months and between 4 and 6 years.[15] The incidence of otitis media dramatically decreases with age and is infrequently seen in adults.

Otitis media often occurs simultaneously with an upper respiratory infection and can be caused by a virus or bacterium. Common bacterial sources for otitis media are *Streptococcus pneumoniae* and *Haemophilus influenzae*.[16]

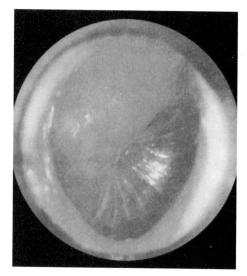

Figure 10-21 Otitis media. (From Seidel HM, Ball JW, Dains JE, Benedict GW. *Mosby's guide to physical examination*, ed 5, St Louis, 2003, Mosby, p 351.)

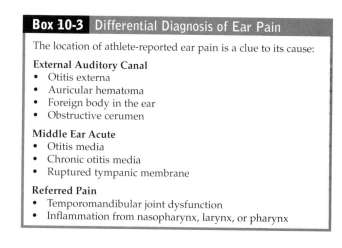

Box 10-3   Differential Diagnosis of Ear Pain

The location of athlete-reported ear pain is a clue to its cause:

External Auditory Canal
- Otitis externa
- Auricular hematoma
- Foreign body in the ear
- Obstructive cerumen

Middle Ear Acute
- Otitis media
- Chronic otitis media
- Ruptured tympanic membrane

Referred Pain
- Temporomandibular joint dysfunction
- Inflammation from nasopharynx, larynx, or pharynx

Signs and Symptoms

Common signs and symptoms of otitis media include earache, fever, a feeling of fullness in the ear, dizziness, tinnitus, and diminished hearing. Typically children are febrile, but adults may not be febrile and may not feel sick.[14,16]

Referral and Diagnostic Tests

Otitis media may be confirmed by physical examination with an otoscope. Visualization of the tympanic membrane may be difficult and painful in the otalgic ear, but the tympanic membrane will appear inflamed and thickened if visualized.[15] A Weber test will confirm a conductive hearing loss in the affected ear.[14] The athlete is referred to a physician for antibiotic treatment as soon as possible.

Differential Diagnosis

The primary differential diagnosis for **otalgia** (ear pain) is otitis media, otitis externa, and temporomandibular joint (TMJ) dysfunction (Box 10-3). People with TMJ problems typically do not have hearing difficulties, and physical examination should rule out otitis externa.

Treatment

The physician generally will prescribe a broad-spectrum antibiotic, such as amoxicillin. For patients who are allergic to penicillin, a cephalosporin or erythromycin may be used.[16] Chapter 3 gives more information about antibiotics. Antihistamines and decongestants have not proven beneficial for managing otitis media.

Prognosis and Return to Participation

After dealing with the discomfort that accompanies otitis media, the athlete who is afebrile may participate in sports. Air travel should be avoided until the middle ear has returned to normal appearance and function because of the increased risk of ruptured tympanic membrane from pressure changes on ascent and descent. Complications of acute otitis media are uncommon but are best recognized early and treated aggressively.[8] These complications may include meningitis, facial nerve paralysis, and neck infections.

Prevention

Avoidance of situations that will introduce bacteria into the ear may help decrease the occurrence of otitis media. Aggressive treatment of upper respiratory infections may also reduce the risk. The efficacy of employing prophylactic antibiotic treatment for upper respiratory infections for those individuals susceptible to otitis media is debatable.

Ruptured Tympanic Membrane

A ruptured tympanic membrane or tympanic membrane perforation (TMP) may occur when there is a sudden change of air pressure caused by a blunt trauma or an infection that inhibits the ability to regulate inner ear pressure.[17] Sticking a sharp object, even a cotton swab, in the ear may also rupture the membrane.

Signs and Symptoms

Signs and symptoms of TMP include audible whistling sounds and decreased hearing. Purulent fluid or bleeding may be noted leaking from the ear. TMP may be painless if not accompanied by infection, typically otitis media. The hearing loss is more severe if the **ossicular chain** is disrupted or the inner ear injured.[8] Vertigo may be present if the inner ear is injured.

Referral and Diagnostic Tests

Radiography and magnetic resonance imaging (MRI) are usually of no use in uncomplicated TMP and are typically not performed.[17] TMP is usually diagnosed with simple history, physical exam, and otoscopy.[7] The presence of a hole or perforation in the tympanic membrane is often visible on exam (Figure 10-22). A **tympanogram** is often performed to determine the integrity of the tympanic membrane. Audiometry is typically performed by the physician to determine the amount of hearing loss and is especially performed before any attempted repair.[17]

Differential Diagnosis

Other causes of hearing loss, otalgia, and **otorrhea** should be ruled out, including otitis media, impacted cerumen, otitis externa, or **infectious myringitis.**[8,17] A TMP can usually be visualized with the use of the otoscope, thus differentiating it from other ear conditions.

Treatment

The tympanic membrane tends to heal itself, and even eardrums that have been perforated multiple times often remain intact.[17] Larger perforations may take 3 to 6 months to heal. The athlete with a small perforation will tend to heal quickly but must be protected from water and debris. Over-the-counter analgesics may be required during the initial healing stages if the athlete is in pain. If the TMP was caused by an infection, the physician will generally prescribe drying agent drops as well as topical and oral antibiotics.[8]

Larger or complicated ruptures may require surgical procedures by an **otolaryngologist** involving a graft of surgical paper, fat, muscle, or other material.[8] These procedures are usually done in the office with the patient under local anesthesia.

Prognosis and Return to Participation

The prognosis for small uncomplicated perforations of the tympanic membrane is very good and should result in minimal time lost, especially in the non-swimming athlete. Larger or multiple perforations may cause scarring of the tympanic membrane and some resultant hearing loss.[17] Divers may be held out of activity longer than swimmers because of the combination of water and pressure changes associated with the sport. Athletes with TMP are more susceptible to middle ear infections so must take special care to keep the ear dry until it heals.

Prevention

Prevention of TMP includes avoidance of foreign objects in the ear, such as sharp objects or cotton-tipped applicators that are inserted too deeply. Treating otitis media aggressively to reduce the pressure on the tympanic membrane will also reduce the chances of TMP. The athlete with otitis media also needs to avoid sudden altitude changes resulting in pressure from air or water pressure. A TMP from a blow to the external ear may be unavoidable unless head or ear protection is worn.

PATHOLOGICAL CONDITIONS OF THE NOSE

Allergic Rhinitis

Allergic rhinitis is a hypersensitivity response to nasally inhaled allergens that causes sneezing, rhinorrhea, nasal pruritus, and congestion (Figure 10-23).[9] It affects 10% to 20% of the U.S. population.[9] Seasonal allergic rhinitis occurs in the spring, summer, and fall and is triggered by pollens, ragweed, or grasses. Perennial rhinitis occurs daily and is typically triggered by dust, animal allergens, smoke, detergents, or soaps.[8,9]

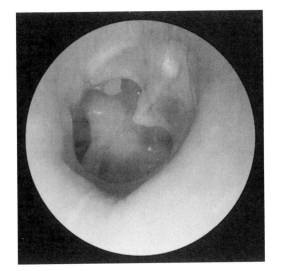

Figure 10-22 View of a large tympanic membrane perforation. (From Epstein O, Perkin GD, Cookson J, de Bono DP: *Clinical examination,* ed 3, Philadelphia, 2003, Mosby, p 93.)

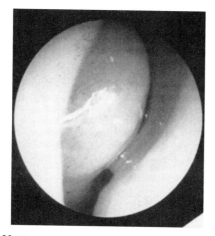

Figure 10-23 Allergic rhinitis. (From Jarvis C: *Physical examination & health assessment,* ed 4, Philadelphia, 2004, WB Saunders, p 397.)

Signs and Symptoms

Allergic rhinitis presents with clear nasal discharge and sneezing, nasal congestion, cough, and sensation of plugged ears accompanied by itchy, watering eyes. The mucosa of the turbinates may appear pale from venous engorgement. The throat may appear erythematous from postnasal drip.[18]

Referral and Diagnostic Tests

Diagnostic tests are often unnecessary; however, a detailed medical history is useful in identifying the irritating allergen. A temperature may be taken to confirm that the patient is afebrile. The athlete with chronic symptoms that affect athletic performance should be referred to the physician, especially if over-the-counter medications have not been effective in the past.[9] The athlete should be referred to a physician if the symptoms persist for more than 7 days. Some patients may benefit from allergy testing.

Differential Diagnosis

Allergic rhinitis must be distinguished from viral, bacterial, or fungal rhinitis as well as influenza. Septal obstruction must also be ruled out as a cause of nasal congestion. In addition, rhinitis medicamentosa from cocaine use or excessive nasal drop usage should be considered.

Treatment, Prognosis, and Return to Participation

Antihistamines are available over the counter and generally relieve symptoms. Most first-generation antihistamines, however, cause considerable drowsiness.

The second-generation antihistamines (loratadine, fexofenadine) are also available over the counter and are nonsedating. Many athletes find that these nonsedating antihistamines provide good results. The physician may choose to treat chronic cases with cromolyn sodium (Nasalcrom). Chapter 3 gives a more complete description of antihistamines.

Most athletes experience considerable relief with avoidance of the allergens and proper use of medications. Athletes may participate in athletics as able.

Prevention

Avoidance of the irritating allergens is the best prevention for patients and athletes with allergic rhinitis. Use of air conditioning and maintaining humidity below 50% may be helpful to prevent episodes of allergic rhinitis. The use of humidifiers and air filters may also be helpful.

Nonallergic Rhinitis

Rhinitis is a viral, bacterial, or vasomotor-related inflammation or infection of the nasal passages that causes excessive mucous production, resulting in nasal congestion and mucous discharge. Vasomotor rhinitis shows exacerbation of symptoms with changes in temperature and humidity or exposure to hot and cold foods.[7]

Signs and Symptoms

Nonallergic rhinitis is similar to perennial allergic rhinitis with symptoms of nasal obstruction, clear rhinorrhea sneezing, watery eyes, and pruritus of the nose, eyes, and palate but fails to show responses on allergy testing.[9]

Referral and Diagnostic Tests

The athlete is referred to a physician for further evaluation if the symptoms persist for more than 7 days. The athlete's temperature may be taken to rule out a fever. Allergy tests may be performed to rule out allergic rhinitis.

Differential Diagnosis

Nonallergic rhinitis is differentiated from allergic rhinitis, sinusitis, nasal obstruction, nasal polyps, and noninflammatory rhinitis. Many nasal conditions result in rhinorrhea. A yellow or brown discharge accompanied by a fever indicates a bacterial or viral condition and not rhinitis (see Table 10-2).

Treatment, Prognosis, and Return to Participation

Rhinitis is usually treated symptomatically with over-the-counter medications. Second-generation antihistamines should be used with athletes because of their nonsedating properties. Adequate hydration should be ensured if the athlete is taking antihistamines because of the drying effects of the medication. Rhinitis is self-limiting, and typically athletes are able to participate in athletics with few limitations. Performance may be affected if the athlete is using sedating antihistamines.

Sinusitis

Sinusitis is an inflammation of the mucous membrane lining of the nasal cavity or one or more of the paranasal sinuses.[18] Sinusitis may be acute, subacute, recurrent, or chronic and may result from bacterial or viral exposure. Sinusitis occurs when mucus or other infectious materials cause blockage within the passageways connecting the sinuses to the nasal cavity. It may follow upper respiratory tract infections; however, less than 1% of upper respiratory tract infections result in the clinical syndrome of acute sinusitis.[18] Most cases of sinusitis are caused by bacterial infections. Besides upper respiratory infections, sinusitis may be caused by dental infections, which are mainly in the maxillary sinus, or by swimming in contaminated water.[9] It is almost always accompanied by inflammation of the nasal mucosa so may be more correctly termed rhinosinusitis. Acute viral infection may be preceded by infection with the common cold or influenza. This is typically followed by mucosal edema and sinus infection. The drainage of thick secretions is decreased, resulting in obstruction of the sinus. This may result in the entrapment of bacteria in the sinuses, resulting in a secondary bacterial infection.

Signs and Symptoms

The athlete typically presents with a history of previous upper respiratory infection with postnasal drip lasting more than 7 to 10 days. Athletes may experience a purulent nasal discharge, facial tightness, nasal obstruction, and headache. They may also complain of point tenderness over the infected sinus and toothache if the maxillary sinus is involved. Occasionally, athletes will present with a cough that is often worse at night.

Referral and Diagnostic Tests

The athletic trainer should refer the athlete suspected of having sinusitis to the physician so that the diagnosis can be confirmed and pharmacological treatment started. Diagnosis is typically done through history and examination. Transillumination of the sinuses may help to confirm if the sinuses are indeed blocked. For chronic conditions that do not improve with medication, radiological examination may be performed, but it is only helpful to rule out, not to confirm, sinusitis.[15,18]

Differential Diagnosis

Because of the facial pain associated with sinusitis, it should be differentiated from migraine headaches and dental infections. Sinusitis should also be differentiated from viral or bacterial rhinitis and influenza.

Treatment

Symptomatic treatment can be initiated for the athlete with mild symptoms using analgesics, antipyretics, decongestants, or **mucolytics.** Saline nasal spray may help clear nasal crusts and thick mucus. Use of topical decongestants, if necessary, should be short term only. Systemic decongestants may also be used to help dry up the sinuses. Because most cases of acute sinusitis have a viral etiology, they will resolve within about 2 weeks without pharmacological treatment. Antibiotics are reserved for severe or chronic cases.[15,18] Nonpharmacological treatments include air humidification, hydration, and application of hot compresses over the sinuses to help promote sinus drainage.

Prognosis and Return to Participation

Acute sinusitis is often self-limiting because of the nasal obstruction, facial pain, headache, and fever and comes to full resolution in 3 to 4 weeks.[7] The athlete who is afebrile and feels well enough may be allowed to participate in athletics. Chronic sinusitis represents a persistent low-grade infection involving the paranasal sinuses with persistent mucosal thickening.[7] More aggressive treatment is often required for chronic sinusitis to prevent long-term complications, and surgical procedures may be utilized to relieve the obstruction.

Prevention

Seventy percent of acute sinusitis is caused by *S. pneumoniae* or *H. influenzae.*[7] Frequent hand washing is one of the best lines of defense when in contact with people who are known to be affected with the pathogens and may drastically reduce the incidence of infection. Rapid treatment of upper respiratory tract infection may decrease the incidence of sinusitis.

Avoidance of swimming in contaminated water will also reduce the incidence.[18]

Deviated Septum

A deviated septum in an athlete typically occurs from trauma, often a blow to the side of the nose (Figure 10-24). It may present with epistaxis and is often associated with nasal fracture.[9] A deviated septum often is discovered well after the initial trauma has healed and may present with only a minor deformity or complaints of chronic nasal obstruction.

Signs and Symptoms

The patient with a deviated septum will typically present with a history of trauma to the nose and initially will have swelling and pain throughout the nose. There may be external nasal deformity. The athlete may complain of a unilateral nasal obstruction often confirmed on examination by visualization of the space between the septum and the lateral nasal wall on the affected and the nonaffected sides. The nasal passage will appear narrow on the side to which the septum is deviated.

Referral, Diagnostic Tests, and Differential Diagnosis

Diagnosis of a deviated septum may be made by the history and physical examination. Visualization of the nasal passage will usually reveal the deviation; radiographs are inconsequential.

When a deviated septum is suspected, both nasal fracture and septal hematoma should be ruled out.

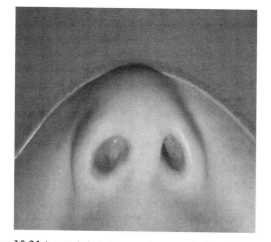

Figure 10-24 A septal deviation may be recognized by the difference between the spacing in the nares and the angulation of the septum. (From Jarvis C: *Physical examination & health assessment*, ed 4, Philadelphia, 2004, WB Saunders, p 382.)

Other causes of unilateral nasal obstruction, such as polyps or a foreign body, must also be eliminated.

Treatment

The acute treatment of nasal trauma involves stopping the epistaxis and minimizing the swelling. If considerable swelling occurs, it may be more difficult to correct the deviation with a minor surgical procedure.[7] The athlete must be seen quickly to prevent long-term complications from septal deviations. Correction of a deviated septum is typically a minor elective surgical procedure that is performed with the patient under local anesthesia.[7] If an external nasal deformity is also present, then a **rhinoplasty** may also be performed to improve both function and cosmetic appearance.

Prognosis and Return to Participation

Early recognition and treatment of the deviated septum may prevent long-term complications, and the athlete should be able to return to play as soon as the septum has been reduced and healed. The physician may allow the athlete to go back sooner if the nose is adequately protected with a mask. If the septum is not treated expediently, the athlete may have chronic unilateral nasal obstruction later in life.

Prevention

The incidence of deviated septum by trauma is drastically reduced in athletes who wear facial protection. Many collision sports require facial protection; however, a large number of traumatic nasal injuries occur in the "noncollision" sports. The unprotected athlete is at risk from contact with another athlete or sports implement (e.g., ball, bat, tennis racket).

Epistaxis

Epistaxis, commonly known as nosebleed, is a prevalent medical disorder among athletes. It is typically associated with trauma to the nose; however, it may occur without trauma. Epistaxis can be divided into anterior bleeds and posterior bleeds depending on where the bleeding originates. More than 90% of all epistaxes occur anteriorly from where Kiesselbach's plexus forms on the septum.[9,19,20] The cause is often an erosion of the mucosa that causes the vessels to become exposed. Anterior bleeds from capillaries and veins provide a constant ooze rather than a profuse pumping of blood observed from an arterial origin.

Posterior epistaxes are usually more profuse and often are of arterial origin. A posterior bleed is a more serious hemorrhage that presents a great risk of airway obstruction and difficulty in controlling bleeding.

Signs and Symptoms

Epistaxis will present with blood coming from the nostrils. The athlete will generally complain of swallowing and spitting blood. Epistaxis may result from local or systemic factors. Local causes generally occur in young children and are usually reported as spontaneous events. Epistaxes resulting from local events are frequently related to nose picking, excessive blowing, sneezing, or rubbing of the nose.[9,19,20] Recurrent bleeding may occur if a scab forms at the bleeding site and becomes dislodged.[7] In adults, bleeding tends to be caused by external trauma to the nose or may be caused by the above mentioned local factors, especially in very dry or high climates in which nasal membranes tend to dry. Systemic epistaxis may be caused by **acquired coagulopathies,** such as hemophilia, the use of blood thinners, or long-term aspirin use.[19] Hypertension is not a cause of epistaxis but may impede clotting.[19,20]

Referral and Diagnostic Tests

Typically the diagnosis of epistaxis is made through the history and physical examination. A nasal speculum is used to visualize the site of bleeding once the active bleeding is slowed. Sinus radiographs are only done when tumors are suspected as the cause of the bleeding.[7]

Differential Diagnosis

It is important to determine the cause of the epistaxis. If it is caused by trauma, a deviated septum, nasal fracture, and septal hematoma must all be ruled out. If the epistaxis is recurrent, a thorough history may reveal information leading to its cause.

Treatment

The management of epistaxis depends on the site of bleeding, the severity, and the etiology. If the athlete presents with active bleeding, necessary treatment may precede the normal history and palpation of a nasal exam. As in all cases in which the athletic trainer is handling body fluids, universal precautions must be followed.

Most anterior epistaxes will stop spontaneously with direct pressure applied to the nose. The athlete should be encouraged to sit with the head elevated but not hyperextended, which may cause bleeding into the pharynx. Digital compression or pinching of the nose should be done for 4 to 5 minutes. In traumatic situations, ice should also be applied. A cotton or gauze plug may be inserted into the nose to absorb the blood.[20]

If direct pressure is not sufficient in the treatment of an anterior bleed, gauze moistened with phenylephrine (Neo-Synephrine) or pseudoephedrine (Afrin) may be placed in the affected nostril to help vasoconstriction.[9,19,20]

For recurrent nosebleeds, conservative treatment, such as improving the humidity of inspired air, using saline nasal drops, and applying antibiotic ointments to the affected area, may be beneficial. Further evaluation by a physician should be sought to determine the etiology of the epistaxis.

Prognosis and Return to Participation

Most cases of anterior epistaxis from Kiesselbach's plexus can be stopped by nasal compression and local vasoconstriction.[9] If there is no indication of nasal fracture, septal deviation, or septal hematoma, the athlete may return to participation once the nose has stopped bleeding. Because minimal aggravation can restart the bleeding, it is important to protect the athlete from trauma to the nose. If possible, strenuous physical activity should be avoided when bleeding is active.[6]

Prevention

Incidence of epistaxis may be decreased by ensuring proper humidity and hydration, especially for athletes in dry environments or high altitudes. Saline nasal drops may be helpful in reducing dryness in the nose. Additional humidification through the use of humidifiers and vaporizers may be needed. Repeated trauma to the nose should be avoided, including foreign bodies, nose picking, and trauma in sports. Those athletes susceptible to epistaxis may need to wear facial protection during athletic participation.

PATHOLOGICAL CONDITIONS OF THE MOUTH AND THROAT

Pharyngitis and Tonsillitis

Pharyngitis is an inflammation of the pharynx. Tonsillitis is an inflammation of the tonsils. Both may be caused by bacteria or a virus. Pharyngitis is most often initially viral but may be followed by a bacterial infection (Figure 10-25, *A*). Tonsillitis is most commonly caused by the beta-hemolytic *Streptococcus* (Figure 10-25, *B*).[18] When caused by *Streptococcus*, pharyngitis is called strep throat.[8,9] Pharyngitis may be

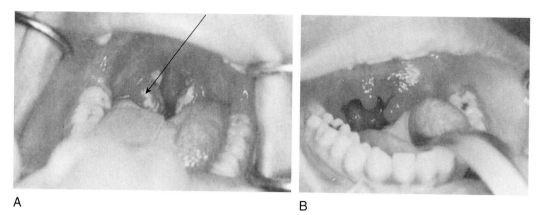

A   B

Figure 10-25 Examination of the mouth and throat may reveal, **A,** tonsillitis and pharyngitis or, **B,** acute viral pharyngitis. (Courtesy Edward L. Applebaum, MD, Head, Department of Otolaryngology, University of Illinois Medical Center, Chicago. From Barkauskas VH et al: *Health and physical assessment,* ed 2, St Louis, 1998, Mosby.)

secondary to sinusitis, tonsillitis, smoking, or alcoholism. Because many of the symptoms are identical, pharyngitis and tonsillitis will be discussed together.

Signs and Symptoms

Common signs and symptoms of pharyngitis and tonsillitis include sore throat, pain with swallowing, hoarseness, and possibly chills or fever. In both viral and bacterial pharyngitis, the mucous membranes may be inflamed mildly to more severely and may be covered by purulent exudates. Tonsillitis will present with red and swollen tonsils, possibly covered in white exudates. Fever and swollen neck lymph nodes are common.

Referral and Diagnostic Tests

The athletic trainer should monitor the temperature of the athlete. The athlete with a persistent fever or symptoms for more than 5 days should be referred to a physician. If the tonsils or pharynx presents with exudates on observation, the athlete needs to be referred. It is difficult for the physician to tell from physical examination alone whether pharyngitis is viral or bacterial.[8] A throat culture is often conducted to determine if the pharyngitis or tonsillitis is indeed caused by the *Streptococcus* strain.[13] Laboratory tests may also include a complete blood count (CBC) that shows a high **leukocyte count,** supporting the diagnosis of bacterial infection.[9]

Differential Diagnosis

When diagnosing pharyngitis or tonsillitis, other conditions that cause throat pain and fever must be ruled out. These include upper respiratory infection, laryngitis, and influenza. Viral infections may present with rhinorrhea, **conjunctivitis,** and cough, whereas patients with bacterial infections will not have these symptoms.

Treatment

The physician will typically prescribe antibiotics for a 10-day course for strep pharyngitis or tonsillitis to prevent complications from the disease.[2,7,8,21] Because viral pharyngitis is typically not treated with antibiotics the throat must be cultured if there is question of the etiology of the disease. Nonpharmacological treatment includes plenty of fluids and saltwater gargles. Acetaminophen is often given for discomfort and reduction of fever.[9]

Prognosis, Return to Participation, and Prevention

The athlete should be afebrile and must be able to tolerate fluids before participation in vigorous athletic activities. Full recovery typically occurs in 7 to 14 days. Several serious complications, such as rheumatic fever, can arise from untreated streptococcus infections.[8]

As with other bacterial and viral conditions, frequent hand washing when in contact with people who are known to be infected with the pathogens may drastically reduce the incidence of infection.

Laryngitis

Inflammation of the larynx is termed **laryngitis.** It often occurs simultaneously with the common cold, bronchitis, pneumonia, or influenza and can be acute or chronic. Laryngitis may also be caused by direct trauma to the throat, **gastroesophageal reflux disease (GERD),** allergies, cigarette smoke, or excessive use of the voice. It may be particularly seen in the athletic population and has been termed **cheerleader's nodules.**[8]

Signs and Symptoms

The athlete will typically experience a hoarse or weak voice and in some cases may be unable to speak.

A constant urge to clear the throat or a tickling may also occur. In more severe cases, fever, **dysphagia, malaise,** and throat pain may occur.[8,18] Edema of the larynx may cause **dyspnea.**

Referral and Diagnostic Tests

The athlete should be referred to a physician if symptoms do not resolve within 5 to 7 days. The physician may perform an **indirect laryngoscopy** that may disclose mild to marked erythema of the mucous membrane. Laryngeal cultures and biopsies may be performed if an etiology other than viral infection or irritation is suspected.[9]

Differential Diagnosis

Other conditions that can cause throat pain and dysphagia should be considered, including viral or bacterial pharyngitis, mononucleosis, or candidiasis. In chronic laryngitis, laryngeal tumors and **papillomatosis** must be ruled out.

Treatment

Voice rest and increasing humidification through a vaporizer may help to relieve symptoms. Acetaminophen or other analgesics for pain may be helpful as may other supporting treatments, such as throat lozenges or sprays. Elimination or treatment of the irritating cause of chronic laryngitis (e.g., GERD, inhaled smoke) may decrease the symptoms dramatically.

Prognosis and Return to Participation

Most symptoms of uncomplicated laryngitis usually resolve within a few days. Athletes with laryngitis may participate as long as they are afebrile and feel well with the exception of the laryngitis.

Prevention

Chronic laryngitis is typically from overuse or exposure to irritants. The athlete susceptible to chronic laryngitis caused by these irritants should try to avoid smoke, air pollution, and straining the voice as in cheerleading or singing.[9]

Oral Mucosal Lesions

Lesions to the mouth and lips are common in athletics and may be caused by local trauma, infectious disease, autoimmune disorders, **neoplastic disease,** and toxic reactions. Identification of atraumatic oral lesions is especially important because it may allow early recognition and referral of oral cancer or infectious disease (Table 10-3). Oral lesions are often the first clinical evidence of human immunodeficiency virus (HIV) infection and acquired immunodeficiency syndrome (AIDS).

Oral lesions may be categorized and described on the basis of clinical appearance similar to skin disorders. They are often described as white or pigmented and vesicular or ulcerated (see Chapter 13). Many oral

Table 10-3	Common Diseases Affecting the Oral Cavity		
Disease	**Cause**	**Symptoms**	**Appearance**
Candidiasis	*Candida albicans*	White to yellow lesions in the cheek, at folds, and on tongue	Soft, white to yellow, slightly elevated plaques; milky curds
Herpes simplex labialis	Herpes simplex virus type 1	Itching, neuralgiform complaints as prodrome, changing to painful when lesions form	Recurrent, episodic eruptions of yellowish, fluid-filled vesicles on upper or lower lip or nose
Herpes zoster	Varicella-zoster virus	Extremely painful; burning pain; fever; malaise	Unilateral vesicles on buccal mucosa, tongue, uvula, pharynx, larynx; erosions noted when vesicles rupture
Leukoplakia	Multifactorial (tobacco use, trauma, lupus, irritative reactions)	Painless, white patch or plaque on surface of mucosa	White patch typically on lips, tongue, palate, floor of mouth, or buccal mucosa
Basal cell carcinoma of the lips	Prolonged exposure to sunlight	Lesion ulcerates, heals over, then breaks down again; history of ultraviolet light exposure	Crusted ulcer with heaped or rolled borders
Squamous cell carcinoma, oral cavity, floor of mouth, anterior tongue	Lack of specific etiology; tobacco, alcohol, poor oral hygiene are implicated as contributors	Usually painless ulcer unless nerves or periosteum involved; fetid breath	Ulcerated lesion with raised borders
Kaposi's sarcoma	HIV infection	Purplish, tender or painful nodules on mucous membrane	Purplish macules; can also be raised, nodular, or ulcerated

lesions will present as a white plaque and can be differentiated depending on their location. White lesions that are easily removed by wiping them off suggest candidiasis, whereas a defect that cannot be wiped away is consistent with precancerous leukoplakia or squamous cell carcinoma.[22] Brown- or black-pigmented **macules** on the oral mucosa may be caused by something as benign as localized melanin production or may be the sign of something much more significant, including malignant melanoma.[18]

Oral Candidiasis

Oral candidiasis is caused by the yeastlike fungus *Candia albicans*. It is called thrush in infants and is the most common white lesion of the oral cavity (Figure 10-26).

Signs and Symptoms

Oral candidiasis presents as a cheesy, curdlike patch on the tongue and buccal mucosa.[3,5,9] It is seen most commonly in newborns and also may occur after the use of antibiotics, in immunosuppressed patients, and in association with corticosteroid treatment.[3]

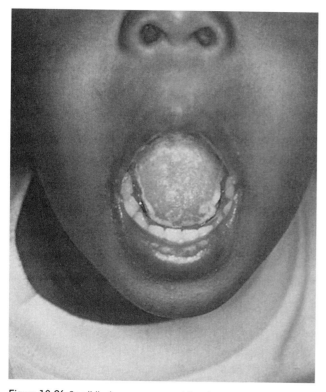

Figure 10-26 Candidiasis appears as a white, cheesy patch on the buccal mucosa or tongue; the plaque may be scraped off the mucosal membranes, revealing a red, raw surface that bleeds easily. (From Jarvis C: *Physical examination & health assessment*, ed 4, Philadelphia, 2004, WB Saunders, p 401.)

Referral and Diagnostic Tests

The white, curdlike patch characteristic of oral candidiasis can be scraped from the tongue or buccal mucosa with a tongue depressor and typically bleeds easily. If the plaque does not easily scrape off the surface, other oral lesions should be considered. In the adult with oral candidiasis, tests should be conducted for HIV infection.

Treatment, Prognosis, and Return to Participation

Candidiasis is typically treated with an oral rinse of nystatin and oral antifungal medications. Antifungals such as fluconazole (Diflucan) are administered for 2 weeks or until symptoms resolve.[22] Candidiasis can often be persistent, requiring treatment for several weeks.

The athlete with oral candidiasis who is otherwise in good health may participate in athletics.

Oral Cancers

Oral cancer is a very serious condition and often involves the tongue, lips, and gums (Red Flags—Early Signs of Lip and Oral Cancer). This form of cancer

> ⏵ **Red Flags for Early Signs of Lip and Oral Cancer**
> - A sore in the mouth that does not heal in 2 to 3 weeks
> - Any sores that are painful or bleed easily
> - Any unusual lumps in the mouth
> - Numbness or pain in the mouth and throat
> - Persistent red or white patches on the oral mucosa
> - A change in voice not associated with a cold or allergies
> - Difficulty chewing or swallowing

From the National Cancer Institute: Oral cancer screening. Available at http://cancer.gov/cancertopics/pdq/screening/oral/HealthProfessional/. Accessed September 2004.

accounts for about 3% of cancers in men and 2% in women.[23] Oral cancer occurs more frequently in African-Americans than in Caucasians.[24] The numerous predisposing risk factors include any type of tobacco use, excessive alcohol use, poor oral hygiene, being over the age of 40 years, and having a family history of oral cancer. Men have twice the risk of women.

Signs and Symptoms

Patients will typically present with red or white lesions or other open wounds in the mouth. They may experience tongue swelling and dysphagia as well as abnormal taste.[22] Crusting lesions of the lips or ulcerated lesions within the mouth are prime suspects of

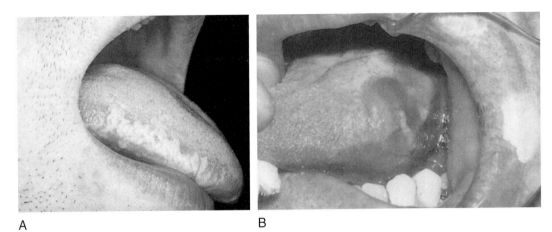

A   B

Figure 10-27 Oral lesions. **A,** Oral hairy leukoplakia on the lateral border of the tongue. **B,** Carcinoma ulcer with rolled edges indurated on the side of the tongue. (A from Noble J: *Primary care medicine,* ed 3, St Louis, 2001, Mosby. B from Jarvis C: *Physical examination & health assessment,* ed 4, Philadelphia, 2004, WB Saunders, p. 403.)

oral cancer. Ninety percent of all oral cancer cells arise on the floor of the mouth, the ventrolateral aspect of the tongue, or the soft palate.[25,26] Treatment, prognosis, and return to participation following oral cancers will be discussed in general.

Leukoplakia

Leukoplakia is a precancerous lesion of the mucosa and is usually found on the sides of the tongue (Figure 10-27) and the floor of the mouth.[22] It appears as a white patch that cannot be removed by scraping. Chewing tobacco and other local irritants can create this lesion. Although considered precancerous, leukoplakia can progress to squamous cell carcinoma if left untreated.[9,22] Not all leukoplakias are precancerous, but biopsy needs to be done, especially if risk factors are present.[27]

Squamous Cell Carcinoma

Squamous cell carcinoma is the most common type of oral cancer. It starts as a nonhealing, painless, red ulceration that may grow rapidly. It may spread from the oral cavity to the cervical and submandibular lymph nodes.[26]

Kaposi's Sarcoma

Unlike leukoplakia, Kaposi's sarcoma is a pigmented lesion that may be either flat or raised and is reddish to purple in color. It is found more often in males than females and is a common manifestation of HIV infection.[28] Kaposi's sarcoma is initially asymptomatic but progresses to a painful lesion that interferes with eating and talking.

Referral and Diagnostic Tests

The athletic trainer should refer any athlete with an unusual skin lesion in the mouth to the physician

for **biopsy.** This includes any lesion that does not heal in a timely manner or heals and then breaks down again. The athletic trainer should be especially suspicious if multifactorial risk factors, such as alcohol, excessive sunlight exposure, and tobacco use, are present.[9,22,25,28]

Treatment

Early cancers of the lip and oral cavity are highly curable by surgery or radiation therapy. The choice of treatment as well as the prognosis often depends on the location of the cancer, how early it is detected, and anticipated functional and cosmetic results of treatment.[29]

Prognosis and Return to Participation

The extent to which the athlete can participate depends largely on the treatment and not necessarily on the disease itself since often the disease goes undetected for a considerable time. For the athlete being treated with radiation therapy or surgery, participation will be determined by the extent of the treatment.

Dental Disease

Numerous conditions may fall under the category of dental disease, but for the purposes of this book only gingivitis and periodontitis will be discussed. **Gingivitis** is an inflammatory condition of the gums caused by bacteria (Figure 10-28). Bacteria are typically a result of food deposits from inadequate brushing and flossing. **Periodontitis** may occur if gingivitis is left untreated. Periodontitis results in a receding gum line and loss of alveolar bone.[2]

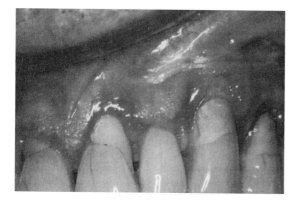

Figure 10-28 Gingivitis presents with swollen, red, painful gums that may bleed easily with brushing. (From Jarvis C: *Physical examination & health assessment*, ed 4, Philadelphia, 2004, WB Saunders, p 400.)

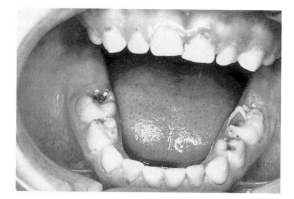

Figure 10-29 Dental caries. (From Jarvis C: *Physical examination & health assessment*, ed 4, Philadelphia, 2004, WB Saunders, p 400.)

Signs and Symptoms

In gingivitis, the gums will often appear red and swollen and the patient will complain that brushing causes pain and bleeding of the gums.[2] The athlete may also have bad breath or a bad taste in the mouth. If the disease progresses to periodontitis, the patient will experience tooth sensitivity; red, swollen gums; pain and bleeding with brushing; and possibly loosening of the teeth.

Referral, Diagnostic Tests, and Differential Diagnosis

Athletes with swollen or bleeding gums are referred to a dentist or **periodontist** for evaluation. Radiographs and observation of the gums will reveal the extent of the disease.

Gingivitis and periodontitis should be differentiated from other conditions that may cause oral pain or sensitivity to hot or cold, including lacerations to the gums, oral lesions, or tooth decay.

Treatment

Treatment of gingivitis includes an aggressive oral hygiene program to stimulate the gingivae. This may include flossing and use of dental picks and oral stimulators. Advanced gingivitis may require treatment with antibiotics, tooth scaling, and removal of plaque below the gum line.

Prognosis and Return to Participation

The athlete with periodontal disease may participate as able. If advanced periodontitis results in loosening of teeth, the athlete participating in contact sports must be cautious and appropriate mouth guards should be used.

Prevention

Prevention of periodontal disease includes frequent brushing and flossing as well as using antibacterial mouth rinses. Regular dental hygiene visits allow periodontal disease to be detected at an early, reversible stage.

Dental Caries

Although dental caries is a common condition, the athlete will typically seek the advice and treatment of a dentist for all dental problems. Tooth decay occurs when bacteria in the mouth form plaque, which collects on the teeth both above and below the gum line.[8] The plaque then produces acids that cause tooth decay. Decay starts at the enamel and may extend into the dentin and even the pulp of the tooth.[8] If the decay is caught early, only the enamel is affected and the condition is fairly easily remedied. If the bacteria reach the pulp, the tooth will die and an abscess may form near the root.[30]

Signs and Symptoms

Decay will initially look white and chalky and later turn brown or black (Figure 10-29). The dental decay may be asymptomatic, however, in advanced stages; the athlete's teeth may be sensitive to hot or cold. Later stages of dental decay may also be accompanied by red, swollen gums. The athlete may note a roughness in the tooth when felt with the tongue. If an abscess forms, the area around the tooth will be painful and the tooth will be sensitive to heat. There will be a fluctuant mass on the buccal side of the tooth.[30]

Referral, Treatment, and Differential Diagnosis

Everyone needs to practice good dental hygiene. An athlete with poor dental hygiene needs to be educated about annual dental health visits. An athlete who presents with tooth decay can be referred to a dentist for treatment. Treatment depends on the severity of the decay. Cavities caused by mild tooth decay are repaired with fillings, whereas more severe tooth decay requires repair with a crown. If the pulp is involved, a root canal treatment may be needed, or in extreme cases the tooth may need to be extracted.[30]

Other conditions that may cause oral pain or sensitivity to hot or cold include gingivitis, periodontitis, fractured teeth, and oral lesions.

Prognosis, Return to Participation, and Prevention

The athlete with dental caries has no restrictions, and participation is self-limiting.

Good dental hygiene and annual dental checkups will help catch dental decay in the early stages in which it can be easily treated. New dental treatments, such as early childhood fluoride and tooth-sealing treatments, have dramatically reduced the frequency of dental caries.

SUMMARY

The athletic trainer will commonly see injuries and conditions of the ears, nose, mouth, and throat as a result of athletic participation, as well as from causes not related to athletics. This chapter reviews the anatomy and evaluation of the ear, nose, mouth, and throat and highlights nontraumatic medical conditions common to these areas. The athletic trainer needs to be able to recognize normal and abnormal conditions in the ear, nose, mouth, and throat and know when to refer the athlete to the physician for more definitive diagnostic testing and treatment.

WEB RESOURCES

National Institute of Dental and Craniofacial Research
http://www.nohic.nidcr.nih.gov/
Provides patient and professional education materials on conditions of the mouth, including a large section on oral cancers; presents a step-by-step examination of the mouth

Medem Medical Library, part of the Medem network
http://www.medem.com/MedLB/articleslb.cfm?sub_cat=554
Offers an online source of comprehensive, peer-reviewed health care information for practitioners as well as easy-to-understand patient handouts

Virtual Hospital, sponsored by the University of Iowa
http://www.vh.org/
Can search for a topic in this indexed digital database; information on many medical disorders cataloged here, especially appropriate for conditions of the ears, nose, mouth, and throat; offers links to other sources

Medline Plus
http://www.nlm.nih.gov/medlineplus/medlineplus.html
Provides a gateway to refereed articles through Medline as well as pictures, medical encyclopedias, and dictionaries; useful for all medical conditions, including those of the ears, nose, and throat

American Academy of Otolaryngology
http://www.entnet.org/
ENTLink provides a searchable database to obtain more information on examination and treatment for conditions of the ears, nose, and throat

Oral Cancer Foundation
http://www.oralcancerfoundation.org/
Provides information on oral cancer screening and diagnosis as well as statistics related to oral cancer

American Dental Association
http://www.ada.org/
Articles and information for the health care professional and the patient on disorders of the teeth and mouth

REFERENCES

1. Seidel HM, Ball JW, Dains JE, Benedict GW: *Mosby's guide to physical examination*, ed 5, Philadelphia, 2003, Mosby.
2. Starkey C, Ryan J: *Evaluation of orthopedic and athletic injuries*, ed 2, Philadelphia, 2002, FA Davis.
3. Jarvis C: *Physical examination & health assessment*, ed 4, Philadelphia, 2004, WB Saunders.
4. Epstein O, Perkin GD, Cookson J, de Bono DP: *Clinical examination*, ed 3, Philadelphia, 2003, Mosby.
5. Potter PA, Weilitz PB: *Mosby's pocket guide to health assessment*, ed 5, St Louis, 2003, Mosby.
6. Nguyen Q: Epistaxis. Available at http://www.emedicine.com/ent/topic701.htm. Accessed August 2004.
7. Noble J: *Textbook of primary care medicine*, ed 3, St Louis, 2001, Mosby.
8. Beers MH, Berkow R: *The Merck manual of diagnosis and therapy*, ed 17, Whitehouse Station, NJ, 1999, Merck Research Laboratories.
9. Ferri FF: *Ferri's clinical advisor 2004: instant diagnosis and treatment*, Philadelphia, 2004, Mosby.
10. Bahalla SK, Garry JP: Otitis externa. May 21, 2002. Available at http://www.emedicine.com/sports/topic161.htm. Accessed August 2004.
11. Braunwald E, Fauci A, Kasper D, et al: *Harrison's principles of internal medicine*, ed 15, New York, 2001, McGraw-Hill.
12. Rosen P, Barkin R, Hayden S: Otitis externa. In *The 5 minute emergency medicine consult*, Philadelphia, 1999, Lippincott Williams & Wilkins.
13. Landry G, Bernhardt D: *Essentials of primary care sports medicine*, Champaign, Ill, 2003, Human Kinetics.
14. Davidson TM, Neuman TR: Managing inflammatory ear conditions, *Physician and Sportsmedicine* 22(8):56-60, 1994.
15. Cotran R, Kumar V, Collins T: *Robbins pathologic basis of disease*, ed 6, Philadelphia, 2001, WB Saunders.

16. Harrison CJ: The laws of acute otitis media, *Primary Care: Clinics in Office Practice* 30(1), 2003.

17. Howard ML: Middle ear, tympanic membrane perforation. Available at http://www.emedicine.com/ent/topic206.htm. Accessed November 2004.

18. Goldman L, Ausielllo D: *Cecil textbook of medicine,* ed 22, Philadelphia, 2004, WB Saunders.

19. Gluckman W, Barricella R: Epistaxis, *eMedicine,* 2003. Available at http://www.emedicine.com/ped/topic1618.htm. Accessed August 17, 2004.

20. Tintinalli JE, Gabor D, Kelen J, Stapczynski JS: *Emergency medicine: a comprehensive study guide,* ed 6, New York, 2004, McGraw-Hill.

21. Shultz S, Houglum P, Perrin D: *Assessment of athletic injuries,* Champaign, Ill, 2000, Human Kinetics.

22. Knight J: Diagnosing oral mucosal lesions, *Physician Assistant* 27(3):34-43, 2003.

23. American Cancer Society. Available at http://www.cancer.org/docroot/STT/stt_0.asp. Accessed September 2004.

24. Ries LA, Kosary CL, Hankey BF, et al: *SEER cancer statistics review 1973-1995,* Bethesda, Md, 1998, National Cancer Institute.

25. National Cancer Institute: Oral cancer screening. Available at http://cancer.gov/cancertopics/pdq/screening/oral/HealthProfessional. Accessed September 2004.

26. Scully C: Cancers of the oral mucosa, August 19, 2004. Available at http://www.emedicine.com/derm/topic565.htm. Accessed September 2004.

27. Lynch D: Oral examination, August 19, 2004. Available at http://www.emedicine.com/derm/topic836.htm. Accessed September 2004.

28. Bickley L: *Bates' guide to physical examination and history taking,* ed 8, New York, 2003, Lippincott.

29. Cummings CW, Harker LA, Krause CJ, et al: *Otolaryngology: head and neck surgery,* ed 3, St Louis, 1998, Mosby.

30. Schneider K, Segal G: Dental abscess, August 5, 2004. Available at http://www.emedicine.com/ped/topic2675.htm. Accessed September 2004.

CHAPTER 11

Systemic Disorders

Richard Figler

OBJECTIVES

At the completion of this chapter, the reader should be able to do the following:

1. Appreciate the complexity of systemic diseases.
2. Recognize signs and symptoms of common systemic ailments.
3. Identify conditions that warrant referral to a physician.
4. Understand the warning signs of lymphatic and colon cancers.
5. Describe prevention strategies for Lyme disease and type 2 diabetes mellitus.
6. Determine and understand diabetic emergencies.

INTRODUCTION

Systemic disorders have shortened the careers of many athletes. The importance of the athletic trainer as a gatekeeper to the health care system for athletes cannot be overlooked because early detection often can prevent permanent disability or deadly consequences. Numerous systemic conditions can affect the general health of the athlete. These medical problems range from vector-borne infections to life-threatening cancers, and typically, systemic disorders cross several body systems and present in multiple fashions.

Because the discussion of systemic conditions covers all body systems, the organization of this chapter differs slightly from that of other chapters. The chapter begins with a review of the anatomy and physiology of the lymphatic system. The anatomy and physiology of the respiratory, cardiovascular, gastrointestinal, genitourinary, gynecological, and neurological systems have already been discussed, and the integumentary and musculoskeletal systems will be covered in Chapters 13 and 14.

The description of specific pathological conditions begins with lymphatic disorders, the lymphomas, to provide continuity. A discussion of Lyme disease, a vector-borne illness, and two cancers with systemic implications follow. In addition, several chronic systemic conditions and endocrine disorders are covered in this chapter.

Chronic systemic conditions can affect athletes as well as the general population. Most are treatable but require special care to ensure the safety of the athlete as well as to optimize athletic performance. Generally the conditions discussed here are not preventable; however, prevention is discussed when applicable.

ANATOMY AND PHYSIOLOGY OF THE LYMPHATIC SYSTEM

The lymphatic system is a collection of capillaries, vessels, valves, ducts, nodes, and organs that maintain internal fluid of the human body (Figure 11-1). It transports fats, proteins, and lymphatic fluid throughout the body. In addition, it restores the majority of the fluid that filters out of the blood during normal homeostasis.

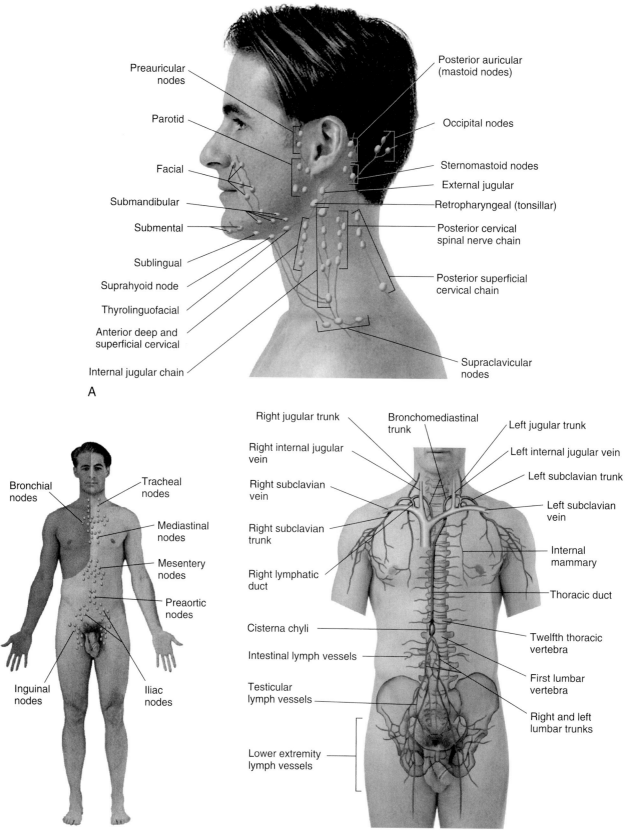

Figure 11-1 The lymphatic system is the core of the body. These figures illustrate the complete lymphatic drainage pathways from the head and neck (A) through the trunk and extremities (B). In the overview, the shaded area is drained through the right lymphatic duct and lymph from the remainder of the body drains via the thoracic duct. The limbs have an extensive drainage system that follows venous return to the heart. (From Seidel HM, Ball JW, Dains JE, Benedict GW: *Mosby's guide to physical examination*, ed 5, St Louis, 2003, Mosby, pp 227, 231.)

The lymphatic system is largely a filter that also produces both lymph and blood cells. This system has accessibility to all organs within the body and can facilitate disease proliferation into other remote areas with ease. Lymph is moved throughout the body within this system through normal muscular movement and respiratory functions. Specific lymph organs are the tonsils, thymus gland, and spleen. Rarely are conditions of the lymphatic system preventable.

PATHOLOGICAL DISORDERS

Lymphatic Disorders

Non-Hodgkin's Lymphoma

Non-Hodgkin's lymphoma (NHL) is a group of malignancies of the **lymphoreticular** system. The lymphoreticular system is a collection of lymphoid tissues formed by several types of immune system cells from both the lymph and reticuloendothelial systems that primarily fight against infection. There are several types of NHL as well as several different classifications. The median age for diagnosis with NHL is 50, and the incidence increases with age. Estimates of more than 54,000 new cases of NHL during 2004 in the United States have been reported, and approximately 19,400 of those patients died of the disease.[1] It is typically among the top six cancers diagnosed in the United States and holds the same ranking for cancer-related deaths.[1]

Signs and Symptoms
Because NHL is a group of lymphatic cancers, patients can present with a variety of symptoms depending on the site affected. The most frequent sites are the abdomen, mediastinum, and neck. If the abdomen is affected, the patient can experience nausea, vomiting, or diarrhea, usually accompanied by abdominal pain and weight loss. The patient may also have an enlarged spleen or liver or a palpable mass in the abdomen. Other general signs include excessive sweating, including night sweats, weight loss, fatigue, and unexplained fevers. When the mediastinum is affected, the disease generally progresses more rapidly (Key Points—The Mediastinum). Presenting symptoms can range from chest pain to severe shortness of breath on exertion. Neck masses and enlarged lymph nodes can also present as NHL. Figure 11-1, *A* shows the location of specific cervical lymph nodes.

Referral, Diagnostic Tests, and Differential Diagnosis
Athletes who have enlarged lymph nodes without apparent cause (e.g., infection distal to the gland), inexplicable chest pain, or dyspnea should be referred to a physician for further evaluation. When NHL is suspected, imaging with computed tomography (CT) or ultrasound can help confirm the presence and size of the affected lymph nodes. The diagnosis is confirmed by sampling of tissue from the enlarged lymph nodes by fine-needle biopsy or removal of the affected lymph node with subsequent analysis by pathologists. If the diagnosis is confirmed by biopsy, referral

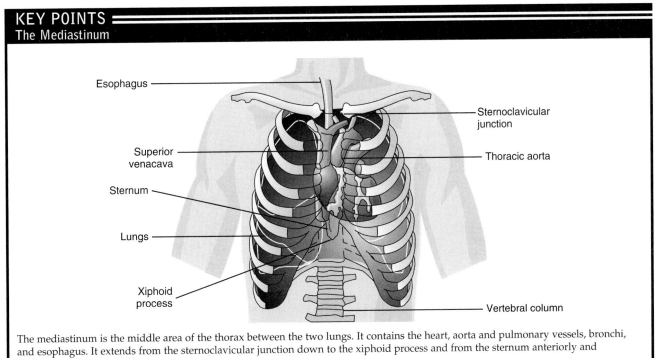

KEY POINTS
The Mediastinum

Esophagus — Sternoclavicular junction — Thoracic aorta — Superior venacava — Sternum — Lungs — Xiphoid process — Vertebral column

The mediastinum is the middle area of the thorax between the two lungs. It contains the heart, aorta and pulmonary vessels, bronchi, and esophagus. It extends from the sternoclavicular junction down to the xiphoid process and from the sternum anteriorly and posteriorly to the vertebral column.

to an oncologist should be initiated for specific treatment.

Patients suspected of having NHL will undergo a complete history and physical exam followed by lab work. Initially, patients may present with a mild anemia and an elevation of lactate dehydrogenase (LDH).[2] A battery of other blood tests is performed to help stage the disease. The cancer staging is accompanied by CT scans of the abdomen and pelvis to assess for spread of the disease (Table 11-1). Other tests can be performed depending on the initial findings.

In patients with enlarged lymph nodes, the differential diagnoses are extensive. Hodgkin's disease, bacterial infections, human immunodeficiency virus (HIV), infectious mononucleosis, and sarcoidosis are just a few that need to be considered. Patients with chest pain or dyspnea would have a differential diagnosis of hypertrophic cardiomyopathy, coronary artery disease, gastrointestinal-esophageal reflux disease, asthma, or influenza.

Treatment, Prognosis, and Return to Participation
The treatment depends on the histological type as well as the stage of NHL. Radiation therapy, chemotherapy, or both can be implemented as treatment and are performed by oncologists.

Prognosis varies widely and depends on the stage, size, and histological type of the disease. Patients with low-grade lymphoma, despite long-term survival of

6 to 10 years,[3] are rarely cured and usually die of lymphoma. Those patients with high-grade or metastasized NHL tend to do better and may achieve a cure with aggressive chemotherapy. The success rate for cure in this case is 35% to 50%.

A decision to return to athletic competition must be made once treatment has ended. Obviously, with NHL's poor prognosis and risks involved with the treatments, athletes should remain out of competition while being treated, and any return to competition must be made after consultation with their physicians.

Hodgkin's Lymphoma

Hodgkin's lymphoma is a malignant disorder of lymphoreticular origin, different histologically from NHL because of the presence of **Reed-Sternberg cells** (multinucleated giant cells).[3] The incidence of the disease increases throughout childhood and into the late teenage years[2] but peaks from age 25 to 30. Hodgkin's disease is rare in children under the age of 5, and children 16 and under account for 10% to15% of the disease. The overall incidence is 4 per 100,000. A second peak in incidence is after 55 years of age. The disease is more common in Caucasians, higher socioeconomic groups, and males; of teens with Hodgkin's, 80% are male.[3]

Signs and Symptoms
Although Hodgkin's lymphoma has several possible presenting signs, the most common initial sign is an enlarged lymph node, typically in the lower anterior neck region. It is usually nontender, discrete, firm, and rubbery; is not fixed to adjacent structures; and can vary in size.[4] Patients with mediastinal chest involvement can present with shortness of breath, chest pain, or cough. Occasionally, enlarged lymph nodes are present in the axillary or inguinal region; Figure 11-2 illustrates the most common sites of Hodgkin's lymphoma. Intense itching and intermittent fevers associated with night sweats are classical symptoms of this disease. Roughly 25% of patients will present with systemic symptoms, including fatigue, fever, weight loss, and night sweats.[5]

Referral, Diagnostic Tests, and Differential Diagnosis
Athletes with persistent neck masses (Figure 11-3) or constitutional symptoms such as night sweats, intermittent fevers, and a weight loss of greater than 10% of total body weight should be evaluated by a physician. If the diagnosis is confirmed, referral to an oncologist is appropriate for further treatment.

If a patient presents with a persistent neck mass that does not respond to antibiotics or is not associated with an infection, an excisional or fine-needle lymph node biopsy is performed. This tissue can then be sent for histological diagnosis. If a persistent cough or other chest symptoms are found, a chest radiograph is taken.

Table 11-1	TNM System for Cancer Staging*
Stage	**Characteristics**
Primary Tumor (T)	
T_x	No primary tumor can be assessed
T_0	No evidence of primary tumor
T_{is}	Carcinoma in situ (i.e., without spread)
T_1, T_2, T_3, T_4	Increasing size and extent of the primary tumor
Regional Lymph Nodes (N)	
N_x	Cannot be assessed
N_0	No regional lymph node involvement
N_1, N_2, N_3	Increasing involvement of regional lymph nodes
Distant Metastasis (M)	
M_x	Presence of metastasis cannot be assessed
M_0	No distant metastasis
M_1	Distant metastasis

Data from the American Joint Committee on Cancer at http://training.seer.cancer.gov/ module_staging_cancer/unit03_sec03_part00_ajcc.html; Maskowski C, Buchsel P: *Oncology nursing assessment and clinical care*, St Louis, 1999, Mosby; Black JM, Hawks JH: *Medical-surgical nursing: clinical management for positive outcomes*, ed 7, St Louis, 2005, Elsevier Saunders.
*The universally accepted TNM system for cancer staging helps to determine the extent or spread of the disease in order to establish treatment decisions and prognosis for recovery. It groups cancers into one of four stages (I to IV) or stage 0 for carcinoma in situ, which means without spread. Higher stages such as stage IV or M_4 represent distant metastasis and the worst prognosis.

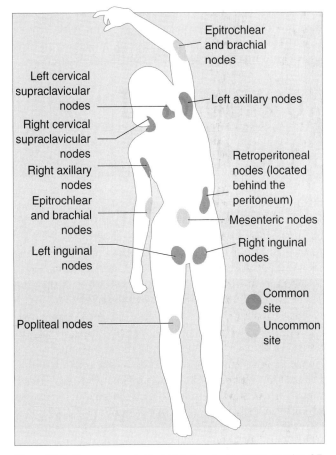

Figure 11-2 Sites common to Hodgkin's lymphoma. (From Huether SE, McCance KL: *Understanding pathophysiology*, ed 2, St Louis, 2000, Mosby.)

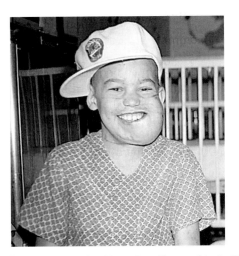

Figure 11-3 A young boy with sublingual swelling consistent with malignant Hodgkin's lymphoma. (From Seidel HM, Ball JW, Dains JE, Benedict GW: *Mosby's guide to physical examination*, ed 5, St Louis, 2003, Mosby, p 246.)

Blood work is performed as well, including complete blood counts, LDH, and an erythrocyte sedimentation rate (ESR). Imaging studies are vital for staging the disease and include CT scans of the chest, abdomen, and pelvis.

In patients who present with enlarged lymph nodes, the differential diagnosis is extensive. Non-Hodgkin's disease, bacterial infections, HIV, infectious mononucleosis, and sarcoidosis are just a few diagnoses that need to be considered.

Treatment, Prognosis, and Return to Participation

Treatment revolves around the histological diagnosis as well as the staging, but Hodgkin's lymphoma generally requires radiation therapy as well as chemotherapy. With recent advances in chemotherapy, Hodgkin's disease can be cured in most patients with both localized and advanced disease.[5] Surgery may be indicated if the disease is extensive.

The overall survival rate for Hodgkin's disease is 60% to 99% at 10 years, depending on the type and involvement.[1] A decision regarding return to competition is made by the athlete's physician, and competition is best avoided during the acute illness as well as during the treatment phase.

Vector-Borne Disease

A vector-borne disease is one that is carried by an infected organism (i.e. tick or mosquito) to a healthy individual. This group of diseases is largely preventable by avoiding the habitats where these organisms live or by applying repellent. Box 8-4 depicts the relationship among vector-borne diseases, carriers, and their hosts.

Lyme disease, the most common tick-borne illness in the United States, was first described in the 1970s in Lyme, Connecticut. It is a multisystem disorder that when left untreated can lead to serious arthritic and neurological symptoms that become increasingly difficult to treat because of permanent tissue damage.[6] The culprit responsible for Lyme disease is the *Borrelia burgdorferi* bacterium that is transmitted to humans from infected ticks.

People most affected by Lyme disease are those bitten by ticks between May and September who spend a large amount of time outdoors in endemic areas, such as New York, New Jersey, Connecticut, Rhode Island, Maryland, Massachusetts, Pennsylvania, or Wisconsin.[7] In 2002, almost 24,000 infections were reported the United States.[8]

Signs and Symptoms

Lyme disease can be broken down into three different categories based on longevity of the symptoms.

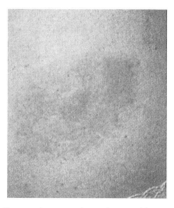

Figure 11-4 Erythema migrans rash consistent with Lyme disease. (From Larson WG, Adams RM, Maibach HI: *Color text of contact dermatitis*, Philadelphia, 1991, WB Saunders, p 191.)

Early localized Lyme disease usually begins as a red, circular rash called **erythema migrans** that enlarges over days (Figure 11-4). This rash can appear anywhere from 1 to 30 days after a tick bite and generally occurs on the trunk of the body. The rash is usually accompanied by a viral-like illness, with symptoms that can include headaches, muscle aches, fevers, joint aches, fatigue, and occasionally a stiff neck. Fewer than 20% recall being bitten by a tick.[6]

Disease that is not treated at the onset of the rash can lead to early disseminated Lyme disease within weeks to months. Patients may present with facial nerve palsies or even meningitis in 10% of cases.[7] Patients who develop lymphocytic meningitis generally have only neck pain and stiffness, but they may not have the typical findings associated with meningitis on physical examination, such as positive **Brudzinski's** and **Kernig's signs** (see Figures 8-12 and 8-13).

The diagnosis of nervous system Lyme disease is confirmed by testing spinal fluid taken from a lumbar puncture (see Box 8-6). Early disseminated Lyme disease can also present with cardiac manifestations occurring anywhere from 1 week to 7 months after the bite and peaking at 1 to 2 months. Affected patients may have a variety of symptoms, including chest pain, palpitations, weakness, fatigue, or shortness of breath. The cause of these symptoms can be a conduction abnormality in the heart, leading to irregular rhythms or abnormal findings on an electrocardiogram. The heart muscle may also become inflamed because of infection of the heart tissue.

Late Lyme disease is characterized by manifestations of the musculoskeletal system or central nervous system. Patients may experience intermittent attacks of brief swelling of the joints followed by chronic pain and arthritic changes. This can occur from weeks to years after the initial tick bite, and its incidence approaches 50% of those who were untreated at the time of infection.[6] Tertiary neuroborreliosis is the name given to a syndrome of progressively worsening cognitive function, which is thought to be caused by infection of the central nervous system by *B. burgdorferi*, the spirochete that is passed on from the infected tick.

Referral and Diagnostic Tests

Athletes who have recently visited wooded areas or have a rash that is suspect of erythema migrans are referred to a primary care physician. Once signs and symptoms of Lyme disease are identified, the diagnosis can only be confirmed definitively with laboratory testing. A positive test without the symptoms does not support the diagnosis of Lyme disease since 3% to 5% of those tested can have false-positive tests. Blood tests routinely used include immunoassays such as the enzyme-linked immunoassay to identify antibodies to *B. burgdorferi*. If this test is positive, it must then be confirmed with a Western immunoblot test.

Despite this information, routine serological testing of those with erythema migrans is not recommended since only one third of those patients with a single lesion will test positive. If several erythema migrans lesions are noted, the number of positive tests jumps to 90%.[7] Those persons with suspected Lyme disease without the rash should have samples taken immediately with repeated sampling in 4 to 6 weeks. Regardless of the laboratory outcomes, if the symptoms are consistent with Lyme disease, treatment needs to be initiated.

If the athlete has a clinical history of a tick bite and central nervous system manifestations or a swollen joint, fluid from the affected area should be taken for analysis. The clinician should remember that all swollen joints are not necessarily caused by trauma or injury, and if the suspicion is high, Lyme arthritis needs to be ruled out to ensure appropriate treatment.[9]

Differential Diagnosis

The differential diagnoses for Lyme disease includes depression, **fibromyalgia,** cellulitis, and **chronic fatigue syndrome.** In athletes with no trauma and a joint effusion, autoimmune, infectious, neoplastic, and other inflammatory processes must also be considered.[9]

Treatment

Early treatment of Lyme disease usually prevents any of the aforementioned complications. For early disease, oral antibiotics, including doxycycline or amoxicillin, are used in a 10- to 21-day course.[6] Cases diagnosed later or that involve the central nervous or cardiac systems typically require intravenous antibiotics. Giving antibiotics to symptom-free people who have been bitten by ticks has not been proven to lessen the disease. The current recommendation is to monitor those bitten by ticks closely for findings of Lyme disease, including erythema migrans, and treat those infected appropriately.

Prognosis, Return to Participation, and Prevention

With appropriate and expeditious treatment of Lyme disease, major late sequelae of the disease can be prevented, including nervous system manifestations, carditis, and recurrent arthritis.[6]

As with any acute illness, an individual assessment of the athlete must be made to determine clearance to play. The majority of patients can return to play when their symptoms have dissipated and proper treatment has been initiated. Transmission of Lyme disease from athlete to athlete cannot occur.

Primary prevention is obviously avoidance of ticks; wearing proper clothing, including long pants tucked into socks; using insect repellent; and routine inspection for ticks after possible exposure. Insect repellent containing the compound N,N-diethyl-3-methyl-benzamide (DEET) has been shown to be especially helpful in deterring ticks.[10] Early removal of ticks is essential (Box 11-1) because transmission of *B. burgdorferi* is rare unless the tick has been attached to the human host for more than 48 hours.[3] After marketing a vaccine for four years from 1998 to 2002, the manufacturer announced that it would no longer be commercially available.[3]

Cancers

The term cancer is a general name for all malignant entities, especially carcinomas and sarcomas. As a group, cancer is the second leading cause of death

---

Box 11-1   Tick Removal

It is important to remove a tick within 48 hours of its attachment to prevent disease. Follow these steps:

- Cleanse the area with a povidone-iodine solution or antibacterial soap.
- Grasp the tick as close to the skin as possible with tweezers, forceps, or gloved fingers.
- Pull up and perpendicular to the skin without twisting or jerking; such movements can break off parts of the insect's mouth and leave them embedded in the skin.
- Take care not to crush, squeeze, or puncture the body of the tick while attached to the skin because it may release infectious fluid into the body.
- Cleanse the area again as above.
- Refer patient to a physician for removal of part of the skin containing the tick with a punch biopsy when part of the tick is left in the skin or if the tick bite occurred in a highly endemic area.
- Send excised tissue to a pathologist when confirmation of tick removal is necessary.

---

in adults.[1] Since the cause of specific cancers is largely unknown, it is difficult to prevent the disease. Cancer occurs when a cell mutates and no longer performs the function for which it was intended. These cells are abnormal in appearance, function, and growth. As the cells divide and multiply, the cancer grows in size, and potentially spreads to local and then remote areas of the body. The lymphatic system is especially well-suited to facilitate the spread of cancer throughout the body and is associated with the metastasis of leukemia and colorectal cancer. Cancers discussed in this chapter have systemic ramifications because they present with vague symptoms and can have whole-body sequelae. Cancers of specific regions of the body are discussed in the chapters devoted to those regions. For example lung cancer is discussed in the respiratory chapter, and breast and testicular cancers are discussed in the genitourinary chapter.

Leukemia

The several different types of **leukemias** have different treatments and prognoses. In general, leukemias are characterized by uncontrolled proliferation of white blood cells in the bone marrow, which accumulate and replace normal blood cells in the marrow. It can then spread to different parts of the body, including the lymph nodes, liver, spleen, and central nervous system. Cancers that start from other places and then spread to the bone marrow are not leukemias.

Nearly 35,000 cases of all types of leukemia are diagnosed in the United States annually. Leukemia is among the top 10 types of cancer in the adults, but it is the most common malignancy in children. In adults, the most common leukemias are **acute myelogenous leukemia** (AML) and **chronic lymphocytic leukemia** (CLL).[11] **Chronic myeloid leukemia** (CML) is about half as common as CLL, affects mostly adults, and is very rare in children. Children, especially between the ages of 1 and 10 years, are most likely to get acute lymphoblastic leukemia (ALL).[2] Of the 3000 to 4000 cases of ALL diagnosed each year, two thirds of them are in children.[1] Leukemia is more common in Caucasians and males, but there is an increasing incidence of AML in African-American men.[11]

The specific etiology of leukemia is unknown; however, several different risk factors are associated with an increased incidence of leukemia. These include prior chemotherapy with certain agents, history of prior radiation therapy, cigarette smoking, genetic syndromes such as Down syndrome, and a family history of leukemia.

Signs and Symptoms

The diagnosis of leukemia is very challenging because the initial symptoms can be very nonspecific and mimic symptoms of a common viral infection. Adults and children can present with generalized fatigue, loss of appetite, fevers, enlarged lymph nodes, and weakness. Additional findings include pallor, **petechiae,** ecchymoses, frequent nose bleeds, and weight loss. An enlarged liver or spleen noted on physical examination can be the explanation for a patient's abdominal pain. If leukemia spreads to the central nervous system, it may cause seizures, blurred vision, headaches, and loss of balance. Some patients are diagnosed on the basis of abnormal findings on a routine complete blood count (CBC) even though their symptoms may be very mild or absent. There are no screening tests for leukemia.

Referral and Diagnostic Tests
Athletes suspected of having leukemia should be referred to a hematologist or oncologist as quickly as possible to allow for initiation of treatment.

Several different findings evident on a CBC are helpful in the diagnosis of leukemia. Patients can have a very low (<5000/mm^3) or very high (>100,000/mm^3) white blood cell count. Table 2-5 gives normal blood values. The CBC may also reveal a low platelet count or anemia, which would explain easy bruising and fatigue, respectively. The key for identifying the type of leukemia is a peripheral blood smear or a bone marrow biopsy, which will show the type of abnormal white blood cells that predominate. Other abnormal lab findings include elevated LDH and uric acid levels. Chest radiographs are routinely performed to rule out mediastinal masses. CT, MRI, or ultrasound of the abdomen is used to check for **hepatomegaly** or **splenomegaly.**[2]

Differential Diagnosis
In children and adults the differential diagnosis is similar. This includes infectious mononucleosis caused by the Epstein-Barr virus or cytomegalovirus, infiltrative diseases of the bone marrow, and aplastic anemia. The biggest differential is the various leukemias, which can usually be proven by bone marrow biopsy or a peripheral blood smear.

Treatment
Treatment varies depending on which type of leukemia has been diagnosed. In general the treatments include radiation, chemotherapy, blood and platelet transfusions, possibly bone marrow or stem cell transplant.

Prognosis and Return to Participation
For ALL, the prognosis is much better in children (80% cure rate) than in adults (40%). The overall 5-year survival rate for ALL is less than 40%.[1] Remission can be achieved in AML in 80% of patients younger than 55 years old. The remission rates in children are even higher. In CLL, the prognosis is related to the stage of the disease at time of diagnosis. When the disease is caught early, the average survival is nearly 10 years; when the disease is caught late, average survival can be only 2 years. The overall 5-year survival for CLL is 60%. The average survival rate for patients with CML is 4 to 6 years.[1]

Avoidance of activity during treatment is essential, and return-to-participation decisions are made under the supervision of the oncologist. Follow up examinations, lab work, and CT scans are essential in the years following treatment to ensure no recurrence of disease.

Colorectal Cancer

The colon represents the final one third of the digestive system and is primarily responsible for reabsorption of fluids and electrolytes (Figure 11-5). The colon, also known as the large intestine, absorbs chloride and sodium while secreting potassium and bicarbonate. Bicarbonate is a buffer accountable for neutralizing gastric acid left over from digestion earlier in the process. Overall, the colon receives approximately 2 liters of fluid per day from the small intestine, and it reabsorbs 1.9 liters back into the body. The colon does not absorb nutrients as does the small intestine. Damage to any portion of the colon can affect fluid homeostasis in a person, which in turn could be problematic in athletic endeavors.

Colon cancer is a neoplasm arising from the lumen of the surface of the large bowel. In the United States, colon cancer is currently the second leading cause of all cancer deaths behind lung cancer. According to the American Cancer Society 145,290 new cases of colorectal cancer will be diagnosed annually, with an expected 56,290 deaths.[1] The frequency of the cancers varies among the sites in the colon. The descending colon accounts for roughly 40% of cancer of the colon, and the rectosigmoid and rectum account for 30%. Roughly 20% of colon cancer arise from the proximal colon, including the cecum and ascending colon. The remaining 10% of colon cancer is found in the transverse colon.[3] Colon cancer incidence increases with age, with a peak incidence in the seventh decade of life.[1]

Numerous risk factors are known to increase the incidence of colorectal cancer. The lifetime risk of sporadic colorectal cancer is 2.5% to 5% in the general population, but it increases to two to three times that for a person with a first-degree relative with colon cancer or an **adenomatous polyp.**[12] Younger patients with colorectal cancer tend to have a more aggressive form of the disease compared with older adult patients. Socioeconomic factors relate to a delay in the diagnosis of colorectal cancer in African-Americans and Hispanics, who are more likely to present with a later stage of the disease. Several other risk factors increase one's likelihood of developing colon cancer, including hereditary

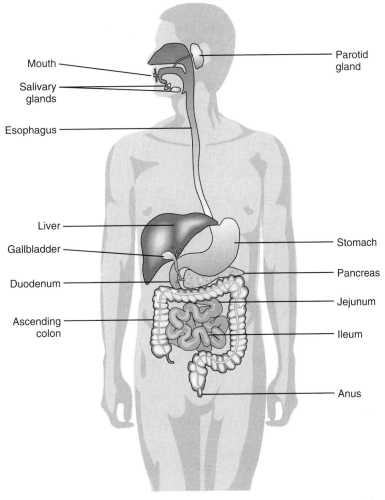

Figure 11-5 The gastrointestinal system emphasizing the anatomical placement of the parotid gland, liver, pancreas, and colon. (From Copstead L E, Banasik J L: *Pathophysiology: biological and behavioral perspectives,* ed 2, St Louis, 2000, WB Saunders, p 795.)

polyposis syndromes, inflammatory bowel diseases such as Crohn's disease and ulcerative colitis, previous other cancers, smoking, lack of physical activity, and dietary factors such as heavy consumption of red meat (Box 11-2).[12]

Box 11-2   Risk Factors for Colon Cancer

The following are risk factors for colon cancer:
- Personal history of colon polyps
- Family history of colon polyps
- Family history of colon cancer
- Inflammatory bowel disease
- High-fat diet, especially high in animal fat
- Low-fiber diet
- Smoking
- Lack of physical activity
- Heavy alcohol use
- Obesity
- Diabetes
- Aging

Signs and Symptoms

The signs and symptoms of colon cancer vary depending on the location and size of the tumor. Tumors in the descending colon usually present with bright red blood in the stool. Colorectal cancer of the ascending and transverse colon tends to present with dark or maroon colored stools. These patients may also have anemia caused by the chronic, slow blood loss from the tumor. Individuals may also describe changes in their bowel habits, including diarrhea and constipation, abdominal pain, weight loss, and palpable masses in the abdomen.[13]

Referral, Diagnostic Tests, and Differential Diagnosis

If colon cancer is suspected, referral should be made to a physician capable of performing flexible sigmoidoscopy or colonoscopy to make a definitive diagnosis. This includes specially trained family medicine physicians, gastroenterologists, or surgeons who specialize in colorectal surgery. After the diagnosis of colon cancer is made, referral should be made to a colorectal surgeon if resection of the colon needs to be performed (Figure 11-6). Referral may also be made to an **oncologist** depending on the stage of the disease.

Several methods are used to diagnose and screen for colorectal cancers. If a patient presents with symptoms that are worrisome for colorectal cancer, such as bleeding from the rectum, direct visualization of the colon is essential. This can be performed with either flexible sigmoidoscopy, that reaches the splenic flexure but does not require sedation, or colonoscopy, which visualizes the entire colon and requires sedation. If polyps, or precancerous growths, are seen, biopsy or entire removal of the polyp can be easily performed and the specimen sent for final pathological diagnosis (Figure 11-7).

The current screening guidelines for colorectal cancer put forth by the American Cancer Society recommend several different techniques (Box 11-3). Those men and women with average risk should start to be screened at age 50 years. Average risk is defined as less than 50 years old with no personal or family (i.e., first-degree relative) history of colorectal cancer or adenomatous polyps, no inflammatory bowel disease, and no genetic

syndrome putting one at increased risk. The screening method chosen should be individualized and take into consideration the patient's comfort, other medical conditions, and the resources available for testing. These methods include fecal occult blood testing for "hidden" blood in the stool, double-contrast barium enema, and flexible sigmoidoscopy or colonoscopy, which allows a direct look at the colon by insertion of a flexible tube with a fiberoptic camera. These tests are performed at variable intervals.

The differential diagnosis to consider with colon cancer includes metastatic cancer from other sites, bowel obstruction, infections of the colon, mesenteric ischemia (caused by blocked blood vessels to the bowel), inflammatory bowel disease, and diverticular disease.

Treatment

The treatment for colorectal cancer depends entirely on the stage of diagnosis. Early cancers that have not spread can be treated with local resection only. Local resection can be just removal of the polyp itself. Occasionally, resection of a part of the colon must be performed. Depending on the individual case, the surgeon may need to place a colostomy bag, which is attached to the abdomen and serves to collect fecal matter by attaching the colon to the abdominal wall. This may be temporary or permanent. More advanced cancers that have spread to local lymph nodes or distant organs involve surgical

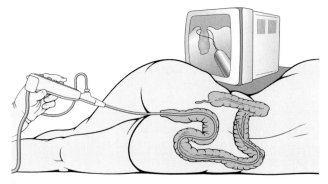

Figure 11-7 Colonoscopy examination. (From Chabner D-E: *The language of medicine*, ed 6, Philadelphia, 2001, WB Saunders.)

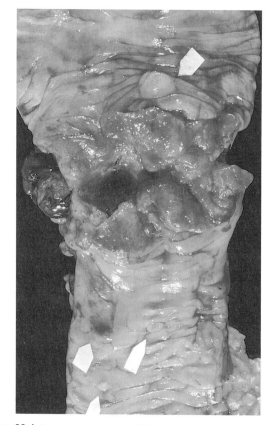

Figure 11-6 An excised carcinoma of the descending colon. (From Cotran RS, Kumar V, Collins T: *Robbins pathologic basis of disease*, ed 6, Philadelphia, 1999, WB Saunders, p 834.)

Box 11-3	Screening for Colon Cancer

Guidelines for screening to promote early detection of colon cancer include the following:
- Beginning at the age of 50 years, in addition to an annual digital rectal exam, follow one of the recommended examination schedules:
  - Fecal occult blood test annually and flexible sigmoidoscopy every 5 years
  - Colonoscopy every 10 years
  - Double-contrast barium enema every 5 to 20 years
- Follow a physician's advice about screening when there is personal or family history of colon polyps or colon cancer

resection as well as adjunctive radiation, chemotherapy, or both.

Prognosis and Return to Participation

The importance of early diagnosis cannot be overemphasized in colon cancer. Colon cancer is divided into four stages. Those that are diagnosed at an early, localized stage have more than a 90% five-year survival rate. Unfortunately, only 39% of colorectal cancers are diagnosed at this stage.[12] Patients with more advanced cancer in the latest stage with distant metastases have a much worse prognosis with a 5-year survival rate of 3% to 5%. These numbers reflect the extreme importance of appropriate screening. If these cancers are caught early, they are curable; if caught late, they are deadly.

Prevention

Prevention is accomplished with vigilant screening techniques. Appropriate screening and removal of precancerous polyps can decrease the risk of colorectal cancer by 80%.[3] As noted previously, the later colorectal cancer is detected, the worse the prognosis. Primary prevention of colorectal cancer is a commonly discussed topic in the news. Regular use of aspirin and other nonsteroidal antiinflammatory drugs has been shown to provide some degree of protection against colorectal cancer, as have the statin medications, which are used commonly to lower cholesterol. Other studies have suggested that diets high in fiber and low in fat, adequate folate, high dietary calcium intake, and increased physical activity all decrease the risk of colon cancer.[1]

Chronic Disorders

Raynaud's Disease

Raynaud's phenomenon is a disorder characterized by vasospasm of the arteries primarily in the hands but it can also affect the feet, nose, and ears (Figure 11-8).

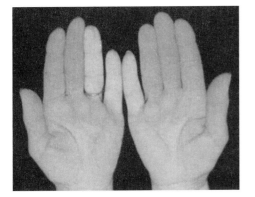

Figure 11-8 Raynaud's phenomenon consisting of pallor on the digits when exposed to cold or stress. (From Jarvis C: *Physical examination & health assessment,* ed 4, Philadelphia, 2004, WB Saunders, p 555.)

Stressors, including cold temperatures and emotional trauma, exacerbate the disease. The two presentations of Raynaud's disease are primary and secondary. Typically, the primary condition is referred to as Raynaud's disease if no other cause can be found. Secondary Raynaud's is caused by an underlying problem and is termed Raynaud's phenomenon. The numerous causes for secondary Raynaud's phenomenon include medications such as oral contraceptives, systemic lupus erythematosus (SLE), rheumatoid arthritis, and tools that cause vibration (Box 11-4).[3]

Raynaud's phenomenon is found in 5% to 20% of the population. Primary Raynaud's is more common than secondary and occurs more commonly in women and in people under 40 years old.

Signs and Symptoms

Patients typically present with a triphasic color response to cold exposure. Pallor, or pale skin, will appear on the digits because of the vasospasm. The skin will then become blue in color from the cyanosis caused by the increase of venous, or deoxygenated, blood in the digits. The final color happens when the vasospasm resolves and a rush of blood enters the digits, turning the digits red and causing pain and numbness. As noted previously, these symptoms can happen in the hands, feet, nose, and ears and usually occur bilaterally. The symptoms generally resolve over minutes, but if they persist, they can lead to ulcerations, gangrene, and dead tissue.[3]

Referral, Diagnostic Tests, and Differential Diagnosis

If a secondary cause of Raynaud's phenomenon is suspected, the appropriate referral should be made depending on the diagnosis. A rheumatologist should be involved for cases with underlying diseases such as **scleroderma** and **systemic lupus erythematosus** (SLE). If patients' symptoms are such that they have the potential to lose digits, referral to a vascular or plastic surgeon is appropriate.

History of the symptoms is usually enough to diagnose Raynaud's phenomenon. Once the diagnosis is made, a good history and physical exam should aid in ruling out secondary causes of Raynaud's phenomenon.

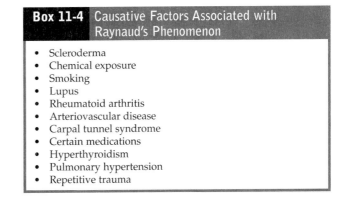

Box 11-4   Causative Factors Associated with Raynaud's Phenomenon

- Scleroderma
- Chemical exposure
- Smoking
- Lupus
- Rheumatoid arthritis
- Arteriovascular disease
- Carpal tunnel syndrome
- Certain medications
- Hyperthyroidism
- Pulmonary hypertension
- Repetitive trauma

If a secondary cause is suggested, the physician will order appropriate blood work. Occasionally, the diagnosis can be "seen" by having the patient expose the fingers to a cold environment, such as ice water, and monitoring the results. No blood tests assist in the diagnosis of Raynaud's, but a CBC, basic electrolytes, kidney and liver function tests, an ESR, and a urinalysis should be ordered to help differentiate this from other diseases.

The differential diagnosis of Raynaud's phenomenon includes those secondary causes listed previously, as well as **CREST** (*c*alcinosis cutis, *R*aynaud's phenomenon, *e*sophageal dysfunction, *s*clerodactyly, *t*elangiectasia) syndrome, scleroderma, carpal tunnel syndrome, and **Buerger's disease.**[3]

Treatment

The simplest of treatments is avoidance of the triggers that propagate Raynaud's, such as avoiding medications that may cause it, staying out of the cold, wearing appropriate protective clothing, and avoiding other triggers such as caffeine and tobacco.[3] For those with no relief from the nonpharmacological approach, medications can be used to decrease symptoms. Calcium channel blockers, such as nifedipine, have proven to be the most effective treatment for Raynaud's disease. Other medications proven helpful include alpha-blockers and to a lesser extent aspirin and topical nitrates.[3]

Prognosis and Return to Participation

Patients with primary Raynaud's phenomenon usually have good control of their problems with nonpharmacological treatments. Unfortunately, for those with secondary Raynaud's phenomenon caused by CREST syndrome, Buerger's disease, or scleroderma, symptoms may be so severe that the disease causes ulcerations, gangrene, and even autoamputations.[3]

Systemic Lupus Erythematosus

SLE is a chronic autoimmune disorder affecting the musculoskeletal, skin, renal, cardiac, and nervous systems. It tends to be an exacerbation-remission disorder with long-term consequences. It affects approximately 1 in 2000 individuals.[14] SLE predominantly affects women, especially during their child-bearing years, and is also more common in African-Americans. Twenty percent of cases are diagnosed before the age of 20 years.[14] Children who are affected tend to have a more severe onset and follow a more aggressive clinical course.

The exact cause of SLE is not known, but the process is the development of autoantibodies that are directed at the nuclei of several different cells. It is a chronic, progressive disorder that can affect several different systems at various times through the course of the disease.

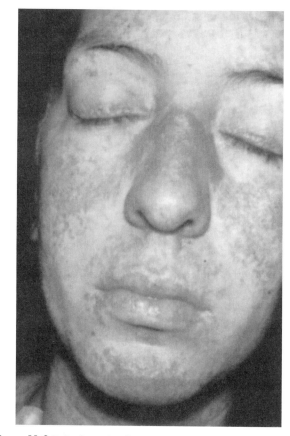

Figure 11-9 Butterfly rash of systemic lupus erythematosus. (From Copstead LE, Banasik JL: *Pathophysiology: biological and behavioral perspectives,* ed 2, St Louis, 2000, WB Saunders, p 1191.)

Signs and Symptoms

SLE is a multisystem disease process; consequently, the patient presents with multiple complaints. At some point during the course of their disease, 90% of patients with SLE will have musculoskeletal complaints. Typically, patients will have numerous muscle aches and pains as well as arthritis or swelling of several joints. Because of the long-term use of corticosteroids to treat many patients with SLE, they have a much higher risk of osteoporosis as well as a high risk of avascular necrosis, typically presenting in the hip. This can affect up to 14% of patients with SLE and typically requires surgery for treatment.[15] Approximately 30% of patients with SLE will also present with fibromyalgia.[15]

The skin is largely affected in patients with SLE. The hallmark sign is a red rash over the malar eminence of the face, sparing the nasolabial folds, called the "butterfly rash" for its typical appearance (Figure 11-9). Patients can also present with hair loss, red and scaly patches that turn to plaques, and oral ulcers, as well as photophobic skin responses to sun.

In addition, the kidneys can be affected, with approximately one half of patients with SLE developing lupus nephritis.[15] This is more common in African-Americans

The presence of four or more of the following indicates SLE:
- Neurological disorder, including seizures or psychosis
- Renal disorder
- Ulcers, either oral or nasopharyngeal
- Butterfly rash
- Skin photosensitivity
- Serositis, including pericarditis or pleurisy
- Hematological disorders including leukopenia (<400/mm³), lymphopenia (<1500/mm³), thrombocytopenia (<100,000/mm³), hemolytic anemia
- Elevated antinuclear antibodies (ANA)
- Discoid rash
- Immunological disorders including anti-DNA antibody, anti-Smith antibody, antiphospholipid antibody, lupus erythematosus cells

Data from Beers MH, Berkow R: *The Merck manual of diagnosis and therapy*, ed 17, Whitehouse Station, NJ, 1999, Merck Research Laboratories; Gladman D, Ginzler E, Goldsmith C, et al: The development and initial validation of the systemic lupus international collaborating clinics/American College of Rheumatology damage index for systemic lupus erythematosus, *Arthritis & Rheumatism* 39(3):363-369, 1996; Ferri F: *Ferri's clinical advisor instant diagnosis and treatment*, Philadelphia, 2004, Mosby; Hildebrand J, Muller D: Systemic lupus erythematosus, *Emedicine*. Available at http://www.emedicine.com/MED/topic2228.htm. Accessed November 2004; Millea P, Holloway R: Treating fibromyalgia, *American Family Physician* 62(7):1575-1582, 2000.

with SLE. Although the treatment for lupus nephritis can keep the kidneys functioning well, kidney problems are a major cause of morbidity and mortality in SLE patients.

The central nervous system effects of SLE are numerous and widely varied. Patients can present with seizures, psychosis, decreased cognitive function, stroke, or even coma.

The heart can also show manifestations of SLE, including premature atherosclerosis of the arteries surrounding the heart that affects 6% to 10% of patients.[15] This, like many of the complications seen in SLE, is thought to be caused by the side effects from long-term corticosteroid use. Blood clots forming in the circulatory system are also seen in SLE because of the production of specialized **antiphospholipid antibodies.** SLE patients also commonly develop anemia and a low platelet count that at times can be severe and require transfusions.[14]

Referral and Diagnostic Tests

Certified athletic trainers who see athletes with unexplained joint pain and swelling, especially if accompanied by a butterfly rash, should refer these athletes to a physician for further testing. Referrals depend on the severity of the disease and the organ systems involved. In addition to a primary care physician, SLE patients need a rheumatologist at the center of their care. Nephrologists should be involved for patients with kidney disorders, hematologists for those with blood manifestations, and if needed, orthopedic surgeons for those with avascular necrosis.

The American College of Rheumatology (ACR) has developed criteria to aid in the diagnosis of SLE (Box 11-5). Four of the eleven criteria must be met for the diagnosis of SLE.[15] In addition to the criteria, several blood tests can be performed to help in the diagnosis of SLE. Antinuclear antibody (ANA), anti-Smith antibody, and anti–double-stranded deoxyribonucleic acid (anti-dsDNA) antibodies are all helpful in the diagnosis.

Differential Diagnosis

Because of its effect on numerous systems, the differential diagnosis of SLE is determined by the symptoms of the presenting patient. In brief, these can include infection, malignancies including lymphoma and leukemia, rheumatoid arthritis, and mixed connective tissue disease.

Treatment

The goal of treatment of SLE is to care for the acute symptoms while avoiding the progression of the damaging effects of the disease in the long term. Photosensitivity for those with skin manifestations can be controlled with the use of sunscreens and avoidance of sunlight. Patients with musculoskeletal symptoms can benefit from nonsteroidal antiinflammatory medications. In more severe cases, antimalarial medications, such as hydroxychloroquine (Plaquenil), have been proven to help and also are effective in treating some skin manifestations. Corticosteroids have been the mainstay of treatment for SLE symptoms affecting the renal, nervous, and hematological systems. Although corticosteroid treatment is extremely beneficial for patients with SLE, its many side effects complicate the disease itself. Patients taking long-term corticosteroids have a higher likelihood of infections, osteoporosis, avascular necrosis, steroid-induced diabetes, and several skin ramifications (see Chapter 3). All of these side effects need to be monitored for and treated appropriately while the patient remains on corticosteroids. The key is to have the patient take the lowest dose possible that controls the disease while limiting the side effects.

Prognosis and Return to Participation

Because patients with SLE tend to have remissions and exacerbations, prognosis is often complicated. Infection from the immunosuppression as a result of not only SLE itself but also the chronic corticosteroid treatment is the leading cause of death in patients with SLE.[3] Other causes of death in patients with SLE include renal and central nervous system involvement. The 10-year survival rate for those with SLE is 75%.[3] The overall challenge of treating SLE is to monitor the patient for exacerbations and new complications of the disease while balancing the potential side effects of treatment.

Fibromyalgia

Fibromyalgia is a chronic, noninflammatory, diffuse pain syndrome characterized by multiple areas of musculoskeletal pain, sleep disturbances, fatigue, and depression. The majority (85%) of those affected are women between the ages of 30 and 50 years.[3] The overall prevalence of fibromyalgia in the United States is 2%, and it affects a total of 3.5% of women and 0.5% of men.[16]

The cause of fibromyalgia remains unknown, but several theories implicate a disturbed sleep pattern and its deleterious effect on the neuorendocrine axis.[17] Although how this process is set in motion in some people and not others is unknown, it is thought that usually a precipitating event, such as extreme weight gain, injury, emotional trauma, withdrawal from medication, or abrupt cessation of exercise, is involved.[16]

Signs and Symptoms

Patients with fibromyalgia typically experience severe musculoskeletal pain that is unrelated to a clearly defined anatomical lesion.[17] The pain is mostly located in the neck and lower back, but it can also affect the extremities. This pain syndrome will wax and wane not only in severity but also in location and may be exacerbated by any emotional or physical trauma.[16] If a patient has any findings consistent with another disease process or injury, such as a swollen joint, warmth or redness over the affected site, or abnormal x-ray findings, a diagnosis other than fibromyalgia should be investigated thoroughly.

Referral, Diagnostic Tests, and Differential Diagnosis

Athletic trainers are mindful to watch for athletes who present with symptoms longer than usual for a given injury or illness. If an athlete has symptoms that are thought to be consistent with fibromyalgia, referral to a primary care physician is appropriate to help with the diagnosis. If needed, referral to a rheumatologist, psychiatrist, physical therapist, or a specialist in fibromyalgia can be made.

The diagnosis of fibromyalgia rests on a thorough history, physical exam, and a set of criteria established by the ACR (Box 11-6). The criteria include widespread, bilateral pain located above and below the waist and pain involving the axial skeleton that has been present for at least 3 months. To meet the diagnosis of fibromyalgia, the patient must also have pain at 11 of 18 sites when the examiner applies pressure equal to the pressure that would make the fingernail blanch with pressing.[17,18] Basic lab evaluations, including a CBC, creatinine kinase, thyroid-stimulating hormone, and ESR, are performed to differentiate fibromyalgia from other diseases that have overlapping symptoms.[19]

| **Box 11-6** | **Diagnostic Criteria for Fibromyalgia** |

The following criteria have been established by the American College of Rheumatology (ACR):
1. History of widespread pain over the four quadrants of the body lasting more than 3 months.
2. Presence of specific tender points. ARC has identified 18 points, and 11 must be tender to confirm a diagnosis; any of nine areas listed below can have pain bilaterally:
    a. Occiput—at the suboccipital muscle insertion
    b. Anterior cervical intertransverse spaces at C5-C7
    c. Trapezius at the midpoint of the muscle
    d. Supraspinatus origin
    e. Second rib—at the costochondral junction
    f. Lateral humeral epicondyle
    g. Gluteal area—upper outer quadrants of the buttocks
    h. Greater trochanter
    i. Medial knee, proximal to joint line

Data from Wolfe F, Smythe H, Yunus M, et al: The American College of Rheumatology 1990 criteria of classification of fibromyalgia, report of the Multicenter Criteria Committee, *Arthritis & Rheumatism* 33(2):160-172, 1990; National Institute of Arthritis and Musculoskeletal Skin Diseases: Questions and answers about fibromyalgia. Available at http://www.niams.nih.gov/hi/topics/fibromyalgia/fibrofs.htm. Accessed November 2004; Millea P, Holloway R: Treating fibromyalgia, *American Family Physician* 62(7):1575-1582, 2000.

The differential diagnosis of fibromyalgia includes many diseases with similar signs and symptoms. These include depression, chronic fatigue syndrome, myofascial pain syndrome, hypothyroidism, rheumatoid arthritis, and SLE.[16]

Treatment

The treatment for fibromyalgia usually incorporates a variety of disciplines. The key element is patient education, which can be accomplished through lectures, handouts, videos, or the Internet.[19] Counseling is also an important aspect of fibromyalgia, especially in those individuals with manifestations of depression or poor coping skills. Exercise has proven to be very beneficial since deconditioning plays a large role in fibromyalgia. Good sleep habits and mild exercise have a positive effect on mood disorders and depression (see Chapter 15).[17] Cardiovascular exercise seems to be of more benefit than stretching and flexibility exercises, and after a 3-month program, some patients can see benefits that last for up to 1 year. Water aerobics, swimming, biking, yoga, and other nonimpact exercises are appropriate.

The patient with fibromyalgia may also benefit from pharmacological treatment. Antidepressants, especially the tricyclic antidepressants such as amitriptyline at low doses, have been shown to help. Not only do they aid with the possible underlying depression, but also their sedative effect makes them ideal, especially when taken before bedtime. Muscle relaxants such as cyclobenzaprine (Flexeril) have shown merit in helping patients with fibromyalgia and also have a sedating side effect. Selective serotonin reuptake inhibitors (SSRIs), such as fluoxetine (Prozac), also have proven beneficial.[17] Nonsteroidal antiinflammatory agents have not proven to be beneficial in patients with fibromyalgia. Several other treatments that may help patients with fibromyalgia include hypnosis, chiropractic treatments, acupuncture, and herbal medications. These modalities need to be further studied to determine their true effectiveness.

Prognosis and Return to Participation

The prognosis of fibromyalgia is uncertain because the symptoms commonly come and go over the course of the disease. Although patients can show improvement, there is no cure for the disease. An aggressive, multifaceted, organized approach to treatment will help lead to a substantial improvement and ideally a remission of symptoms. Participation in athletic events is determined on an individualized basis. Most athletes can function as long as their symptoms are well controlled.

Chronic Fatigue Syndrome

Chronic fatigue syndrome (CFS) is an often-disabling illness with the primary symptom being persistent severe fatigue. This is often accompanied by several other symptoms involving the musculoskeletal, immunological, and neurological systems. People of all races and ages can be affected.

There is no known cause of CFS, and no specific diagnostic tests are available. It is likely a spectrum of illnesses sharing a common pathogenesis with varying degrees of fatigue and associated symptoms.[20]

Signs and Symptoms

The primary presenting symptom for CFS is persistent fatigue. Several other symptoms can be present as well; however, these vary widely and are mainly used to differentiate CFS from other causes of persistent fatigue.

Referral and Diagnostic Tests

The diagnosis of CFS is one of exclusion. Because of the overlapping symptoms CFS has with several other diseases, including depression, fibromyalgia, and infectious mononucleosis, to name just a few, several criteria must be met in order to diagnose a person with CFS. A complete history and physical exam are mandatory to help exclude other disease processes. Lab tests include a standard CBC, but other lab tests are ordered depending on the patient's symptoms. The Centers for Disease Control and Prevention have established diagnostic criteria for CFS that include persistent severe fatigue lasting for at least 6 consecutive months, no definable organic disease, and associated physical symptoms.[20] A host of diseases needs to be excluded before giving the diagnosis of CFS (Box 11-7).

> **Box 11-7 Differential Diagnoses for Chronic Fatigue Syndrome**
>
> Differential diagnoses for chronic fatigue syndrome may include the following:
> - Mononucleosis
> - Anemia
> - Leukemia
> - Depression
> - Systemic lupus erythematosus
> - Human immunodeficiency virus
> - Multiple sclerosis
> - Myasthenia gravis
> - Thyroiditis
> - Hypothyroidism
> - Hypopituitarism
> - Lyme disease
> - Chronic hepatitis B or C
> - Rheumatoid arthritis
> - Tuberculosis
> - Fibromyalgia
> - Diabetes mellitus
> - Pregnancy
> - Sleep apnea
> - Narcolepsy
> - Medication reaction

Treatment, Prognosis, and Return to Participation

The optimal treatment of CFS includes a multifactorial approach aimed at managing the disease and its manifestations. Since there is no definitive cure for CFS and each individual may present with a variety of symptoms, the treatment needs to be tailored toward the individual. Basic tenets of treatment currently employed seem to have a beneficial effect in managing the disease. Suggested management includes a graded exercise program, proper nutrition, improved sleep, an antidepressant such as one of the tricyclic antidepressants or SSRIs, and behavioral therapy to include counseling.[20] Counseling is very important in the athletic setting since CFS can hamper an individual's performance substantially, making return to competition at any level quite challenging.

Treatment of any other coexistent disorders, such as depression, fibromyalgia, panic disorders, and irritable bowel syndrome, is also very important in the overall approach to patients with CFS.

The prognosis for people with CFS is unknown because there is no definitive cure for the disease. The hope with a multidisciplinary approach is to allow the athlete to return to the previous level of competition; however, this may take months to years to accomplish.

Endocrine Disorders

Endocrine glands secrete hormones directly into the blood stream, allowing specific body functions to occur. The disorders discussed here are related to the pancreas (see Figure 11-5), a gland with both exocrine and endocrine functions, and the thyroid. The pancreas lies with its ends laterally touching the spleen (see Figure 6-1) and the duodenum of the small intestine medially. The chief functions of the pancreas are to secrete bicarbonate to protect the duodenum from gastric acid and to produce insulin, glucagons, and somatostatin from the endocrine glands, called islets of Langerhans.[21] The normal pancreas has between 500,000 and several million islets. The islets comprise four cell types, but only the two primary cells types, alpha and beta, are discussed here. Alpha cells produce glucagon, whereas beta cells secrete insulin.

When serum glucose or blood sugar is high, the beta cells are stimulated to produce insulin. The secreted insulin then allows muscle, blood, and fat cells to absorb glucose out of the blood, effectively lowering blood sugar to normal ranges. The alpha cells of the islets of Langerhans secrete glucagon, which has the opposite effect of insulin. If blood sugar is low, glucagon is secreted where it has the most effect on the liver. Glucagon stimulates liver cells to break down stored glycogen into glucose and release it into the blood stream, increasing serum levels of glucose. Glucagon also stimulates muscle to manufacture glucose from stored protein by means of gluconeogenesis. The human body functions best when glucose levels are relatively constant within the blood stream. Because most body functions rely on glucose in some form, severely fluctuating levels can have profound sequelae.

Pancreatitis

Acute pancreatitis is an inflammatory process of the pancreas with intrapancreatic activation of enzymes. In 90% of cases, it is caused by blockage of the biliary tract by gallstone formation or from alcohol abuse. Several medications have been implicated in pancreatitis as well. This condition is more common in urban settings, thought to be because of the higher rate of alcoholism.

Signs and Symptoms
Patients typically present with abdominal pain located in the epigastric area and occasionally radiating to the back. They may have severe nausea and vomiting. Some patients report weight loss as well. On exam, patients are typically guarding their abdomen because of the extreme pain associated with palpation of this area. Patients' bowel sounds will be hypoactive, and they may have signs of fluid or blood in their abdominal cavity, such as abdominal rigidity and guarding; Chapters 2 and 6 present basic assessment of the abdomen. These patients may also have fever, confusion, elevated heart rate, or jaundice.

Referral, Diagnostic Tests, and Differential Diagnosis
Athletes with nontraumatic abdominal swelling, pain, or jaundice should be referred to a physician for further evaluation. Patients often require hospitalization for pain control and treatment of the pancreatitis.

History and physical examination are paramount in the assessment of these patients. Inclusion of alcohol intake history is very important to help elucidate a cause for the inflamed pancreas. Pancreatitis will present with elevated enzymes produced by the pancreas, including lipase and amylase. Of the two enzymes, lipase is more sensitive. Further testing, including blood count, liver enzymes, and glucose and serum calcium levels, is important in the initial work-up. Abdominal radiographs, ultrasound, or CT scans are appropriate for diagnosis. These studies help to evaluate not only for inflammation of the pancreas but also for any potentially obstructing stones or cancers.

Several diseases can present with abdominal pain. These include peptic ulcer disease, intestinal obstruction, early acute appendicitis, pneumonia, and heart attack. The history, physical exam, and lab work will help differentiate these problems.

Treatment
Treatment of pancreatitis is performed in the hospital. Food is avoided since it may irritate the pancreas and therefore slow the healing. Maintenance of intravascular volume with intravenous fluids is paramount because these patients tend to have a total body water deficit. Pain control is provided with medications such as meperidine (Demerol). Surgical consultation may be warranted if there is evidence of gallstone pancreatitis.

Prognosis and Return to Participation
Prognosis varies with the severity of the illness. Severe disease has an overall mortality for acute pancreatitis that approaches 5% to 10% of patients.[3] Individuals with a history of alcohol abuse commonly have recurrent bouts of pancreatitis, leading to chronic pancreatitis.

Athletes with pancreatitis will need to refrain from competition until the acute phase has resolved, since the pain associated with pancreatitis is so great it will not allow one to make any sudden movements. Once the cause of pancreatitis is identified, it should be treated appropriately.

Diabetes Mellitus

Diabetes mellitus (DM) is a disease in which the body is unable to produce or use insulin effectively. Diabetes mellitus affects 7% of the population, or roughly 18 million people, in the United States.

Of these, 5 million are unaware that they have the disease.[22] Type 1 diabetes, formerly insulin-dependent diabetes mellitus (IDDM), is characterized by the body's inability to produce insulin, which is needed for the proper use and storage of carbohydrates. Type 1 DM accounts for roughly 10% of the total number of cases, and its onset usually occurs in people under the age of 20 years old.[23] Type 2 DM, formerly non–insulin-dependent diabetes mellitus (NIDDM), makes up the remaining 90% of cases. This form of DM is related to the body's inability to use insulin effectively because of a combination of resistance to insulin as well as an overall decreased production of insulin.

The incidence of diabetes is known to increase with age. It is the leading cause of end-stage renal disease in the United States and is a primary cause of blindness and foot and leg amputations in adults. Individuals with diabetes are twice as likely as persons without diabetes to develop cardiovascular disease.[3]

Type 1 DM is caused by autoimmune-mediated destruction of beta cells in the pancreas that are responsible for producing insulin.[24] There appears to be a hereditary link in people with type 1 DM. Other factors have been postulated to induce type 1 DM, including viral infections, toxins, and other environmental factors. Although there is a genetic predisposition for developing type 2 DM, several physical factors also put an individual at increased risk for the disease. Type 2 DM results more from an insulin resistance syndrome that is felt to be exacerbated by excess body fat linked primarily to a sedentary lifestyle and an excess consumption of calories.[25] Women can also be affected by gestational diabetes, usually occurring in the third trimester of pregnancy and typically resolving in the postpartum period. These individuals are more likely to develop type 2 DM later on in life. Other causes of type 2 DM are Cushing's syndrome, pancreatic disorders such as pancreatitis, or prolonged medication usage, including glucocorticoids.[3]

Signs and Symptoms

There is usually a prolonged, albeit unknown, period of time when persons with type 2 diabetes have hyperglycemia but do not have any clinical symptoms. Later in the disease process, as the body can no longer compensate for the elevated sugar load, symptoms begin. The most common initial symptoms include **polyuria** (increased urination), **polydipsia** (excessive thirst), **polyphagia** (persistent hunger), weight loss, and occasionally blurred vision.[26] All these symptoms are due to an elevated glucose level in the bloodstream. Also, certain risk factors predispose a person to diabetes (Box 11-8). Sometimes the symptoms of early diabetes are repeated episodes of hyperglycemia. Overtreatment of diabetes or inadequate food intake can cause hypoglycemia.

Box 11-8   Risks Factors for Diabetes

Regular screening is recommended for individuals at risk for developing diabetes including the following individuals:
- Over 45 years old
- Obese (BMI > 25)
- Blood relatives with diabetes
- History of gestational diabetes (women)
- High blood pressure
- High cholesterol
- Elevated triglycerides
- Belong to certain ethnic populations that are at increased risk for diabetes, including Native Americans, African-Americans, Asian-Americans, and Hispanic-Americans

---

Referral, Diagnostic Tests, and Differential Diagnosis

Athletes with signs or symptoms consistent with diabetes or those who have risk factors are referred to a physician. Three tests of blood glucose levels can be performed to confirm the diagnosis of type 1 and type 2 DM (Table 11-2). The first test requires 8 hours of fasting before blood glucose is measured, and a result equal to or greater than 126 mg/dl indicates disease. The second requires 2 hours of fasting, and a blood glucose level greater than or equal to 200 mg/dl is significant. The final test is performed without regard to food intake on a random basis, and a blood glucose level equal to or greater than 200 mg/dl associated with weight loss, polyuria, and polydipsia indicates DM.[24] All three of these criteria can diagnose diabetes, but one positive test needs to be confirmed on the following day by another one of the tests.[26] A fasting blood glucose level between 100 to 125 mg/dl is consistent with the diagnosis of prediabetes.

Once the diagnosis is confirmed, those caring for individuals with diabetes, especially athletes, need to be well versed in the signs and symptoms of hyperglycemia and hypoglycemia. A comparison of symptoms for hypoglycemia and hyperglycemia is found in Box 11-9. Although exercise is paramount in treating and controlling diabetes, there are also inherent risks for persons with diabetes who do exercise. Hypoglycemia, or low blood sugar, defined as less than 60 mg/dl, usually presents several hours after exercise but can happen during competition as well or as a result of an overuse of insulin (Red Flags—Diabetes). The symptoms are numerous and include sweating, palpitations, hunger,

---

Table 11-2   Normal Blood Glucose Levels

Take Measurement	Blood Serum Levels
After fasting for 8 hr	60-80 mg/dl*
2-3 hr after eating	100-140 mg/dl
Random and unplanned	<126 mg/dl

*mg/dl = milligrams of glucose in 100 milliliters (1 deciliter) of blood; hypoglycemia is defined as <70 mg/dl and hyperglycemia is defined as >180 mg/dl.

Box 11-9 Compared Signs and Symptoms for Hypoglycemia and Hyperglycemia

Hypoglycemia (<60 mg/dl)
Palpitations
Tachycardia
Anxiety
Hyperventilation
Blurred vision
Shakiness
Diaphoresis
Weakness
Hunger
Nausea
Confusion
Behavior changes
Hallucinations
Hypothermia
Seizures
Coma

Hyperglycemia (>180 mg/dl)
Weakness
Polyuria
Altered vision
Weight loss
Dehydration
Polydipsia
Hyperventilation
Stupor
Coma
Hypotension
Cardiac arrhythmias

Red Flags for Diabetes

Untreated hypoglycemia is dangerous because it can result in coma, convulsions, permanent brain injury, and possible death. Recognizing the following symptoms, particularly when presenting together, can lead to early diagnosis:
- Sweating
- Palpitations
- Hunger
- Tremors
- Confusion
- Nausea
- Headaches
- Fatigue
- Slurred speech
- Inappropriate behavior
- Incoordination

tremors, confusion, nausea, headaches, fatigue, slurred speech, inappropriate behavior, and incoordination.[24] It is important to recognize these symptoms because if left uncorrected, hypoglycemia can result in coma, convulsions, permanent brain injury, and possibly death. Hyperglycemia is another risk factor for persons with diabetes; it has a variety of symptoms, such as polyuria, polydipsia, fatigue, nausea, and an elevated blood sugar.

The differential diagnosis of diabetes includes diabetes insipidus, stress hyperglycemia, and diabetes secondary to medications, pancreatic disease, and possible hormonal excess.

Treatment
Patients with diabetes, whether type 1 or 2, need to be under the care of a physician because of the high number of complications that can arise if diabetes is not controlled. Because there are so many individuals with diabetes in the United States, most primary care physicians can manage the disease without the assistance of specialists. If referral is needed, as may be the case with most people with type 1 diabetes, an endocrinologist or diabetologist would be appropriate. The care of the person with diabetes requires a multidisciplinary approach. Patients may be referred for nutritional counseling, exercise prescriptions, yearly eye examinations by an eye specialist, and routine podiatric care.

The overall goal in the treatment of diabetes is to decrease the end-stage effects, such as renal disease and failure, coronary artery disease, blindness, and stroke. In addition to medications, diet, and exercise to improve glucose control, treatment of other conditions common to people with diabetes, including hypertension, elevated cholesterol and triglycerides, and tobacco abuse, needs to be addressed.

If further complications arise, nephrologists, cardiologists, podiatrists, or other appropriate specialists are called on.

Type 1 Diabetes Mellitus. The treatment for diabetes is multifactorial. At the cornerstone of therapy is education about the disease, sound nutrition, and increased physical activity. Lifestyle modification has been shown to delay or prevent the onset of diabetes.[25] The goal of therapy is to have a normal blood sugar and prevent the multiple complications that can occur if blood sugar remains elevated. This is accomplished with insulin in persons with type 1 diabetes because of the decreased production of insulin. Numerous types of insulin are available for treatment of type 1 diabetes; some are long acting and some shorter acting. Active onset of insulin can range from 15 minutes to 8 hours, with duration lasting from 3 hours to longer than 36 hours. The type of insulin used needs to be tailored to each individual. This is commonly based on eating habits, exercise schedule, and convenience.

Athletes with type 1 diabetes need to carry testing strips and a glucometer to measure their blood sugar levels. In addition, they must carry their own insulin at all times. The athletic trainer must have a full appreciation and understanding of the athlete's regular insulin schedule and dosage, as well as proper storage and disposal of insulin and needles. It is common for some athletic events to take an entire day (e.g., volleyball, softball, baseball, swimming, and track events) and for

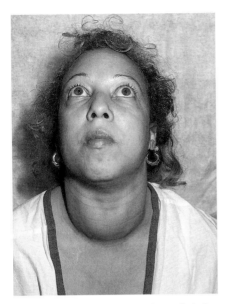

Figure 11-12 Hyperthyroidism, which is also called Graves' disease. Note the swelling in the thyroid region as well as the exophthalmos of the eyes. (From Jarvis C: *Physical examination & health assessment,* ed 4, Philadelphia, 2004, WB Saunders, p 295.)

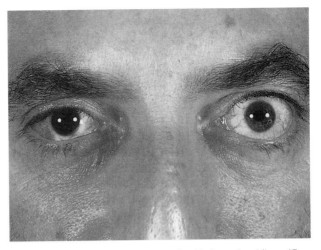

Figure 11-13 Exophthalmos associated with hyperthyroidism. (From Epstein O, Perkin GD, Cookson J, de Bono DP: *Clinical examination,* ed 3, Philadelphia, 2003, Mosby, p 30.)

Signs and Symptoms. The signs and symptoms of hyperthyroidism are vast. Common symptoms include an increased heart rate, heart palpitations, difficulty concentrating, shakiness, nervousness, gastrointestinal disturbances (excess gas, frequent normal bowel movements, or diarrhea), eyelid retraction, depression, menstrual irregularities, panic or anxiety attacks, weight loss despite a good appetite, and increased sweating. Athletes can also present with fatigue and muscle weakness leading to impaired performance.

The physical findings of hyperthyroidism include brisk reflexes, tremors, anxiety, reddening of the palms, an elevated heart rate, and occasionally an irregular heart rhythm such as atrial fibrillation. Patients will also usually have an enlarged or swollen thyroid gland. Because of swelling that accumulates behind the globe of the eye, patients may present with **exophthalmos** or a bulging out of the eyes (Figure 11-13). Other eye symptoms include diplopia and blurred vision.

Referral, Diagnostic Tests, and Differential Diagnosis. Athletes who appear to have an enlarged thyroid gland, bulging eyes, and symptoms associated with hyperthyroidism are referred to the team physician. Individuals with hyperthyroidism can be initially evaluated by their primary care physician and then referred to an endocrinologist who specializes in diseases of the thyroid if needed. A surgical referral may be needed if part of the treatment would require removal of the thyroid gland. A patient who presents with an acute exacerbation of thyroiditis may need to be admitted to the hospital for further management.

The diagnosis of hyperthyroidism is usually made by a complete history, physical exam, and a simple blood test to check TSH. If TSH is elevated, additional testing can be done including a free T_3 index and a free T_4 index. These tests measure the thyroid hormone that is not bound to protein and is typically elevated in patients with hyperthyroidism.

Imaging studies also can be performed to help differentiate types of hyperthyroidism. The test most often used is a 24-hour radioactive iodine uptake (RAIU) scan. The radioactive iodine will be taken up by the thyroid gland and will have different appearances on the scan to help determine the underlying cause for the hyperthyroidism.

The differential diagnosis of hyperthyroidism includes anxiety, diabetes mellitus, myasthenia gravis, premenopausal state, metastatic neoplasms, and pheochromocytoma.

Treatment. The treatment for hyperthyroidism centers on controlling the patient's symptoms and slowing the overactive thyroid gland. To control symptoms, especially the increased heart rate and tremors associated with hyperthyroidism, patients are typically given beta-blocker medications, also commonly used to treat hypertension. These medications are used in the acute presentation and are usually withdrawn after definitive treatment of the overactive thyroid.[29] Those taking care of athletes must be aware that beta blockers are banned substances in several governing bodies for sports such as archery and shooting. The three ways to manage the thyroid gland are medications, radioactive iodine, and thyroid surgery.

The medications typically used to treat hyperthyroidism include propylthiouracil (PTU) and methimazole.

These medications act to inhibit the production of thyroid hormone. They are usually given for 6 to 24 months and are usually used as adjunctive therapy before thyroid surgery or radioactive iodine treatment. While the patient is taking this medication, free T_3 and T_4 are checked to determine how well the medication is working. Radioactive iodine ablation of the thyroid is a common, effective, and safe treatment for those patients who are not pregnant. A single dose of radioactive iodine will put roughly 80% of patients into a normal state.[3] Thyroid surgery is usually limited to those with very large goiters that may be causing obstruction, abnormal appearing thyroid nodules, or pregnant women. It is rarely used in the United States because the aforementioned treatments are effective and, in general, have fewer adverse effects.

Prognosis and Return to Participation. After successful treatment of hyperthyroidism, many individuals will need to take lifelong thyroid replacement therapy because the gland itself may be rendered incapable of producing thyroid hormone. Patients with a history of treated hyperthyroidism must be checked annually with blood tests to determine the functional status of their thyroid. Return to full participation is generally not problematic.

Hypothyroidism

Hypothyroidism is a metabolic condition caused by a thyroid hormone deficiency. It ranks second to diabetes mellitus as the most common endocrine disorder in the United States.[30] It is more prevalent in women, and its frequency increases with age.

Of the numerous causes of hypothyroidism, 95% are classified as primary hypothyroidism. In this group, the most common is an inflammatory disorder of the thyroid gland called **Hashimoto's thyroiditis.** Hashimoto's is the most frequent cause of goiter in the United States and is characterized by a lymphocytic infiltration of the thyroid gland.[30]

Other common causes of hypothyroidism include previous treatment for hyperthyroidism, such as radioactive iodine ablation or surgery to remove the thyroid. These treatments lead to intentional destruction of the thyroid gland, which then requires supplemental thyroid hormone replacement. Medications such as lithium and interferon can cause hypothyroidism. The thyroid gland can be infiltrated by abnormal tissue caused by diseases such as sarcoidosis and **amyloidosis,** which can then result in hypothyroidism. Causes of secondary hypothyroidism include cancers of the pituitary or hypothalamus, as well as a decreased blood supply to the pituitary gland that leads to a necrosis of the gland. This necrosis of the pituitary gland is known as **Sheehan's syndrome** and is only seen in pregnant women after delivery.

Signs and Symptoms. Hypothyroidism usually presents with signs and symptoms that develop over a prolonged period and represent a slowed metabolic state. The most common symptoms include weakness, fatigue, dry or coarse skin, cold intolerance, weight gain, and swelling of the tongue leading to thickened or slurred speech (Figure 11-14). Other symptoms include coarse, dry hair; hair loss; constipation; depression; a hoarse voice; carpal tunnel syndrome; and memory impairment.[30,31]

Active patients, especially those involved with athletics, may prove particularly difficult to diagnose in the early stages of hypothyroidism because of common muscle fatigue and overuse injuries that may be attributed to delayed-onset muscle soreness.

Physical findings in hypothyroidism are nonspecific and include a bradycardia (slow heart rate), low blood pressure, hair loss—especially outer thirds of eyebrows, dry skin, and decreased reflexes.[30] The thyroid gland may feel enlarged on palpation (Box 11-10).

Referral, Diagnostic Tests, and Differential Diagnosis. An athlete who has numerous musculoskeletal complaints, does not respond to typical treatments in

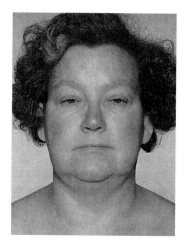

Figure 11-14 Hypothyroidism is associated with edema, puffy eyes, dry skin, and coarse hair. (From Jarvis C: *Physical examination & health assessment,* ed 4, Philadelphia, 2004, WB Saunders, p 295.)

Box 11-10 Signs and Symptoms of Hypothyroidism
The following are signs and symptoms of hypothyroidism: • Bradycardia • Cerebellar ataxia • Hearing impairment • Poor memory • Muscular weakness • Thickened tongue • Slow-moving, thick lips • Brittle or coarse hair • Hair loss, especially lateral third of eyebrow • Dry, sallow skin • Edema in the skin

an expected time frame, and experiences persistent, unexplained fatigue should be referred to a physician to rule out hypothyroidism.[31]

Because of the vague symptoms present in the initial stages of hypothyroidism, athletic trainers need to be suspicious of the possibility for this disease if no other plausible explanations exist for the symptoms. Evaluation for an elevated TSH level is the first laboratory test for hypothyroidism. In addition, Knopp and colleagues[31] suggest collecting a free T_4 level to help aid the diagnosis and differentiate between primary and secondary hypothyroidism. There are no imaging studies that aid in the diagnosis of primary hypothyroidism, but evaluation of the pituitary gland with an MRI or ultrasound is appropriate when a secondary cause is suspected.

The differential diagnosis for hypothyroidism is primarily based on the symptoms and includes depression, fibromyalgia, chronic fatigue syndrome, anemia, and viral infections such as infectious mononucleosis.

Treatment. When diagnosis is made, treatment can start with replacement of thyroid hormone with levothyroxine. The initial starting dose is based on the patient's weight, age, and other medical problems. The dose can then be titrated as needed with the goal of returning TSH levels to normal ranges. Blood samples to check the TSH levels should be drawn every 4 to 6 weeks to help with the titration. The medication is generally safe but will need to be monitored, especially in the older adults and in those with heart conditions since too much medication can elevate the heart rate and have deleterious effects on certain heart conditions.

Prognosis and Return to Participation. The prognosis and return to activity for primary hypothyroid patients is excellent because the symptoms associated with the disorder improve immensely, if not completely, with medication. Follow-up to ensure proper dosages of the levothyroxine is imperative. The prognosis for patients with secondary hypothyroidism depends on the underlying cause.

SUMMARY

Systemic disorders are not uncommon in the general population and are often accompanied by general maladies, such as body aches and fatigue. The challenge in active people is to distinguish body aches associated with increased activity from something more ominous. Persistent fatigue, body aches, weight loss, or slower than typical healing must alert the athletic trainer to conditions that may warrant referral to a physician. Many systemic disorders, once correctly diagnosed, can be effectively treated, allowing the athlete to continue participation in sports.

REFERENCES

1. American Cancer Society: Cancer facts and figures, 2004. Available at http://www.cancer.org/docroot/STT/stt_0.asp. Accessed November 2004.
2. Young G, Torestsky J, Campbell A, Eskenazi A: Recognition of common childhood malignancies, *American Family Physician* 61(7):2144-2154, 2000.

3. Ferri F: *Ferri's clinical advisor: instant diagnosis and treatment*, Philadelphia, 2004, Mosby.

4. Twist C, Link M: Assessment of lymphadenopathy in children, *Pediatric Clinics of North America* 49:1009-1025, 2002.

5. Yung L, Linch D: Hodgkin's lymphoma, *Lancet* 361: 943-951, 2003.

6. Verdon M, Sigal L: Recognition and management of Lyme disease, *American Family Physician* 56(2):439-440, 1997.

7. Edlow J: Lyme disease and related tick-borne infections, *Annals of Emergency Medicine* 30:680-693, 1999.

8. Centers for Disease Control and Prevention: Lyme disease. Available at http://www.cdc.gov/ncidod/dvbid/lyme/. Accessed November 2004.

9. Wang D, Goodman J: Joint pain and swelling: could it be Lyme arthritis? *Physician and Sportsmedicine* 25(2):320-326, 1997.

10. Anderson A: Arthropod pests and the diseases they carry: prevention in community and athletic settings, *Athletic Therapy Today* 9(3):16-21, 2004.

11. Murphy-Ende K, Chernecky C: Assessing adults with leukemia, *Nurse Practitioner* 27(11):49-60, 2002.

12. Rudy D, Zdon M: Update on colorectal cancer, *American Family Physician* 61(6):1759-1770, 1773-1774, 2000.

13. *Professional guide to diseases*, ed 7, Springhouse, Pa, 2001, Springhouse.

14. Klein-Gitelman M, Reiff A, Silverman E: Systemic lupus erythematosus in childhood, *Rheumatic Diseases Clinics of North America* 28(3):561-577, 2002.

15. Petri M: Treatment of systemic lupus erythematosus: an update, *American Family Physician* 57(11):2753-2760, 1998.

16. Gremillion R: Fibromyalgia: recognizing and treating an elusive syndrome, *Physician and Sportsmedicine* 26(4):55, 1998.

17. Millea P, Holloway R: Treating fibromyalgia, *American Family Physician* 62(7):1575-1582, 2000.

18. Wolfe F, Smythe H, Yunus M, et al: The American College of Rheumatology 1990 criteria of classification of fibromyalgia. Report of the Multicenter Criteria Committee, *Arthritis & Rheumatism* 33(2):160-172, 1990.

19. Goldenberg D: Office management of fibromyalgia, *Rheumatic Diseases Clinics of North America* 28(2):437-446, 2002.

20. Craig T, Kakumanu S: Chronic fatigue syndrome: evaluation and treatment, *American Family Physician* 65(6):1083-1090, 2002.

21. Epstein O, Perkin DF, Cookson J, de Bono DP: *Clinical examination*, ed 3, Philadelphia, 2003, Mosby.

22. American Diabetes Association: All about diabetes. Available at http://www.diabetes.org/about-diabetes.jsp. Accessed November 2004.

23. Draznin M: Type I diabetes and sports participation: strategies for training and competing safely, *Physician and Sportsmedicine* 28(1):49-56, 2000.

24. Birrer R, Sedaghat V: Exercise and diabetes mellitus: optimizing performance with patients who have type I diabetes, *Physician and Sportsmedicine* 31(5):85-86, 2003.

25. Colberg S, Swain D: Exercise and diabetes control: a winning combination, *Physician and Sportsmedicine* 28(4): 63-81, 2000.

26. American Diabetic Association: Report of the Expert Committee on the Diagnosis and Classification of Diabetes Mellitus Expert Committee on the Diagnosis and Classification of Diabetes Mellitus, *Diabetes Care* 26: S5-S20, 2003.

27. Birrer RB, Sedaghat VD: Exercise and diabetes mellitus, optimizing performance in patients who have type 1 diabetes, *Physician and Sportsmedicine*, 31(5): 29-33, 37-41, 2003.

28. Beers MH, Berkow R, editors: *The Merck manual of diagnosis and therapy*, ed 17, Whitehouse Station, NJ, 1999, Merck Research Laboratories.

29. Wang D, Koehler S, Mariash C: Detecting Graves' disease: presentations in young athletes, *Physician and Sportsmedicine* 24(12):35, 1996.

30. Hueston W: Treatment of hypothyroidism, *American Family Physician* 64(10):1717-1724, 2001.

31. Knopp W, Bohm M, McCoy J: Hypothyroidism presenting as tendonitis, *Physician and Sportsmedicine* 25(1): 47, 1997.

CHAPTER 12

Infectious Diseases

Katie M. Walsh

OBJECTIVES

At the completion of this chapter, the reader should be able to do the following:

1. Understand common infection transmission routes and their prevention.
2. Realize the importance of maintaining immunization against those diseases for which there is vaccine.
3. Describe the signs and symptoms of common infectious diseases.
4. Recognize common childhood diseases and how to prevent them.
5. Appreciate the necessity of universal precautions in the prevention and transmission of infectious disease.

INTRODUCTION

In 2002 there were approximately 53 million deaths worldwide, and of these, one third were attributed to infectious disease.[1] Nearly every chapter in this text addresses an infectious condition: meningitis in the chapter on neurological disorders; sinusitis in the chapter on disorders of the ear, nose, throat, and mouth; urinary tract infection in the chapter on genitourinary and gynecological disorders; and pneumonia in the chapter on respiratory disorders. This chapter provides an overview of the infectious disease process that includes common transmission mechanisms and routes as well as preventive measures that can be used to stop the infectious cycle and protect athletes and the population at large. The conditions discussed in this chapter encompass many common childhood diseases. In addition, hepatitis, streptococcal infections, staphylococcal infections, and sexually transmitted diseases (STDs) and infections are discussed.

TRANSMISSION

Most infections arise from one of four transmission routes: airborne, direct contact, blood borne, or water and food borne.[2-5] Infectious organisms from someone who is sick can be spread via these pathways, and sanitary precautions are the most important line of defense in retarding many illnesses found in otherwise healthy adults (Key Points—Nosocomial Infections). The healthy human lives in harmony with microbial flora that protect against the invasion of disease-causing microorganisms.[6] These flora reside in specific organs of the body, such as the skin, respiratory system, and gastrointestinal tract and provide assistance in safeguarding these organs' natural environment. Certain medications can disrupt this balance, as can repeated exposure to infectious organisms in an overtrained athlete. Many flora protecting humans can also do a turnabout and invade their hosts given certain conditions. Specific disease transmission routes are discussed within the appropriate section on the disorder.

KEY POINTS
Nosocomial Infections

A nosocomial infection is one that is acquired in the athletic training room or medical facility and that is unrelated to the athlete's purpose for the visit. Many infections and illnesses discussed in this text can be acquired in the athletic training setting from other athletes or caregivers. They include influenza, sinusitis, conjunctivitis, and certain staphylococcal and streptococcal infections.

PREVENTION

Practicing universal precautions and sanitation measures (see Chapter 1) can prevent the transmission of most infectious diseases. In addition, immunization has eradicated the spread of many adult and childhood diseases, such as the MMR vaccine for measles, mumps, and rubella (Key Points—Importance of Immunization).

KEY POINTS
Records of Immunization

Immunization records with proof of vaccination against communicable diseases are required for entrance into most public schools and colleges. Recently, some colleges have required proof of vaccination against meningococcal infections that tend to affect colleges students living in dormitories.

Immunizations are also available against meningitis, and college freshmen are encouraged to take the vaccine before moving into dormitories. An annual influenza shot for those working in the field of health care, older adults, children, and those with weakened immune systems has become an important health care benchmark each fall.[7]

Some adults missed the window of opportunity for certain immunizations because they were born before these immunizations became available. For example, an effective vaccine for hepatitis B virus (HBV) was not established until 1982. Adults who were not immunized as children and who have no history of a particular disease should be vaccinated as adults, especially if they work in areas where they would be susceptible to the disease. Tables 12-1 and 12-2 provide the recommended schedules for vaccination for children and adults.

Children are no longer routinely vaccinated for smallpox because this disease has not been found in humans for more than a generation. Other communicable diseases, such as typhus, botulism, *Escherichia coli*, polio, and anthrax, are not common but are extremely dangerous if contracted.[8] The danger with rare and extinct diseases is that they do still live in some laboratories, and recent events have made many people aware that releasing these organisms could initiate global germ warfare. Since few individuals are currently

Table 12-1	Recommended Childhood Immunization Schedule
Vaccine	**Age Administered**
Hepatitis B	First dose: birth–2 mo Second dose: 1-4 mo Third dose: 6-18 mo
DPT	First dose: 15-18 mo Second dose: 11-16 yr
Influenza B	12-15 mo
Poliovirus	6-18 mo
MMR	12-15 mo Again at 11-12 yr if necessary
Varicella	12-18 mo

DPT, Diphtheria, tetanus, pertussis; *MMR*, measles, mumps, rubella.

Table 12-2	Adult Immunization Schedule*
Disease	**Indications for Immunization**
Tetanus	All adults every 10 yr
Diphtheria	All adults every 10 yr
Hepatitis A	Travelers to endemic countries; people who work with hepatitis A–infected primates; chronic liver disease; illegal drug users; homosexual men; recipients of clotting factors
Hepatitis B	Unvaccinated health care workers potentially exposed to blood; client and staff of developmentally disabled living quarters; household and sexual partners of hepatitis B patients; people with sexually transmitted diseases (STDs); travelers to countries with high incidence of hepatitis B
Influenza	Adults under 65 yr; medical personnel; pregnant women in third trimester during flu season
Meningococcal disease	College freshmen living in dorms
Pneumococcal disease	Adults under 65 yr; those with cardiovascular disease, pulmonary issues, diabetes, alcoholism, Hodgkin's lymphoma, chronic renal failure

*For adults who have had all scheduled childhood vaccines.

vaccinated against these dormant, yet deadly, diseases, their rapid spread is plausible.[8]

As previously mentioned, airborne contact and direct contact are two methods of infecting others with communicable diseases. The close surroundings of athletic huddles, time-outs, locker rooms, and team buses afford these two methods many opportunities to spread infections among team members.[2,9] Numerous precautions, however, can help prevent infections from being transmitted. The basic practices of personal hygiene are underappreciated in the fight against the spread of disease. Simple habits of frequent hand washing (Figure 12-1), covering one's mouth or nose when coughing or sneezing, showering with quality antibacterial soap, and protecting the skin, including good foot care, are all examples of personal

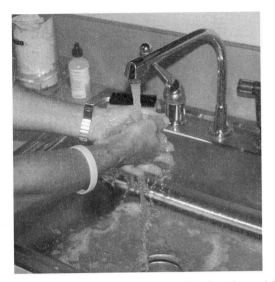

Figure 12-1 Hand washing, properly performed, is the primary defense against infection.

responsibility in hygiene.[9] Athletes with infections are isolated while contagious, and any equipment or clothing that they have worn is sanitized before the next use.

Methods of protection against disease that could affect the whole team include safeguarding the water source and containers and sanitizing surfaces that athletes have contact with, such as treatment tables, mats, and rehabilitation equipment. Certain states have regulations about the type of hose that may be used to draw potable (i.e., drinkable) water. These regulations may be found on the particular state health website or U.S. Occupational Safety and Health Administration (OSHA) website. When sanitizing equipment, surfaces, and water containers such as coolers, ice containers, and water bottles, a solution of 1 part bleach to 9 parts water is effective as a germicidal agent.[9]

Prevention of many infectious diseases discussed in this chapter is easily attainable. Compliance with preventive immunization programs when available can be followed up with good hygiene, sanitation, and practicing universal precautions.

PATHOLOGICAL CONDITIONS

Infectious Mononucleosis

Infectious mononucleosis (mono) has also been called the kissing disease because it is easily transmitted via oropharyngeal contact. Caused by the Epstein-Barr virus (EBV), mononucleosis is a common occurrence in college-aged athletes, but 50% of children have also had the infection by the age of 5 years. There is some speculation that **chronic fatigue syndrome** is

associated with a chronic EBV infection, but little evidence supports this theory.[6]

The EBV is a herpesvirus that attacks lymphocytes and nasopharyngeal cells. It is found in oropharyngeal saliva secretions of up to 50% of healthy, nonsymptomatic adults.[10] Ninety percent of adults over the age of 50 years have serological evidence of the disease, but few have had a full clinical presentation.[11] Although a tainted blood transfusion is not a common transmission pathway for EBV, it is possible.[10] Despite its reputation as the kissing disease only 5% of patients have a recent history of contact with an infected person, and it is not a particularly contagious disease. For reported direct exposure, the incubation period is 10 to 50 days.[11] Nevertheless, athletes are warned to avoid sharing drinking cups and putting their mouths on common water bottle spouts.

Signs and Symptoms

The chief signs and symptoms of infectious mononucleosis consist of fatigue, pharyngitis, fever, and **lymphadenopathy,** but not all signs and symptoms are present in every patient. Often the first complaint is overwhelming fatigue and the inability to get enough sleep (Figure 12-2). The athlete will feel run down or experience sore throat symptoms. Other manifestations include hepatitis, renal failure, pulmonary involvement, cough, encephalitis, dyspnea, and a maculopapular rash.[12]

Splenomegaly, or an enlarged spleen, is a worrisome side effect of mononucleosis; the spleen is forced down from its generally protected space behind the rib cage and is readily palpated during the course of the disease (Red Flags—Splenomegaly). Splenomegaly is present

> **⊘ Red Flags for Splenomegaly**
>
> Splenomegaly is a possible side effect of mononucleosis, which causes the spleen to protrude out from under the normal protection of the lower left ribs. Unprotected, the spleen is susceptible to injury and rupture from athletic activity. An unrecognized ruptured spleen is life threatening.

in 50% of cases and is most prevalent in the second and third weeks of the disease.[6] When enlarged, the spleen is more susceptible to injury, since swelling causes it to protrude below the left costal margin (Figure 12-3). A blow to the left ribs in an athlete with splenomegaly can rupture the spleen, causing a life-threatening emergency if the injury is not quickly recognized and treated.

Although 10% of patients experience hepatomegaly, or an enlarged liver, with infectious mononucleosis, it does not carry the severe ramifications that splenomegaly does in athletics.[11] There are hepatic complications, however, because hepatocellular enzyme levels are elevated two to three times normal in 95% of patients

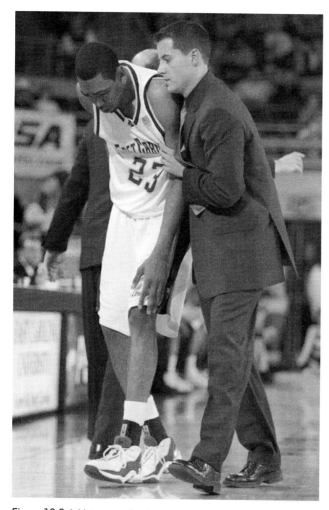

Figure 12-2 Athletes experiencing overwhelming fatigue or a run-down feeling need referral to a physician for evaluation to rule out underlying illnesses or diseases.

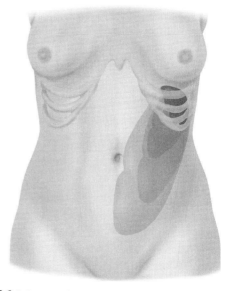

Figure 12-3 Splenomegaly, an enlargement of the spleen, is sometimes associated with acute infections, such as mononucleosis. (From Jarvis C: *Physical examination & health assessment,* ed 4, Philadelphia, 2004, WB Saunders, p 599.)

and can take as long as 1 month to return to preinfection rates.

Other potential complications are related to the central nervous system (CNS), including seizures, peripheral neuropathy, aseptic meningitis, cranial nerve palsy, and Guillain-Barré syndrome.

Referral, Diagnostic Tests, and Differential Diagnosis

An athlete who presents with a history of **malaise** combined with a sore throat and a fever should be referred to a physician, especially if the symptoms are present for a number of days.

Athletes suspected of having infectious mononucleosis will often present with mild **leukocytosis,** which is also common in a number of other illnesses.[6] Specifically, a strong indicator for EBV includes a blood count representing **lymphocytosis** of 50% or greater including at least 10% atypical cells.[10,11]

A more specific blood test, the Monospot, is based on agglutination, or clumping, of erythrocytes. This test is

reliable in up to 90% of patients and is usually positive within 4 weeks of onset.[11,12] False-positive Monospot tests can occur in other diseases, such as lymphoma, autoimmune disease, and hepatitis.[13]

Group A beta-hemolytic streptococci, cytomegalovirus (CMV), hepatitis B, rubella, and primary human immunodeficiency virus (HIV) infection are all options to consider and rule out when diagnosing mononucleosis.

Treatment

The standard treatment for mononucleosis is rest and hydration although complete bed rest is not recommended.[13] More than 95% of patients recover with symptomatic treatment alone.[12]

Research has shown that there is no specific pharmacological treatment promoting recovery from infectious mononucleosis.[6] However, if the pharyngitis is such that it warrants medication, corticosteroids have been shown to relieve pain and prevent airway compromise from swelling. To assist in the management of body aches and fever, acetaminophen is preferred over aspirin because of aspirin's association with **Reye's syndrome.**[6] In addition, athletes would be wise to avoid prolonged use of nonsteroidal antiinflammatory drugs (NSAIDs) during the illness because of hepatic complications already associated with mononucleosis.

Prognosis, Return to Participation, and Prevention

Infectious mononucleosis is a self-limiting disease associated with obvious symptoms for 2 weeks to 2 months; the most acute phase lasts 2 weeks. Research shows that

20% of military and university patients return within 1 week, and 50% return within 2 weeks.[6] In athletics, special care must be taken to be sure the athlete is reconditioned for sport before full return. Athletes involved in contact or collision sports may need 1 month or more to recover sufficiently to allow the spleen to again fit behind the rib cage for adequate protection. Physicians need to consider each athlete individually along with the sport involved before allowing full return to activity. Whereas a swimmer may return to full activity rather quickly, a diver may still be in danger of spleen injury with a premature return to activity.

Mononucleosis has a mortality rate of less than 1% because of complications from the disease, namely encephalitis, splenic rupture, or airway obstruction from severe pharyngitis.[6] It is prevented by proper hygiene and not sharing eating or drinking dishes or materials with infected people. Infectious mononucleosis is not a nationally reportable disease.

Mumps

Mumps is a contagious viral disease that manifests with enlarged parotid and salivary glands and on occasion involves the sublingual or submaxillary glands as well. It presents as an acute epidemic that peaks in late winter or early spring and chiefly involves 5- to 15-year-old children. Children younger than 2 years are typically immune.[6]

Mumps has a 2- to 3-week incubation period and is spread through the air via infected droplets as well as through direct contact with contaminated saliva. It has been found in saliva 1 to 6 days before onset and up to 9 days after glandular swelling. It has also been found in the urine 6 days before **parotitis** (i.e., inflammation of the parotid salivary glands) and 15 days afterward. In addition, the virus may be isolated in symptomatic patients' blood.[6]

Signs and Symptoms

The chief signs and symptoms of mumps include parotitis, headache, low-grade fever, malaise, anorexia, vomiting, and **nuchal rigidity** in the posterior neck. Common symptoms also include pain with chewing and swallowing, especially swallowing acidic drinks or foods such as orange juice, pickles, or lemons. Within 24 hours of onset of the aforementioned signs and symptoms, the parotid glands swell and become sensitive to palpation (Figure 12-4). Initially, is it not unusual for only one gland to become swollen, with the second following about 2 days later.[14] An athlete generally presents with asymmetry in the face and jaw caused by the unilateral swelling of the parotid gland. The enlargement of the glands can extend from in front of to below

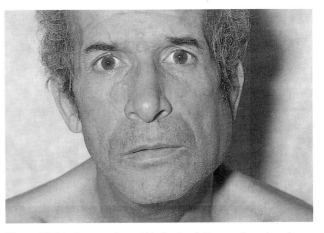

Figure 12-4 Salivary and parotid glands of the mouth and neck can become rapidly and painfully inflamed as a result of mumps; note the swelling anterior to the lower ear lobe. (From Jarvis C: *Physical examination & health assessment,* ed 4, Philadelphia, 2004, WB Saunders, p 292.)

the ear, and the associated skin can become tight and shiny because of the pressure of the swelling.[6]

The complications of mumps include orchitis, oophoritis, **meningoencephalitis,** and pancreatitis. Postpubertal males may experience testicular inflammation, which is typically unilateral. Although this can occur in 20% to 30% of the adult males with mumps, it is rarely associated with infertility, but it can lead to testicular atrophy in 50% of the cases.[10] Epididymitis precedes **orchitis** in 85% of the cases.[15]

In females, **oophoritis** occurs in 50% of postpubertal women and is more difficult to diagnose yet rarely results in fertility issues.[15] Exposure to mumps within the first trimester of pregnancy may induce spontaneous abortion.[1]

Because the patient with mumps has a headache, stiff neck, and sometime low (20 to 40 mg/dl) cerebrospinal fluid (CSF) glucose levels, it is often mistaken for bacterial meningitis. Fifty percent of the patients affected have the mumps infection of the CNS, but only 1% to 10% manifest symptoms. Although permanent damage such as deafness or facial paralysis is unusual, it may result from mumps with CNS involvement.[6] Another rare association with mumps is encephalitis, which is more serious than viral meningitis.[14] Encephalitis is thought to be an autoimmune response producing demyelination and has an onset 7 to 10 days following parotitis.

Referral, Diagnostic Tests, and Differential Diagnosis

Athletes who present with swollen saliva glands, malaise, or a low-grade fever are referred to a physician. The diagnosis is largely based on signs and symptoms coupled with a history of recent exposure. Atypical presentations require laboratory confirmation, usually by culturing the mumps virus or discovering the mumps immunoglobulin M (IgM) antibody.[1]

The differential diagnoses for mumps include streptococcal throat infection, diphtheria, dental caries, typhoid, influenza A, diabetes mellitus, **Mikulicz's syndrome,** leukemia, **lymphosarcoma,** malignant and benign tumors of the salivary glands, and an obstructed duct in the parotid gland.

Treatment, Prognosis, and Return to Participation

An athlete with mumps should be isolated from others until parotid swelling returns to normal. Treatment of the disease is based on the athlete's symptoms. The athlete uses over-the-counter analgesics or antipyretics as necessary to alleviate headache and fever and avoids acidic foods and beverages, maintaining a soft diet to lessen **mastication.** Because mumps is typically a self-limited disease, most patients recover without pharmacological intervention.[16]

Because most of the symptoms (e.g., fever, malaise, vomiting, nuchal rigidity, parotitis) seem to resolve within 3 to 10 days, long-term absence from athletic participation is not typical. Of greater importance is the prevention of spread of infection.

Prevention

A vaccine for mumps is available that entails only one injection and causes little systemic reaction. The live virus vaccine was introduced in the United States in 1967 as either a single dose or in combination with rubella and measles (MMR) viruses. It is generally administered anytime after the first year of life but most typically between 12 to 15 months of age.[10] Current recommendations suggest a second dose between ages 4 and 6 years. This childhood vaccination is intended to be lifelong, but no studies have supported this claim. Postexposure vaccination will not necessarily prevent subsequent onset from that exposure.[6]

Rubeola

Also known simply as "measles" or "red measles," **rubeola** is one of the most highly communicable infectious diseases. Before immunization was available, more than 90% of the population was infected by the age of 20 years.[10] Following immunization, measles cases have dropped 99%, with the residual attributed to unimmunized or underimmunized children who have had only one shot.

Measles is spread through airborne droplets via nasal or throat secretions of infected people. A lesser means of transmission is through direct contact with soiled articles such as towels, which may contain secretions from those already sick. The incubation period is typically 10 days but can range from 7 to 18 days.[10] Measles is most contagious just before the rash erupts through 4 days following eruption.

Signs and Symptoms

Most often, a rash is the manifestation of the disease, and it appears following a **prodromal** fever, most often in the third to seventh day of the disease. The erythematous rash begins on the face before spreading to the body proper and lasts approximately 4 to 7 days (Figure 12-5). The athlete is contagious before eruption of the rash and for up to 4 days following the rash appearance. Other signs and symptoms of measles include conjunctivitis, cough, leukopenia, headache, fever, and sore throat. **Leukopenia** will be present beginning with the onset of the rash largely because of a decrease in lymphocytes.[1] Complications arising from the disease include otitis media, pneumonia, encephalitis, diarrhea, and laryngotracheobronchitis, or croup.[10]

Referral, Diagnostic Tests, and Differential Diagnosis

Athletes with a rash indicative of measles are referred for further evaluation. Likewise, athletes with signs or symptoms of measles before the onset of the rash, such as sore throat, fever, cough, conjunctivitis, or recent exposure, need to be referred to a physician. A recent history of measles vaccine does not preclude one from contracting measles. Therefore a recently immunized athlete who shows signs or symptoms of the disease needs to be referred immediately to a physician.

A specific diagnosis of measles can be confirmed by presence of a certain IgM antibody in the blood,

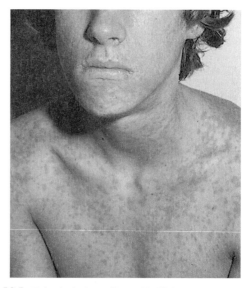

Figure 12-5 Rubeola lesions. (From Zitelli BJ, Davis HW: *Atlas of pediatric physical diagnosis,* ed 3, St Louis, 1997, Mosby.)

which presents itself 3 to 4 days following onset of the measles rash. A nasopharyngeal swab is also used to identify the antigen but is less common than the blood test.

Many childhood diseases have similar presentations and are often the differential diagnoses of each other. Table 12-3 compares several childhood diseases. Specific differential diagnoses for rubeola are rubella, mononucleosis, influenza, Rocky Mountain spotted fever, and allergic rhinitis.

Treatment, Prognosis, and Return to Participation

Because no antiviral remedy for measles is currently available, the best treatment is supportive and symptomatic care. Rubeola is largely a self-limiting disease, but analgesics and antipyretics may help alleviate symptoms associated with the illness.[16] If the patient has accompanying bacterial complications, such as conjunctivitis, otitis, sinusitis, or pneumonia, antibacterial therapy may be warranted.

Mortality rates for measles are low, but pneumonia and encephalitis are complications of the disease in children under the age of 5 years. For athletes, activity during the contagious stages is discouraged.

Prevention and Public Health Implications

Individuals born after 1957 are encouraged to be immunized for measles. A single injection of the live measles virus is often administered in conjunction with two other live viruses, mumps and rubella, and reduces susceptibility to measles by 94% to 98%, whereas a second dose may elevate immunity to 99%.[1,6,16] The two-dose vaccine is recommended to ameliorate the possibility of immunization failure. Most often, the MMR initial dose is given at 12 to 15 months of age, with the second dose administered at the onset of school (4 to 6 years), although if

exposure risk is high, the second dose can be delivered as soon as 4 weeks following the first.

Measles is defined as a class 2A reportable disease. Reporting to the local agency as early as within 24 hours of diagnosis can provide greater control over the spread of the disease. Typically, patients are not quarantined, but isolating school-aged children and athletes while contagious is advisable.

Rubella

Rubella, also known as German measles, is an acute contagious virus that has mild symptoms in children and adults but can cause death or profound congenital defects in infants born to mothers infected during the first trimester of pregnancy.

Rubella is acquired through the upper respiratory tract or through placental blood exchange with a mother infected in early pregnancy. Exposure to rubella during pregnancy can cause abortion or stillbirths or profoundly affect the fetus.[13] Congenitally acquired rubella can result in deafness in 85% of children, intrauterine growth restriction (70%), **retinopathy** (35%), in utero death (20%), mental retardation (up to 20%), behavior disorders (20%), bone radiolucencies (10% to 20%), diabetes mellitus (up to 20% by age 35 years), and cardiac defects.[15] Obviously, great care must be taken to ensure pregnant women are safeguarded from exposure (Red Flags—Rubella).

> **▶ Red Flags for Rubella**
>
> Rubella is profoundly dangerous to expectant mothers because exposure during the first trimester of pregnancy can cause the following for the fetus:
> - Abortion
> - Intrauterine death
> - Stillbirth
> - Intrauterine growth retardation
> - Mental retardation
> - Behavior disorders
> - Bone radiolucencies
> - Diabetes mellitus
> - Cardiac defects

Signs and Symptoms

Rubella has a 12- to 24-day incubation period, and infected patients present with low-grade fever that is often transient, a mild rash, lymphadenopathy, conjunctivitis, cough, headache, and joint pain (i.e., arthralgia). The rash usually lasts about 3 days and is a blotchy eruption that has its origin on the face and spreads to the trunk and limbs (Figure 12-6).[15] At the onset of the rash, the patient appears to have a brightly flushed face that may be mistaken for scarlet fever. Mild rose-colored spots may appear on the palate; and although the pharynx may be bright red, the throat is

Table 12-3	Comparison of Childhood Infectious Diseases		
Disease	Incubation	Transmission	Duration of Symptoms
Mononucleosis	2-3 wk	Saliva, air droplets	Up to several months
Mumps	2-3 wk	Air droplets, saliva	Up to 10 days
Rubeola	1-2 wk	Airborne, direct contact	4-7 days
Rubella	2-3 wk	Respiratory secretions, placental blood	3 days
Varicella	2-3 wk	Direct contact, respiratory secretions	1 wk

not typically sore. Swelling of specific glands, including the suboccipal, postauricular, and postcervical, precedes the rash by 5 to 10 days and may be first noted when washing hair or putting on a helmet.[12] On occasion, the patient has splenomegaly and hepatitis in conjunction with the rash. Arthritis can be involved as a complication, especially in adult females.[10]

Referral, Diagnostic Tests, and Differential Diagnosis

Any unimmunized athlete with a history of exposure to rubella who presents with symptoms of the disease is referred to a physician for confirmation. Diagnosis of rubella is often made on the basis of the combination of glandular swelling and onset of facial rash. A history of immunization or recent exposure may expedite disease confirmation or rule it out. Serological testing

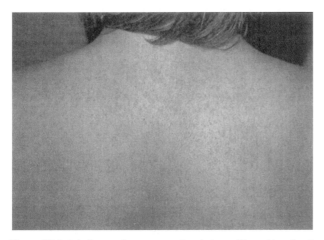

Figure 12-6 Rubella, or German measles, lesions. (From Hurwitz S: *Clinical pediatric dermatology: a textbook of skin disorders of childhood and adolescence,* ed 2, Philadelphia, 1993, WB Saunders, p 356.)

can confirm the disease by a fourfold increase in specific antibodies.[6]

Differential diagnoses of rubella include allergic reactions, scarlet fever, secondary syphilis, infectious mononuclear viral infections, and **Kawasaki disease.**

Treatment, Prognosis, and Return to Participation

There is no known antiviral treatment for rubella after the disease is present. Most patients do well with supportive care.

Rubella is a mild illness, and symptoms rarely last more than 3 to 4 days.[12] However, the athlete is contagious from the seventh day of exposure through the twenty-first day after the last known exposure and should be isolated from pregnant women.

Prevention and Public Health Implications

The MMR immunization provides protective antibodies to 90% to 95% of those immunized at 1 year of age, with 99% protected by the second vaccination. Also, adult women should practice birth control for at least 3 months following administration of the vaccine.[12] Congenital rubella has been a reportable disease in the United States since 1966.

Chickenpox and Shingles

Chickenpox, or varicella, is a viral, readily communicable disease (Figure 12-7, *A*). It is one of the most common childhood diseases, and children tend to contract the disease before beginning school.[1] Ninety percent of cases of varicella happen within 10 to 20 days of exposure.

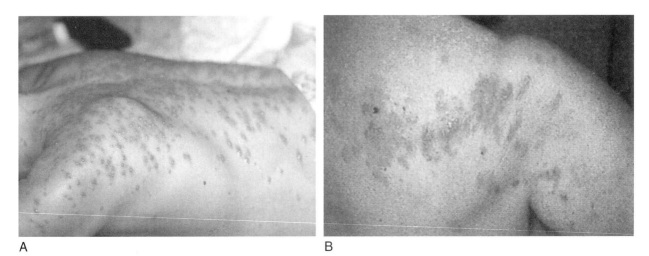

A   B

Figure 12-7 A, Varicella, or chickenpox, lesions. **B,** Herpes zoster, or shingles, lesions. (**A** from McKinney ES, Ashwill JW, Murray SS, et al: *Maternal-child nursing,* Philadelphia, 2000, WB Saunders, p 1043; **B** from Moschella SL, Hurley HJ: *Dermatology,* ed 3, Philadelphia, 1992, WB Saunders, p 219.)

Shingles, also known as herpes zoster (Figure 12-7, *B*), is a reactivation of varicella disease in the dorsal ganglia. Both diseases are problematic to the **immunosuppressed** patient. Ninety percent of unvaccinated contacts become infected, making varicella an extremely contagious disease to the unprotected individual.[15]

Although both varicella and zoster have similar methods of transmission, varicella is much more contagious. These infections are spread by direct person-to-person contact; by respiratory secretions, which are seen in varicella only; by direct contact with vesicle fluid; or indirectly via vesicle fluid on soiled articles (e.g., towels or jerseys). Scabs themselves are not transmittable sources of the infection.

Signs and Symptoms

Chickenpox begins rapidly with a headache and a **maculopapular rash** that gives rise to vesicles within hours of onset. The subsequent vesicles last 3 to 4 days and represent the time of highest contagiousness. Whereas lesions may occur anywhere on the body, they tend to cluster on covered, rather than exposed, parts of the body. Lesions begin on the trunk and face, eventually spreading to the extremities; but it is also common to find lesions on the scalp, buccal mucous membrane, conjunctiva, and axilla. Other findings include fever, chills, malaise, and backache.[15]

As with chickenpox, herpes zoster presents with a vesicular rash. However, in zoster, these vesicles follow one or more sensory nerve roots. They give rise to patterns following specific dermatomes and most often are unilateral (see Box 8-2). In zoster patients, severe pain and paresthesia along the rash increase with the age of the patient.

Patients are typically contagious from a few days before the rash until the vesicles have scabbed over.

Referral, Diagnostic Tests, and Differential Diagnosis

The initial presentation of chickenpox is a headache, fever, chills, and the ensuing rash. Symptoms tend to be more severe in adults, and intense pruritus accompanies the rash. Athletes who present with these complaints are referred to a physician. In general, laboratory tests are not warranted, but a complete blood count (CBC) may reveal leukopenia and **thrombocytopenia**.[15] The differential diagnoses for varicella and zoster include impetigo, scabies, urticaria, smallpox, and an allergic drug rash.[15]

Treatment

The drugs vidarabine and acyclovir are both used to treat varicella and herpes zoster, but acyclovir is considered the preferred treatment for varicella. If acyclovir is administered within 24 hours of initial rash, it alleviates and shortens symptoms associated with the diseases. Other treatments for varicella combat pruritus and superinfection.[16] Simple calamine lotion is an excellent agent to diminish itching associated with this disease, as is a colloidal starch bath.

Prognosis and Return to Participation

Athletes may return to sport activity when fully asymptomatic and engage in noncontact (and nonswimming) activities as long as they have no vesicles and feel good. Activities in the water should be avoided until athletes are cleared by a physician.

Prevention and Public Health Implications

In 1995, the varicella virus vaccine (Varivax) was recommended as a single dose to protect children aged 12 to 18 months and for immunization of children up to 12 years old. Studies have demonstrated that this one-time immunization has an effectiveness of 70% to 90% complete prevention and 100% prevention of moderate to severe outbreak.[10] Immunization within 3 days of exposure will lessen symptoms and duration of the disease

Varicella is not a reportable disease, but varicella-related deaths are reportable under class 3A as of 1999.[10] Affected children must be isolated from school, the public, and medical offices until the lesions have scabbed over. Likewise, adults must not have contact with others until their vesicles dry. Extra caution is maintained with athletes involved in contact or collision sports because vesicles can "unroof" and secrete fluid infected with the virus.

Hepatitis A to D

The liver is the largest organ in the body and functions primarily as the central organ of glucose homeostasis. It lies protected chiefly by the lower right ribs in the upper right abdominal cavity (Figure 12-8). This four-lobe organ secrets bile to facilitate digestion of fats and has metabolic functions as well. The liver also assists in amino acid and carbohydrate metabolism, fat-soluble vitamin storage (A, D, E, K), phagocytosis, and detoxification of potentially harmful substances. Damage to the liver has profound repercussions to many body functions.

Hepatitis literally translated means inflammation of the liver, and in particular it is characterized by diffuse necrosis affecting the smallest secretory units of the liver.[6,17] The many varieties of the disease are differentiated by letters, mechanisms of acquisition, and lasting sequelae. Table 12-4 compares the common hepatitis viruses. In 2002, more than 50,000 new cases of hepatitis

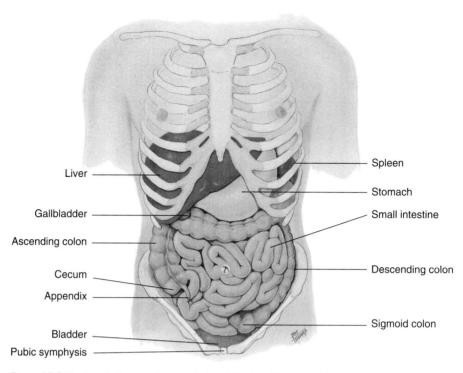

Figure 12-8 The liver in its normal anatomical position is well protected by the lower right ribs. (From Jarvis C: *Physical examination & health assessment,* ed 4, Philadelphia, 2004, WB Saunders, p 563.)

Table 12-4   Comparison of Hepatitis Viruses

Disease	Incubation	Transmission	Notes
Hepatitis A	30 days	Oral-fecal contact; crowding; poor sanitation; contaminated food or water	Clinical illness more severe in adults than children
Hepatitis B	6 wk–6 mo (average 12-14 wk)	Infected blood and blood products; sexual contact; virus is present in saliva, semen, and vaginal secretions	Chronic HBV is a high risk for cirrhosis and liver cancers
Hepatitis C	6-7 wk	Intravenous drug use, body piercing, multiple sex partners	High coinfection with HIV patients; highest mortality
Hepatitis D	30-150 days	In the United States, primarily intravenous drug users	Best prevented via HBV vaccine

HBV, Hepatitis B; *HIV,* human immunodeficiency virus.

were reported in the United States; 32% were hepatitis A (HAV), 43% hepatitis B (HBV), 21% hepatitis C (HCV), and 4% unidentified.[18] The emphasis here is on hepatitis A, B, C, and D; hepatitis E and hepatitis G typically do not affect the athletic population, occurring more often in endemic countries or **immunocompromised** patients.

In general, hepatitis can be caused by certain bacteria or viruses in addition to some drugs, toxins, and excessive alcohol abuse. Hepatitis A and hepatitis E are infectious and highly contagious forms of the disease associated with poor sanitation and fecal-oral transmission. Hepatitis B, hepatitis C, and hepatitis D are varieties of serum hepatitis and transmitted via parenteral (i.e., blood) or sexual contact; these forms can lead to chronic conditions.[19]

Signs and Symptoms

Viral hepatitis has an incubation period of 2 weeks to 6 months and has several phases, each marked by specific signs and symptoms. In the prodromal stage, the athlete could experience malaise, fatigue, upper respiratory infection (URI), anorexia, nausea and vomiting, mild abdominal pain, myalgia, or arthralgia. Some patients have accompanying headaches, fever, and a rash. When jaundice occurs, it typically manifests 5 to 10 days after the prodromal symptoms present and peaks within 1 or 2 weeks. Following the jaundice, a 2- to 4-week recovery phase is marked by a state of well-being, return of appetite, and disappearance of fatigue and pain. General recovery is based on the specific virus, but the acute illness typically subsides within 2 to 3 weeks. Some patients have few of these signs but instead experience a lingering, unexplainable fatigue.

Referral, Diagnostic Tests, and Differential Diagnosis

Athletes with unexplainable fatigue are referred to a physician for further evaluation. Physical findings include an enlarged liver and jaundice, but, if this occurs, it is later in the progression of the disease. Blood and urine tests will reveal a normal to low white blood cell (WBC) count, mild proteinuria, and bilirubinuria in patients with jaundice.[1,21]

Differential diagnoses may include EBV, herpes simplex, URI, influenza, and infectious mononucleosis.

Treatment

Hepatitis typically resolves spontaneously within 4 to 8 weeks but can have lasting sequelae. Until the patient has completely recovered, alcohol is avoided and sex partners are limited. To prevent possible spread of the disease, household members receive immune globulin and initiation of vaccine as appropriate.[1] Physician follow-up of hepatitis requires thorough management to ensure complete resolution of the disease.

Prognosis and Return to Participation

HCV is the most likely hepatitis virus to fluctuate for several months or years, and HBV is more likely to have a higher mortality rate than HAV or HCV. Chronic hepatitis occurs more often with HBV; 5% to 10% of patients have persistent inflammation and cirrhosis and are subclinical chronic carriers.[6]

Athletes who participate in collision sports may need additional laboratory tests to determine any residual effects of the disease before resuming full activity of the sport.

Prevention and Public Health Implications

HAV and HBV can be prevented by vaccine and good personal sanitation measures, such as hand washing following bowel movements and after contact with contaminated linens, clothing, patients, or utensils.[20] The athletic trainer must routinely adhere to universal precautions when working with athletes with open wounds or cleaning up body fluid spills. In addition, sexually transmitted hepatitis can be prevented by using prophylactic barriers.

All cases of acute hepatitis need to be reported to local or state health agencies following diagnosis.[1]

Hepatitis A

In the United States, approximately 30% of the population have serological evidence of previous infection with HAV.[12,13] HAV is caused almost exclusively by poor sanitation because it is transmitted via the oral-fecal contact. Outbreaks occur most often in crowded areas and through contaminated food or water. Transmission of HAV through food is typically via milk, sliced meat, shellfish, and salads. HAV is the only hepatitis infection accompanied by a high fever, yet two thirds of the cases are asymptomatic. Although the acute phase of the disease lasts up to 3 weeks, the convalescence is prolonged.[14] HAV is a self-limiting disease that rarely causes death.

Hepatitis B

HBV is a hearty virus that can live an extended time outside the human host. It is approximately 100 times easier to contract than human immunodeficiency virus (HIV).[20] The chronic version of the disease affects nearly 400 million people worldwide[12] and has been demonstrated to be transmitted among football players and sumo wrestlers.[5,21] Those infected with HBV include 33% who have severe hepatitis and 5% to 10% who become chronically infected with the virus.[22] Complications of chronic HBV can lead to cirrhosis or liver cancer. The 1982 licensure of the HBV vaccine has made a considerable difference in the spread of HBV (Key Points—Hepatitis B Immunization); in 1996, the

---

KEY POINTS
Hepatitis B Immunization

Hepatitis B vaccine is given as a series of three shots over 9 months and is highly recommended for all health care workers.

United States recommended vaccination to adolescents who missed the immunization as a child.[23-27]

Transmission of HBV is primarily via sexual activity, with 33% acquired through heterosexual activity and 17% by homosexual activity.[20] High-risk activities include multiple sex partners, intravenous drug use, men who have sex with men, and piercing or tattooing.[1] HBV is spread through blood and body fluids or via the mother to her unborn child.

HBV symptoms are unremarkable, and patients are often asymptomatic. Those who develop symptoms will see their symptoms resolve over 4 to 6 months.[13] Individuals with HBV and HCV, however, are more susceptible to chronic infection, cirrhosis, and liver cancer than those with other types of hepatitis.[15]

Most athletes in noncontact sports who contract acute HBV are allowed to participate in athletics depending on clinical signs and symptoms. In the absence of fever or fatigue, there is no evidence that intense training is contraindicated.[22] In close-contact sports, such as wrestling or boxing, however, athletes with acute HBV need to refrain from participation until they are not infectious.[22] The risk of transmission to others is very limited, but it is a higher risk than with HIV.[4,5,21, 28-30] As a precaution against infecting others, athletes who develop chronic HBV should not participate in close-contact, combative sports.[22,29]

Hepatitis C

Although HCV is less prevalent than HBV, approximately 50% to 84% of the patients remain chronic carriers of the virus.[14,15] HCV is a dangerous variety of the virus and the cause of liver disorders. Close to 20% of chronic HCV carriers will develop cirrhosis over 20 to 30 years; of these cases, up to 2.5% will also develop hepatocellular carcinoma.[15]

Common transmission routes for HCV come from injection drug use (60%) or multiple sex partners (15% to 20%); the remainder comes from needle sticks, maternal-infant transmission, or unknown etiology.[21] Coinfection with HIV occurs in 30% to 50% of HCV patients.[1,12] Currently, there is no known prevention for HCV other than avoidance of at-risk behaviors.

Hepatitis D

HDV, or delta virus, is linked to HBV and therefore is similar in nature to the B virus. It is sexually transmitted and associated with injected drug use. Those at particular risk are the recipients of blood products, health care workers handling needles, and chronic carriers of HBV.[21] As a separate disease, HDV presents with more severe symptoms and has a 2% to 20% mortality rate.[14] HDV patients are more prone to develop chronic versions of hepatitis and eventually liver cirrhosis. HBV immunization also prevents HDV disease.

Streptococcal Infections

Streptococci (strep) are small, spherical, gram-positive chains of bacteria found quite often in human tissue as a normal state. Various types of streptococci are typically found in the gastrointestinal tract, throat, respiratory system, vagina, and skin. It is important to note that the presence of bacteria does not in itself indicate a streptococcal infection. These infections are, however, among the most common, yet dangerous infections known to humans. Table 12-5 compares the various streptococcal bacteria, their normal habitat, and related illnesses.

Streptococcal infections are a group of microbially similar pathogens that have unique characteristics. They are categorized into groups A, B, C, D, and G, with groups A, B, and D being most common (Box 12-1). Certain streptococci in groups C and G are resistant to bacitracin therapy and are naturally found in human intestinal tract, skin, pharynx, and vagina. These can attack their host and cause a variety of problematical responses, including pneumonia, cellulitis, impetigo, sepsis, and pharyngitis. This chapter provides an overview of groups A, B, and D; most common streptococcal infections are discussed in chapters covering the system related to infection.

As a class, streptococcal infections have three states of infection: carrier or nonactive, acute, and delayed nonsuppurative complications.[31] The term **carrier state** is used to refer to the presence of streptococci in tissues that have no sign of infection, although this term is usually specific to the vagina and pharynx. Those with acute infections show physical signs of streptococcal bacteria invading tissues, and the delayed state becomes apparent approximately 2 weeks after an overt streptococcal infection.

Group A Streptococcal Infections

Infections and diseases caused by group A beta-hemolytic streptococci (*Streptococcus pyogenes*) fall into two categories: suppurative and nonsuppurative.[17] **Suppurative** infections are derived from invading bacteria that produce necrosis and cause acute inflammation, whereas **nonsuppurative** diseases occur in tissues remote from the original bacterial attack. Examples of the former are tonsillitis, streptococcal pharyngitis (i.e., strep throat), impetigo, myositis, pneumonia, toxic shock syndrome, and cellulitis. Nonsuppurative infections include rheumatic fever and acute poststreptococcal glomerulonephritis.

Table 12-5	Comparison of Streptococcal Infections	
Bacterium	**Normal Location**	**Diseases or Illnesses Caused**
Streptococcus agalactiae	Raw milk	Meningitis in newborns, endometritis and fever in postpartum women
Streptococcus bovis	Alimentary tract of cattle	Endocarditis
Streptococcus equisimilis	Upper respiratory tract	Pneumonia, osteomyelitis, endocarditis, bacteremia
Streptococcus mutans	In dental cavities	Dental caries, endocarditis
Streptococcus pneumoniae	Has more than 80 serological varieties	Pneumonia, meningitis, conjunctivitis, endocarditis, periodontitis, otitis media, septic arthritis, osteomyelitis
Streptococcus pyogenes	Group A beta-hemolytic streptococci	Scarlet fever, septic sore throat
Streptococcus viridans	Upper respiratory tract	Endocarditis

Box 12-1	Categories of Common Streptococcal Infections
Group	**Common Streptococcal Infections**
A	Pharyngitis, impetigo, wound infections, rheumatic fever, scarlet fever, necrotizing fasciitis
B	Neonatal, maternal, and cutaneous infections in persons with diabetes
C and G	Respiratory infections, pneumonia, cutaneous infections
D	Bacteremia associated with gastrointestinal cancer, urinary tract infection, endocarditis, meningitis, otitis media, pneumococcal pneumonia

Recent interest in a group A streptococcal gangrene called **necrotizing fasciitis,** or "flesh-eating bacteria," has been generated because infection in previously healthy individuals can rapidly become critical, requiring hospitalization and surgical debridement of the infected skin. Other names for this affliction are hemolytic streptococcal gangrene, acute dermal gangrene, suppurative fasciitis, and synergistic necrotizing cellulitis.[31]

Necrotizing fasciitis is a rare, severe, and potentially fatal condition whereby an infection progressively invades the skin, fascia, and blood supply (Red Flags—Necrotizing Fasciitis). Although the mortality rate is as

> **Red Flags for Necrotizing Fasciitis**
>
> Necrotizing fasciitis has a mortality rate as high as 80%. Signs and symptoms include the following:
> - Pain disproportionate to the severity of injury or wound
> - Rapid deterioration of the wound over the first 24-48 hours
> - Rapidly changing skin surface over the injury or wound (e.g., color, integrity)
> - Fever
> - Respiratory difficulty or failure
> - Possible mental confusion

high as 80%, this rate drops drastically with early recognition and interventions using surgery, antibiotics, and hyperbaric oxygen therapy.[31] The main symptom associated with necrotizing fasciitis is disproportionate pain for the size and apparent severity of the wound or incision combined with rapid degeneration within the first 24 to 48 hours. Over several days, a local erythema quickly changes from red to blue and progresses to purple with fluid-filled blisters. By the tenth day, necrotizing skin has separated from the erythema, exposing the underlying trauma. Accompanying signs include fever and respiratory difficulty, and on occasion, the patient presents in a delirious or confused state.[31]

Group B Streptococcal Infections

Group B beta-hemolytic streptococci (*S. agalactiae*) contain bacteria causing infections, endocarditis, septic arthritis, postpartum sepsis, and neonatal pneumonia. These infections in general are uncommon in adults; however, they are also opportunistic in nature and occur in patients with lowered resistance.[10,17] Group B streptococci are indigenous to the upper respiratory, gastrointestinal, and female genitourinary tracts.

Group D Streptococcal Infections

Group D includes two distinct bacteria: enterococcal and nonenterococcal species. These streptococci are commonly found in the gastrointestinal system (*S. bovis*) but also can be the culprit in bacterial endocarditis, urinary tract infections, abdominal sepsis, cellulitis, and wound infections.

Signs and Symptoms

Because streptococci can attack almost any system, the signs and symptoms are not unique to this specific group of infections but to the individual body system affected. For example, pneumonia will have signs and symptoms unique to that infection, as will cellulitis; both are vastly different in presentation yet both are caused by the streptococcal infection. The most common streptococcal presentation is pharyngeal infection from group A; strep throat presents with a bright red pharynx, fever, sore throat, lymphadenopathy, and tonsillar exudates.

Referral and Diagnostic Tests

Athletic trainers refer an athlete exhibiting any signs of infection, such as fever, malaise, pain, local swelling, and heat, to a physician. It is important to note that patients may present with symptoms or signs remote from the origin of the infection, as is the case in nonsuppurative infections. Laboratory blood tests showing a WBC count of 12,000 to 20,000 with 75% to 90% neutrophils indicate a streptococcal infection. Table 2-5 gives normal CBC values. A sample cultured overnight and evaluated under microscopic examination provides confirmation, whereas the absence of streptococcal bacteria indicates other pathology.

Treatment

Penicillin or erythromycin is the best medicinal treatment for most streptococcal infections. Patients are counseled to complete the course of their medication for complete effectiveness. Depending on the disease, isolation may be required (i.e., scarlet fever), and to prevent all types of streptococci from spreading, any materials soiled with residue from the infection or infected person are handled as infectious waste.

Prognosis, Return to Participation, and Prevention

The prognosis for return to activity following a confirmed streptococcal infection depends on the severity and duration of the symptoms, the tissues involved, and the progression of the disease. Certain streptococcal infections, such as impetigo, require absence of participation until the skin has completely healed (see Chapter 13).

Prevention of streptococcal infections includes proper sanitation, personal hygiene, and isolation of contagious persons until the period of communicability has passed.

Staphylococcal Infections

Staphylococcal infections are found on the skin of 20% of healthy adults and in the nares of 30%. Staphylococcal organisms are grapelike clusters of gram-positive bacteria that cause a tremendous number of infections in nearly every human body system. Table 12-6 compares staphylococcal infections, their normal environment, and the body systems most often attacked. Immunocompromised patients, especially those with influenza, chronic pulmonary disorders, chronic skin conditions, diabetes mellitus, and surgical incisions, are prone to staphylococcal infections.[15] Transmission is commonly through hand-to-hand contact during patient care and airborne spread. In athletics, the biggest culprits are postsurgical infections and those associated with seemingly benign skin wounds.

Certain types of staphylococcal infections are caused by ingestion of infected or undercooked food. Toxic shock syndrome, made infamous because of an epidemic surge of cases in menstruating women during the 1980s and associated with the use of high absorbancy feminine hygiene tampons, is another result of a staphylococcal infection. Women using tampons and barrier contraceptive devices are at risk. Five percent of all cases are fatal.

Methicillin-Resistant Staphylococcus Aureus

A recent problem with staphylococcal infections is the impediment to treatment using antibiotics, specifically the methicillin-resistant *Staphylococcus aureus* (MRSA). The first report of MRSA infection in athletes was in 1998, but such reports have steadily risen since then.[32] A low estimate is 100,000 people treated annually for MRSA.[33]

Signs and Symptoms
Most MRSA infections begin as a small lesion similar to a pimple, as a mosquito bite, as a recent injury or abrasion, or from surgery. The wound quickly enlarges and becomes inflamed and quite painful. Athletes may run a low-grade fever that progresses to higher temperatures as the body fights the infection. It is not unusual for breakouts to occur among teammates.[32]

Referral and Diagnostic Tests
An athlete who presents with a wound that shows signs of infection, such as heat, swelling, and redness, and that is accompanied by pain is referred to a physician. Wounds that rapidly deteriorate or become enlarged are suspect. Any athlete with a postoperative wound needs to be especially diligent in cleaning and inspecting the wound and immediately report any increase in pain, swelling, or fever. Current medical treatment of choice is trimethoprim with sulfamethoxazole (TMP-SMZ) or a member of the tetracycline family because these medications have proven effective for athletes with MRSA.[32] Hospitalization may be required for the athlete with high fever and pain unmanageable with outpatient medications.

Treatment
If an infection is detected and the athlete referred early enough in the infection's history, a physician may be able to drain it to prevent further problems. The release of infectious materials coupled with an antibiotic and proper hygiene may be enough to prevent MRSA. If the athlete is a staphylococcal carrier or has a history

Table 12-6	Comparison of Staphylococcal Infections	
Bacterium	**Normal Location**	**Diseases or Illnesses Caused**
Staphylococcus aureus	Skin, mucous membranes (nose, mouth) Produces golden-yellow pigment	Boils, carbuncles, internal abscesses, toxins (food poisoning, toxic shock syndrome)
Staphylococcus aureus— methicillin resistant (MRSA)	Same as above	Resistant to many penicillin drugs
Staphylococcus aureus— vancomycin resistant	Becomes serious in nosocomial infections	Resistant to many vancomycin drugs
Staphylococcus epidermidis	Skin	None
Staphylococcus hominis	Frequently recovered in skin	Causes no known diseases
Staphylococcus saprophyticus	Newly identified	Urinary tract infection

of resistance to penicillin treatment, other medications may be required to eradicate the infection.

Prognosis, Return to Participation, and Prevention

An athlete confirmed to have MRSA cannot engage in contact athletic activity until proven infection free. Communal areas, including the weight rooms and athletic training clinics, need to be sanitized after every patient use.

Soap and water go a long way in the initial cleaning and disinfecting of wounds (Box 12-2). Athletes must clean abrasions or turf burns as soon as possible after they occur and follow up with hot water and soap in a shower; finally, the wounds are covered with a sterile dressing. Daily cleaning and inspection of wounds will indicate if an athlete may be slower to heal or prone to infection.

Sexually Transmitted Diseases and Infections

Sexually transmitted diseases and infections (STDs) are a group of infectious diseases transmitted through body secretions from an infected partner. There are documented rare occasions in which an STD may be contracted in a nonsexual fashion, such as through occupational hazard (i.e., needle stick) or dental care (i.e., an infected health care provider); and infants can acquire an STD through the maternal placenta before or during birth (Table 12-7).

The presentation and detection of STDs differ for each gender. Males tend to come forth more regularly with signs and symptoms of a STD, whereas women do not, chiefly because their anatomy precludes obvious symptoms (see Chapter 7). Many women may forgo medical evaluation and self-treat if they think they have a urinary tract infection. General signs and symptoms of STDs are similar in both genders: dysuria (i.e., painful urination), urge to void but production of small volume, urethral discharge, itching, and burning.

Catchall terms associated with STDs are **nongonococcal** or **nonspecific urethritis** (NGU or NSU). Both occur in men and women and are caused by organisms that are not necessarily sexually transmitted. The signs and symptoms of these are similar to other STDs in that patients present with dysuria, frequent need to void, and discharge. These symptoms are less intense than those of gonorrhea and occur up to 6 weeks after exposure, unlike the 2- to 8-day incubation period of gonorrhea. A large number of causative agents include *E. coli,* herpes simplex, trauma, chemical contact, or chlamydia. NGU is not a true sexually transmitted infection. Undetected, this infection can spread to the testes, epididymis, prostate, and seminal vesicles in males.[11] In females, the inflammation can spread to the labia, ovaries, uterus, and fallopian tubes, producing

---

Box 12-2 Wound Care

Whether wounds that break the skin result from turf or trail abrasions during high-impact sports, the difference between successful healing and infection can be attributed to diligent use of soap and water and daily follow-up cleaning and inspection of the skin involved.

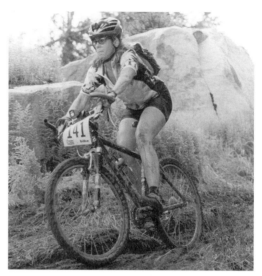

A postsurgical fasciotomy for thigh compartment syndrome could make a perfect entryway for methicillin-resistant *Staphylococcus aureus* (MRSA).

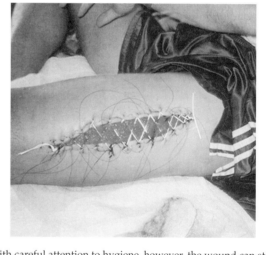

With careful attention to hygiene, however, the wound can stay infection free. Note how this wound is clean and free of drainage or other signs of infection. Inspection of the incision and changing the dressing in sterile conditions are paramount to prevent infection.

---

pelvic inflammatory disease (PID). **Reiter's disease** is a rare syndrome that may be a sequela of NGU or NSU. It is manifested by inflammation of mucous membranes, joints, and the cardiac lining.

Prevention

Most STDs can be prevented by using barrier protection such as a condom during sexual intercourse, knowing

Table 12-7   Sexually Transmitted Diseases and Infections

Disease	Incubation	Transmission	Signs and Symptoms	Treatment	Long Term
HIV	1-6 mo	Sexually transmitted	Malaise, fever	ZDU for maintenance	AIDS
HPV	1-6 mo	Sexually transmitted	Genital warts	Symptomatic	Chronic carrier
Syphilis	1-13 wk	Sexual contact	Chancre, dermatological signs, constitutional symptoms	Penicillin	Incapacitating cardiovascular disease, often has neurological signs
Gonorrhea	Men: 2-14 days Women: 7-21 days	Sexually transmitted	Dysuria, discharge, frequency of voiding	Ceftriaxone, doxycycline	Hydrocele and abscesses in men, salpingitis in women
Chlamydia	7-28 days	Sexually transmitted	Dysuria, meatal itching, asymptomatic	Tetracycline or doxycycline	Untreated: pelvic inflammatory disease
Herpes 2	4-7 days	Contact	Lesions	Acyclovir	Chronic carrier

HIV, Human immunodeficiency virus; *HPV*, human papillomavirus; *ZDU*, Zidovudine; *AIDS*, acquired immunodeficiency syndrome.

the medical history of the sex partner, and avoiding risky behaviors that include multiple sex partners, unsafe sexual practices, and excessive drinking of alcohol, which may lead to risky behaviors. Some STDs, such as herpes, can be contagious even if there is a barrier because the barrier must completely cover the lesion to deter the infection.

Athletes must understand that having an STD does not provide immunity to another infection in the manner seen with childhood diseases discussed earlier. The only certain method to avoid STDs is to abstain from sexual relations or to maintain mutually monogamous sexual intimacy with a partner who has proven to be uninfected. An infected person needs to abstain from sexual contact until the course of treatment has been completed and all lesions have completely healed.[36]

Concerns with Adolescents and Public Health Implications

Athletes under the age of 18 years who are sexually active and report their anxiety about a possible STD to the athletic trainer are of special concern. In addition to state statutory rape laws, each state has specific laws regarding the reporting of this type of medical information to a parent or guardian. The athletic trainer should consult the school counselor or nurse about applicable laws. The health of the athlete is of utmost importance. The treating physician has the obligation to report infectious diseases to the appropriate agency, but athletic trainers need to be aware of the ramifications of children with STDs.

Human Immunodeficiency Virus and Acquired Immunodeficiency Syndrome

Human immunodeficiency virus (HIV) is the precursor for acquired immunodeficiency syndrome (AIDS) for which there is no known cure. AIDS is the late-stage result of HIV infection but may lay dormant for years following HIV infection. It is estimated that 90% of those infected with HIV will eventually develop AIDS if left untreated.[10]

HIV is transmitted through body fluids from an infected person through sexual contact, shared use of contaminated needles or inadvertent needle sticks from contaminated needles, transfused blood bearing the disease, infants born to infected mothers, or transplantation of infected organs.[3,6,10,35] Transmission via saliva, urine, tears, or bronchial secretions has not been recorded, but the virus has been found in these fluids. Transmission of HIV through sexual contact is much rarer than HBV because HIV is not as hardy, but that should not preclude caution. The presence of a concurrent STD increases the likelihood of acquiring HIV.[10]

The incubation period for HIV can last several months or years before onset of symptoms, but most infected individuals will test positive for the virus within 6 months. Some patients develop a self-limiting mononucleosis-like illness weeks to months following exposure to HIV, but the acute illness lasts only a few weeks and is often dismissed.[10]

Signs and Symptoms

Following infection, a broad variety of clinical issues may occur. AIDS-related complex (ARC) is the term used for HIV-positive patients who have not yet developed opportunistic infections that are associated with AIDS. General signs and symptoms of ARC include malaise, intermittent fever, diarrhea, anemia, weight loss, lymphadenopathy, **hairy leukoplakia,** and **thrush.** Some life-threatening cancers, including **Kaposi's sarcoma** (Figure 12-9), non-Hodgkin's lymphoma, and lymphoma of the brain, may actually be acquired through AIDS-related infection in patients who never manifested ARC symptoms.[6]

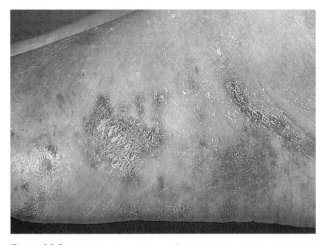

Figure 12-9 Kaposi's sarcoma is a life-threatening cancer associated with diabetes, malignant lymphoma, or AIDS. It begins as discolored papules on the feet, spreads to the skin, and metastasizes to the lymphatic system. (From Cotran RS, Kumar V, Collins T: *Robbins pathologic basis of disease*, ed 6, Philadelphia, 1999, WB Saunders, p 536.)

The AIDS virus itself is considered an opportunistic infection, settling on whole body systems or organs. Signs and symptoms are chiefly presented via other known pathologies but are in fact caused by AIDS. Associated illnesses include encephalitis, meningitis, tuberculosis, CNS infections, vascular and digestive complications, peripheral neuropathies, and renal pathologies.

Referral, Diagnostic Tests, and Differential Diagnosis
Athletes who present with unexplainable fatigue or slow-healing wounds are referred to a physician for further evaluation. If an athlete has reason to warrant HIV testing, a blood test is necessary to confirm the disease. Serological testing (e.g., enzyme-linked immunosorbent assay [EIA]) for HIV antibodies has been available to the public since 1985, but, although detectable antibodies typically appear within 1 to 3 months of exposure, they can be delayed as much as 6 months or more.[10] False-positive test results are known to occur, so reactive tests are supplemented by additional studies, such as the **Western blot** or the indirect fluorescent antibody (IFA) test.

Because HIV/AIDS can manifest as a multi–organ system problem, the differential diagnoses for these diseases are lengthy, ranging from malaise and simple gastrointestinal disturbances to pneumonia, cancer, or reflex sympathetic dystrophy.

Treatment, Return to Participation, and Public Health Implications
There is no vaccine to prevent HIV; however, the drug zidovudine (ZDU), which was originally called Azidothymidine (AZT) has proven helpful in the management of HIV and in delaying the onset of AIDS.

An HIV-positive athlete is not banned from sport, and as long as health care providers practice approved blood-borne pathogen policies, the chance of transmission via sport is negligible. The illnesses associated with AIDS may preclude athletic endeavors, but that is up to the individual athlete and physician. Since HIV attacks the immune system, infected athletes would be wise to keep their distance from sick teammates.

The National Collegiate Athletic Association (NCAA) does not require that HIV-positive college athletes report or acknowledge infection to the organization or on health screenings. HIV is, however, reportable to the local health authority; and it is mandatory to report AIDS in the United States and most countries.[10]

Genital Warts

Genital warts are caused by human papillomavirus (HPV) and are typically acquired via sexual contact. They are also called venereal warts or condylomata acuminata and result in a fibrous overgrowth of the dermis. There are more than 60 identified strains of HPV, any of which can cause genital warts. These warts tend to grow rapidly in areas of heavy perspiration or poor hygiene and often accompany other sexually transmitted infections.[31] It is disconcerting to note that in the past decade, the prevalence of HPV has increased to twice the rate of genital herpes in the United States because HPV has an association with cancer that herpes does not share.[6] The incubation period for HPV is 1 to 6 months.

Women who have a history of specific types of genital warts need to be monitored over time because these warts can develop into an invasive cervical carcinoma. In addition, some types have developed into bladder cancer.[6] Genital warts are not common before puberty or following menopause.[31] HPV also causes nongenital warts, such as the common and plantar warts (see Chapter 13).

Signs and Symptoms
Genital warts appear as the common wart, typically painless, minute, pink or red, soft, moist outgrowths that can appear in clusters. They can resemble cauliflower and are found in warm, moist areas of the body. In women, they are found on the vulva, vaginal walls, cervix, and perineum. Males with HPV may present with warts in the urethra or penile shaft and in the perianal area or rectum in homosexual men. Genital warts do not resemble acne nor do they express any discharge.

Referral, Diagnostic Tests, and Differential Diagnosis
Athletes with wartlike genital growths are referred to a physician for assessment. Genital warts are diagnosed by their appearance; however, they must be differentiated from secondary syphilis through biopsy on lingering or unusual warts. Women with cervical warts must

obtain a clear pap smear before undergoing any further diagnostic tests on the warts. Differential diagnoses for genital warts include secondary syphilis, cervical cancer, and skin tags.

Treatment, Prognosis, and Return to Participation
Although genital warts are typically removed by electro-cauterization, cryotherapy, laser, or, if necessary, surgical excision, these remedies are not infallible. Early treatment consists of topical medication application using trichloroacetic acid or podophyllin, but these agents must be reapplied often over weeks to months and are typically not effective. When the warts appear in the urethra, thiotepa is an effective treatment as well as topical 5-fluorouracil for men. Alternative urethral wart treatments are removed via resectoscope with the patient under general anesthesia and circumcision in males to prevent recurrence. Urethral lesions also need to be monitored for the rare occasion of urethral obstruction. Direct injection of interferon alpha may remove genital warts that have returned after previous removal but will not reduce the rate of return. HPV and genital warts do not prohibit sports participation.

Syphilis

Syphilis is a sexually acquired disease caused by the organism *Treponema pallidum* that has systemic ramifications. The disease has been called the "great imitator" because so many of its symptoms reflect other diseases.[34] Although syphilis is a preventable and curable affliction, new cases are seen in the United States each year. The most recent report shows a trend upward with 32,000 reported cases, including nearly 7000 primary and secondary cases in 2002.[36] More than one half of the new cases were reported from 28 counties clustered in the southeastern United States.[34,37] The CDC has an "Eliminate Syphilis" campaign that intends to reduce syphilis to fewer than 1000 cases nationwide and increase the syphilis-free counties to 90% by the year 2005.[37] Although no particular group is without representation, homosexual men are the fastest growing population with new diagnoses; the disease rate among African-Americans and women has decreased.[36]

Syphilis presents with a series of clinical manifestations interrupted by years of latency. No body system is protected from the disease, and it can be transmitted to the fetus from an infected mother. Acquired, not congenital, syphilis is discussed here. Unlike HBV, *T. pallidum* is an unstable organism that cannot live long outside its human host. Transmission occurs from person to person via direct contact with a syphilis sore.[34] Syphilis has an incubation period of 1 to 13 weeks, but it is more typical to develop signs and symptoms between weeks 3 and 4. Within hours of exposure, *T. pallidum* infiltrates the lymphatic system and subsequently moves throughout the entire body. The CNS is affected during the secondary stage of the disease.

Signs and Symptoms
Box 12-3 gives the four distinct stages of syphilis; signs and symptoms depend on the stage of the disease. Primary syphilis begins with a chancre or sore at point of contact with the infected person. This occurs most often on the external genitalia and mouth.[34] The chancre may be a single firm, round, painless sore or multiple sores. This sore forms a painless ulcer and exudes a clear serum. More often than not, the person with the disease is unaware of it, because many patients are asymptomatic for years. Typically, chancres persist 3 to 8 weeks and resolve without treatment.[6,36] Without treatment, however, the syphilis infection progresses to the secondary stage.

Signs of secondary syphilis include skin rash and mucous membrane lesions that can appear 6 to 12 weeks after infection. Although most rashes are antipyretic, they are rough and red with reddish brown spots. Some secondary rashes may appear on the palms (Figure 12-10, *A*) or soles, but they can appear anywhere on the body and may be so subtle that they are overlooked (Figure 12-10, *B*). These rashes often heal spontaneously, only to reappear. Other signs and symptoms associated with the secondary stage include fever, lymphomegaly, pharyngitis, myalgia, malaise, headache, weight loss, and patchy hair loss.[6,34] Again, if left untreated, secondary syphilis progresses to latent-stage syphilis.

The latent period of disease may last the remainder of the patient's life or may spontaneously relapse.

Box 12-3   Stages of Acquired Syphilis

Primary Stage
- Chancre
- Lymphadenopathy
- Infectious

Secondary Stage
- Dermatological presentations, including rash and mucous membrane erosion
- CSF abnormalities

Latent Stage
- 2 or more years
- Reappearance of infectious lesions
- Contagious while lesions are active
- May never progress to late stage

Late, or Tertiary, Stage
- Symptomatic but not contagious
- Cardiovascular syphilis marked by aortic insufficiency, coronary stenosis, aortic aneurysm
- Neurosyphilis marked by personality changes, hyperactive reflexes, decreased memory, slurred speech, optic atrophy, seizures, hemiparesis

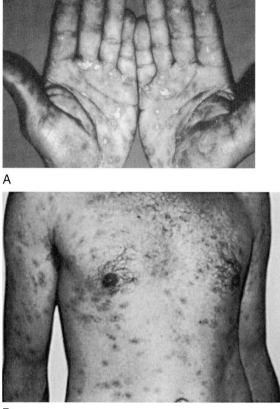

A

B

Figure 12-10 Skin lesions or rash is typically associated with secondary syphilis. A, On the palms of the hands. B, On the chest. (A from Goldstein BG, Goldstein AO: *Practical dermatology*, ed 2, St Louis, 1997, Mosby; B from Gorbach SL, Bartlett JG, Blacklow NR: *Infectious diseases*, ed 2, Philadelphia, 1998, WB Saunders, p 981.)

This period begins approximately 2 years following infection and may be treated by penicillin given for another reason than the syphilis.

Tertiary or late-stage syphilis is the final stage of this devastating disease. When other body systems are affected by the syphilis infection, profound sequelae, including cardiovascular, neurological, musculoskeletal, and visual system deterioration, occur. The outcomes of untreated syphilis can cause death.[34,36,37] In addition, there is a fivefold increased risk of acquiring the HIV infection in patients who have syphilis.[34]

Referral and Diagnostic Tests
Primary syphilis is diagnosed from exudates removed from the chancre followed by serological workup if the results are unremarkable

The serological test for syphilis (STS) is the most common screening tool used for diagnosis. This test is often utilized by allied health workers to determine if subsequent evaluation is warranted. Two other tests, the Venereal Disease Research Laboratory (VDRL) and rapid plasma reagin (RPR), are also common screening tools for syphilis. Because CSF shows abnormal

findings in less than 30% of patients, it is sometimes used as an indicator of the disease.[6]

Differential Diagnosis
The differential diagnoses for primary syphilis include genital herpes, scabies, ulceration, and trauma. Alternative diagnoses for secondary syphilis, which presents primarily as a dermatological reaction, include dermatitis, drug reaction rash, rubella, mononucleosis, ringworm, warts, and fungal infection. Latent-stage syphilis is more troublesome because it can manifest in any body organ or system and not be identified as the initial culprit until serological tests for *T. pallidum* have been performed.

Treatment and Public Health Implications
Treatment for primary and secondary syphilis includes a full sexual history from the patient that includes all sexual partners during the past 3 months in the case of primary syphilis and during the past 12 months for secondary infections.

Penicillin is the appropriate medication for all forms of syphilis, and a single intramuscular injection of penicillin will cure a patient who has had syphilis less than 1 year.[34] If the patient is allergic to penicillin, erythromycin or tetracycline can be administered with a dosage of 500 mg every 6 hours for 15 days (see Chapter 3).

Syphilis is a reportable disease, and sexual partners of the infected person must be notified by the reporting agency, tested, and given treatment.

Gonorrhea

Gonorrhea is a sexually transmitted disease caused by a gram-negative organism, *Neisseria gonorrhoeae*. It can affect the epithelium of the urethra, cervix, rectum, pharynx, and conjunctiva. Greatest incidence occurs in people 15 to 29 years old, and the infection has a relatively short incubation period of 2 to 21 days.[12] Transmission almost always is via direct sexual contact, with the rare exceptions of infants during vaginal birth and health care personnel through broken skin.

If gonorrhea is left untreated, serious, gender-related complications may include male postgonococcal urethritis, epididymitis, and prostatitis; women can develop PID or **salpingitis,** an inflammation of the fallopian tube, and both of these can lead to acute pain, infection, possible tubal scarring and adhesions, and resultant infertility (Figure 12-11).

Both men and women may develop systemic or disseminated gonococcal infection (DGI), which presents with malaise, mild febrile illness, pustular lesions, and arthritis. Systemic disease is associated with bacteremia that may manifest in ocular infections, septic arthritis, skin lesions, and tenosynovitis.

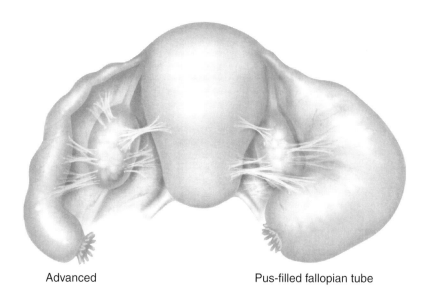

Advanced   Pus-filled fallopian tube

Figure 12-11 Salpingitis is an inflamed or infected fallopian tube that can result from unresolved gonorrhea. (From Seidel HM, Ball JW, Dains JE, Benedict GW: *Mosby's guide to physical examination,* ed 5, St Louis, 2003, Mosby, p 644.)

Signs and Symptoms

Men and women have differing presentations and complications with this disease. Women may not seek treatment as soon as men because their symptoms are mild and may be more easily dismissed.[6] In men, the symptoms begin as a discomfort in the urethra, moving quickly to dysuria and a purulent, yellow-green urethral discharge.[6,15] Women's symptoms include dysuria, frequency of voiding, and vaginal discharge.

Referral, Diagnostic Tests, and Differential Diagnosis

Athletes manifesting symptoms consistent with gonorrhea are immediately referred to a physician. A patient suspected of having gonorrhea is also tested for syphilis (STS) before initiating treatment. Gonorrhea may occur concurrently with other STDs; it is important to treat them all. Specific tests for gonorrhea include a urethral swab of the discharge, which confirms the disease in 90% of infected men but only 60% of infected women.[6] Culture with exudates from the urethra, cervix, rectum, and pharynx can confirm diagnosis.

Differential diagnoses for gonorrhea include syphilis, chlamydia, urinary tract infection, injury, or infection related to a lost tampon in women.

Treatment and Public Health Implications

Because strains of drug-resistant gonorrhea have emerged, the use of penicillin has been challenged.[6] The current drug of choice is ceftriaxone (125 mg intramuscularly), but since this STD often occurs in conjunction with chlamydia, it also must be treated.[6] The referring physician will typically use a combination of medications, keeping in mind the complexity of treating two STDs and the challenge of drug resistance.

All the patient's sexual contacts, just as with syphilis, must be located, cultured, and treated.[15]

Chlamydia

Chlamydia includes all members of the genus *Chlamydia,* gram-negative bacteria with a unique developmental cycle within host cells.[12] Almost every species of bird and mammal is infected with chlamydia, which because of its parasitic reproductive process is capable of producing a broad spectrum of disease. It causes many different diseases in the human, largely in the eye, respiratory system, and genital tract. The strain of chlamydia most commonly associated with a sexually transmitted infection is *Chlamydia trachomatis.*[14] Chlamydial infection is the most common STD in the United States and tends to be linked with other STDs such as gonorrhea, NGU, and syphilis.[15] Approximately one half the NGU cases are caused by *C. trachomatis,* which has an incubation period of 2 to 3 weeks.

The primary danger from chlamydia is the possible repercussions from untreated disease (Red Flags—Chlamydia). Female sequelae include risk of infertility, ectopic pregnancy, and chronic pelvic pain.[6,10]

▶ Red Flags for Chlamydia

Chlamydia is the most common sexually transmitted infection in the United States and often concurrently linked with other STDs. Untreated, it can cause the following:
- Infertility
- Ectopic pregnancy
- Chronic pelvic pain
- Epididymitis
- Reiter's syndrome
- Male urethral infections

Males risk urethral infection, epididymitis, infertility, and Reiter's syndrome.[6,10]

Signs and Symptoms

The signs and symptoms of chlamydia are consistent with other STDs. It presents with urethral discharge, dysuria, fever, and meatal itching. The disease may be asymptomatic in up to 25% of sexually active men and in up to 70% of sexually active women.[10]

Referral, Diagnostic Tests, and Differential Diagnosis

Diagnosis of chlamydia is based on cultured secretions obtained from the infected area by swab. Physicians have found little benefit from serology for this diagnosis.[14]

Other STDs, such as gonorrhea and NGU, need to be ruled out when chlamydia is suspected. In addition, differential diagnoses include urinary tract infection, yeast infection, and dermatitis.

Treatment and Public Health Implications

Because chlamydia is often concurrent with gonorrhea and tends to persist after gonorrhea is successfully treated, it is important that the physician evaluates and provides remedies for both diseases. Chlamydia is resistant to penicillin and cephalosporins and must be treated by tetracycline, erythromycin, or doxycycline to be eradicated. Chlamydia is also a disease that must be reported to the local health authority in most states.[10]

 WEB RESOURCES

Centers for Disease Control
www.cdc.gov
Facts and surveillance of infectious diseases

National Institutes of Health
http://www.nih.gov
Information on health issues and prevention of disease

CDC National Prevention Information Network
http://www.cdcnpin.org/scripts/index.asp
Sexually transmitted diseases and human immuno-deficiency virus (HIV) information

American Social Health Association (ASHA)
http://www.ashastd.org/
Information on sexually transmitted diseases (STDs) and harmful consequences

---

SUMMARY

Infectious diseases commonly attack every system in the human body, but most are largely preventable. Individuals who take advantage of immunizations, follow universal precautions, and practice safe sex will protect themselves from most common infectious diseases. The athletic trainer must consider infectious diseases when working with an athlete who has fever,

unexplained fatigue, or a skin abrasion that does not heal in order to ensure that person access to the best care possible and to protect other athletes who may also have been exposed to the infectious agent.

REFERENCES

1. Goldman L, Ausiello D: *Cecil textbook of medicine,* ed 22, Philadelphia, 2004, WB Saunders.
2. Walsh K, Raedeke S: Infection and disease transmission in the athletic training setting, *Athletic Therapy Today* 9(3):11-15, 2004.
3. Sepkowitz K: Occupationally acquired infections in health care workers—part 1, *Annals of Internal Medicine* 125(10): 826-834, 1996.
4. Sepkowitz K: Occupationally acquired infections in health care workers—part 2, *Annals of Internal Medicine* 125(11): 917-924, 1996.
5. Tobe K, Matsuura K, Ogura T, et al: Horizontal transmission of hepatitis B virus among players of an American football team, *Archives of Internal Medicine* 160:2541-2545, 2000.
6. Beers M, Berklow R, editors: *The Merck manual of diagnosis and therapy,* ed 17, Whitehouse Station, NJ, 1999, Merck Research Laboratories.
7. Strikas R, Schmidt J, Weaver D, Wolfe C: Immunizations. Recommendations and resources for active patients, *Physician and Sportsmedicine* 29(10):33-48, 2001.
8. Sifton D, editor: *PDG guide to biological and chemical warfare response,* ed 1, Montvale, NJ, 2002, Thompson.
9. Howe W: Preventing infectious disease in sports, *Physician and Sportsmedicine* 31(2):23-29, 2003.
10. Chin J: *Control of infectious diseases manual,* ed 17, Washington, DC, 2000, American Public Health Association.
11. Brettle R, Thompson M: *Infection and communicable diseases,* London, 1984, William Heinemann Medical Books.
12. Tierney L, McPhee S, Papadakis M, editors: *Current medical diagnosis and treatment,* ed 43, New York, 2004, Lange Medical Books/McGraw-Hill.
13. Bryan C: *Infectious diseases in primary care,* Philadelphia, 2002, WB Saunders.
14. Ellner P, Neu H: *Understanding infectious disease,* St Louis, 1992, Mosby.
15. Ferri F: *Ferri's clinical advisor: instant diagnosis and treatment,* Philadelphia, 2004, Mosby.
16. Rakel RE, Bope ET: *Conn's current therapy 2004,* Philadelphia, 2004, WB Saunders.
17. Rubin E, Gorstein F, Rubin R, et al: *Rubin's pathology: clinicopathologic foundations of medicine,* ed 4, Philadephia, 2005, Lippincott Williams & Wilkins.
18. Holcomb S: An update on hepatitis, *Dimensions of Critical Care Nursing* 21(5):170-179, 2002.
19. Cotran RS, Kumar V, Collins T: *Robbins pathologic basis of disease,* ed 6, Philadelphia, 1999, WB Saunders.
20. Buxton B, Daniell J, Buxton B, et al: Prevention of hepatitis B virus in athletic training, *Journal of Athletic Training* 29(2): 107-112, 1994.
21. Kashiwagi S, Hayashi J, Ikematsu H, et al: An outbreak of hepatitis B in members of a high school sumo wrestling club, *JAMA* 248(2):213-214, 1982.
22. Bubb R: *NCAA 2003 wrestling rules and interpretations,* Indianapolis, 2003, National Collegiate Athletic Association.

23. Arnot R: The evolving efforts to control hepatitis B virus, *Pediatric Infectious Disease Journal* 17(7):S26-S29, 1998.
24. Cassidy W: School-based adolescent hepatitis B immunization programs in the United States: strategies and successes, *Pediatric Infectious Disease Journal* 17(7):S43-S46, 1998.
25. Moore-Caldwell S, Werner M, Powell L, Greene J: Hepatitis B vaccination in adolescents: knowledge, perceived risk, and compliance, *Journal of Adolescent Health* 20:294-299, 1996.
26. Osterholm M: Hepatitis B infection in Minnesota: a case for universal immunization, *Pediatric Infectious Disease Journal* 17(7):S30-S34, 1998.
27. Lancman H, Pastore D, Steed N, Maresca A: Adolescent hepatitis B vaccination—comparison among 2 high school-based health centers and an adolescent clinic, *Archives of Pediatric Adolescent Medicine* 154:1085-1088, 2000.
28. Harmon K, Rubin A: Preventing infectious disease in sport, *Physician and Sportsmedicine* 31(2):23-29, 2003.
29. Klossner D, editor: *2004-2005 NCAA sports medicine handbook,* Indianapolis, 2004, National Collegiate Athletic Association.
30. Mast E, Goodman R: Prevention of infectious disease transmission in sport, *Sports Medicine* 24(1):1-7, 1997.
31. *Professional guide to diseases,* ed 7, Springhouse, Pa, 2001, Springhouse.
32. Schnirring L: MRSA infections, *Physician and Sportsmedicine* 32(10):12-17, 2004.
33. Division of Healthcare Quality Promotion: MRSA—methicillin-resistant Staphylococcus aureus fact sheet. Available at http://www.cdc.gov/ncidod/hip/Aresist/mrsafaq.htm. Accessed October 2004.
34. National Center for HIV, STD and TB Prevention: STD prevention: syphilis fact sheet. CDC. Available at http://www.cdc.gov/std/Syphilis/STDFact-Syphilis.htm#WhatIs. Accessed September 2004.
35. Cates J, Weinstock H, Chesson H, DiClemente R: Communicating the facts and figures on sexually transmitted diseases in youth. Paper presented at 2004 National STD Prevention Conference, September 2004.
36. National Center for HIV, STD and TB Prevention: *US syphilis rates climb for the second consecutive year,* Atlanta, November 20, 2003, Centers for Disease Control and Prevention.
37. National Center for HIV, STD and TB Prevention: Syphilis elimination: history in the making. CDC. Available at http://www.cdc.gov/stopsyphilis/. Accessed September 2004.

SYSTEMIC DISORDERS AND INFECTIOUS DISEASES

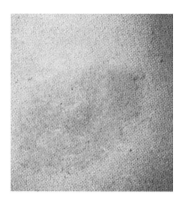

Figure 11-4. Prominent radiating lesion of Lyme disease

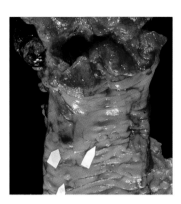

Figure 11-6. Carcinoma of the descending colon

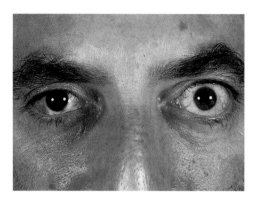

Figure 11-13. Graves' disease, unilateral exophthalmos

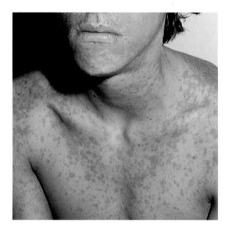

Figure 12-5. Rubeola rash

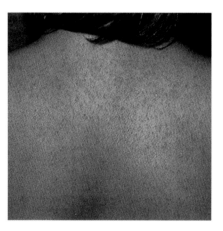

Figure 12-6. Rubella

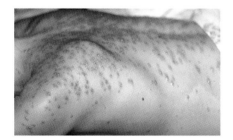

Figure 12-7, A. Chickenpox

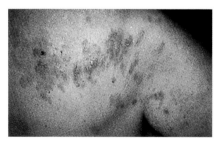

Figure 12-7, B. Shingles

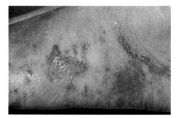

Figure 12-9. Kaposi sarcoma

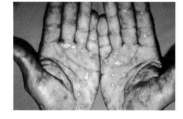

Figure 12-10, A. Rash associated with secondary syphilis

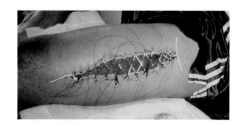

Box 12-2, Figure 2. Page 307. Postsurgical fasciotomy

THE SKIN

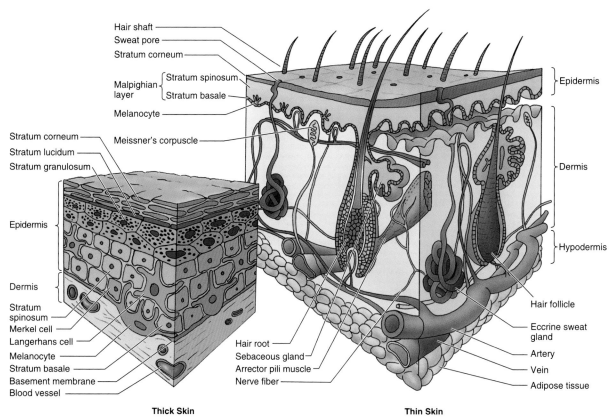

Figure 13-1. Anatomy of skin

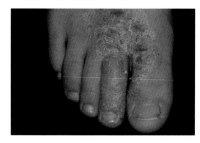

Figure 13-3. Urticaria reaction to exercise

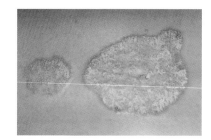

Figure 13-5. Cholinergic urticaria

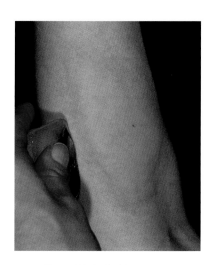

Figure 13-6. Cold urticaria

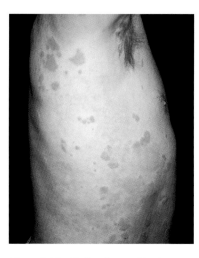

Figure 13-8. Eczema

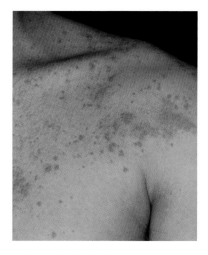

Figure 13-9. Psoriasis

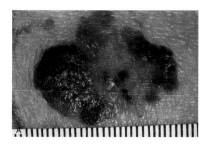

Figure 13-11. Melanoma

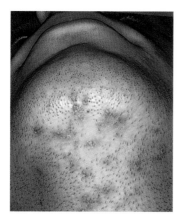

Figure 13-13. Folliculitis in a beard

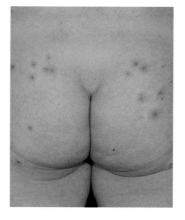

Figure 13-14. *Pseudomonas* folliculitis resulting from hot tub use

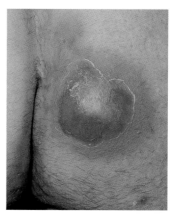

Figure 13-15. Furuncle

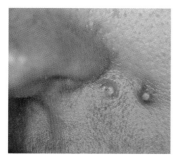

Figure 13-16, A. Acne

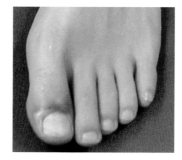

Figure 13-17. Paronychia surrounding great toe

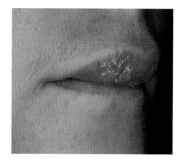

Figure 13-18. Herpes simplex or cold sore

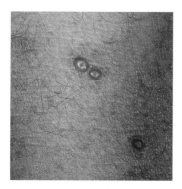

Figure 13-19. Molluscum contagiosum

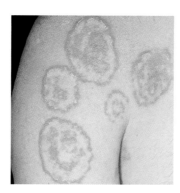

Figure 13-21. Tinea corporis

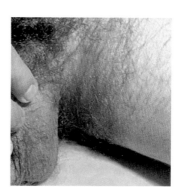

Figure 13-22. Tinea cruris or jock itch

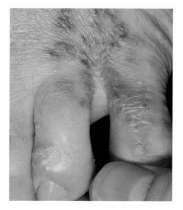

Figure 13-23. Tinea pedis or athlete's foot

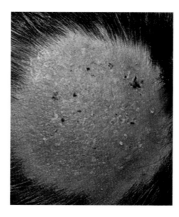

Figure 13-24. Tinea capitis

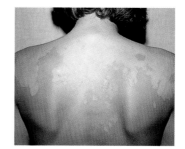

Figure 13-25. Tinea versicolor

THE SKIN

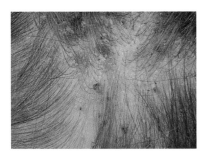

Figure 13-26. Pediculosis in the hair

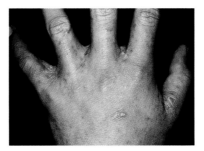

Figure 13-27. Scabies on the dorsum of hand

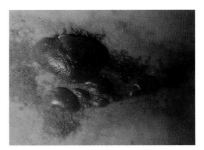

Figure 13-29. Severe reaction to Brown Recluse spider bite

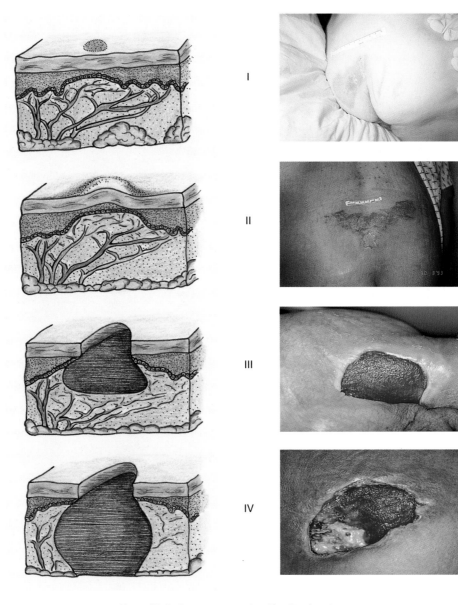

I

II

III

IV

Figure 16-3. Pressure sore classification by stages

CHAPTER
13

Dermatological Conditions

Patrick Sexton and
Todd Kanzenbach

OBJECTIVES

At the completion of this chapter, the reader should be able to do the following:

1. Understand the anatomy of the integumentary system.
2. Recognize signs and symptoms of common skin conditions.
3. Appreciate the differences among viral, fungal, and bacterial skin disorders.
4. Refer an athlete with a problematic skin disorder to the appropriate health care provider.
5. Differentiate which acute skin conditions are contraindicated for certain athletic participation.

INTRODUCTION

Dermatological conditions in athletes are common in a variety of settings and are a major reason that many athletes miss practice or competition. The National Collegiate Athletic Association (NCAA) Injury Surveillance System indicates that dermatological conditions account for at least 15% of practice time–loss injuries in wrestling.[1] Although most dermatological conditions are the result of skin-to-skin contact and resultant transmission, some may involve respiratory or airborne transmission. Others may result from allergic reactions, cancer, or insect bites. The five main types of dermatological conditions are general, bacterial, viral, fungal, and parasitic. This chapter reviews pertinent anatomy and discusses clinical presentation, diagnosis, treatment, and the criteria for return to participation related to simple dermatological conditions.

OVERVIEW OF ANATOMY AND PHYSIOLOGY

The skin or integument, is the largest organ of the body and can be divided into three layers: the epidermis, the dermis, and the subcutaneous tissue or hypodermis (Figure 13-1). The epidermis itself is composed of up to five layers from deep to superficial: stratum basale; stratum spinosum; stratum granulosum; stratum lucidum, found only in the soles of the feet and palms of the hands; and stratum corneum.[2]

Each layer of the epidermis except for the stratum basale is composed of dead cells (Box 13-1). The epidermis provides the primary protective shield for the body through the constant formation of new cells and the sloughing of old cells and through the production of pigment known as melanin. The dermis, which is composed of a papillary layer and a reticular layer, contains a variety of vascular and sensory structures, hair follicles, sebaceous or sweat glands, and nails. Finally, the hypodermis or the subcutaneous layer is made up of connective tissue, which binds the dermis to the deeper structures, and adipose, which provides insulation and cushioning. Together the epidermis, the dermis, and the hypodermis make up the integumentary system.[2]

The integumentary system serves as the interface between the body and the external environment. It is a dynamic system that serves as a protective barrier against invading organisms and outside influences such as ultraviolet radiation, toxic chemicals, thermal changes, and penetrating forces. However, at the same time, the integumentary system allows people to sense and to adapt to the environment in terms

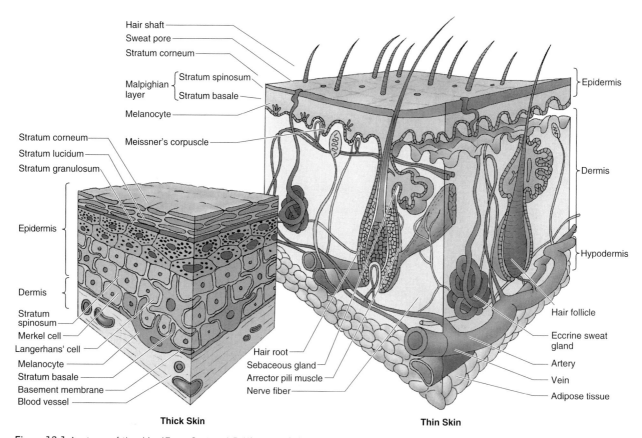

Figure 13-1 Anatomy of the skin. (From Gartner LP, Hiatt JL: *Color textbook of histology*, ed 2, Philadelphia, 2001, WB Saunders, p 326.)

Box 13-1	Layers of the Epidermis

- Stratum corneum—consists of many layers of keratinized, dead cells that are flattened and nonnucleated; cornified
- Stratum lucidum—a thin, clear layer found only in the epidermis of the palms and soles
- Stratum granulosum—composed of one or more layers of granular cells that contain fibers of keratin and shriveled nuclei
- Stratum spinosum—composed of several layers of cells with centrally located, large, oval nuclei and spinelike processes; limited mitosis
- Stratum basale—consists of a single layer of cuboidal cells that undergo mitosis; contains pigment-producing melanocytes

From Van De Graaff K, Fox S: *Concepts of human anatomy and physiology,* ed 3, Dubuque, Iowa, 1992, William C Brown, p 149.

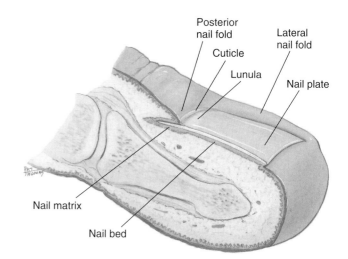

Figure 13-2 Anatomy of the nail. (From Jarvis C: *Physical examination & health assessment*, ed 4, Philadelphia, 2004, WB Saunders, p 223.)

of thermoregulation, fluid loss, proprioception and kinesthesis, force dissipation, cutaneous absorption of gases, ultraviolet light, toxins, and synthesis of vitamin D. Finally, the skin plays an important role in human communication by helping people to convey emotions through changes in skin color and texture as well as through facial expression.[2]

Nails are made up largely of keratin and are found on the dorsal surfaces of all fingers and toes (Figure 13-2). The nail is a hard, clear surface that presents a pink

color from the underlying highly vascular epithelial cell layer. The lunula lies at the proximal end of all nails. It is a moon-shaped, white opaque layer that protects the nail matrix, which in turn produces new keratinized cells. The nail fold surrounds the lateral and proximal nail and hooks onto the nail bed. It is in this area that certain bacterial conditions arise.

PATHOLOGICAL CONDITIONS

The athletic trainer is usually the first clinician to evaluate a dermatological **lesion** on an athlete. Lesions are typically in the very early stages of development and quite difficult to differentiate without microscopic or laboratory testing. Since these types of diagnostic procedures are beyond the scope of athletic training, the athletic trainer must utilize sound clinical judgment when determining the appropriate course of action for athletes with dermatological conditions.

When referral to a medical doctor for evaluation and treatment is necessary, the athletic trainer must understand the patient's signs and symptoms and be able to effectively describe findings to the physician using dermatographical nomenclature. The appropriate use of terminology to describe the appearance of a lesion or condition is very specific. The athletic trainer must have the knowledge and resources necessary to make these distinctions. It is much easier and more efficient to describe the lesion as a "fissure" rather than as a "linear loss of epidermis and dermis with sharp defined borders." In addition, the athletic trainer must understand that these terms are important to the description and not a specific diagnosis (Table 13-1).

Dermatitis, for example, is an inflammation of the skin or dermal layers and can be the result of a variety of dermatological conditions with various causes. Whereas the term dermatitis merely indicates a general inflammation of the skin, **contact dermatitis** indicates an inflammation of the skin caused by direct contact with a specific allergen and **actinic dermatitis** indicates inflammation of the skin from exposure to sunlight or another irritating light source. Thus the term dermatitis is a general descriptor whereas contact dermatitis and actinic dermatitis indicate specific conditions and constitute a particular diagnosis.

Another way to describe dermatological conditions is by referencing the area of skin affected. Most physicians use millimeters (mm) to describe the width or breadth of a particular condition, but centimeters (cm) are used in larger surface areas. As a point of reference, 1 inch is equal to 25.40 mm or 2.54 cm.

Table 13-1 Common Skin Lesions

PRIMARY LESIONS

NONPALPABLE

 Macule: A spot, circumscribed, up to 1 cm; not palpable; not elevated above or depressed below surrounding skin surface; hypopigmented, hyperpigmented, or erythematous.
Example: freckles. Referred to as **patch** if greater than 1 cm.
Examples: café au lait spots, mongolian spots.

PALPABLE, SOLID

 Papule: A bump, palpable and circumscribed, elevated and less than 5 mm in diameter; may be pigmented, erythematous, or flesh-toned.
Example: elevated nevus (mole).

 Nodule: A lesion similar to a papule, with a diameter of 5 mm to 2 cm; may have a significant palpable dermal component.
Examples: fibroma, xanthoma, intradermal nevi.

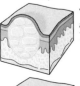 **Tumor:** Any mass lesion; generally larger than a nodule; may be either malignant or benign.
Example: lipoma.

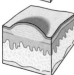 **Plaque:** Usually well-circumscribed lesion with large surface area and slight elevation.
Examples: psoriasis, lichen planus.

 Wheal: An elevation in the skin, with a smooth surface, sloping borders, and (usually) light pink color; caused by acute areas of edema in the skin; may appear, disappear, or change form abruptly within minutes or hours; size ranges from 3 mm to 20 cm.
Example: mosquito bite.

PALPABLE, FLUID-FILLED

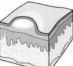 **Vesicle:** A small blister (up to 5 mm in diameter); fluid collection may be subcorneal, intraepidermal, or subepidermal.
Example: herpes simplex (early stages).

 Bulla: A blister larger than 5 mm; fluid may be located at various levels.
Examples: pemphigus, pemphigoid.

 Pustule: An elevated, well-circumscribed lesion containing purulent exudate.
Example: acne vulgaris.

From Copstead LEC, Banasik JL: *Pathophysiology: biological and behavioral perspectives,* ed 2, Philadelphia, 2000, WB Saunders, pp 1184-1185.

Continued

Table 13-1   Common Skin Lesions—cont'd

SECONDARY LESIONS

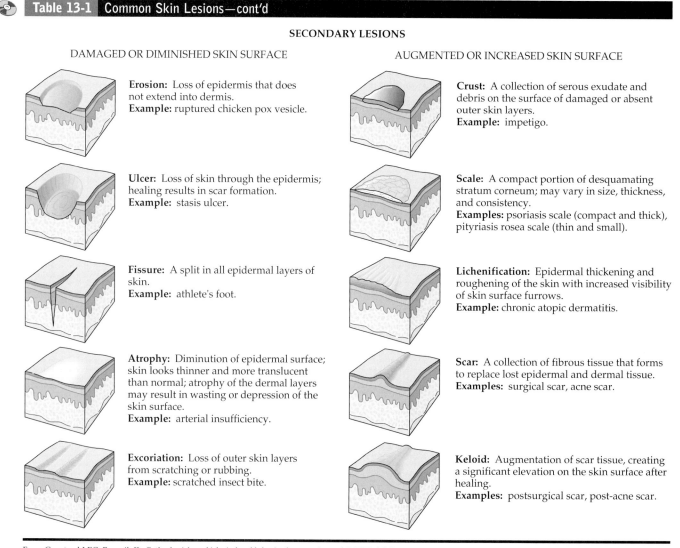

DAMAGED OR DIMINISHED SKIN SURFACE

Erosion: Loss of epidermis that does not extend into dermis.
Example: ruptured chicken pox vesicle.

Ulcer: Loss of skin through the epidermis; healing results in scar formation.
Example: stasis ulcer.

Fissure: A split in all epidermal layers of skin.
Example: athlete's foot.

Atrophy: Diminution of epidermal surface; skin looks thinner and more translucent than normal; atrophy of the dermal layers may result in wasting or depression of the skin surface.
Example: arterial insufficiency.

Excoriation: Loss of outer skin layers from scratching or rubbing.
Example: scratched insect bite.

AUGMENTED OR INCREASED SKIN SURFACE

Crust: A collection of serous exudate and debris on the surface of damaged or absent outer skin layers.
Example: impetigo.

Scale: A compact portion of desquamating stratum corneum; may vary in size, thickness, and consistency.
Examples: psoriasis scale (compact and thick), pityriasis rosea scale (thin and small).

Lichenification: Epidermal thickening and roughening of the skin with increased visibility of skin surface furrows.
Example: chronic atopic dermatitis.

Scar: A collection of fibrous tissue that forms to replace lost epidermal and dermal tissue.
Examples: surgical scar, acne scar.

Keloid: Augmentation of scar tissue, creating a significant elevation on the skin surface after healing.
Examples: postsurgical scar, post-acne scar.

From Copstead LEC, Banasik JL: *Pathophysiology: biological and behavioral perspectives,* ed 2, Philadelphia, 2000, WB Saunders, pp 1184-1185.

Urticaria

Urticaria, or hives, is a common skin condition that is often seen in athletes. When histamine is released from mast cells, it produces a characteristic triple response: vasodilation causing local erythema, erythematous flare beyond the local erythema, and leakage of fluid causing local tissue edema (Figure 13-3). The majority of cases are acute and can last up to a few weeks. The causes of urticaria are wide ranging and include allergies to foods such as shellfish, nuts, and eggs; food additives such as salicylates, dyes, and sulfites; drugs such as penicillin, aspirin, and sulfonamides; bacterial, viral, and fungal infections; and allergens such as pollens, mold, and animal dander. Internal disease; physical stimuli such as dermatographism, exercise, cholinergic agents, cold, and sun; skin diseases; hormones as seen during pregnancy; and genetic predisposition can also trigger urticaria.

A typical hive is an intensely itchy erythematous or white edematous area. A discussion of general urticaria and specific conditions follows.

Signs and Symptoms

General urticaria may develop at any age and is extremely common. The characteristic appearance described previously is fairly easy to diagnose, and most cases are self-limiting lasting from a few hours to a few weeks. The lesions are usually very itchy or **pruritic,** but the intensity may vary. Also, the size may range from small 2 mm lesions to very large areas.

Referral and Diagnostic Tests

Referral to a physician is appropriate if the symptoms persist for an extended period and they are interfering with daily activities. Immediate referral to a medical facility is necessary if an athlete shows signs or symptoms of **anaphylactic shock,** which may include

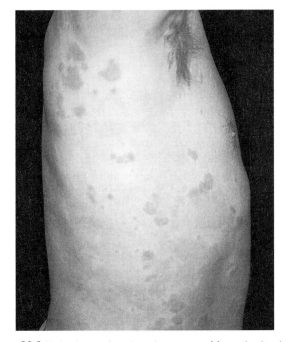

Figure 13-3 Urticaria seen here in various stages of formation is a local erythema reaction to exercise, temperature changes, drugs, or allergies. (From Habif TP: *Clinical dermatology e-dition*, ed 4, St Louis, 2004, Mosby, p 130.)

Box 13-2   Sedating Antihistamines

The following antihistamines have a sedating effect that may be counterproductive to athletic participation:
- Diphenhydramine (Benadryl)
- Hydroxyzine (Atarax)
- Dimenhydrinate (Dramamine)
- Promethazine (Phenergan)
- Brompheniramine (Dimetapp Allergy)
- Chlorpheniramine (Chlor-Trimeton)
- Clemastine (Tavist)
- Cyproheptadine (Periactin)

---

facial edema, swollen tongue, difficulty breathing, difficulty talking, hoarseness, or having near-syncopal or syncopal episodes (Red Flags—Anaphylactic Shock).

Red Flags for Anaphylactic Shock

General urticaria may also indicate anaphylactic shock. Any athlete with the following signs or symptoms should be referred to a medical facility immediately:
- Facial edema
- Swollen tongue
- Difficulty breathing
- Difficulty talking
- Difficulty swallowing
- Hoarseness
- Syncope or near syncope

Diagnostic testing to determine the exact cause of urticaria can be extremely expensive and endless, commonly with no resolution.

Treatment

The most effective treatment is to determine and eliminate the cause, but this is often extremely difficult. Most athletes will need an oral nonsedating antihistamine, such as loratadine (Claritin) or fexofenadine (Allegra), since the sedating antihistamines may impair performance. Another popular antihistamine commonly used for urticaria is cetirizine (Zyrtec), but it also has mild sedative properties although not as severe as the sedating antihistamines listed in Box 13-2.

If the aforementioned antihistamines are unsuccessful, the use of glucocorticoids (steroids) has been effective. In emergent situations, in which the athlete's airway is compromised, use of epinephrine (EpiPen) injection prescribed for that athlete may be warranted. Chapter 3 describes the correct use of an EpiPen.

Prognosis, Return to Participation, and Prevention

Most cases resolve spontaneously and have a good prognosis. The athlete may return to participation if stable and comfortable. The best prevention for most urticaria conditions is to determine and eliminate the cause or allergen if possible.

Dermatographism

Dermatographism is hives induced by rubbing or stroking the skin or rubbing of the skin with clothing. As many as 2% to 15% of the population may be dermatographical.[3] The exact cause is unknown, but recent infections or medications appear to be the most common cause. The hives develop within 1 to 3 minutes of stroking the skin and resolve in 30 to 60 minutes. The patients affected will go through periods of reactivity during their lifetimes, but dermatographism is more common in younger patients.

Signs and Symptoms

Dermatographism presents with blanching and associated linear edema and erythema (Figure 13-4). It can be on any part of the body because it does not matter if the skin is covered by clothing or equipment.

Referral, Diagnostic Tests, and Treatment

If an athlete presents with signs of dermatographism, referral may be warranted when the reaction is either severe or prolonged. The common test for this condition is to use a tongue blade to draw a line on the area to see the response. Any raised or discolored reaction is considered positive for dermatographism. No other diagnostic tests are needed. Treatment ranges from conservative use of topical agents to the use of oral antihistamines as described with general urticaria.

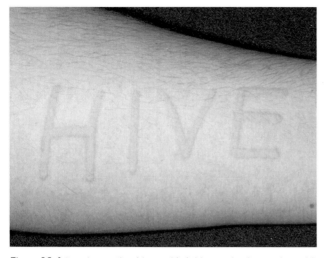

Figure 13-4 Drawing on the skin provided this reaction in a patient with dermatographism. (From Habif TP: *Clinical dermatology e-dition*, ed 4, St Louis, 2004, Mosby, p 143.)

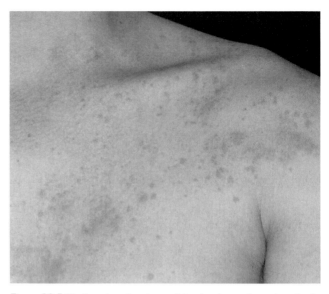

Figure 13-5 Cholinergic urticaria consists of red, round papular wheals. (From Habif TP: *Clinical dermatology e-dition*, ed 4, St Louis, 2004, Mosby, p 145.)

Prognosis and Return to Participation

The prognosis is excellent for dermatographism, and sports participation is not restricted. If the allergen is associated with the uniform or equipment necessary to participate, it would be wise to alter the allergen within safety rules to prevent recurrence. Another means of preventing dermatographism is to wear a barrier between the allergen and skin.

Cholinergic Urticaria

Cholinergic urticaria usually develops in younger patients between ages 10 and 30 years old and resolves spontaneously in only a small percentage of these patients. This reaction consists of 2 to 4 mm hives with surrounding erythema that occur during or shortly after the patient experiences an exposure to heat or overheating of the body during exercise, stress, or submission to heat (Figure 13-5). This reaction typically occurs within 2 to 20 minutes of exposure but may be delayed for up to 1 hour. Signs and symptoms are induced by the parasympathetic nervous system's release of acetylcholine and may last up to 3 hours.[3]

Signs and Symptoms

Symptoms of cholinergic urticaria include itching, burning, tingling, warmth, or irritation of the skin and may last from minutes to hours. Systemic symptoms of wheezing, **angioedema,** or hypotension may also occur. The athlete will have a higher core temperature than is normal.

Referral and Diagnostic Tests

The athletic trainer refers the athlete with symptoms of cholinergic urticaria to a physician for definitive diagnosis, which is typically by history and clinical examination. The patient may also exercise in place or on a stationary bicycle for about 10 to 15 minutes while being observed for the development of hives over 1 hour's time. This exercise will help to establish the diagnosis and is done only under the supervision of a physician at a medical facility.

Treatment

Treatment consists of limiting strenuous exercise, stressful environments, and hot showers. Antihistamines may help before exercise, but most often a strong sedating antihistamine is needed. Also, the athlete may shower with hot water to induce a reaction and deplete the histamine stores to begin a refractory period of about 24 hours. Athletes known to be reactive should always exercise with someone else in case exercise anaphylaxis occurs.

Prognosis and Return to Participation

Only a few cases of cholinergic urticaria spontaneously resolve because most of these patients will have persistent symptoms. Return to participation depends on the development of any additional symptoms, especially exercise-induced anaphylaxis.

Cold Urticaria

Cold urticaria occurs often in athletes since ice baths and ice therapy are a common treatment modality. Hives occur with exposure to cold objects such as ice or cold temperatures. The initial episode may occur after infections, medications, or emotional stress and is most commonly seen in 18- to 25-year-old patients. The recurrences will spontaneously resolve, typically

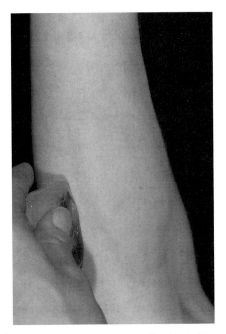

Figure 13-6 Cold urticaria hive reaction produced by holding an ice cube on this ankle. (From Habif TP: *Clinical dermatology e-dition*, ed 4, St Louis, 2004, Mosby, p 146.)

within 1 to 2 years, but some patients will have recurrences for 10 years or more.

Signs and Symptoms
An athlete will usually develop hives within 5 minutes of exposure to ice, cold water, or a sudden drop in the air temperature. These lesions may last 1 to 2 hours after removal of the stimulus. Systemic symptoms of generalized urticaria, angioedema, or anaphylaxis may also develop.

Referral, Diagnostic Tests, and Differential Diagnosis
The athletic trainer refers any athlete with extreme reactions to cold to a physician for definitive diagnosis and evaluation for other systemic symptoms. Diagnosis is made in the physician's office by applying ice to the skin for 1 to 5 minutes or exposing the forearm to water of 0° to 8° C (32° to 46° F) for 5 to 15 minutes and monitoring for hives (Figure 13-6). This is recommended only under the supervision of a physician in a medical facility since systemic symptoms and anaphylaxis may develop. Urticarial vasculitis, cholinergic urticaria, Raynaud's phenomenon, and dermatographism are all differential diagnoses for cold urticaria.

Treatment
Treatment consists of avoidance of sudden decreases in temperature and exposure to cold water or ice.

The antihistamine cyproheptadine and the tricyclic antidepressant doxepin have been shown to help suppress this reaction.[4-6]

Prognosis, Return to Participation, and Prevention
Symptoms in the majority of patients will eventually spontaneously resolve. Return to participation depends on the development of any other symptoms, such as angioedema, general urticaria, or anaphylaxis. If the reaction is local, the athlete may return if no other symptoms have developed within the following 1 to 2 hours. If generalized symptoms develop, return to participation should be determined by a physician. Prevention of cold urticaria includes reducing exposure to ice, cold objects, and sudden decreases in temperature.

Solar Urticaria

Solar urticaria is a condition manifested by hives that occur within minutes of exposure to ultraviolet (UV) light and resolve within 1 to 3 hours. The range of the electromagnetic spectrum, or UV light, that causes the hives is between 290 and 500 nm.[3] Systemic reactions such as syncope have occurred but are rare. Syncope typically occurs in young adults and more commonly in females shortly after sun exposure.

Referral, Diagnostic Tests, and Differential Diagnosis
The diagnosis of solar urticaria is based on the obvious hive or wheal formation and quick resolution. Further diagnostic testing includes photo testing and UV sleeve testing. UV sleeve testing exposes a section of skin to a given amount of UV light. The reaction determines if the patient is reactive to that range of UV light. Polymorphous light eruption, sunburn, and photo-allergic drug reaction are the differential diagnoses for solar urticaria.

Treatment, Prognosis, and Return to Participation
Treatment consists of antihistamines, liberal use of sunscreens, hats, long-sleeved clothing, and graded exposure to UV light. Prognosis is unknown, but immediate return to play is reasonable if no systemic symptoms, such as angioedema, syncope, or anaphylaxis, have occurred. Also, the athlete may return to outdoor activity with use of appropriate sunscreens.

Prevention
Prevention of solar urticaria consists of decreasing the amount of sun-exposed skin; using sunscreens; and wearing long sleeves, pants, and hats when possible. Most sunscreen agents absorb the ultraviolet B (UVB) radiation (290 to 320 nm) responsible for the development of hives; however, sunscreens that contain avobenzone (also known as Parasol 1789) will absorb

UVA I and UVA II wavelengths (340 to 400 nm and 320 to 340 nm, respectively), and sunscreens containing menthyl anthranilate and oxybenzone will absorb UVA II wavelengths.[7] All are responsible for the development of hives and other skin injuries related to sun exposure.[7]

Sebaceous Cysts

Sebaceous cysts, also known as epidermal or **keratinous cysts,** are very common in young people to middle-aged adults. These cysts have a thin wall filled with a white keratin material produced by the skin epithelium. They are slow growing, movable, and nontender (Figure 13-7).

Signs and Symptoms

Sebaceous cysts may occur anywhere on the body; however, the most common sites are the face, back, ears, chest, and scrotum. The cysts range in size from a few millimeters to several centimeters. They are usually soft, round, mobile, and smooth and have some communication with the surface. Some originate from comedones and are usually found on the back. The cyst wall may rupture, and the keratin creates an inflammatory reaction within the dermis. Sebaceous cysts may reabsorb or recur. They do not itch nor do they cause a localized increase in temperature.

Referral, Diagnostic Tests, and Differential Diagnosis

The athletic trainer refers an athlete who has skin swelling contained within a specific area or one that does not diminish in size or is problematic because of its location to a physician. No specific diagnostic tests are needed, but referral is necessary so that the physician can incise and drain the cyst. The differential diagnoses for sebaceous cysts include abscess, acne, boil, and skin tumor.

Treatment

Sebaceous cysts should be opened and drained by a physician, although some cysts require excision. The physician opens cysts with a no. 11 blade, and the keratin material is expressed through the opening. A no. 1 curette is then used to remove the remaining excess material, and the wall is removed by either expressing the cyst edges or grasping the wall with a small forceps. Infected cysts may require placement of a gauze drain following excision; the drain remains in place for 7 to 10 days. An oral antibiotic regimen may also be prescribed.

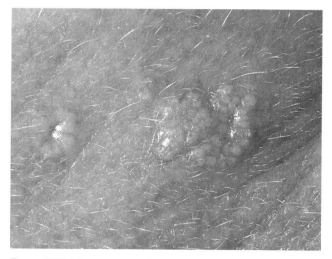

Figure 13-7 Sebaceous cyst. (From Habif TP: *Clinical dermatology e-dition,* ed 4, St Louis, 2004, Mosby, p 721.)

Prognosis and Return to Participation

Sebaceous cysts often recur. Sports participation is not restricted other than prevention of secondary infection.

Dermatitis

The term dermatitis is used loosely. Dermatitis means inflammation of the skin, and the large variety of causes is beyond the scope of this chapter. This chapter discusses two conditions: eczema and psoriasis.

Eczema

Eczema is often used synonymously with dermatitis and is the most common inflammatory skin disease. Whereas eczema itself often indicates vesicular dermatitis, some refer to it as chronic dermatitis.[8] It consists of three components: erythema, scales, and vesicles. The many causes of eczema include a contact allergic reaction such as to poison ivy, topical medicines including neomycin, atopic dermatitis, fungal infections, **dyshidrosis,** and habitual scratching. If left alone, most eczematous lesions will resolve, but patients are rarely able to avoid scratching.

Signs and Symptoms

Eczema consists of three stages: acute, subacute, and chronic. The acute stage consists of a red swollen plaque with small tiny vesicles. These lesions are very itchy, appear within days after exposure, and last for days to weeks. The subacute stage consists of **erythema** and scales of various degrees, which may also itch. The chronic stage consists of thickened skin with increased skin markings and moderate to intense itching (Figure 13-8).

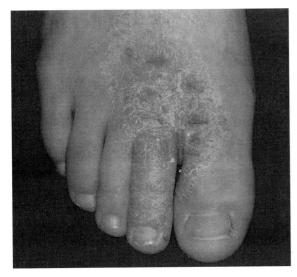

Figure 13-8 Chronic eczema of the feet. (From Callen JP, Jorrizzo JL, Greer KE, et al: *Color atlas of dermatology*, Philadelphia, 1993, WB Saunders, p 192.)

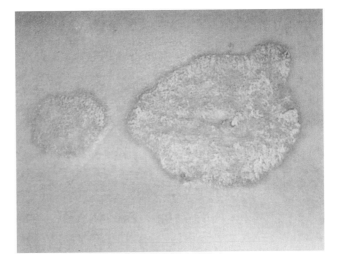

Figure 13-9 Psoriasis illustrated is in scaly erythematous patches with silvery scales on the top. (From Jarvis C: *Physical examination & health assessment*, ed 4, Philadelphia, 2004, WB Saunders, p 262.)

Referral and Diagnostic Tests

Referral to a physician is warranted for an athlete exhibiting increasing or persistent symptoms consistent with eczema. Diagnostic tests may include microscopic examination with a **potassium hydroxide (KOH)** preparation. Patch testing may be needed to determine specific allergens. Patch testing involves covering the skin with various patches of allergens for 1 to 2 days to determine which ones cause an allergic response.

Differential Diagnosis

Differential diagnoses for eczema include bacterial infection, fungal infection, herpes simplex virus (HSV) infection, psoriasis, atopic dermatitis, asteatotic dermatitis, habitual scratching, scabies, seborrheic dermatitis, contact dermatitis, systemic lupus erythematosus (SLE), or discoid lupus erythematosus.

Treatment, Prognosis, and Return to Participation

The most important treatment for eczema is removal from the allergen if possible. The acute stage is treated with cool compresses changed every 30 minutes, with or without Burow's (aluminum sulfate) solution. Oral steroids may be needed to control the inflammation. Antihistamines may be used to reduce itching, and antibiotics should be started if there are signs of infection.

The subacute stage is treated by eliminating wet dressings and using topical steroids, ointments, creams, or lotions. Oral antibiotics may be necessary when signs of infection are present. The chronic stage is similar to the subacute stage, but stronger topical steroids are necessary and steroid injections may also be required. Prognosis of eczema depends on the severity of the reaction. Unless the reaction is severe

or a significant infection has developed, the athlete may return to play without restriction.

Psoriasis

Psoriasis is a genetic, chronic, and recurring disorder that usually begins during childhood. It is a scaling, papular infection similar to eczema but without the epithelial eruptions, wet areas, and crusts.[8] In some cases, a streptococcal infection may precipitate the onset of the disorder. Psoriasis affects an estimated 4% of the population worldwide.[8] Psoriasis has a gradual onset and usually has chronic remission and recurrence states that vary in frequency and duration, but permanent remissions are rare.[8]

A small percentage of patients with psoriasis also experience psoriatic arthritis.[8] The exacerbation-remission cycle common to the skin disorder may coincide with the arthritic component. Most often, the distal interphalangeal joints of the fingers and toes are affected. Unlike rheumatoid arthritis (RA), psoriatic arthritis tends to be in remission more frequently and rapidly than RA, and it lacks the typical joint nodules associated with RA. The psoriatic arthritic patient may progress to chronic, disabling arthritis, so complaints of joint pain in the psoriatic person must not be overlooked.[8]

Signs and Symptoms

The distinctive lesion of psoriasis is a silvery white plaque with surrounding erythema with distinct borders (Figure 13-9). The lesions usually begin as small, red, scaly papules that coalesce into round or oval plaques except in the skinfolds, where they appear as deep red, macerated plaques. These lesions are most common on the extensor surfaces, such as

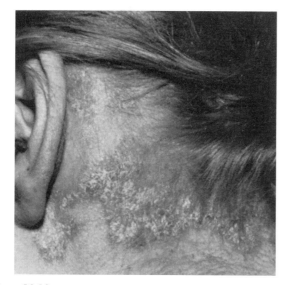

Figure 13-10 Psoriasis is common on the elbows, knees, neck, and low back. (From Arnold HL, Odom RB, James WD: *Andrew's diseases of the skin: clinical dermatology,* ed 8, Philadelphia, 1990, WB Saunders, p 200.)

the elbows and knees, but are also very common on the scalp, fingernails, toenails, gluteal clefts, and previous sites of trauma (Figure 13-10).

Forms of psoriasis may develop other than the general chronic plaque type just described. Another common form is scalp psoriasis. The scalp, which may be the only site affected, has a thick erythematous silvery scale in multiple areas. This lesion may extend onto the forehead. Psoriasis of the nails is another type and is demonstrated by pitting of the nails.

Referral and Diagnostic Tests

Any athlete suspected of having psoriasis is referred to a physician for medical evaluation and initiation of treatment. The clearly defined, dry, and silvery scales are quite distinguishable and unique to psoriasis. Although diagnosis is rarely difficult, testing includes a complete blood count (CBC) and a streptococcus screen.

Differential Diagnosis

Streptococcal infections; pityriasis rosea; SLE; seborrheic dermatitis; **lichen simplex chronicus;** squamous cell carcinoma; secondary syphilis; candidiasis; drug eruptions generally caused by beta-blockers, gold, or methyldopa; and pancreatic tumor are all differential diagnoses for psoriasis.

Treatment

Treatment for psoriasis is very complicated and involves the use of topical steroids such as calcipotriol (Dovonex), anthralin ointment, UV light, and steroid injections. Lubricating creams, including hydrogenated vegetable oil, white petrolatum, and crude coal tar,

combined with exposure to UV light (280 to 320 nm) have been effective.[8] The prescription of oral steroids is contraindicated because of the drug's side effects, which include severe exacerbations of psoriasis.

Prognosis and Return to Participation

The prognosis for psoriasis is determined by the extent of the disease and whether the arthritic component is present. Traditionally, more severe attacks coincide with an earlier onset of the disease. Return to participation depends on whether arthritis is involved and the degree of debilitation. Most likely the athlete will have no restrictions, but close follow-up is recommended to prevent flare-ups.

Melanoma

Mention of melanoma in this chapter is not intended to provide definitive diagnosis but to encourage an appreciation of suspicious lesions so timely recognition and referral are made (Red Flags—Melanoma).

▶ Red Flags for Melanoma

Moles: A mole is a benign skin tumor. Certain types of moles increase a person's chance of getting melanoma. People with many moles and those who have some large moles have an increased risk for melanoma.

Fair skin: People with fair skin, freckling, light hair, or blue eyes have a higher risk of melanoma, but anyone can get melanoma.

Family history: Around 10% of people with melanoma have a close relative (e.g., mother, father, brother, sister, child) with the disease. A strong family history of breast and ovarian cancer could mean that certain gene changes or mutations are present. Men with this gene change have a higher risk of melanoma.

Immune suppression: People who have been treated with medicines that suppress the immune system, such as transplant patients, have an increased risk of developing melanoma.

Ultraviolet (UV) radiation: Too much exposure to UV radiation is a risk factor for melanoma. The main source of such radiation is sunlight. Tanning lamps and booths are another source.

Age: About one half of melanomas occur in people over the age of 50 years, but younger people are also susceptible.

Gender: Men have a higher rate of melanoma than women.

Xeroderma pigmentosum (XP): XP is a rare, inherited condition. People with XP are less able to repair damage caused by sunlight and are thus at greater risk of melanoma.

Past history of melanoma: A person who has already had melanoma has a higher risk of getting another melanoma.

From the American Cancer Society website @ http://www.cancer.org/docroot/ CRI/content/CRI_2_2_2X_What_causes_melanoma_skin_cancer_50.asp?sitearea=.

Melanoma is a very dangerous skin disorder and may produce a lifetime risk of more than 1 in 79 Caucasian Americans.[9] This number will surely grow with the increasing number of people exposed to UV light from either the sun or tanning booths. The rate of malignant melanoma has increased by an alarming 1900% since the 1930s, has tripled since 1980,

Table 13-2	The ABCDs of Skin Cancer	
	Descriptor	Parameters
A	Asymmetry	A melanoma lesion cannot be "folded in half"; in other words, the lesion does not have equal right and left sections or top and bottom sections.
B	Border	Benign lesions have a sharp distinct border that can easily be traced, whereas malignant lesions may have borders that can fade off and be difficult to trace.
C	Color	Benign lesions have a uniform tan, brown, or black color, whereas malignant lesions may have variegated or multiple (i.e., red, white, and blue) color patterns. In addition, a sudden darkening in color or spreading into normal skin suggests a malignant lesion.
D	Diameter	Benign lesions usually have a diameter of less than 6 mm, whereas malignant lesions usually have a diameter greater than 6 mm.

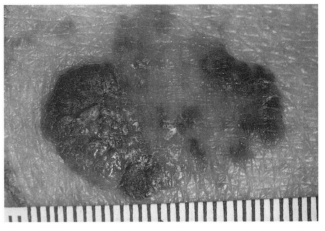

Figure 13-11 Melanoma is characterized by asymmetry, border irregularity, and color differences within its borders. (From Cotran RS, Kumar V, Collins T: *Robbins pathologic basis of disease*, ed 6, Philadelphia, 1999, WB Saunders, p 1179.)

and is growing at more than 9% per year.[10] The American Cancer Society[11] estimates that in 2004, 55,100 new cases of melanoma will be diagnosed in the United States and 7900 people will die annually. The most susceptible individuals have fair skin and blue eyes, sunburn easily, had multiple sunburns at an early age, and have a personal or family history of skin cancer.[9,11] Since 40% to 50% of malignant melanomas arise from pigmented moles, people with moles or freckles should be especially cautious.[8]

Signs and Symptoms

The athlete should note any changes in a skin mole or lesion. Although it is important to be cognizant about all changes that occur in skin, athletes must also be aware of alterations that are suspicious. Both the American Academy of Dermatology and the American Cancer Society use the ABCD acronym to assess skin changes: A for asymmetry, B for border irregularity, C for color, and D for diameter (Table 13-2). A mole or lesion should have clear, definitive borders. If it does not, the lesion is suspicious and needs to be evaluated by a physician. The mole should not be larger than 0.6 mm, or the diameter of a pencil eraser, nor should it grow. The athletic trainer needs to refer any athletes with changes in shape, border, or size of a mole or lesion or the development of ulceration or bleeding, all of which are suggestive of melanoma, to a physician for assessment (Figure 13-11).

Referral, Diagnostic Tests, and Treatment

Although benign moles, freckles, and age spots may provoke suspicion, it is wise to refer any questionable lesion to a medical doctor for inspection and likely a biopsy. If caught early, surgically removed melanoma has a high cure rate, but once it metastasizes to the lymph nodes, the 5-year survival rate drops to 30% to 40%.[9] If organ involvement has occurred through this spread, the survival rate drops again to 12%.[9] Excision includes removing at least 1 cm lateral to the tumor.[8] Large surgical areas may require skin grafts or loss of underlying tissue that could result in deformity of the area involved.

Prognosis and Return to Participation

Prognosis for the athlete with melanoma depends on the thickness of the tumor involved. Tumors less than 0.76 mm have a 98% to 100% 5-year survival rate, whereas tumors greater than 3.0 mm thick have approximately a 46% survival rate for the same period.[8] The more tissue involved, the longer an athlete will need to recover.

Prognosis and return to participation also relate to the tumor's growth to other areas or tissues. An athlete with a melanoma contained within one mole will have a return-to-participation rate that is based on the sutures and the location of surgery as well as any additional treatment, such as chemotherapy. Melanoma involving organs or the lymphatic system most likely will require cessation or at least great reduction of activity until the cancer is fully under control.

Prevention

People can be genetically predisposed to melanoma.[9,11] Overexposure to UV light, even for brief periods, can cause a two-fold increase in incidence of melanoma, so protection from the sun is paramount.[9] The liberal use of sunscreens with at least an SPF 30 rating and those effective against UVA and UVB can greatly reduce exposure. Darker skinned athletes are not immune to melanoma and should be encouraged to follow these precautions as well (Key Points—Proper Sunscreen Application).

KEY POINTS
Proper Sunscreen Application

- Apply sunscreen at least 20 to 30 minutes before exposure.
- Use a sunscreen with a high SPF (sun protection factor), as well as one that has waterproof capabilities.
- Apply liberally to all exposed areas, including ears, back of the neck, and posterior aspect of legs.
- Reapply often (at least every hour) and after drying off from water activities.
- Realize that the sun does not need to be shining for one to be dangerously exposed to UVA or UVB light so make using sunscreen a daily habit.
- Use sunscreen even when in the shade; sunlight reflected off water can also cause damage to skin.

UVA, Ultraviolet A; *UVB*, ultraviolet B.

Other protection from the sun includes hats with wide brims that can increase coverage to the face, neck, and portions of the shoulders. Long-sleeved shirts and pants aid in protection, as does wearing gloves when possible during gardening, golf, or cycling. Sunglasses with UVA or UVB protection help protect the eyes from not only direct sun but also reflective sunlight.

Educating athletes to be proactive in regular self-screening of their skin for the basic ABCDs may help determine if lesions need further evaluation. Benign lesions usually appear early in life, and malignant lesions typically arise from preexisting moles or appear spontaneously later in life. If these characteristics are recognized in evaluation or normal daily interaction with athletes, referral to a physician for follow-up evaluation is in order.

Bacterial Conditions

Bacterial skin disorders include impetigo, abscesses, folliculitis, furuncles or boils, carbuncles, and paronychia or onychia. The healthy skin typically has many different bacterial and fungal organisms that are usually held in check and do not cause infection. The bacteria, often *Staphylococcus aureus* or *Streptococcus pyogenes*, are introduced into a break in the skin where they begin to secrete toxins or interfere with cellular function, thereby producing symptoms.

S. aureus and *S. pyogenes* are responsible for the vast majority of bacterial dermatological conditions. One must also realize that bacterial and viral conditions may coexist within the same infection and therefore complicate the diagnosis and treatment. Finally, it is important to note that an individual is not necessarily immune from a particular bacterial infection

---

Box 13-3 NCAA Participation Regulations for Wrestlers

The following regulations apply to participation with the bacterial conditions of impetigo, folliculitis, furuncles, carbuncles, and staphylococcal diseases:
- Completion of at least 72 hours of antibiotic therapy
- No new lesions for 48 hours
- No moist, draining, or exudative lesions
- Active lesions may *not* be covered to participate

From National Collegiate Athletic Association (NCAA): *2005 NCAA wrestling rules and interpretations*, Indianapolis, 2004, NCAA.

---

after recovery. Given the right conditions, infection is possible again.

The NCAA has specifically singled out the bacterial infections of impetigo, folliculitis, furuncles, carbuncles, **cellulitis,** and staphylococcal diseases for particular restrictions (Box 13-3). Wrestlers, especially, must have successfully completed 72 hours of antibiotic therapy, have no new lesions for 48 hours, and have no moist, draining, or **exudative** lesions at time of participation. In addition, the covering of any active infections is not allowed for participation.[12] Although these rules are especially for wrestlers, they may apply to all athletes, from swimmers to football players. Protection of others from infection is paramount along with the health and welfare of the infected athlete. These guidelines will be reiterated under each bacterial infection discussed.

Impetigo

Impetigo is a highly contagious skin disorder caused by either *S. aureus* or *S. pyogenes* bacteria, with *S. aureus* accounting for the majority of the infections. It is common in warm temperatures and humid areas and usually occurs in areas of previous skin disease or injury, such as eczema or abrasion. Earlier damage to the skin by abrasion opens a pathway for bacteria to invade, leading to impetigo.[13] Impetigo is transmitted by contact, with combative sports having a higher incidence of transmission than other activities.[14] Each year, it easily prevents a large number of athletes from participating. Impetigo is a self-limiting disease that heals without scarring, but it can have life-threatening sequelae in acute poststreptococcal **glomerulonephritis.**[15]

Signs and Symptoms
Athletes with impetigo generally are afebrile but may have localized **lymphadenopathy.**[13] The two types of impetigo are nonbullous and bullous. The nonbullous form typically appears as a yellow or honey-colored, crusted lesion on an erythematous base (Figure 13-12). Bullous impetigo first presents with moist, red skin that resembles an actual burn and progresses to flaccid small to large vesicles that appear filled with clear or

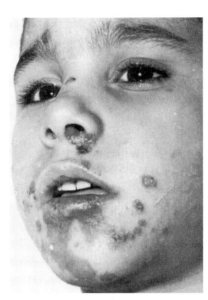

Figure 13-12 Impetigo presents with a honey-yellow crust covering the lesion. (From Arnold HL, Odom RB, James WD: *Andrew's diseases of the skin: clinical dermatology*, ed 8, Philadelphia, 1990, WB Saunders, p 275.)

yellow fluid.[15] Both forms have lesions that may be small and pea shaped or large and blisterlike in appearance or circinate ribbonlike strands of the bacteria.[8]

Lesions of impetigo eventually erupt, leaving **purulent** discharge to dry on the skin. They are painless yet pruritic, which exacerbates and spreads the infection to other regional areas.[15] The face, arms, legs, and trunk are the most common sites for impetigo.

Referral, Diagnostic Tests, and Differential Diagnosis
The athletic trainer who suspects an athlete may have impetigo should remove the athlete from activity immediately to prevent the spread of the infection to others and make a referral to a physician. Diagnosis is mostly by clinical examination, but a culture may be obtained if the diagnosis is unclear.[13] In this case, the patient is treated for both impetigo and herpes simplex until the cultures return. Differential diagnosis for impetigo includes HSV, varicella-zoster virus (VZV), and tinea infections.

Treatment
Treatment for a small area of impetigo consists of a topical antibiotic such as mupirocin (Bactroban) applied three times daily for 10 days or until the lesion has cleared. Larger areas of impetigo are generally treated with oral antibiotics that cover both *S. aureus* and *S. pyogenes*, such as penicillin, erythromycin, cephalexin (Keflex), and dicloxacillin.

The athlete washes the area with soap and water three times daily, removes the crusts before application of a topical antibiotic, and is not allowed to participate in contact activity until the lesions have completely cleared.

Prognosis and Return to Participation
The athlete may return to play on complete resolution of the crusted, infected, exposed areas. In wrestling, the NCAA recommends that the athlete not return until there have been no new lesions over the last 48 hours and the athlete has been taking antibiotics for the last 72 hours. Active lesions are not to be covered to allow for competition. Any nonactive lesions, however, are covered with a nonpermeable barrier sturdy enough to remain in place during aggressive participation.[12]

Prevention
When impetigo recurs multiple times, family members or close contacts may need to have nasopharyngeal cultures because 30% to 40% may be asymptomatic carriers of the causative bacteria (*S. aureus*).[13] If this proves to be the case, the carrier will need to apply mupirocin ointment to the nasal passages twice daily for 5 days.[13,16]

Equipment that may have come in contact with athletes who have lesions must be sanitized on a daily basis to prevent the spread of infection or recurrence. Equipment in this case includes all mats, towels, protective gear, water bottles, clothing, and uniforms.[1]

Folliculitis

Folliculitis is another common bacterial skin infection. There are two types of bacteria that cause folliculitis: *S. aureus* and *Pseudomonas aeruginosa*, which is often associated with infections picked up in hot tubs.

Folliculitis is an inflammatory reaction in the hair follicles and most commonly occurs in the hair follicles on the face, chest, axilla, buttocks, groin, and legs. The most common cause is shaving with a razor blade. When a razor blade nicks the skin the opening produced allows bacteria to be introduced into the tissue (Figure 13-13). Folliculitis may also be caused from friction by helmets, equipment padding or straps.

The other common bacterial cause of folliculitis is *Pseudomonas*, which is commonly referred to as hot tub folliculitis (Figure 13-14). This type usually appears 2 or 3 days after exposure to water contaminated with *P. aeruginosa*. The most common conduits are poorly maintained hot tubs, pools, baths, water slides, and contaminated waters. There does not appear to be any skin-to-skin transmission.

Signs and Symptoms
Clinical presentation of folliculitis demonstrates small, tender, red papules or bumps in the hair follicles with a hair shaft within the papule. These lesions tend to occur in multiples and are often pruritic.[15] The typical

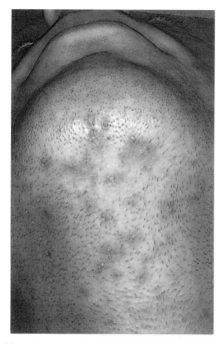

Figure 13-13 Folliculitis in a beard, characterized by superficial infection of hair follicles. (From Jarvis C: *Physical examination & health assessment*, ed 4, Philadelphia, 2004, WB Saunders, p 267.)

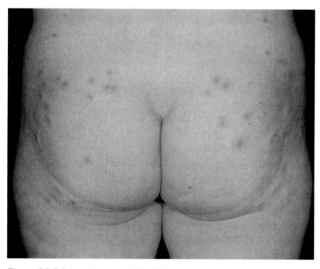

Figure 13-14 *Pseudomonas* folliculitis reaction resulting from exposure to a hot tub; the rash appears in areas covered by a swimsuit. (From Habif TP: *Clinical dermatology e-dition*, ed 4, St Louis, 2004, Mosby, p 291.)

presentation of hot tub folliculitis consists of itchy red papules around hair follicles in many areas of the body but most commonly under areas covered by the swimming suit.

Referral, Diagnostic Tests, and Differential Diagnosis
The athletic trainer refers athletes with persistent symptoms despite conservative treatment or those with an unusual presentation. Physician diagnosis is made on the basis of clinical examination, but a Gram stain and culture may be obtained if the exam is questionable or persistent. Differential diagnosis for folliculitis includes *Pityrosporum* folliculitis, dermatophytic folliculitis, gram-negative folliculitis, HSV, acne, pityriasis rosea, molluscum contagiosum, and syphilis.

Treatment
Treatment for folliculitis includes topical or oral antibiotics that provide coverage for both *S. aureus* and *S. pyogenes*. Warm saline compresses and a topical antimicrobial ointment such as bacitracin may also benefit the athlete.[15] The athlete washes the area with an antibacterial soap and water two or three times daily, changes razors after each use, and uses single-edge razors until the infection is healed. In cases of recurrent folliculitis, the athlete may benefit from a nasal culture for *S. aureus*.[15] Treatment of *Pseudomonas* is not needed because this type of folliculitis usually resolves spontaneously in 7 to 10 days as long as there is no additional exposure. Sometimes antibiotic treatment is required. The athlete may return to participation immediately and without restrictions.

Prognosis and Return to Participation
An athlete may return to participation when the lesions of folliculitis begin to heal. In wrestling, the NCAA recommends that the athlete not return until there have been no new lesions for the last 48 hours and the athlete has been taking antibiotics for the last 72 hours. As with impetigo, nonactive lesions must be covered with durable, nonporous bandaging for participation.[12] The amount of time it takes for these lesions to heal may depend on their location; some areas, such as the beard, take much longer to heal. The athlete with *Pseudomonas* may participate without restriction.

Abscess, Furuncle, and Carbuncle

Furunculosis is similar to folliculitis but occurs when lesions are deeper in the hair follicle cavity and contain pus.[13] These lesions are also bacterial skin infections but are caused by *S. aureus* and include abscesses, furuncles, and carbuncles, which are a conglomeration of multiple furuncles. An **abscess** is a collection of pus that arises in a variety of locations. A **furuncle**, or boil, is a walled-off abscess containing pus that usually develops in a preexisting site of folliculitis. Boils commonly occur at site of trauma or friction, such as a belt line, waistline, axilla, groin, thigh, and buttocks, and are more common after puberty.[13]

A **carbuncle** is a collection of several coalescing furuncles. Carbuncles are common among wrestlers and readily transmitted by skin-to-skin contact. New strains of *S. aureus*, such as methicillin-resistant

S. aureus (MRSA), have recently appeared that are resistant to certain commonly used medications.[17] These strains are difficult to treat and eradicate. This becomes especially problematic in athletics where athletes are allowed to participate as long as they are receiving medical treatment. One study on high school wrestlers noted that 22% of furuncles contained methicillin-resistant strains of *S. aureus*.[18] Resistant strains cause the athlete to sustain the effects of the infection for a longer period of time, allow more opportunity to spread the disease, and may result in severe systemic illness.

Signs and Symptoms

The lesion usually begins with a tender, deep, firm, erythematous papule that enlarges and becomes painful and fluctuant over a period of days (Figure 13-15). The abscess remains deep, reabsorbs, or drains through the skin.

Referral, Diagnostic Tests, and Differential Diagnosis

The athletic trainer refers an athlete who presents with an elevated temperature, malaise, vomiting, and persistence of furuncles following conservative treatment to a physician. Diagnostic tests include a Gram stain for gram-positive cocci and a culture to determine the organism involved, but a culture is usually reserved for persistent infections that do not respond to treatment. A blood culture with antibiotic sensitivities may be obtained with symptoms of a systemic infection, such as fever and malaise. Differential diagnosis includes folliculitis, sebaceous cyst, skin cancer, severe HSV infection, **hidradenitis suppurativa** if located in the axilla or groin, and **pilonidal** cyst if the furuncle is located in the gluteal cleft.

Treatment and Prevention

Treatment of furuncles consists of warm moist compresses applied frequently throughout the day (Red Flags—Contagion). If this fails, a physician incises and

> **Red Flags for Contagion**
>
> Moist compresses or heat packs used on infectious skin disorders MUST be disinfected before use on another patient!

evacuates the abscess. Antibiotics are usually not effective once the abscess has developed, although they are still frequently prescribed.

An athlete who develops frequent episodes of furuncles may need topical antibiotic ointment for the nasal passages to eradicate a carrier state as discussed with impetigo. Return to sport with protection is allowed when the infection begins to heal. In wrestling, however, the NCAA recommends that an athlete not return until there have been no new lesions for the

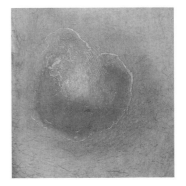

Figure 13-15 A furuncle or boil is an enlarged swollen purulent mass. (From Habif TP: *Clinical dermatology e-dition,* ed 4, St Louis, 2004, Mosby, p 284.)

last 48 hours and the athlete has been taking antibiotics for the last 72 hours. As with the other bacterial infections, active lesions should not be covered to allow for participation.[12]

Preventive measures include treating the athlete and close contact members for *S. aureus* carrier states for recurrent infections. Other prevention techniques mentioned with folliculitis and impetigo will also assist in retarding the spread of furuncles.

Acne

Acne is a common problem among adolescents, but very little information exists regarding acne and sports participation. **Acne** is a condition of the pilosebaceous unit and most commonly occurs where the concentration of sebaceous or sweat glands is the greatest, such as on the face, neck, chest, and back (Figure 13-16). The condition is common in both males and females.

Signs and Symptoms

Acne consists of inflammatory and noninflammatory lesions. Inflammatory lesions are composed of erythematous papules, pustules, or deep cysts; noninflammatory lesions are made up of open and closed comedones. **Open comedones** are commonly referred to as blackheads, and **closed comedones** are commonly referred to as whiteheads.

The bacteria involved is *Propionibacterium acnes* and not *S. aureus* or *S. pyogenes*. The follicular shaft becomes plugged, and the proliferation of *P. acnes* secondarily increases keratin formation. This is known as a noninflammatory reaction, but when white blood cells are attracted to these lesions, the acne becomes inflammatory. Symptoms range from a few open or closed comedones on the face or another area to multiple comedones, pustules, and deep, large, painful cysts.

Differential Diagnosis

Differential diagnosis for acne includes bacterial folliculitis, *Pityrosporum* folliculitis, pseudofolliculitis, perioral dermatitis, **human papillomavirus** (HPV), HSV infections, and **contact dermatitis.**

Treatment and Prognosis

Depending on the type, acne responds well to a variety of agents. Noninflammatory acne responds well to

topical adapalene (Differin), tretinoin (Retin-A, Avita), azelaic acid (Azelex, Finevin), and tazarotene (Tazorac). Benzoyl peroxide is an antibacterial agent but also works well for noninflammatory acne. Inflammatory acne responds well to topical benzoyl peroxide either alone or in combination with an antibiotic as well as topical and oral antibiotics. For resistant or severe cystic acne, isotretinoin (Accutane) is used but has a significant number of side effects. The athletic trainer and physician counsel athletes during acne treatment about the side effects of some acne medications; these medications may cause sensitivity to sunlight and, as a result, may increase likelihood of sunburn.

Acne is not considered contagious or counterproductive to activity, so athletes are allowed to participate without restrictions.

Paronychia or Onychia

Paronychia is an infection that affects the proximal or lateral nail fold that separates the skin from the nail, and **onychia** is an infection of the nail matrix (see Figure 13-2). The infection may occur after manipulation, other infection, or trauma. The organism usually involved is *S. aureus* but can also be a fungal infection if the athlete is immunocompromised. Other obscure causes include prolonged water exposure, herpes simplex, or candidal vaginitis.[8]

Signs, Symptoms, Referral, and Diagnostic Tests

A paronychia is a bright red swelling of the nail fold, which may show an accumulation of purulent material (Figure 13-17). Onychial infection is deeper and proximal to the nail instead of a superficial location in the nail fold.

Athletes with infected nail beds are referred when conservative care is not effective. Referral is also indicated for immunocompromised patients or persistent

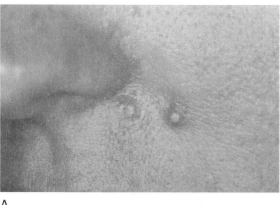

A

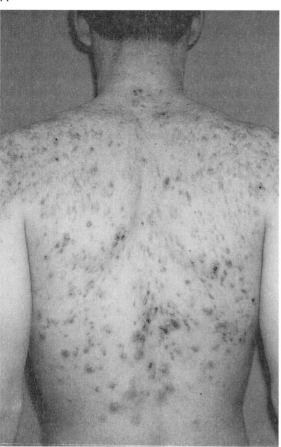

B

Figure 13-16 Acne is typical among adolescent athletes and common on the, **A**, face and chin, and, **B**, shoulders and back. (From Callen JP, Jorrizzo JL, Greer KE, et al: *Color atlas of dermatology*, Philadelphia, 1993, WB Saunders, p 178.)

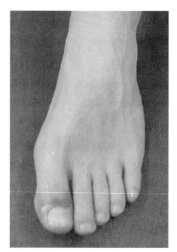

Figure 13-17 Paronychia surrounding a great toe.

worsening symptoms. If the patient is immunocompetent, no further diagnostic testing is needed unless the symptoms persist, and then a Gram stain, KOH preparation, and culture of the fluid are obtained.

Differential Diagnosis and Treatment

Differential diagnosis for paronychias includes bacterial infections, fungal infections, *Pseudomonas,* and trauma. Conservative treatment consists of warm to hot soaks and acetaminophen (Tylenol) for mild pain. If the infection is large, especially painful, or disabling, a small incision into the corresponding location will relieve the pressure by draining the infection. Sometimes antibiotics are needed if incision and drainage are inadequate.

Prognosis, Return to Participation, and Prevention

Participation is not restricted with a paronychial infection, and the prognosis following treatment is good. If the area was drained, the athletic trainer should follow basic wound care protocol to prevent further infection.

Prevention of paronychial or onychial infections consists of good nail and skin hygiene and limited manipulation with careful nail cutting. Keeping fingers and toes clean and dry will retard these infections.[8]

Viral Conditions

Viral infections represent one of the most difficult and challenging problems in athletes, especially wrestlers. The viruses presented in this section include herpes simplex (HSV), varicella-zoster (VZV), molluscum contagiosum, and human papillomavirus (HPV).

Herpes Simplex

HSV is an extremely contagious viral infection and presents as cold sores or fever blisters, genital herpes, and herpes gladiatorum. There are more than 80 types of HSV, but the most common types are HSV-1, which typically occurs above the waist, and HSV-2, which typically occurs below the waist. Both types, however, can be found on both areas, and typing may only be significant for future outbreak prediction and response to treatment.

It is estimated that 1 in 5 people in the United States ages 12 years and older (22%) is infected with HSV-2, and 80% to 90% of the population are infected with HSV-1.[19] Not everyone develops symptoms once infected, and each person experiences a different rate of recurrence. HSV enters the skin through a site of previous injury, such as a cut or abrasion, or damage, such as eczema, and follows the nerve root to the dorsal root ganglion in the spinal cord. An individual may not develop symptoms or a rash during the primary infection.

At various times, HSV will follow the nerves back to the skin and produce symptoms along the dermatomal distribution. HSV is never eradicated, but symptoms present in varying degrees. One study of genital herpes suggests that approximately 70% of genital herpes is transmitted by asymptomatic shedding of the virus in people who report never having had the infection.[20]

When HSV occurs on the face and trunk, it is commonly known as **herpes gladiatorum.** Estimates indicate that 2.6% of high school and 7.6% of collegiate wrestlers have been infected with HSV, and approximately 20% to 40% of NCAA Division I wrestlers have been infected.[21] These numbers probably underestimate the problem because some lesions remain unrecognized. Spread of infection is typically the result of direct skin-to-skin contact with an infected person. Outbreaks are usually found on the head and trunk but are not limited to these areas.

Complications of HSV are numerous and include chronic recurrences, skin lesions, possible scarring, eye or corneal scarring, and blindness. **Herpes keratoconjunctivitis** is a highly infectious condition of the cornea of the eye that may lead to corneal damage, scarring, or even blindness.[22] HSV keratoconjunctivitis is the leading infectious cause of blindness in the United States.[22-24] The infection may be either by direct contact or reactivation of HSV through the ophthalmic branch of the trigeminal nerve.

So-called fever blisters or cold sores are also caused by HSV, and people with active lesions can transmit the virus to otherwise healthy body areas (Figure 13-18). Also known as herpes labialis, cold sores can be exacerbated by UV light from the sun and cold stress.[25]

Signs and Symptoms

Typical symptoms for the primary HSV infection mimic the flu and include fever, sore throat, lymphadenopathy, malaise, and vesicles on an erythematous base.

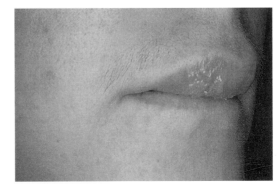

Figure 13-18 Herpes simplex, also called a cold sore, presents as tight vesicles that develop into pustules and ulcers. (From Jarvis C: *Physical examination & health assessment,* ed 4, Philadelphia, 2004, WB Saunders, p 262.)

Recurrent HSV infection symptoms include vesicles of the same shape and age on an erythematous base. Occasionally, tingling or pain precedes the outbreak.

Outbreaks may present in many ways, however, and do not always present as the typical vesicles on an erythematous base. In the early stages they are often easily confused with ringworm, impetigo, acne, and eczema. Sometimes wrestlers break open the vesicles, cover the rash with makeup, sandpaper the rash, or even use bleach to alter the rash in order to continue to wrestle. Obviously, diagnosis is then even more difficult and the infection can spread more easily to others.

Referral, Diagnostic Tests, and Differential Diagnosis

The clinical diagnosis in many cases of HSV is made on the basis of symptoms and exposure. The most definitive method of diagnosis is to unroof an intact moist vesicle and culture the base for HSV. This method may take 4 to 5 days to yield results and is only about 70% to 80% accurate, so once a diagnosis is suspected, the athlete should be kept out of contact with other athletes.[25] A relatively new test, polymerase chain reaction (PCR), is accurate and fast but expensive. Withholding an athlete from contact activity before a culture is taken and medications are started is absolutely necessary to prevent spread of the disease. Differential diagnoses for HSV include bacterial infections such as impetigo, acne, various types of folliculitis; viral varicella-zoster; and fungal tinea infections.

Treatment

Oral antiviral medications include acyclovir, zovirax, valacyclovir (Valtrex), and famciclovir (Famvir). Doses differ depending on whether the condition is a primary or recurrent outbreak. For wrestlers, prophylactic medications should be continued after the outbreak for the remainder of the wrestling season. Prophylactic doses are acyclovir, 400 mg two times daily; valacyclovir, 1000 mg daily; and famciclovir, 250 mg daily. The athlete must shower with antibacterial soap and launder all towels and uniforms daily. Although drug reactions with antiviral medications are rare, dehydration is a possible concern in wrestlers or in someone who has poor renal function, and can lead to severe kidney problems.[25] Athletes taking antiviral medications are encouraged to increase fluid intake for the duration of the medical course.

Prognosis and Return to Participation

Current NCAA recommendations require the athlete to be withheld from contact sports until the athlete is asymptomatic, no new lesions are seen for the previous 3 days, the athlete has been taking medications for the previous 5 days, and there is a firm, adhered crust on each lesion.[12] Once these four criteria are met, the athlete may return to competition.

New unpublished data suggest the virus is detected 6.5 days after starting antiviral medications such as valacyclovir and recommends that the athlete may return on the seventh calendar day after starting medication provided the other three criteria are met.[26] The Minnesota State High School League has also adopted the recommendation of no contact until the seventh calendar day after starting antiviral medications if the previous three criteria have been met.[27]

Varicella-Zoster

VZV, otherwise known as chicken pox for the initial infection with the varicella virus and shingles for reactivations with the herpes zoster virus, is another common viral infection.

Varicella

As presented in Chapter 12, chickenpox is a common childhood disease with some cases presenting in adolescence or adulthood. This infection is very contagious and is spread by respiratory droplets or direct skin-to-skin contact. Patients are contagious from about 2 days before the onset of the rash until all lesions have crusted over.[28]

Symptoms include low-grade fever, headache, and malaise before the rash begins; the patient will develop a papular or vesicular rash that begins on the trunk and spreads to the extremities and face. The rash is described as a "dew drop on a rose petal," or a vesicle on an erythematous base. New lesions will develop over about 4 days and start as erythematous papules progressing to vesicles. These lesions are of varying size, shape, and age and will quickly rupture to form crusts. The patient will usually have a combination of papules, vesicles, and crusts at once.

Young children may get few or no lesions at all whereas older children and adults may get a more extensive eruption. Typically, older individuals experience a more severe course of the illness. Intense itching is often secondary to the rash. Complications include secondary bacterial skin infection, encephalitis, seizures, hepatitis, pneumonia, and even death. Now that most infants receive the VZV vaccine, the illness may be less common in the future.

Herpes Zoster

Herpes zoster, or shingles, is a reactivation of the VZV involving the skin along its dermatomal distribution. It occurs at all ages but increases in frequency with advancing age. Reactivation may result from advancing age, immunosuppression, lymphoma, stress, and radiation therapy.[28] Shingles most commonly is the result of reactivation from a previous VZV infection, not from direct contact with someone with shingles.

Typical symptoms of shingles include pain, tingling, burning, or itching before the onset of the rash along a single dermatome and may present along more than one dermatome or cross the midline. These symptoms may mimic myocardial infarction, pleurisy, acute abdomen, or migraine headaches depending on the location of the outbreak.

The patient may also have fever, malaise, headache, and lymphadenopathy preceding the outbreak. The rash usually presents as an erythematous plaque with the eruption of vesicles of various sizes, as opposed to HSV where the vesicles are all the same size and age. Vesicles may form over the next 7 days before crusting over and falling off. The most common complication is postherpetic neuralgia (PHN), which may require strong analgesic medications to control the pain.

Differential Diagnosis and Treatment

Differential diagnoses for **varicella** include herpes simplex, bullous impetigo, various types of folliculitis, and contact dermatitis; for herpes zoster they include migraine, myocardial infarction, acute abdomen, HSV infection, contact dermatitis, erysipelas, bullous impetigo, and necrotizing fasciitis.

Treatment for varicella is symptomatic and includes lotions and antihistamines to reduce the itching. Antibiotics also may be needed to help prevent secondary bacterial infections. Many physicians prescribe the antiviral medication acyclovir, 800 mg four times per day for 5 days initially, to help prevent complications from varicella. Valacyclovir and famciclovir have not been approved for varicella. Pediatric doses may vary depending on the age and weight of the patient.

Treatment of herpes zoster differs slightly because antiviral medications at high doses should be given within 72 hours of onset. Acyclovir, valacyclovir, and famciclovir are used to help reduce the viral shedding, pain, and frequency of PHN. Sometimes prednisone is prescribed to reduce the chance of PHN. Narcotic analgesics are also used to help with pain control.

Prognosis, Return to Participation, and Prevention

Athletes may return to participation when all lesions have a firm, adhered crust and there is no evidence of a secondary bacterial infection. The best prevention for chickenpox is the varicella vaccine at 12 months of age. Limited exposure at a young age to known cases will prevent contracting the condition later in life when the disease presents more dramatically.

Molluscum Contagiosum

Molluscum contagiosum is a viral infection commonly found in children and in sexually active adults. It most commonly appears on the face, trunk, arms, legs, and genital areas. Palms and soles are usually not involved. It is caused by a virus in the Poxviridae family and is more common in swimmers, wrestlers, and gymnasts.[25]

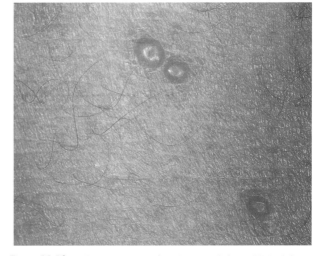

Figure 13-19 Molluscum contagiosum. (From Habif TP: *Clinical dermatology e-dition,* ed 4, St Louis, 2004, Mosby, p 379.)

Signs, Symptoms, and Differential Diagnosis

Molluscum contagiosum presents as a small, skin-colored, sometimes erythematous, smooth, dome-shaped papule with a central punctum (Figure 13-19). It is very contagious and is spread by **autoinoculation** and direct skin-to-skin contact. The lesions usually spontaneously resolve in 6 to 12 months. Differential diagnoses include HPV, sebaceous hyperplasia, squamous cell or basal cell carcinoma, and rare fungal infections in immunocompromised patients.

Treatment

Conservative treatment of molluscum contagiosum is effective for most patients, but wrestlers and those in other contact sports may require aggressive therapy sooner. Lesions may be treated by freezing each one with liquid nitrogen or curetting with a comedones extractor or small needle, although slight scarring is possible with these two procedures. After these treatments the lesions are no longer contagious.

Prognosis and Return to Participation

If the lesions are solitary or grouped, they can be covered with a gas-permeable membrane such as Op-Site, Tegaderm, or Bioclusive followed by pre-wrap and stretch tape so that participation can be allowed. If the lesions are too numerous or cannot be covered, then all lesions must be curetted or frozen before return is allowed.

Human Papillomavirus

HPV or warts are most common in children and young adults but may occur at any age. More than 65 types of HPV have been identified and can be seen at any site on the skin. Some warts may spontaneously resolve in less than 2 years, but others last a lifetime. Warts are spread by skin-to-skin contact and usually

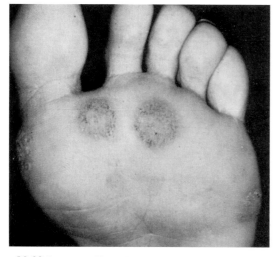

Figure 13-20 Human papillomavirus is the cause of plantar warts on the bottom of this patient's foot. (From Arnold HL, Odom RB, James WD: *Andrew's diseases of the skin: clinical dermatology*, ed 8, Philadelphia, 1990, WB Saunders, p 470.)

occur at sites of trauma, abrasion, or eczema, most commonly on the hands and feet.

Signs and Symptoms

The diagnostic feature of warts is their distortion or obscuring of the normal skin lines (Figure 13-20). Warts present as small, smooth, skin-colored papules that may progress to a rough surface, a flat top surface, or a deep calluslike lesion. Some warts have small black dots, which represent thrombosed capillaries. These dots are often considered a diagnostic sign of warts.

Referral, Diagnostic Tests, and Differential Diagnosis

No specific tests are needed unless the diagnosis is very atypical. In rare cases, a biopsy may aid in the diagnosis. Referral is indicated when conservative treatment has failed or when symptoms interfere with daily activities. Differential diagnoses include molluscum contagiosum, seborrheic keratosis, actinic keratosis, squamous cell and basal cell carcinoma, corns, and calluses.

Treatment, Prognosis, Return to Participation, and Prevention

The many treatments for warts include salicylic acid, liquid nitrogen, and podophyllin. Blunt dissection and laser treatment are reserved for resistant cases. Imiquimod (Aldara) has been approved for genital and perianal warts, and research shows it may have some merit in treating common warts.[14]

Prognosis is generally very good because most lesions do eventually resolve spontaneously. Return to participation for an athlete recovering from warts is unlimited. In wrestling, however, competitors with multiple facial digitate warts will be disqualified if the warts cannot be covered with a mask. Wrestlers with multiple flat warts and common warts should cover them adequately before competition. Acid or freezing treatment of warts may result in a blood-tinged blister that eventually resolves into a scab. While the blister is present, it should be covered during participation. The best prevention of HPV is good skin hygiene that will help prevent transmission through damaged skin areas.

Fungal Conditions

Only 150 of the identified 250,000 species of fungi are known to cause problems in humans. Recently, nosocomial fungal infections have greatly increased, which has been largely attributed to use of certain medications and intravascular devices.[15]

Fungal infections are also extremely common in athletes, especially wrestlers. Fungal infections are common on skin, hair, and nails, with the most common infection sites being the scalp, face, extremities, trunk, groin, and feet.

Those discussed here are topical, or surface, fungal conditions and include tinea corporis, tinea cruris, tinea unguium, tinea pedis, tinea capitis, and tinea versicolor. Tinea infections are named according to the affected body area. All are true fungal infections except for tinea versicolor, which is categorized as a yeast disorder. Table 13-3 lists the common tinea infections, their location on the body, and typical treatment. As a group, these conditions tend to be transmitted person to person or animal to person. Most respond well to topical antifungal ointments, but newer systemic oral medications have recently proven good alternatives to their topical counterparts.[8]

Fungal infections are usually diagnosed by appearance alone, but each can be distinguished by microscopic examination with a KOH stain. Athletes who have recently used a topical over-the-counter antifungal medication may present with a false-negative KOH stain.[29] Generally, medical treatment is continued for at least 2 weeks following resolution of the lesions.[30]

Preventive measures for all fungal infections include keeping wet materials away from the body; fully drying clothing, towels, and uniforms before using them; and allowing light and air exposure to the skin as practical.[30] Additional measures include good personal hygiene; not sharing clothing, towels, or personal items such as grooming accessories; and wearing foot protection when using common shower facilities. Showering with hot water and soap and washing hair with shampoo immediately following practices or athletic events will help prevent fungal and skin diseases in general.[31]

Table 13-3 Comparison of the Tinea Fungi

Name	Body Part Affected	Signs and Symptoms	Treatment
Tinea corporis	Ringworm on the body or face	Scaling, deep erythema; well-defined margins; pruritic	Topical antifungal agents; difficult or recurrent cases may need griseofulvin or oral terbinafine
Tinea pedis	Athlete's foot	Within the interdigital web spaces, maceration, pruritic	Topical cream–based antifungals such as Tinactin (tolnaftate) or Lamisil (terbinafine) are often used; oral antifungals may be necessary in difficult cases
Tinea unguium	Nails of the hands or feet	Nail thickening, multiple nails involved, hyperkeratosis	Griseofulvin, terbinafine, itraconazole (topical antifungal agents not effective)
Tinea capitis	Scalp	Scaly, patchy alopecia; pruritic	Oral antifungal agents; antibiotics if necessary; oral steroids to prevent scarring, hair loss
Tinea cruris	Jock itch, primarily in the groin	Scaly, erythematous rash; pruritic	Same as tinea corporis
Tinea barbae	Beard or base of neck	Inflammatory folliculitis on face, often scars	Oral terbinafine

Unless specifically addressed in the categories that follow, unexposed tinea infections have no restrictions and the athlete is allowed to participate as tolerated. Whereas all active lesions and capitis infections have specific constraints, the NCAA has given expressed permission to the examining physician or certified athletic trainer to determine participation of athletes with tinea on an individual basis.[12]

Tinea Corporis

Tinea corporis, otherwise known as ringworm, is caused by the *Trichophyton, Microsporum,* and *Epidermophyton* species. The most common organism identified is *T. tonsurans.*[5]

Tinea corporis is common in wrestling and is spread mostly by skin-to-skin contact. Wrestlers develop mat burns, abrasions, and scrapes during competition that provide easy entry for fungal infection. Fungus also develops best in dark, damp, and humid conditions. Sites inside shoes or in damp clothing that has not been properly laundered and is hung in a dark, enclosed locker are particularly favorable. There is little evidence that fungus is transmitted from wrestling mats; in fact, one study failed to isolate any fungus from wrestling mats.[32]

Signs and Symptoms

The lesions of tinea corporis are erythematous, scaly areas of varying size and may have a central clearing in the center (Figure 13-21). The active areas of infection are at the border, and the central clearing develops as the fungus digests cells as it moves away from the center. Tinea corporis may be itchy or asymptomatic. It is important to also check the feet of someone with tinea because this may be the original source.

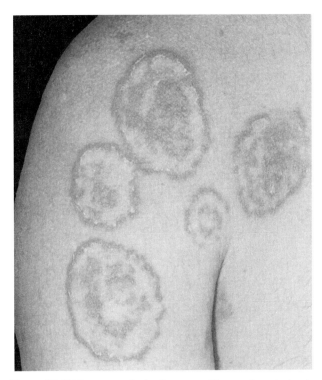

Figure 13-21 Tinea corporis is ringworm with a red, scaly border. (From Habif TP: *Clinical dermatology e-dition,* ed 4, St Louis, 2004, Mosby, p 420.)

Referral, Diagnostic Tests, and Differential Diagnosis

Diagnosis is determined by clinical and microscopical examination. The lesion is scraped onto a slide and examined with a KOH stain under a microscope. Multiple hyphae are seen on active lesions. Athletes with extensive skin involvement, persistence of symptoms despite treatment, and any lesions that are questionable are referred to a physician. The differential diagnoses for tinea corporis include contact dermatitis, psoriasis, atopic dermatitis, seborrheic dermatitis, pityriasis alba, pityriasis rosea, pityriasis versicolor, subacute lupus erythematosus, and erythema migrans.[8]

Treatment

Treatment employs topical or oral antifungal medications. The most commonly used medications are the topical antifungal creams. Typical treatment with topical antifungal medication for noninflammatory tinea corporis includes twice-daily treatment for 1 to 4 weeks depending on the type of cream. Each antifungal is different and is individually dose adjusted. Occasionally, the lesions are too extensive for topical treatment, and oral medications such as terbinafine, itraconazole, and fluconazole are used. Typically doses of these medications must be taken for up to 4 weeks to be fully effective.[33]

In addition, athletes should shower and clean the affected area daily. Clothing needs to be laundered after each practice or competition; and sweaty clothes or towels should not be left in a dark locker.

Prognosis and Return to Participation

The prognosis for tinea corporis is very good if the athlete uses the treatment as directed. If infection recurs, then either the fungus is resistant to the medication used, the treatment was not administered properly, or another source of infection exists that has not been detected. Athletes, especially wrestlers, may return to activity after 3 days of topical antifungal treatment for tinea corporis. Small local lesions are treated by washing with an antifungal shampoo (selenium sulfide or ketoconazole), applying a fungicidal cream (terbinafine or naftifine), covering with a semipermeable membrane (Op-Site or Bioclusive), and wrapping with a prewrap followed by flexible tape. This process is repeated after each practice or match to allow the lesion to air dry.[2] Prophylactic therapies are currently being investigated, especially with oral medications. Available research suggests using itraconazole, 200 mg twice daily for 1 day every 2 weeks,[34] and fluconazole, 100 mg once weekly,[32] to decrease recurrences.

Prevention

Many isolated cultures from the lesions are the same species as those cultured from the scalp.[5] Therefore it may be beneficial to have athletes, especially wrestlers, shampoo with an antifungal shampoo such as Head & Shoulders or Nizoral, both of which are active against *T. tonsurans*. Mats need to be cleaned daily and allowed to dry before storing.

Many wrestlers use wipe-on foams such as Kenshield or KS Skin Protection before practice and competition to provide a barrier against fungal and bacterial infections. Limited research evaluates the efficacy of these products and has not yet demonstrated them to be beneficial. They may, in fact, have an adverse impact by giving a false sense of security, allowing less strict adherence to hygiene.[35]

Tinea Cruris

Tinea cruris, or jock itch, is another common fungal infection. This infection usually occurs in the warm summer months. Although it is more common in men, women may experience this fungal infection as well. It affects the inner thigh, perineum, and perianal regions, with the scrotum, penis, and vagina typically not affected.[15] Women may acquire it on the waistline area.

Signs, Symptoms, and Referral

Signs and symptoms of jock itch are similar to other fungal infections. It presents with a well-demarcated, scaly, erythematous rash that tends to be pruritic.[15] As previously noted, it is localized regionally to the groin area (Figure 13-22). Athletes who complain of symptoms from tinea cruris are referred to a physician if conservative over-the-counter treatment fails.

Differential Diagnosis, Treatment, and Prevention

The differential diagnoses for tinea cruris include heat rash, Candidiasis, erythasma dermatitis from clothing or soap, or skin abrasion from clothing. If the lesions

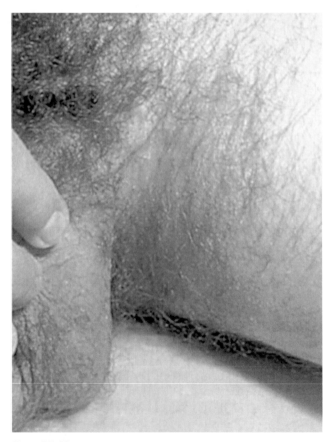

Figure 13-22 Tinea cruris is also known as jock itch. (From Lookingbill DP, Marks JG: *Principles of dermatology,* ed 2, Philadelphia, 1993, WB Saunders.)

appear with a beefy red color and involvement of the scrotum, most likely the condition is Candidiasis and not tinea cruris. Treatment includes completely drying off after showering and applying antifungal ointment. Loose-fitting clothing will hasten the treatment, as will maintaining proper hygiene. Changing clothes frequently and laundering them in hot water also help break the cycle.[30] Since tinea cruris thrives in moist, dark areas, the athlete needs to completely dry following showers and wear loose-fitting clothing whenever possible. Anti-fungal powders and sprays may also be effective in preventing tinea cruris; however, creams are more effective treatments.

Tinea Unguium

Tinea unguium is also known as ringworm of the nails. It can occur in both the fingernails and toenails but is more common in the fingernails.[8]

Signs, Symptoms, and Referral

The most telling signs of tinea unguium are thickening and a lusterless, opaque coloring of the nail. As the condition progresses, the nail plate separates from the nail bed, and the nail itself may be destroyed. Athletes who present with thickened, yellowish nails are referred to a physician for medication to treat the fungus causing the problem.

Differential Diagnosis and Treatment

The differential diagnosis for tinea unguium is injury to the nail. Treatment of this condition is an especially tedious and lengthy process. Topical antifungal treatment is typically ineffective. Instead, oral systemic medication taken twice daily is required for up to 4 months. Unlike antibiotics, this medication does not necessarily need to be taken until all signs of the fungus are gone. The systemic drugs bind to the nail plate and continue to work after oral administration is complete.[8]

Prognosis, Return to Participation, and Prevention

As with many of the tinea infections, participation is not limited for athletes with tinea unguium. Certain conditions, however, make athletes more prone to tinea unguium. These include wearing hand protection covering their nails (i.e., soccer goalkeepers). The dark, moist environment is an excellent place for this fungus to flourish. Equipment, especially equipment used in the summer or during twice-daily practices, is not always allowed to completely dry before reuse.

Using open-finger gloves such as in cycling and weight lifting is one way to prevent risk of infection, but this is not possible in some sports. Athletes would be wise to be aware of the warm, moist, dark conditions that encourage tinea infections and take measures to prevent such situations, including keeping fingers and toes clean and dry; removing socks, shoes, and hand wear immediately after practice; allowing hand wear to completely dry before wearing again; and always wearing clean, dry socks.

Tinea Pedis

Tinea pedis, also known as athlete's foot, is the most common site for **dermatophyte** infections since shoes promote dark and moist conditions.

Signs, Symptoms, Referral, and Diagnostic Tests

The most common sites for tinea pedis are between the toes and on the lateral areas of the feet and soles. The area between the toes is usually macerated and scaly (Figure 13-23). The foot may also demonstrate the classic ringworm pattern of tinea corporis. The lateral edges and soles usually demonstrate dry, scaly, erythematous areas, and these lesions are usually, but not always, itchy. It is not uncommon for cracks or fissures to develop in the macerated skin.[15] Diagnostic tests include scraping the scales for a microscopic evaluation with a KOH preparation. The athlete is referred to a physician if symptoms persist despite treatment.

Differential Diagnosis, Treatment, and Prevention

Differential diagnoses for tinea pedis include impetigo, erythrasma, pitted keratolysis, *P. aeruginosa* infection, psoriasis, allergic dermatitis, dyshidrosis, and contact dermatitis. Treatment consists of topical antifungal creams first with application twice daily for 2 to 4 weeks. If the infection does not respond, another antifungal drug family is tried.

Athletes can help prevent tinea pedis fungal infections by wearing wicking socks, wearing sandals,

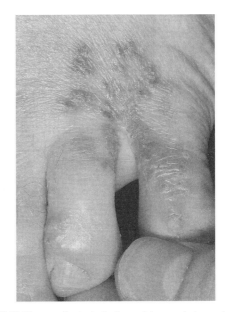

Figure 13-23 Tinea pedis starts in the moist areas between toes and is shown here spreading to the top of the foot. (From Habif TP: *Clinical dermatology e-dition*, ed 4, St Louis, 2004, Mosby, p 414.)

or frequently removing their shoes to allow their feet to dry. Wearing sandals in public showering facilities will also help prevent transmission of the fungus.

Tinea Capitis

Tinea capitis or scalp ringworm occurs commonly in children and is spread by pets or other infected individuals. The most common causative organism in the United States is *T. tonsurans*.[8] Tinea capitis has several varieties with slight differences in presentation.

Generally the infection starts in the scalp and moves into the hair shaft. Black dots on the scalp where the follicle has broken or small semibald patches surrounded by lusterless hairs may be present.[8,15] Often, there is a raised inflammatory response to the fungus, resembling an abscess that quickly heals. The fungus may be limited to a small area in the hair, or it may persist, affecting the entire scalp.[8]

Signs and Symptoms

The tinea capitis infection may be either inflammatory or noninflammatory. Most commonly, identifiable areas of hair loss, scales, and broken hair shafts are seen in the scalp (Figure 13-24). Sometimes the infection causes an exaggerated inflammatory response and produces one or more inflamed, boggy, tender areas on the scalp called *kerions.* Because of this the patient may present with low-grade but persistent inflammation.[8] The hair shafts are usually destroyed, and scarring is common after the kerion resolves.

Referral, Diagnostic Tests, and Differential Diagnoses

Athletes who experience patchy hair loss, who have been exposed to tinea capitis, or who have signs of tinea capitis are referred for medical treatment. Diagnosis is determined by clinical and microscopic examination. Hairs easily removed are examined with a KOH stain under a microscope. Multiple spores are seen either inside or outside infected hair shafts. A **Wood's lamp** has demonstrated a green fluorescence in the past, but fluorescence has not been common recently since *T. tonsurans* does not fluoresce. The differential diagnoses for tinea capitis include **alopecia areata,** psoriasis, atopic dermatitis, and seborrheic dermatitis.

Treatment

Topical antifungal medications are not as effective with tinea capitis, and oral antifungal medications are often needed. Griseofulvin is the most common medication used in the treatment of tinea capitis. The NCAA recommends the systemic or oral antifungals itraconazole or terbinafine as effective treatment for tinea capitis.[12] Treatment is continued until 2 weeks after KOH preparations are negative. Prednisone and systemic antibiotics may also help treat tinea capitis.

Prognosis, Return to Participation, and Prevention

The NCAA recommends 2 weeks of systemic or oral antifungal medications for tinea capitis before return to wrestling is allowed.[12] Return to other sports is up to the discretion of the treating physician and may be less of an issue in noncontact sports or sports with helmets.

Since tinea capitis is very easily transmitted via inanimate objects, all combs, brushes, hats, and other headgear worn by the athlete must be cleaned. Spores of tinea are shed into the air around infected persons and their clothing, so preventive measures must include laundering bed linens, towels, and clothing. Roommates or family members of affected athletes should also be examined for tinea capitis.[30]

Tinea Versicolor

Tinea versicolor is a very common yeast infection seen in adolescents and young adults. This infection is not contagious and is common in high humidity environments and sometimes in areas of prolonged use of topical corticosteroids. It may go unnoticed for months to years and usually produces very few symptoms, if any.

This yeast is part of the normal skin flora but can produce an infection that is mostly found on the trunk, arms, neck, abdomen, and sometimes the groin. It is more common on the face and forehead in children but not in adults.

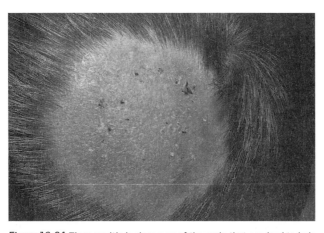

Figure 13-24 Tinea capitis is ringworm of the scalp that can lead to hair loss. (From Callen JP, Jorrizzo JL, Greer KE, et al: *Color atlas of dermatology,* Philadelphia, 1993, WB Saunders, p 106.)

Signs and Symptoms

Versicolor starts as multiple, small, round, scaly macules that enlarge radially. They may present as

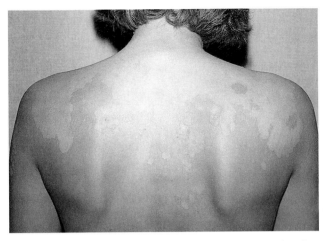

Figure 13-25 Tinea versicolor is often first noted as an area that does not tan. (From Habif TP: *Clinical dermatology e-dition,* ed 4, St Louis, 2004, Mosby, p 451.)

white, brown, or pink areas of the skin that increase and may or may not cause itching (Figure 13-25). These areas typically will not tan when exposed to the sun or ultraviolet light.[8]

Referral, Diagnostic Tests, and Differential Diagnosis
Athletes who have patchy areas that do not tan, who have varying pigment, or who do not respond to conservative treatment are referred to a physician. Scraping the scales onto a slide and examining them microscopically confirm a diagnosis. The microscopic examination with KOH staining demonstrates a spaghetti and meatballs appearance. Wood's light may demonstrate a pale yellow, white, or even a blue-green fluorescence pattern.[8]

The differential diagnoses for versicolor include **vitiligo,** postinflammatory hypopigmentation, pityriasis alba, pityriasis rosea, nummular eczema, guttate psoriasis, seborrheic dermatitis, and tinea corporis.

Treatment and Prevention
Versicolor is treated in many ways. The most common treatment is with a selenium sulfide 2.5% lotion (Selsun Blue shampoo), which is applied for 10 minutes and then washed off. Alternatively, the shampoo may be applied at bedtime to all body areas except the scrotum and washed off in the morning. The typical course of treatment is 7 days.[8]

Another treatment is ketoconazole cream or shampoo (Nizoral) applied once daily for 2 weeks. For resistant cases, both cream and oral antifungal medication may be prescribed.

Prevention of reinfection includes ketoconazole or selenium sulfide treatments once weekly or every other week. Using a salicylic acid, sulfur, or pyrithione zinc bar may also be helpful.

Parasitic Conditions and Bites

Parasitic infestations and insect bites are common causes of skin inflammation and infection. A wide range of insects can cause skin eruptions. The most common infections caused by parasites are pediculosis and scabies. **Pediculosis,** an infection caused by lice, occurs in three forms: head lice, body lice, and pubic lice. **Scabies** is caused by the mite *Sarcoptes scabiei.*

Head Lice

It is estimated that 6 to 12 million people are infested annually with head lice.[36] These tiny insects are about $1/10$ to $1/8$ inch long and live on the human scalp while feeding on human blood. They multiply rapidly and lay small gray-white eggs that are glued to the base of the hair shafts. The lice themselves are hard to see, but the nits can be seen at the hairline behind the ears or on the base of the scalp (Figure 13-26). Both forms of lice are transmitted by contact with a person who is already infested through sharing personal items such as combs, towels, bedding, hats, helmets, or other clothing. Lice cannot survive without a human host for longer than 48 hours.

Signs, Symptoms, and Referral
Clinical presentation consists of intense itching of the scalp and the observation of nits. The itching may not start for several weeks after infestation. An athlete who shows signs of lice is referred to a physician for confirmation of infestation.

Treatment
Treatment consists of application of topical medications, including Nix, RID, malathion (Ovide), or lindane (Kwell). Nix and RID are the initial treatments of choice because lindane has been associated with neurological toxicity in some cases. The lice are usually killed with one treatment, but a second treatment may be needed 7 to 10 days later. After the first treatment, a nit comb is used to remove the eggs. Any nits found that are greater than $1/2$ inch on the hair shaft are old and dead; nits remaining less than $1/4$ inch on the hair shaft after 1 week of treatment may be new and necessitate retreatment. The person needs to be checked for lice every 2 or 3 days for 2 weeks.

It is also important to wash all bedding and recently worn clothing in hot water at a temperature greater than 130° F (54° C) and dry them on a hot cycle for at least 20 minutes.[37] Nonwashable clothing is dry-cleaned. Items that cannot be washed or dry-cleaned, such as helmets, headgear, and shoes, can be placed in a double plastic bag for 2 weeks. Vacuuming the floor and furniture completes the extermination procedure.

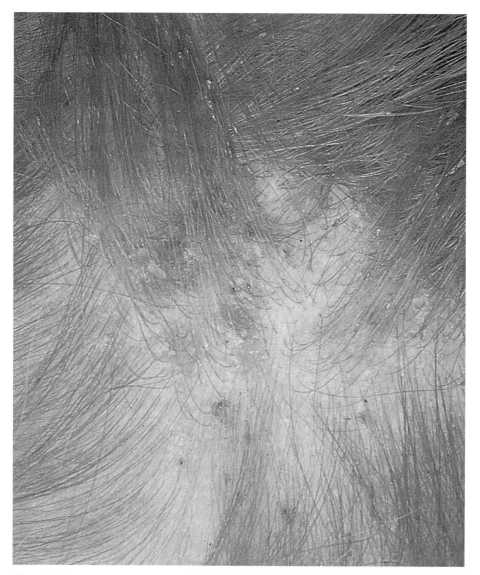

Figure 13-26 Pediculosis capitis. (From Habif TP: *Clinical dermatology e-dition,* ed 4, St Louis, 2004, Mosby, p 507.)

Prognosis, Return to Participation, and Prevention

Athletes are allowed to resume normal activity levels when all lice and nits are confirmed gone. However, the NCAA recommends that athletes be treated with pediculicide and reexamined for complete extermination of lice before resumption of sport activity.[12] Practicing good hygiene and avoiding exposure to infected individuals and their personal items are the best preemptive tools against lice infestation.

Body Lice

Body lice are found on the body as well as in the clothing and bedding of infested humans; the nits typically are attached to the seams of clothing and bedding or body hair. Infestation usually occurs when poor hygiene and crowded environments necessitate frequent close contact with others. Homeless populations without regular access to bathing facilities or clean clothes are particularly vulnerable. People who bathe regularly are seldom infested.

The usual clinical presentation is itching and a rash, usually around the waist, groin, and thighs. Body lice are treated by changing clothes regularly, bathing regularly, washing all clothing in hot water at a temperature above 130° F (54° C), drying it in a hot dryer for at least 20 minutes, and using RID or Nix shampoo applied to the body.[37]

Pubic Lice

Pubic lice, commonly referred to as crabs, are usually found in the genital area but may also be seen on the legs, axilla, mustache, beard, eyebrows, and eyelashes. These lice are usually spread through sexual contact rather than through contact with infested towels, clothing, or bedding. Therefore pubic lice seen in a child may indicate sexual abuse or sexual activity.

Clinical presentation is usually the result of intense itching in the genital area. The lice and nits are much easier to identify than head or body lice. Treatment for crabs is with RID, Nix, or lindane shampoos, followed by removal of nits with fingernails or nit combs. Clothing is washed in hot water at a temperature greater than 130° F (54° C), dried in a hot dryer, and changed regularly; sexual partners need to be informed and treated as well and sexual activity avoided until appropriate treatment has successfully eradicated the infestation.

Scabies

The other common parasite associated with skin infection is the mite *S. scabiei,* which causes scabies. The first exposure does not usually cause symptoms for several weeks, but subsequent infections can produce symptoms within 24 hours. Spread is usually the result of direct contact, sexual contact, or sharing of infested clothes or bedding. These mites are able to survive away from the host for 48 to 72 hours and therefore can be more challenging to eradicate than lice.[38]

Signs, Symptoms, and Diagnosis
Intense itching that interferes with sleep is commonly associated with scabies. The wrists, fingers, and ankles are the most obvious sites, but the itching may occur anywhere on the body with the head and neck usually spared. The patient develops small red bumps that may be arranged in a linear fashion after itching (Figure 13-27). Diagnosis is usually made through clinical examination; however, finding a mite is extremely difficult and requires scraping the skin

for a sample that is then examined under a microscope for a live mite.

Treatment and Return to Participation
Treatment is with permethrin cream (Kwell) applied to the body from the neck down and washed off in 8 to 14 hours or 1% lindane per 1 oz of lotion or 30 g of cream applied from the neck down and washed off after 8 hours. Ivermectin taken orally is an alternative treatment. The patient will likely need an antihistamine because itching may last for at least 2 weeks after initiating treatment. All bedding and recently worn clothing needs to be laundered in hot water above 130° F (54° C) and dried on a hot cycle for at least 20 minutes[37]; nonwashable clothing needs to be dry-cleaned. Items that cannot be washed or dry-cleaned, such as helmets, headgear, and shoes, can be placed in a double plastic bag for 2 weeks. As with lice, all floors and furniture must be vacuumed. The infected person needs to review close and sexual contacts within the past 30 days and notify those individuals for treatment as necessary.[39]

The NCAA Wrestling Rules stipulate that athletes who have had scabies must have and present a negative prep for scabies before being allowed to resume participation.[12]

Insect Bites

Dermatological reaction to insect bites is extremely common. These bites also can lead to anaphylaxis, which causes 90 to 100 deaths in the United States each year.[40] Therefore, exposure to insects becomes a possibility for athletes, coaches, and athletic trainers during outdoor practice and events.

Chiggers, ticks, mosquitos, wasps, bees, and spiders can produce particularly bothersome reactions. Bites and stings can cause direct irritation from the insect's body parts or secretions, immediate or delayed hypersensitivity responses, or specific effects from venoms, or they can serve as vectors for secondary invaders (see Box 8-4).[41]

The incidence of anaphylaxis related to insect sting ranges from 0.3% to 3% in the general population with yellow jackets being the most common cause of allergy.[42] Common reactions may be localized or spread across a larger part of the body and include redness, pain, and swelling that may last as long as 10 days. Individuals with a prior history of allergic reaction to specific insect bites or stings can be extremely vulnerable and often carry an EpiPen when participating in outdoor activities.

The brown recluse spider has received wide attention because of the possible dramatic reaction associated with its bites. **Necrotic arachnidism** is the condition that results when this type of spider deposits venom within a host that leads to tissue necrosis.[43] The brown recluse, also called the fiddle-back spider,

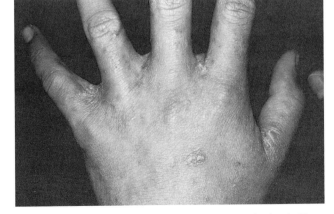

Figure 13-27 A pruritic infestation of scabies on the hand. (From Callen JP, Jorrizzo JL, Greer KE, et al: *Color atlas of dermatology,* Philadelphia, 1993, WB Saunders, p 193.)

is very small at about 1.5 cm long and has a characteristic dark, violin-shaped marking on its dorsum with the broad base of the marking or violin located near the head and the narrow stem pointing toward the abdomen. The brown recluse spider is most prevalent in the southern half of the United States and prefers dark, quiet spaces under porches, woodpiles, and rocks or inside closets, barns, picture frames, and basements. It has also been found in dormitories, and it bites when a person is putting on clothing or rummaging through other materials where the spider resides.

Signs, Symptoms, and Referral

Insect bites can range from a nuisance to an emergency (Red Flags—Insect Bites). Chigger bites can

> **Red Flags for Insect Bites**
> * Take the bites of any venomous insect seriously because the secretions, venom, and insect body parts can provoke dramatic or life-threatening reactions in sensitive individuals.
> * Be aware of the insect varieties common to the geographical location.
> * Recognize and refer athletes with signs and symptoms of anaphylaxis: agitation, chills, facial edema, swollen tongue, wheezing, difficulty breathing, flushing, generalized urticaria, hoarseness or difficulty talking, palpitations, near-syncopal or syncopal episodes, profuse sweating, palpitations, cardiovascular collapse.
> * Have epinephrine on hand for emergency use in the event of a severe reaction.

cause extreme discomfort for days (Figure 13-28) and possibly lead to secondary lesions with bacterial infection as a result of scratching. Wasp and bee stings can be extremely dangerous when the person stung has an allergic reaction, which may quickly progress to anaphylaxis in sensitive individuals; therefore first aid kits should be equipped with EpiPens for emergencies. Symptoms for tick bites that can result in Rocky Mountain spotted fever or Lyme disease do not develop immediately, often making diagnosis a challenge.

A brown recluse bite can produce a dramatic and prolonged reaction. The initial bite produces a bee sting–like pain and often only a mild erythema and swelling; but these spider bites have the potential to develop a severe reaction and may become necrotic within 6 hours.[43] In some cases the wound begins to ache and becomes pruritic over the first 8 hours and subsequently a rapid blue-gray macular halo develops around the bite that represents local hemolysis; the area may become oblong or irregular and result in a sudden increase in pain. Then the macule widens and sinks below the level of intact skin and may advance to necrosis into underlying muscle and over broad areas of skin or even an entire extremity. In such cases, when the dead tissue sloughs, a large ulcer persists, resulting in significant scarring and prolonged healing (Figure 13-29). Systemically, patients with severe reactions often experience fever, chills, nausea, vomiting, myalgias, and weakness. These reactions are rare

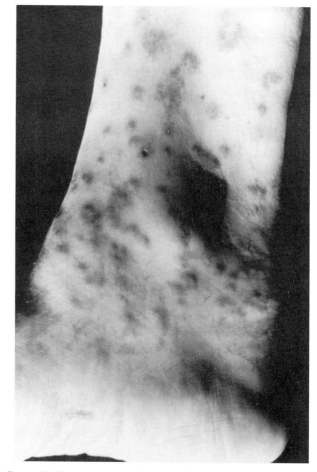

Figure 13-28 Chigger bites. (From Arnold HL, Odom RB, James WD: *Andrew's diseases of the skin: clinical dermatology*, ed 8, Philadelphia, 1990, WB Saunders, p 529.)

and generally limited to children. An athlete who presents with a history of a bite with associated local severe reaction, fever, or systemic manifestations is referred to a physician immediately.

Treatment and Prevention

Insect bites usually are treated conservatively with ice and elevation of the affected extremity. Strenuous exercise, heat, and surgery are avoided.[43] Topical antibiotic ointment may be applied under a sterile dressing to retard infection. Antibiotics for *S. aureus* or *S. pyogenes* may be initiated, and a tetanus booster should be administered by a physician if the term of the vaccine has lapsed. Serious bites become evident in the first 24 to 48 hours; in this event, the athlete is referred for medical treatment immediately.[28]

Prevention of most insect bites can be achieved by avoiding the insects' habitat, wearing protective clothing, or using chemical repellants. When putting on shoes, socks, and other apparel that have been left unattended outdoors, athletes must completely shake them out and exercise caution during storms and floods that may drive insects from their normal habitat.

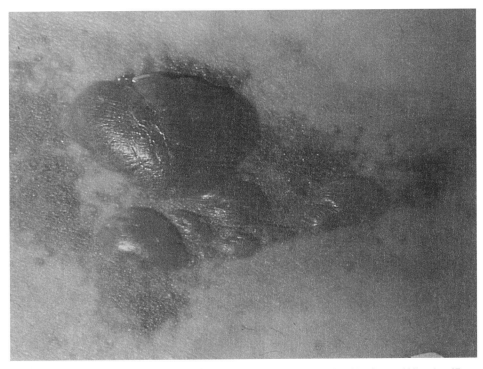

Figure 13-29 This severe reaction to a brown recluse spider bite shows infarction, bleeding, and blistering. (From Habif TP: *Clinical dermatology e-dition*, ed 4, St Louis, 2004, Mosby, p 515.)

WEB RESOURCES

American Academy of Dermatology
  http://aad.org
  Information on various dermatological conditions

American Cancer Society
  http://cancer.org
  Cancer information

National Collegiate Athletic Association
  http://www.ncaa.org
  College athlete sports medicine guidelines

JAMA Archives of Dermatology
  http://archderm.ama-assn.org/
  Archives of this journal

Loyola University Dermatology
  http://www.meddean.luc.edu/lumen/MedEd/medicine/
  dermatology/melton/atlas.htm
  Atlas of photos on skin disorders

Dermatology Image Bank
  http://medlib.med.utah.edu/kw/derm/
  Photos of skin disorders

Dermatology Online Journal
  http://dermatology.cdlib.org/
  An on-line journal covering a variety of skin disorders

Electronic Textbook of Dermatology
  http://www.telemedicine.org/stamford.htm
  An on-line journal covering a variety of skin disorders

Atlas of Dermatology
  http://www.dermis.net/doia/mainmenu.
  asp?zugr=d&lang=e
  Photos of skin conditions

SUMMARY

This chapter is an introduction to the pathology of common skin conditions for athletic trainers, educators, and students. It is not intended as a diagnostic and treatment guide. Signs, symptoms, diagnostic tests, treatment, and suggestions concerning appropriate times to seek referral for dermatological disorders are discussed. The NCAA guidelines determining when an athlete with a given skin condition may be allowed to participate have been presented. These regulations may differ or vary from various school district guidelines, amateur sport organization regulations, or the rules of other governing entities. Readers need to become familiar with the rules overseeing their particular athletic interest and remain abreast of changes as they occur.

Because these recommendations may be revised as research is conducted and made public, health care practitioners should continue to seek out new information as it becomes available. A prudent athletic trainer continues to educate athletes about their personnel responsibility for skin care, hygiene, and prevention with regard to transmission of infectious skin disorders.

REFERENCES

1. Klossner D, editor: *2004-2005 NCAA sports medicine handbook*, Indianapolis, 2004-2005, National Collegiate Athletic Association.

2. Van De Graaff K, Fox S: *Concepts of human anatomy and physiology,* ed 3, Dubuque, Iowa, 1992, William C Brown.
3. Frank M: Urticaria and angioedema. In Goodman L, Ausiello D, editors: *Cecil textbook of medicine,* ed 22, Philadelphia, 2004, WB Saunders.
4. Grandel K: Association for platelet-activation factor with primary acquired cold urticaria, *New England Journal of Medicine* 313:405-409, 1984.
5. Sigler R: The role of cyproheptadine in the treatment of cold urticaria, *Journal of Allergy and Clinical Immunology* 65:309-312, 1980.
6. Neittaanmaki H, Myohanen T, Franki J: Comparison of cinnarizine, cyproheptadine, doxepin, and hydroxyzine in idiopathic cold urticaria: usefulness of doxepin, *Journal of the American Academy of Dermatology* 11:483-489, 1984.
7. Prevention and treatment of sunburn, *The Medical Letter,* June 7, 2004. Available at http://www.medicalletter.org/scripts/search.cgi. Accessed October 2004.
8. Beers M, Berklow R, editors: *The Merck manual of diagnosis and therapy,* ed 17, Whitehouse Station, NJ, 1999, Merck Research Laboratories.
9. American Academy of Dermatology: Basic facts about melanoma. Available at http://www.skincarephysicians.com/melanomanet/basic_facts.ht. Accessed September 2004.
10. Dewald L: The ABCDs of skin cancer: a primer for athletic trainers and therapists, *Athletic Therapy Today* 7(3):29-32, 2002.
11. American Cancer Society: Learn about skin cancer—melanoma. Available at http://www.cancer.org/docroot/lrn/lrn_0.asp. Accessed September 2004.
12. National Collegiate Athletic Association: *2005 NCAA wrestling rules and interpretations,* Indianapolis, 2004, NCAA.
13. Levy J: Common bacterial dermatoses protecting competitive athletes, *Physician and Sportsmedicine* 32(6):33-39, 2004.
14. Adams B: Sports dermatology, *Adolescent Medicine* 12(2):305-322, 2001.
15. Bryan C: *Infectious diseases in primary care,* New York, 2002, WB Saunders.
16. Bikowski J: Disease in wrestlers and other athletes. I. Bacterial infections, *Athletic Therapy Today* 1(5):23-26, 1996.
17. Schnirring L: MRSA infections, *Physician and Sportsmedicine* 32(10):12-17, 2004.
18. Lindenmayer J, Schoenfeld S, O'Grady R: Methicillin-resistant *Staphylococcus aureus* in a high school wrestling team and the surrounding community, *Archives of Internal Medicine* 158(8):895-899, 1998.
19. Fleming D, McQuillan G, Johnson R: Herpes simplex virus type 2 in the United States, 1997 to 1994, *New England Journal of Medicine* 337(16):1105-1111, 1997.
20. Mertz G, Benedetti J, Ashley R: Risk factors for the sexual transmission of genital herpes, *Annals of Internal Medicine* 116:197-202, 1992.
21. Becker T: Herpes gladiatorum: a growing problem in sports medicine, *Cutis* 50:150-152, 1992.
22. Landry G, Chang C: Herpes and tinea in wrestling, *Physician and Sportsmedicine* 32(10):34-42, 2004.
23. Cook S: Herpes simplex virus in the eye, *British Journal of Ophthalmology* 76:365-366, 1992.
24. Nesburn A: Recurrent herpes simplex infection: pathogenesis and treatment. In Binder P, Buxton J, editors: *Symposium on medical and surgical diseases of the cornea,* St Louis, 1980, Mosby.
25. Cyr P: Viral skin infections. Preventing outbreaks in sports settings, *Physician and Sportsmedicine* 23(7):33-38, 2004.
26. Anderson B: Valacyclovir to expedite the clearance of recurrent herpes gladiatorum. Personal communication from the author, 2004.
27. Minnesota State High School League: Protocol for blood exposure, bites and skin infections in wrestling [website]. Available at http://www.mshsl.org/mshsl/activitypage.asp?actnum=424. Accessed February 2005.
28. Habif T: *Clinical dermatology: a color guide to diagnosis and therapy,* ed 3, St Louis, 2004, Mosby.
29. Winokur R, Dexter W: Fungal infections and parasitic infestations in sports, *Physician and Sportsmedicine* 32(10):23-33, 2004.
30. *Professional guide to diseases,* ed 7, Springhouse, Pa, 2001, Springhouse.
31. Landry G, Chang C, Mees P: Treating and avoiding herpes and tinea infections in contact sports, *Physician and Sportsmedicine* 32(10):43-44, 2004.
32. Kohl T, Martin D, Nemeth R: Fluconazole for the prevention and treatment of tinea gladiatorum, *Pediatric Infectious Disease Journal* 19:717-722, 2000.
33. Kohl T, Lisney M: Tinea gladiatorum: wrestling's emerging foe, *Sports Medicine* 29(6):439-447, 2000.
34. Hazen P, Weil M: Itraconazole in the prevention and management of dermatophytosis in competitive wrestlers, *Journal of the American Academy of Dermatology* 36:481-482, 1997.
35. Hand J, Wroble R: Prevention of tinea corporis in collegiate wrestlers, *Journal of Athletic Training* 35(4):427-430, 1999.
36. Centers for Disease Control and Prevention: Division of parasitic diseases. Available at http://www.cdc.gov/ncidod/dpd/parasites/lice/default.htm. Accessed July 2004.
37. Minnesota Department of Health: Lice. Available at http://www.health.state.mn.us/divs/idepc/diseases/headlice/index.html. Accessed February 2005.
38. Centers for Disease Control and Prevention: Scabies fact sheet [website]. Available at http://www.cdc.gov/ncidod/dpd/parasites/scabies/factsht_scabies.htm. Accessed July 2004.
39. Morbidity and Mortality Weekly Report: Sexually transmitted diseases treatment guidelines 2002, *MMWR Recommendations and Reports* 51(RR-6):1-78, 2002.
40. Lyon, W: Bee and wasp stings [website]. Available at http://ohioline.osu.edu/hyg-fact/2000/2076.html. Accessed February 2005.
41. Kumar V, Abbas AK, Fausto N: *Robbins and Cotran pathologic basis for disease,* ed 7, Philadelphia, 2005, Elsevier Saunders.
42. Black JM, Hawks JH: *Medical-surgical nursing: clinical management for positive outcomes,* ed 7, St Louis, 2005, Elsevier Saunders.
43. Auerbach P, Donner H, Weiss E: Bites and stings from arthropods. In *Field guide to wilderness medicine,* Philadelphia, 2003, Mosby.

CHAPTER 14

Musculoskeletal Disorders

Larry Collins

OBJECTIVES

At the completion of this chapter, the reader should be able to do the following:

1. Describe the anatomy of synovial joints.
2. Recognize and identify common inflammatory musculoskeletal conditions in the child and adult athlete.
3. Understand the underlying pathology of common inflammatory rheumatologic disorders.
4. Differentiate between the various inflammatory rheumatologic disorders.
5. Outline treatments plans and goals for inflammatory rheumatologic disorders.

INTRODUCTION

This chapter describes the underlying pathology of common conditions that may affect the musculoskeletal system but does not specifically address acute, traumatic musculoskeletal injuries. Other excellent resources are available that focus on the acute or traumatic musculoskeletal injury in the athlete. The conditions discussed here are seen in both physically active and nonactive populations. Many may be familial, metabolic, and degenerative in nature, and the athletic trainer needs to be familiar with them as well as acute focal injuries.

OVERVIEW OF ANATOMY AND PHYSIOLOGY

Synovial joints are the most common type of articulation within the human body. They are freely moveable joints characterized by the presence of a closed space or cavity between the articulating surfaces of the bones (Figure 14-1).

The articulating surfaces at the ends of the bones are covered by a thin layer of hyaline cartilage, also called articular cartilage, and are lubricated by synovial fluid, which is secreted by the synovial membrane lining the joint cavity. This fluid is composed of mucopolysaccharides, is highly viscous, and reduces friction between the articulating surfaces.

The articular capsule is a thick, double-layered membrane enclosing the joint cavity. The outer layer is a tough membrane of dense collagen fibers firmly attached to the surface of the bones near the metaphyseal-epiphyseal junction. It is continuous with the periosteum of the bone. The deeper layer of the capsule is the synovial membrane, which produces the synovial fluid that lubricates the joint.[1-4]

Ligaments are bands of dense connective tissue attaching one bone to another and adding to the stability of the synovial joint. Ligaments may be an intrinsic part of the fibrous capsule of the joint, (e.g., glenohumeral ligaments), or separate distinct structures (e.g., lateral collateral ligament [LCL]). Ligaments may be extracapsular (e.g., ulnar collateral ligament of the elbow) or intracapsular (e.g., ACL). Extracapsular ligaments are separate and distinct from the fibrous capsule and are found outside the joint capsule, whereas intracapsular ligaments lie within the capsule. These intracapsular ligaments are actually covered with synovial membrane; therefore they do not lie within the joint cavity.

Some synovial joints, such as the knee and shoulder, may also contain fibrocartilage disks within the synovial cavity. These disks help to spread synovial fluid within the joint and help provide stability and shock absorption to the joint.

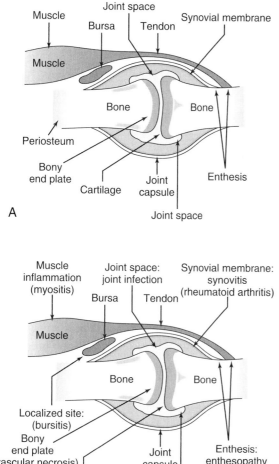

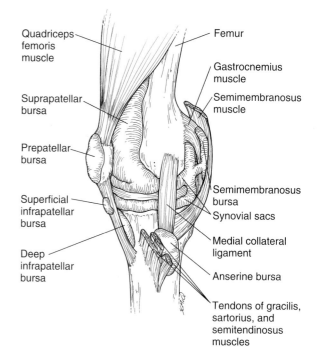

Figure 14-2 Bursae of the knee. (From O'Donoghue DH: *Treatment of injuries to athletes,* Philadelphia, 1984, WB Saunders.)

Figure 14-1 **A,** A synovial joint. **B,** The sites and types of rheumatic pathophysiology. (From Goldman L, Bennet JC: *Cecil's textbook of medicine,* ed 21, Philadelphia, 2000, WB Saunders, p. 1473.)

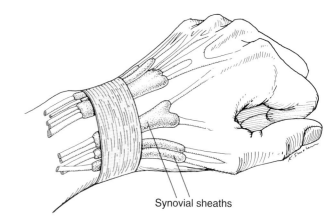

Figure 14-3 Extensor tendons of the wrist with surrounding synovial sheaths. (From Resnick D: *Diagnosis of bone and joint disorders,* ed 4, Philadelphia, 2002, WB Saunders, p. 703.)

Synovial bursae are partially collapsed, balloon-like structures that are lined with a synovial membrane on the inside and have an external fibrous membrane. They are filled with synovial fluid and are found in the vicinity of joints where movement between two adjacent tissues might otherwise result in excessive friction. The bursae are located between bone, tendon, muscle, or skin, and they shield these structures from undue friction (Figure 14-2).

Tendon sheaths are similar to bursae, except they form around the length of a tendon, performing the same function as the bursa[4] (Figure 14-3).

ASSESSMENT OF THE MUSCULOSKELETAL SYSTEM

Athletic trainers are well educated and skilled in the assessment of orthopedic injuries, therefore this chapter will focus on the key points of musculoskeletal evaluation for nontraumatic disorders. The typical assessment includes the HIPS/HOPS method of history, inspection/observation, palpation, and special tests. The patient history will typically include a description of the present problem, including onset, duration, and characteristics of the symptoms. The athletic trainer should ask what aggravates the condition, what relieves it, how long the pain lasts, and whether morning pain and stiffness are present. Knowing specific details about the onset, duration, and presenting characteristics may help to differentiate between underlying musculoskeletal conditions.

The athletic trainer asks about past traumatic injury to the joint or joints involved. In addition, the number of different joints involved and whether or not the symptoms occur bilaterally are noted (Key Points—Terms for Musculoskeletal Involvement). The patient's medical history, as well as any family

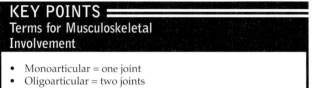

KEY POINTS
Terms for Musculoskeletal Involvement

- Monoarticular = one joint
- Oligoarticular = two joints
- Polyarticular = three or more joints

history of musculoskeletal conditions, is also important. When assessing adolescent conditions, especially in throwing athletes, the athletic trainer attempts to determine the amount and type of repetitive activities and any recent increase in the intensity of workouts for the athlete.

The physical examination typically includes a comparison of joints bilaterally and any other joint involvement. Observing for swelling, symmetry, redness, deformity, and atrophy of the surrounding musculature is important. In adolescents, any pain localized to the growth plates must be noted.

Range of motion and strength assessment is performed to determine loss of function and restriction of movement. When a neurological condition is suspected, a neurological examination is performed (see Chapters 2 and 8). When appropriate, special tests to determine the integrity of the ligamentous structures of the joint are performed.

PATHOLOGICAL CONDITIONS

Musculoskeletal pathology may be divided into eight categories that are grouped according to the type of pathology or the action on the musculoskeletal system. Table 14-1 lists the general classifications and examples of disorders that fit into each category.

Apophysitis

The apophysis is a portion of a bone that contributes to growth and is the attachment site for a tendon. The epiphyseal plate or cartilage, also called the growth plate, separates the metaphysis from the epiphysis or the apophysis. This cartilage plate is responsible for the majority of longitudinal growth of the long bones.

Apophysitis refers to inflammation of the apophysis and is sometimes referred to as **osteochondrosis.** It may be accompanied by widening or separation of the apophysis.[5] It is typically caused by repetitive stress or traction on the apophysis. Normal physiological stresses on bone stimulate tissue breakdown and repair that are kept in balance. However, when activities increase, or rest is not adequate, the breakdown processes may overwhelm the repair process and lead to an inflammatory response with an eventual onset of symptoms. This increased stress may lead to delays or breakdowns in ossification with fragmentation of the apophysis and widening of the epiphyseal cartilage. Such fragmentation and widening can sometimes be seen on a plain radiograph (Figure 14-4). Apophysitis is often identified in relation to a specific body part

Table 14-1   Pathophysiology of Orthopedic Diseases

Category	Pathophysiology	Characteristics	Common Disorders
Synovitis/synovium	Trauma, foreign matter, autoimmune	Swelling is hallmark characteristic	Synovitis, rheumatoid arthritis
Enthesopathy/enthesitis	Familial	Commonly occurs in 20-30 yr olds; inflammation where ligament transitions to bone	Ankylosing spondylitis, spondyloarthropathy
Cartilage degeneration	Familial, traumatic, degenerative	Exposure of subchondral bone; pain but not characterized by swelling	Osteoarthritis
Crystal induced (metabolic)	Metabolic	Monoarticular or oligoarticular; acute; hot, red joint	Gout, pseudogout
Infection	Bacterial, viral	Usually monoarticular; acute; hot, red joints; swelling	Staphylococcus, gonococcal arthritis
Myositis or myalgia	Autoimmune	Polyarticular; weakness; no history of trauma	Polymyalgia rheumatica, dermatomyositis
Focal conditions	Trauma, acute onset	Acute onset of pain and inflammation at one site	Bursitis, tendinitis, tendinosis, strains, sprains
General conditions		Normal tests; ambiguous pain; high emotional, psychological component	Chronic fatigue syndrome, fibromyalgia

or location. The following conditions are all considered apophysitis but are discussed according to their more common names.

Little League Shoulder

Also called proximal humeral **epiphysiolysis**, little league shoulder was first described by Dotter in 1953.[6] It is a stress fracture of the proximal humeral epiphyseal plate, which usually affects overhead

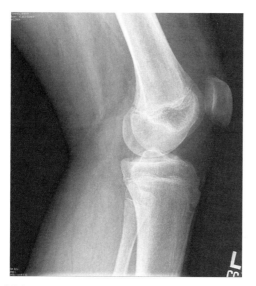

Figure 14-4 Radiograph of a 14-year-old with proximal tibia pain and swelling. Note the widening of the apophysis and small calcifications.

throwers between the ages of 12 and 15 years, although it is now being seen in younger athletes. The exact etiology of this condition is not known, but repetitive overload on the epiphyseal plate is thought to be the common underlying cause.[7]

Signs and Symptoms
The athlete usually presents with gradual onset of increasing shoulder pain, sometimes associated with a recent exacerbation as a result of a specific throw or pitch. Pain is generally localized to the upper arm.

Physical examination is usually consistent with that seen in impingement syndrome in the older population, including pain with full elevation and at extremes of internal and external rotation of the shoulder. Generalized weakness and limited active range of motion, especially in abduction and internal-external rotation, may also be present.[8,9] The positive Neer's impingement sign (Figure 14-5, *A*) and the alternative Hawkins' impingement test (Figure 14-5, *B*) generally reproduce pain, although probably from rotational forces on the proximal humerus as opposed to impingement of the rotator cuff. Pain is usually localized to the proximal lateral humerus.

Referral and Diagnostic Tests
Comparison radiographs often show widening of the proximal humeral epiphyseal plate and sometimes show fragmentation (Figure 14-6). Magnetic resonance imaging (MRI) is usually not necessary but will rule

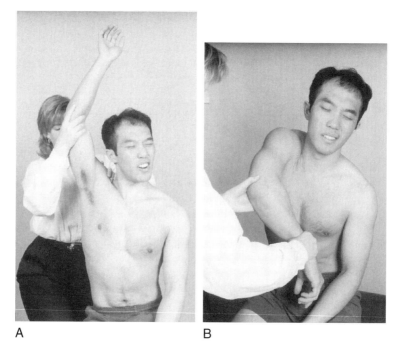

A   B

Figure 14-5 Tests for shoulder impingement. **A,** Neer's sign is positive if pain is reproduced when the arm is forcibly flexed, jamming the greater tuberosity against the antero-inferior surface of the acromion. **B,** Hawkins' test forcibly medially rotates the proximal humerus with the arm forward flexed to 90 degrees, reproducing pain. (From Magee DJ: *Orthopedic physical assessment,* ed 4, Philadelphia, 2002, WB Saunders, p. 263.)

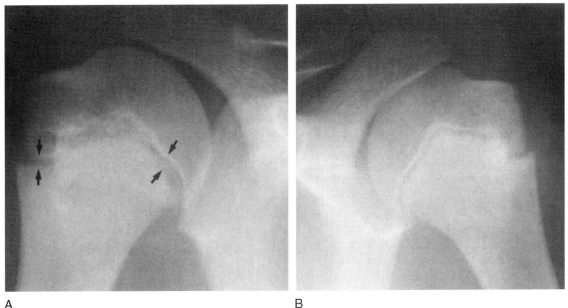

Figure 14-6 Little league shoulder in a 13-year-old elite pitcher. **A,** The arrows on the radiograph show a widening of the physis. **B,** The normal left side for comparison. (From DeLee JC, Drez D: *DeLee and Drez's orthopaedic sports medicine: principles and practice*, ed 2, Philadelphia, 2003, WB Saunders, p 1136.)

Table 14-2	Recommended Limits for Youth Pitchers' Pitch Counts			
Age	Pitches per Game	Pitches per Wk	Pitches per Season	Pitches per Yr
9-10 yr olds	50	75	1000	2000
11-12 yr olds	75	100	1000	3000
13-14 yr olds	75	125	1000	3000

Data from Andrews JR, Fleisig GS: How many pitches should I allow my child to throw? *USA Baseball News* April 1996; Lyman S, Fleisig GS, Andrews JR, et al: Effect of pitch type, pitch count, and pitching mechanics on risk of elbow and shoulder pain in youth baseball pitchers. *American Journal of Sports Medicine* 30(4): 463-468, 2002; USA Baseball Medical and Safety Advisory Committee Position Statement on Youth Baseball Injuries. Available at http://www.usabaseball.com/med_position_statement.html. Accessed February 11, 2005.

out rotator cuff pathology and may demonstrate edema at the epiphysis.

Differential Diagnosis
Differential diagnosis includes humeral stress fracturer, rotator cuff strain or tear, impingement syndrome, glenohumeral instability, labral tear, and infection.[5,10,11]

Treatment
Rest is the hallmark treatment for little league shoulder. Typically the athlete must refrain from throwing for up to 3 months. Usually absolute rest is recommended for 2 to 6 weeks, followed by a conditioning program focusing on range of motion, rotator cuff strengthening, and scapular stabilization. As strength increases and symptoms decrease, a gradual return to throwing is begun following a specific timetable based on strength and absence of symptoms. Nonsteroidal antiinflammatory drugs (NSAIDs) may be used to help decrease symptoms in the early stages of recovery.[7]

Prognosis and Return to Participation
Most individuals with little league shoulder will make a full and complete recovery if allowed to rest appropriately. Adequate rest is necessary for complete healing of the fracture. Following the initial rest period, focus is placed on regaining the athlete's normal range of motion and strength. After the athlete's strength and range of motion are within normal limits, a graduated return to throwing focusing on proper mechanics, including scapular stabilization will help prevent a relapse of the condition.

Prevention
Because the symptoms of little league shoulder are often brought about by an increase in throwing intensity or duration, it is imperative that pitch counts are monitored and regulated in youth baseball (Table 14-2). Gradual introduction of new pitches and increased number of pitches is paramount in the prevention of apophysitis of both the shoulder and the elbow.

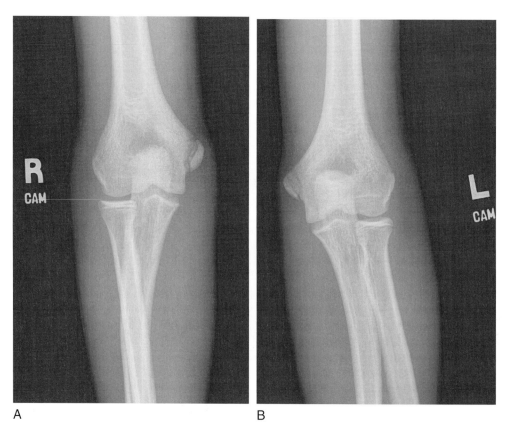

A   B

Figure 14-7 Radiographs showing (A) epiphyseal widening in little league elbow, and (B) normal opposite side for comparison.

Little League Elbow

Medial humeral epicondyle apophysitis, or little league elbow, is often caused by repeated tensile stresses on the medial epicondyle.[12] The apophysis of the medial epicondyle is typically the weak link in adolescents when compared with the ulnar collateral ligament (UCL) or the flexor pronator mass. The specific etiology of medial humeral epicondyle apophysitis is still unclear; however, the traction forces of the UCL on the apophysis are the prime suspect. The highest levels of stress are created during the late cocking and early acceleration phases of throwing and may be significantly higher in the side-arm thrower.[13,14]

Signs and Symptoms

Physical examination usually reveals pain and swelling over the medial epicondyle. Pain may be exacerbated with grip, resisted pronation, or wrist flexion. Valgus stress of the elbow may also increase the pain. Full extension of the elbow may be limited because of pain and muscle contracture. Pain occurs both during and after throwing. The athlete may also complain of pain on lifting objects with the affected arm.

Referral and Diagnostic Tests

Radiographs may reveal a widening or fragmentation of the epiphyseal plate of the medial humeral epicondyle when compared with the contralateral elbow (Figure 14-7).

Differential Diagnosis

Other conditions about the elbow that must be ruled out include osteochondrosis of the humeral capitellum or Panner's disease, olecranon stress fracture, and ulnar nerve entrapment. In addition, ulnar collateral ligament sprain, flexor pronator strain, osteochondritis dissecans, synovitis, and infection must be ruled out.[15]

Treatment

Treatment consists of rest, ice, compression, and elevation (RICE) followed by a gradual initiation of conditioning exercises for range of motion and strengthening. Usually several weeks of rest and avoidance of throwing are necessary to allow for proper healing and resolution of symptoms. It is imperative to focus on throwing technique and proper mechanics as the symptoms improve. As with other inflammatory conditions, NSAIDs may be used to help decrease symptoms in the early stages of recovery. Temporary splinting or casting the elbow may be warranted for displaced avulsions. Rarely, open reduction and internal fixation (ORIF) may be indicated if the apophysis is significantly displaced or there are numerous fragments or **nonunion** of the apophysis.

Prognosis and Return to Participation

Similar to little league shoulder, the prognosis for medial epicondyle apophysitis is good. With adequate rest, followed by an appropriate strengthening program and gradual return to throwing, most athletes will return to their previous level of competition.

Prevention

Prevention of little league elbow also follows the same guidelines for gradual introduction of new pitches and increase in number of pitches thrown per season. Proper throwing mechanics must be stressed with the young thrower. Avoidance of side-arm throwing as well as not allowing early introduction of breaking balls in a young pitcher's repertoire will decrease the chances of medial humeral epicondyle apophysitis (Key Points—Prevention of Little League Shoulder and Elbow).

KEY POINTS
Prevention of Little League Shoulder and Elbow

- Emphasize proper mechanics to young throwers.
- Avoid side arm pitches.
- Pay strict attention to pitch counts and number of days of throwing when supervising young throwers.
- Refer to recommended little league pitch counts (see Table 14-2).

Osgood-Schlatter Disease

Osgood-Schlatter disease is one of the most common causes of anterior knee pain in the adolescent athlete. Other common terms for this condition include epiphyseal aseptic necrosis of the tibial tubercle, osteochondritis of the tibial tuberosity, or patellar tendinitis. This condition was first described by American orthopedist Robert B. Osgood and Swiss physician Carl B. Schlatter.[3] It typically affects adolescents 10 to 15 years of age with the onset of symptoms usually associated with active periods of growth and/or rapid changes in activity levels.[16-23] Explosive and eccentric activities are particularly aggravating to Osgood-Schlatter disease. It is often bilateral and may occur at an earlier age in girls than in boys. Osgood-Schlatter disease may occur once and resolve with appropriate measures or may present as recurring episodes associated with growth spurts throughout adolesence.[3,15] Once the condition is resolved, the athlete may have a more prominent tibial tubercle.

Signs and Symptoms

Examination reveals point tenderness and swelling directly over the usually prominent tibial tubercle. Quadriceps and hamstring tightness is often present, and pain is exacerbated with resisted knee extension, eccentric quadriceps loading, or pressure directly on the tibial tubercle.

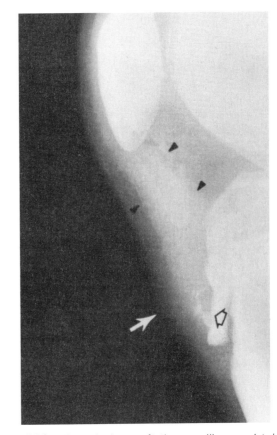

Figure 14-8 Radiograph shows soft tissue swelling associated with Osgood-Schlatter disease. (From Resnick D: *Diagnosis of bone and joint disorders*, ed 4, Philadelphia, 2002, WB Saunders, p 3717.)

Referral and Diagnostic Tests

Diagnosis is usually determined by history and physical exam. A radiograph is often normal but may show fragmentation and separation of the apophysis (Figure 14-8).

Differential Diagnosis

Osgood-Schlatter disease should be differentiated from patellar tendinitis, prepatellar bursitis, patellar fracture, patellar tendon rupture or avulsion, and iliotibial band tendinitis.

Treatment

The treatment of Osgood-Schlatter disease consists of limitation of aggravating activities to diminish symptoms along with cross-training to maintain conditioning. The condition is often self-limiting. Casting or immobilization is only used in severe cases that have not responded to conservative treatments or cases in which the apophysis has separated from the tibia.

The treatment should focus on improving flexibility and the gradual return to conditioning exercises as the symptoms allow. Ice may be used to control pain and swelling. NSAIDs may be very helpful in alleviating symptoms in the acute phases of the condition. Orthoses such as counterforce braces or neoprene

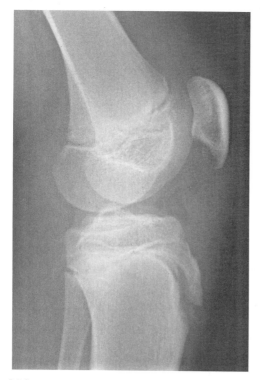

Figure 14-9 Radiograph of a patient who was diagnosed with Osgood-Schlatter disease that progressed to a complete avulsion of the apophysis through continued high demand activities.

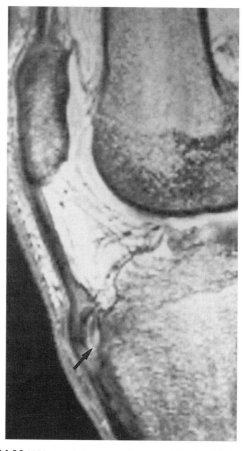

Figure 14-10 MRI reveals bony ossicles around the tibial tubercle with symptoms presenting as Osgood-Schlatter disease. (From Resnick D: *Diagnosis of bone and joint disorders,* ed 4, Philadelphia, 2002, WB Saunders, p 3719.)

knee sleeves have some limited benefit in controlling symptoms in some patients. A simple knee pad may provide protection from pain caused by bumping the hypersensitive area around the tibial tubercle.

Surgery is rarely indicated in acute cases unless complete avulsion of the apophysis has occurred (Figure 14-9). In some cases, individuals may have anterior pain localized to the tubercle that does not resolve and may be a result of bony ossicles that have not completely fused (Figure 14-10). Surgery is sometimes indicated in these individuals if conservative treatment is not successful in decreasing their symptoms.

Prognosis and Return to Participation
Athletes with Osgood-Schlatter disease typically do very well with conservative treatment. A short period of modified activities with instruction in appropriate stretching and strengthening exercises usually will allow the athlete to return to unrestricted activities.

Prevention
Prevention of symptoms related to Osgood-Schlatter disease is accomplished by minimizing risk factors for excessive stress on the extensor mechanism. Gradual increases in activity level with appropriate rest intervals and adequate stretching routines combined with proper warm-up and cool-down are usually sufficient to minimize symptoms.

Sever's Disease

Also known as calcaneal apophysitis, Sever's disease occurs as a result of inflammation of the growth plate at the insertion of the Achilles tendon on the posterior calcaneus. Sever's disease is usually a result of repetitive activities causing inappropriate stress on the growth center (similar to other apophysitis conditions) and typically occurs in children ages 8 to 14 years. Occasionally it worsens as a result of specific trauma.[3,24]

Signs and Symptoms
Examination reveals pain and swelling directly over the insertion of the Achilles tendon on the calcaneus. The pain is generally aggravated by passive ankle dorsiflexion or resisted plantar flexion. Performing a single-leg heel raise is usually difficult and reproduces pain. Achilles tendon tightness is typically pronounced.[24]

Referral and Diagnostic Tests
Radiographs are often normal but may reveal fragmentation or widening of the apophysis (Figure 14-11) compared with the unaffected side.

Differential Diagnosis

Other conditions that may present with similar signs and symptoms are plantar fasciitis, heel contusions, mild ankle sprains, and Achilles tendinitis.

Treatment

Rest remains the key to treatment. Icing and NSAIDs are helpful in decreasing inflammation. Gel heel inserts may help with the daily symptoms by decreasing the tension of the Achilles tendon on the calcaneous. Occasionally a walking boot may be used to help with severe symptoms and still allow for mobilization and stretching. For displaced avulsions or severe symptoms, casting or splinting may be indicated. Range of motion and stretching exercises should be initiated early on with avoidance of explosive and eccentric activities.[5,24]

Prognosis and Return to Participation

With adequate rest and a gradual increase in activities, a full return to participation is expected.

Prevention

Prevention of symptoms is best achieved through a gradual increase in activity levels with appropriate rest intervals and adequate stretching routines as part of the warm-up and cool-down.

Scheuermann's Disease

Scheuermann's disease, also known as juvenile **kyphosis,** is a deformity affecting the thoracic or thoracolumbar spine of adolescents. Patients typically present with poor posture or deformity with or without back pain and stiffness. Scheuermann's disease is thought to be a result of osteochondrosis of the anterior vertebral growth plate of the vertebral bodies and is most common in young males. This causes a narrowing of the anterior portion of the vertebral body causing wedge-shaped vertebrae. It is seen most commonly in the lower thoracic spine from T7 through T9 and usually involves several vertebral bodies but may involve the entire thoracic and lumbar spine.[3,25,26]

Signs and Symptoms

Physical examination usually reveals a kyphotic (humpback) deformity of 20 to 25 degrees that does not change when the athlete bends forward in a flexed position (Figure 14-12). The kyphosis is commonly accompanied by scoliosis and a decrease in flexibility because of the structural nature of the deformity.

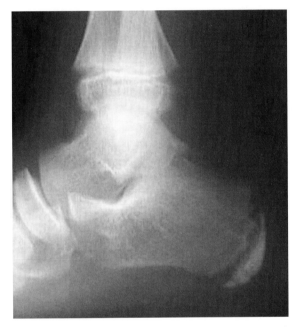

Figure 14-11 Radiograph reveals fragmentation of calcaneal apophysis in a child diagnosed with Sever's disease.

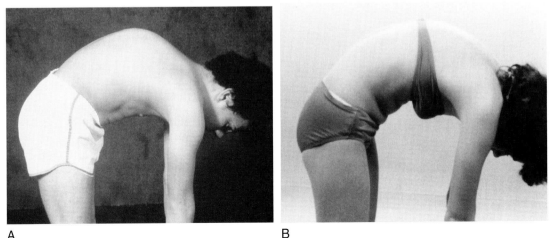

A   B

Figure 14-12 Clinical presentation of, A, Scheuermann's disease as compared with, B, postural kyphosis. (From Canale ST, editor: *Campbell's operative orthopaedics,* ed 10, St Louis, 2003, Mosby, p 1879.)

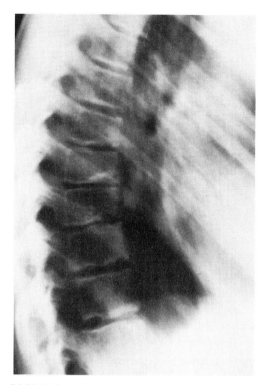

Figure 14-13 Radiographic appearance of Scheuermann's disease. (From Magee DJ: *Orthopedic physical assessment,* ed 4, Philadelphia, 2002, WB Saunders, p 461.)

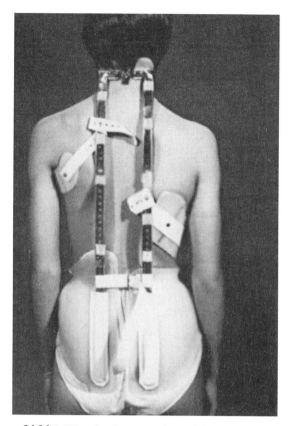

Figure 14-14 A Milwaukee brace may be used for bracing a patient's spine in Scheuermann's disease or other conditions of scoliosis or kyphosis. (From Herkowitz HN, Garfin SR, Balderston RA, et al: *Rothman-Simone: the spine,* ed 4, Philadelphia, 1999, WB Saunders, p 352.)

Athletes will usually have tenderness to palpation around the kyphosis. As with lower spine conditions, hamstring tightness is common. Although neurological complications are rare, a thorough neurological examination is essential (see Chapter 8).

Referral and Diagnostic Tests

Radiographs and MRI scans are helpful to rule out other conditions. Radiographs may reveal decreased disk space anteriorly, irregularly shaped vertebral end plates, and the presence of **Schmorl's nodes** (Figure 14-13).

Differential Diagnosis

Differential diagnosis includes scoliosis, congenital kyphosis, multiple compression fractures, tumor, infection, tuberculosis, skeletal dysplasia, ankylosing spondylitis, and herniated nucleus pulposus.

Treatment

Core strengthening and trunk stabilization exercises remain controversial in individuals with Scheuermann's disease. Some feel that because this condition is usually self-limiting, no treatment is necessary.[25,26] Others recommend strengthening to prevent associated back pain and stiffness.[25,26] In more extreme cases, casting or bracing is appropriate (Figure 14-14). Orthotic management typically requires 12 to 24 months of treatment to show significant improvement and is done to prevent worsening of the condition as opposed to actually correcting the deformity.

NSAIDs are helpful for exacerbations, and activity restrictions to prevent hyperextension of the spine may be indicated. Surgery is rarely indicated and typically is for intractable pain or unacceptable cosmetic deformity.[25,26]

Prognosis and Return to Participation

Because Scheuermann's disease usually occurs in the thoracic spine, which normally has limited motion, most individuals do well with conservative management. In skeletally mature athletes, the kyphosis is usually not progressive. This differs from adolescent scoliosis, which can continue to progress into adulthood (if the deformity is more than 50 degrees). For adults, the treatment is usually observation, antiinflammatory drugs, or reconstructive surgery, depending on the severity of the symptoms. Common complications associated with Scheuermann's disease include chronic back pain, progressive deformity, and neurological deficits. Patient education is essential to help improve posture and overall body mechanics with daily activities.

Avascular Necrosis

Avascular necrosis (AVN) is a condition resulting from the temporary or permanent loss of the blood supply to a bone. With the blood supply gone, the cells within the bone die, eventually causing the bone to collapse. This may lead to collapse of the overlying articular surface of the bone and subsequently to arthritis (Figure 14-15). AVN is also referred to as osteonecrosis, subchondral bone avascularity, ischemic necrosis, or aseptic necrosis.

Avascular necrosis may affect one bone or more than one bone at the same time or over a period of time.[3] The etiology of AVN is most commonly traumatic. Several risk factors are known and listed in Box 14-1. AVN may affect any bone, but is most commonly seen in the carpal scaphoid due to its recurrent blood supply. In bones with recurrent blood supply, the arterial supply passes the bone and its nourishment is supplied in a distal to proximal fashion. The scaphoid is an excellent example of this since a proximal fracture eliminates the possibility of blood supply to the injured area.

Up to 20% of individuals who sustain a femoral head or neck fracture develop AVN. In adults, presentation is typically seen in the 4th and 5th decades. High-dose corticosteroid use is associated with up to 35% of all cases of AVN, and alcohol abuse is also correlated with an increased risk of developing AVN.[2-4] In children, AVN of the femoral head is termed **Legg-Calvé-Perthes disease** or coxa plana (Figure 14-16). Children with Legg-Calvé-Perthes disease are usually

between 4 and 14 years old, and present with increasing hip pain and often no history of injury or trauma.

Signs and Symptoms

Patients typically present with gradually increasing joint pain that may be associated with loss of motion. Patients are often asymptomatic for a significant period before the process starts to affect joint mechanics. As the disease progresses, they begin to experience increasing joint pain with activity and eventually even experience pain at rest.

Physical examination will usually reveal pain with joint motion and restricted range of motion depending on the progression of the disease.

Box 14-1	Risk Factors for Developing Avascular Necrosis

Traumatic
- Fractures
- Dislocations

Atraumatic
- High-dose or long-term use corticosteroids
- Alcohol abuse
- Caisson disease (seen in deep-sea divers)
- Arterial disease
- Radiation or chemotherapy
- Sickle cell disease
- Gaucher's disease
- Lipid disturbances
- Blood-clotting disorders
- Pancreatitis
- Kidney disease
- Liver disease
- Lupus
- Smoking

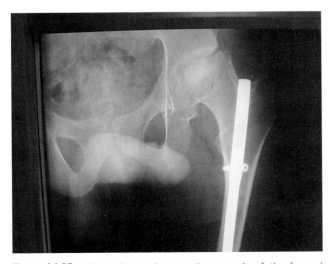

Figure 14-15 Radiograph reveals avascular necrosis of the femoral head in an 18 year old with previous femur fracture fixed with intramedullary rod.

Figure 14-16 Radiograph shows Legg-Calvé-Perthes disease. (From Resnick D: *Diagnosis of bone and joint disorders*, ed 4, Philadelphia, 2002, WB Saunders, p 3693. (Courtesy R Freiberger, MD, New York.)

Referral and Diagnostic Tests

Radiographs are often normal when patients initially present but may show signs of early bone loss in aggressive cases (Figure 14-17). An MRI study is usually ordered for patients with suspected AVN because it is much more sensitive in detecting the disease in its early stages (Figure 14-18). The MRI is able to detect changes in the bone marrow and provides the physician with a better indication of the extent of the affected area. MRI has replaced the bone scan and computed tomography (CT) scan as the diagnostic study of choice for evaluating AVN.[4]

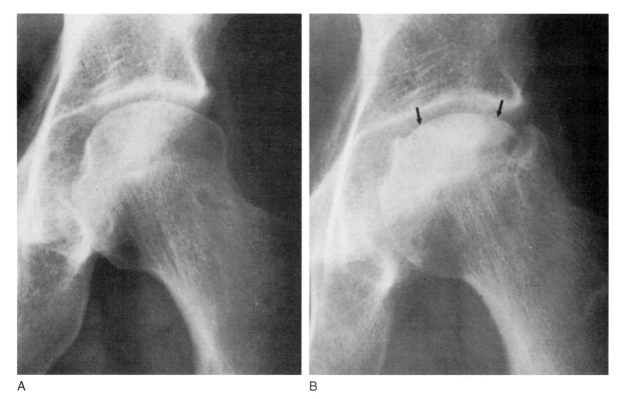

A   B

Figure 14-17 Two radiographs show the progression of avascular necrosis. **A,** Initial radiograph of a 35-year-old man complaining of hip pain. **B,** Seven months later a repeat radiograph shows significant collapse of the superolateral aspect of the femoral head. (From Resnick D: *Diagnosis of bone and joint disorders,* ed 4, Philadelphia, 2002, WB Saunders, p 3616.)

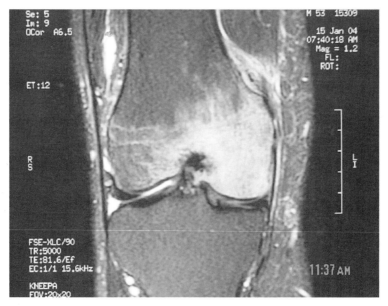

Figure 14-18 Magnetic resonance imaging (MRI) reveals avascular necrosis of the medial femoral condyle of the knee.

Box 14-2	Surgical Procedures for Avascular Necrosis and Other Degenerative Joint Diseases

- **Core Decompression and Bone Grafting:** A surgical procedure that involves drilling into the affected area of the bone and removing a portion of the bone, thereby decreasing pressure within the bone. Healthy bone from another area of the body is sometimes placed in the defect, such as a bone graft, to help support the articular surface and to prevent further collapse. Core decompression may help improve blood flow to the bone and, eventually, allow more blood vessels to form. Core decompression works best in people who are in the earliest stages of avascular necrosis (AVN) before the collapse of the articular surface has begun. This procedure can reduce pain and slow the progression of bone and joint destruction in these patients. Activity is limited for a short time after surgery; normal daily activities are resumed gradually, but high-impact activity is avoided.
- **Osteotomy:** A surgical procedure that involves cutting the bone away from the damaged area and realigning the bone to decrease stress on the affected joint. There is a lengthy recovery period; the patient's activity is very limited for 3 to 12 months after an osteotomy. This procedure is reserved for younger patients with advanced AVN limited to a specific area.
- **Arthroplasty or Total Joint Replacement:** A surgical procedure that is the definitive treatment for late-stage AVN when the joint is completely destroyed in the older adult patient. Arthroplasty involves removing the diseased bone and replacing it with artificial components.

Treatment

Once diagnosed, treatment is designed to prevent or slow progression of the disease. Activity modifications are initiated to limit impact-loading activities. If possible, contributing factors such as steroids, alcohol, or smoking are eliminated. NSAIDs or narcotic analgesics are used for pain control as needed.

As the disease progresses and function begins to be compromised, surgical procedures are available to retard the progression of the disease or replace the damaged joint if necessary (Box 14-2).

Prognosis and Return to Participation

AVN can be a devastating disease with typical progression and eventual destruction of the joint. Activities usually need to be restricted on a permanent basis depending on the extent of the progression and the patient's symptoms. In some cases spontaneous remission occurs, after which the individual is allowed to return to activities as tolerated.

Prevention

Prevention of AVN is based on the elimination or limiting of risk factors (i.e., alcohol use, steroid use, cigarette smoking). Of course, many other risk factors including trauma and **caisson disease** are inherent in certain sports or activities, and these risks need to be assessed by each individual.

Arthritides

Gout

Gout is one of the more painful of the rheumatic arthritides. The ancient Greeks first described it in the fifth century BC. It is usually acute in onset and is associated with pain, erythema, and warmth in one joint (monoarticular). It is a potentially disabling form of arthritis that results from the deposition of uric acid crystals within a joint, in the connective tissues surrounding a joint as deposits called tophi, or a combination of the two.

Pseudogout is sometimes confused with gout because it produces similar symptoms of inflammation. However, in this condition, also called chondrocalcinosis, deposits are made up of calcium pyrophosphate dihydrate crystals, not uric acid.[1,27,28] Pseudogout typically affects the knee, whereas gout most commonly affects the great toe but may affect any joint.

Uric acid is a nitrogen-based substance that is the end product of purine metabolism. Uric acid is primarily excreted through the kidneys and eliminated in the urine and gastrointestinal tract. **Hyperuricemia** results from either the increased production of uric acid or the decreased elimination of uric acid by the kidneys. Hyperuricemia itself is not a disease and does not cause symptoms. However, if excess uric acid crystals form as a result of hyperuricemia, the clinical presentation of gout may develop. The presence of uric acid crystals in the joint activates a number of inflammatory pathways.[1,2] Clinical gout presents if uric acid crystals from hyperuricemia are formed and deposited within the joint cavity, inducing a number of inflammatory responses.

Gout may be considered a continuum ranging from asymptomatic hyperuricemia to the acute gouty flare-up to formation of tophi (deposits of uric acid crystals in soft tissue). Hyperuricemia occurs when an individual has elevated levels of uric acid in the blood but no other symptoms. Acute gout, or acute gouty arthropathy, occurs when the hyperuricemia has caused the deposition of uric acid crystals into the joint space. This leads to a sudden onset of pain and localized swelling in the joint. The joint is also usually very warm, red, and tender. Acute gouty arthropathy often occurs at night and may be triggered by several risk factors (Box 14-3). Flare-ups usually subside within 5 to 10 days, even without treatment, and subsequent episodes may not occur for months or even years.

Interval or intercritical gout is the period between acute flare-ups. During this time, the individual is usually asymptomatic. Prophylactic medications may be used to prevent flare-ups.

Chronic tophaceous gout is the most disabling stage of gout and usually develops over several years of recurrent flares. Tophi is a term used to describe the deposition of uric acid crystals in soft tissue, typically found in the pinnae of the ears, around the interphalangeal (IP) joints, Achilles tendon, and olecranon bursa (Figure 14-19). The disease may cause permanent damage to the affected joints and sometimes to the kidneys. With proper treatment, most people with gout do not progress to this advanced stage.[1,27,28]

Signs and Symptoms
The patient usually presents with the sudden onset of a severe, painful, swollen joint (Figure 14-20). Physical examination confirms the extremely tender, erythematous, inflamed joint. The pain is often worsened with motion or direct pressure. Motion is often restricted because of the swelling.

Referral and Diagnostic Tests
The athlete with atraumatic, sudden onset of pain and swelling in a joint, especially the great toe, is referred for diagnostic tests to confirm the presence of gout. A definitive diagnosis is made by joint aspiration and evidence of uric acid crystals in the joint fluid (Figure 14-21). The fluid is usually evaluated for evidence of infection since this could be an additional cause of joint pain and swelling. Blood uric acid levels may be elevated but this is often transient. Radiographs are often normal in acute flare-ups but may show

characteristic findings of joint erosion or tophaceous deposits in chronic cases of gout (Figure 14-22).

Differential Diagnosis
Initial onset of gout may be confused with other orthopedic conditions that cause sudden onset of a painful swollen joint. Gout is atraumatic, which can differentiate it from joint sprains or fractures. Other conditions that may present with similar signs and symptoms are pseudogout, septic arthritis, cellulitis, acute rheumatic fever, juvenile rheumatoid arthritis, and palindromic rheumatism.[1,27,28]

Treatment
Treatment consists of trying to decrease the pain and inflammation while restoring normal uric acid levels to avoid the formation of tophi and kidney stones. NSAIDs are very beneficial, and analgesics are sometimes needed as well.

Colchicine is a very effective drug, especially if it is started within the first 12 to 24 hours of an attack; however, it has frequent side effects and is often not well tolerated. Corticosteroids are also used to treat gout attacks and can be given orally or by injection during joint aspiration.

For patients who have had multiple episodes, therapy should be directed at normalizing uric acid levels in the blood as a prophylactic measure. Uricosuric agents (probenecid, sulfinpyrazone) lower the serum concentration of uric acid by increasing excretion. Drugs such as allopurinol help slow the production of uric acid and may be used alone or in combination with a uricosuric agent.[1,2,28]

Prognosis and Return to Participation
Patients whose symptoms associated with gout are adequately controlled with diet and oral medications have a very good prognosis, and no restrictions on activities are necessary. Athletes who continue to have

Box 14-3	Risk Factors for Gout

- Foods: high in purines (red meat; shellfish)
- Medications: diuretics, salicylates, niacin, cyclosporine, levodopa
- Family history: males, postmenopausal females, African-Americans
- Medical conditions: diabetes, kidney disease, obesity, hypertension, hyperlipidemia, sickle cell anemia
- Other factors: dehydration, trauma, surgery, alcoholism

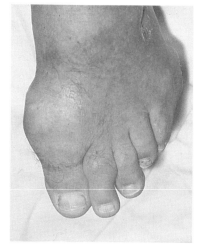

Figure 14-19 Gouty tophi involving the first and fifth metatarsals. (From Klippel JH, Dieppe PA, editors: *Rheumatology,* ed 2, St Louis, 1998, Mosby, p 8.14.3.)

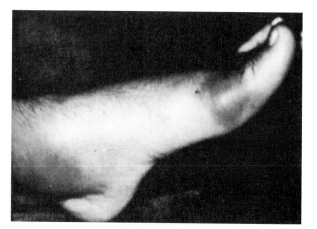

Figure 14-20 Local signs of gout in the great toe. (From Prior JA, Silberstein JS: *Physical diagnosis: the history and examination of the patient,* ed 6, St Louis, 1981, Mosby.)

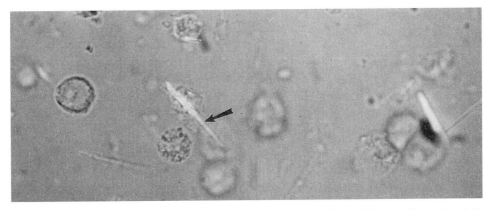

Figure 14-21 Evidence of uric acid crystals in the joint fluid is a definitive diagnosis for gout. (From Resnick D: *Diagnosis of bone and joint disorders,* ed 4, Philadelphia, 2002, WB Saunders, p 1522.)

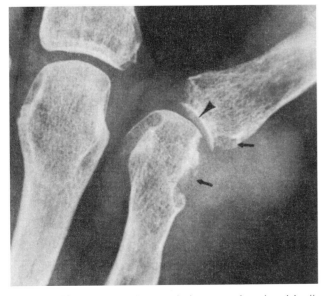

Figure 14-22 Radiograph shows articular space is only minimally narrowed *(arrowhead)* despite the presence of nodular soft tissue masses and osseous erosion *(arrows)*. (From Resnick D: *Diagnosis of bone and joint disorders,* ed 4, Philadelphia, 2002, WB Saunders, p 1525.)

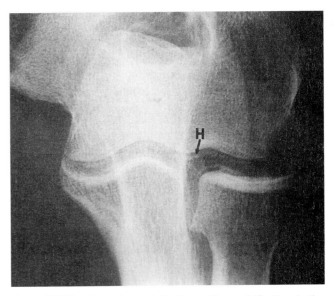

Figure 14-23 Radiograph reveals hyaline cartilage calcifications in the elbow. *H,* Pseudogout. (From Resnick D: *Diagnosis of bone and joint disorders,* ed 4, Philadelphia, 2002, WB Saunders, p 1579.)

flare-ups despite medications and lifestyle changes, however, may need to modify their activities.

Prevention

The athletic trainer can counsel the individual with gout about lifestyle issues that may be contributing to the flare-ups, including the avoidance of fad diets, foods high in purines, alcohol use, and the use of certain medications. Maintaining adequate hydration, especially in times of increased exercise, can also help limit flare-up of symptoms.

Pseudogout

Pseudogout refers to a condition that closely resembles gout, except the crystals are composed of calcium pyrophosphate dihydrate (CPPD). Patients present in a similar fashion to gout. However, aspiration reveals CPPD deposits as opposed to uric acid crystals in

the joint. Chondrocalcinosis is the term used to describe the calcium-containing deposits that are found in cartilage and are usually visible on joint radiographs (Figure 14-23).

The etiology of pseudogout is unknown. There may be a familial predisposition or an association with thyroid or parathyroid gland disorders. NSAIDs, corticosteroid injections, and colchicine are successful in shortening the course of flare-ups and may be effective in preventing attacks. No treatments are available to dissolve the crystal deposits. Controlling inflammation helps to halt the progression of joint degeneration that often accompanies pseudogout.[1,27,28]

Rheumatoid Arthritis

Rheumatoid arthritis (RA) is a systemic autoimmune inflammatory disease that typically causes symmetrical joint pain, swelling, and stiffness and eventually

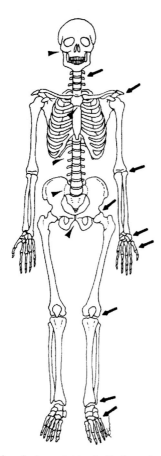

Figure 14-24 Although rheumatoid arthritis is most prevalent in wrists and hands it may also involve the feet, knees, ankles, elbows, glenohumeral and accromioclavicular joints. Rheumatoid arthritis may also affect the hips and the axial skeleton (especially the cervical spine). (From Resnick D: *Diagnosis of bone and joint disorders*, ed 4, Philadelphia, 2002, WB Saunders, p 895.)

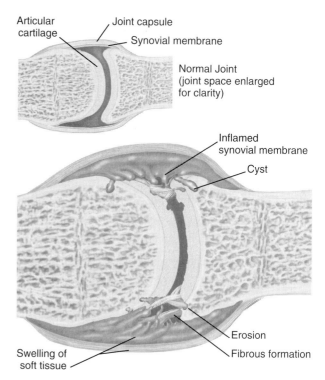

Figure 14-25 Schematic representation of rheumatoid arthritis compared with a normal joint. (From Jarvis C: *Physical examination & health assessment*, ed 4, Philadelphia, 2004, WB Saunders, p 648.)

results in loss of motion and decreased function. Morning joint stiffness that may last for hours is a hallmark of the disease. Although RA may affect any joint, it most commonly presents in the wrists and carpometacarpal (CMC) and IP joints (Figure 14-24). Patients with RA may also experience systemic symptoms, including generalized fatigue, malaise, and fever. Other systemic effects may include ocular dryness, skin ulcerations, **neutropenia,** or **splenomegaly.** These systemic symptoms associated with RA are (also) called **Felty's syndrome.** RA can affect individuals transiently or in cycles with periods of remission and flare-ups that progressively worsen over time. RA affects women more commonly than men and occurs in all races and ethnic groups. RA typically begins in middle age and occurs with increased frequency in older people.

An identical disease that occurs in children is known as juvenile chronic arthritis (juvenile rheumatoid arthritis). Juvenile rheumatoid arthritis can interfere with growth and lead to joint deformities as a result of chronic joint inflammation. Another common progression of juvenile rheumatoid arthritis is the inflammation of the iris in the eye that can lead to permanent eye damage.[1,27,29,30]

The cartilage damage seen in RA is thought to be a result of lymphocytic infiltration of the neutrophils in synovial fluid, chondrocytes, and hypertrophic synovium, which destroy articular cartilage.[30] The exact mechanism for the initiation of these processes is not clear (Figure 14-25).

Signs and Symptoms

Physical examination usually reveals symmetrical, tender, warm, swollen joints. Range of motion begins to be limited as the disease progresses. Eventually, joint deformities may develop, including ulnar drifting of the metacarpophalangeal (MCP) joints (Figure 14-26, *A*), boutonnière and swan neck deformity of the IP joints (Figure 14-26, *B*). Rheumatoid nodules may also develop on the extensor surface of the digits and upper extremities. Rheumatoid nodules are small subcutaneous areas of fibrous necrosis surrounded by epithelial cells. In rare cases, these nodules may also be found systemically within the heart or lungs.[1]

Referral and Diagnostic Tests

Athletes with oligo- or polyarticular symptoms raise special concern for systemic evolvement. Laboratory tests typically reveal elevated levels of rheumatoid factors (immunoglobulin M) and antinuclear antibodies (ANAs). RA frequently causes chronic anemia, the

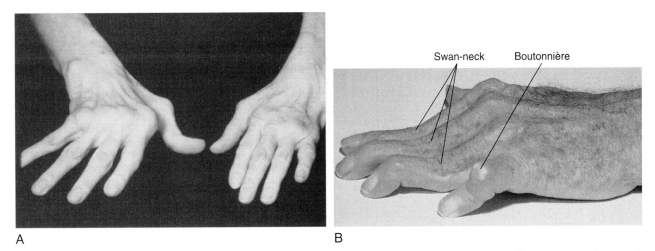

A   B

Figure 14-26 Conditions caused by chronic rheumatoid arthritis. A, Ulnar drifting of metacarpophalangeal (MCP) joint. B, Boutonnière and swan-neck deformities. (From Jarvis C: *Physical examination & health assessment*, ed 4, Philadelphia, 2004, WB Saunders, p 652.)

severity of which often parallels the course of the disease. Erythrocyte sedimentation rates (ESRs) and C-reactive proteins (CRPs) are usually elevated because of the systemic inflammatory response.

Radiographs typically reveal osteoporosis and soft tissue swelling in the early stages. As the disease progresses, joint space narrowing and eventually erosion of the articular surfaces of the joint will be evident on radiographs (Figure 14-27). Radiographs of the wrists, hands, and feet are usually the most dramatic.[1,27]

Differential Diagnosis

RA should be differentiated from other orthopedic conditions, such as osteoarthritis, psoriatic arthritis, gout, Lyme disease, and fibromyalgia.

Treatment

There is no known cure for RA so treatment focuses on reducing pain, restoring joint motion, and improving overall function to allow the individual to lead a normal life. The most important aspect of management is to educate the patient about the condition and to begin a regular exercise program with appropriate periods of rest. Exercise helps to maintain muscle strength and joint mobility and function and prevent osteoporosis. Medications may be used for pain relief and to reduce inflammation. NSAIDs, corticosteroids, and disease-modifying agents (DMARDs) are classes of medications used to treat RA. Newer medications may be used to attempt to modify the disease itself.

Surgery is available to patients with severe joint damage. As with other treatments, the goals of surgery are to reduce pain, improve the affected joint's function, and restore the patient's ability to perform daily activities. Surgery is usually not performed on a pain-free functional joint regardless of the cosmetic deformity.[29]

Prognosis and Return to Participation

Although there is no cure for RA, most individuals do very well with a combination of treatments. Some individuals will continue to have certain level of symptoms despite aggressive therapy. These individuals must rest joints during flare-ups and maintain a regular, nonimpact exercise program.

Osteoarthritis

Osteoarthritis (OA) is probably the most common of the rheumatologic disorders and affects almost every individual to some extent by the sixth or seventh decade in life. Although commonly known by the term degenerative joint disease, OA is actually a complicated process that involves damage to the underlying collagen structure and increasing water content in articular cartilage[30] (Figure 14-28). There is an increase in chondrocytes, which results in an increase in degradative enzymes that shift the homeostasis of the joint from a status of repair to one of breakdown[30] (Figure 14-29). This probably has a greater effect on the articular surface than mechanical degeneration. Several factors have been shown to hasten this degradative process including trauma, ACL deficiency, and joint malalignment.

Other risk factors include obesity, a positive family history, and performing heavy labor for a living. Interestingly, long distance runners show no increased risk of developing OA. OA is seen primarily in the IP and first CMC joints of the hand, cervical and lower lumbar spine, hips, knees, and the first metatarsophalangeal (MTP) joint but may affect any joint.[1,4,27]

Signs and Symptoms

The most common presenting complaint is pain that typically is worse with activity and resolves with rest.

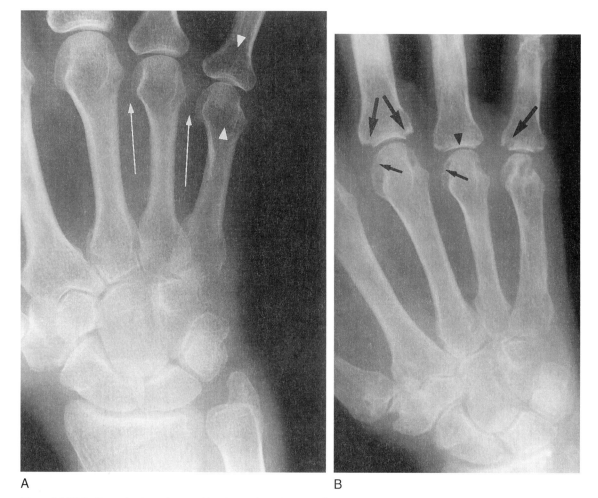

A   B

Figure 14-27 Radiographs show rheumatoid arthritis. **A,** Early stage. **B,** Later stage. Note the symmetrical joint space narrowing and erosion of the joint in the later stage when compared with the early stage. (From Noble J, editor: *Textbook of primary care medicine,* St Louis, 2002, Mosby, p 1117.)

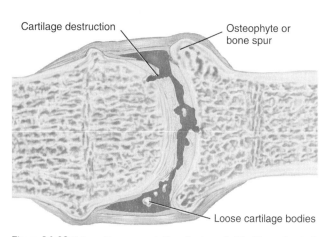

Figure 14-28 Schematic representation of osteoarthritis. (From Jarvis C: *Physical examination & health assessment*, ed 4, Philadelphia, 2004, WB Saunders, p 648.)

However, pain at night and following prolonged immobilization is also common. The symptoms are usually monoarticular or localized to one joint but may affect any number of joints. Joint stiffness in the morning and following rest or inactivity are common but usually resolve quickly unlike RA, the stiffness of which may last for several hours. Patients often experience soreness associated with changes in the weather, especially with barometric changes and cold temperatures.[31]

Physical examination of the knee usually reveals joint crepitus, tenderness, and enlargement of bony prominences because of osteophyte formation. Knee pain may also be noted in the proximal tibia.

Examination of the hands reveals enlargements around the IP joints, which are known as **Heberden's nodes** when distal and **Bouchard's nodes** when proximal (Figure 14-30). As osteophytes progress, joint stiffness and mechanical loss of motion begin to occur.

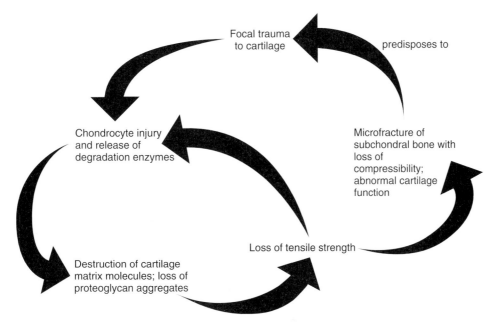

Figure 14-29 Pathogenesis of osteoarthritis. (From Noble J, editor: *Textbook of primary care medicine,* St Louis, 2002, Mosby, p 1235.)

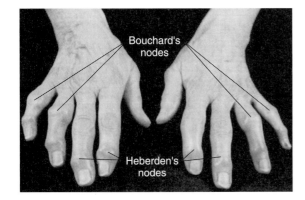

Figure 14-30 Hand showing Heberden's nodes (distal interphalangeal [DIP] joints) and Bouchard's nodes (proximal interphalangeal [PIP] joints). (From Jarvis C: *Physical examination & health assessment,* ed 4, Philadelphia, 2004, WB Saunders, p 653.)

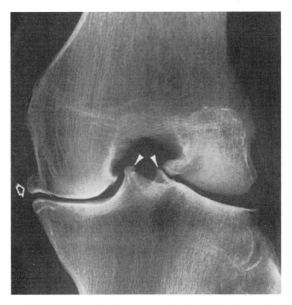

Figure 14-31 Radiograph shows osteoarthritis of the knee with joint space narrowing, enlarged bony prominences and osteophyte formation. (From Resnick D: *Diagnosis of bone and joint disorders,* ed 4, Philadelphia, 2002, WB Saunders, p 1349.)

OA in the hip typically presents as groin pain but may also present as buttock, thigh, or even knee pain. Internal rotation of the hip usually reproduces symptoms.

Lower lumbar OA typically produces buttock or thigh pain. Cervical OA usually produces pain that radiates into the shoulder and arm. In the cervical and lumbar regions the radiated pain is a result of nerve root impingement.

Referral and Diagnostic Tests
Radiographs confirm the diagnosis, although in early cases these films may show very minimal joint destruction. Eventually loss of joint space and osteophyte formation occur (Figure 14-31). Weight-bearing films are recommended to get a true sense of joint height (Figure 14-32). Subchondral bone cysts and irregularities in the intraarticular joint surface begin to appear in the later stages of the disease. Laboratory tests are usually normal.

Differential Diagnosis
OA should be differentiated from other orthopedic conditions, such as RA, psoriatic arthritis, gout, Lyme disease, and fibromyalgia.

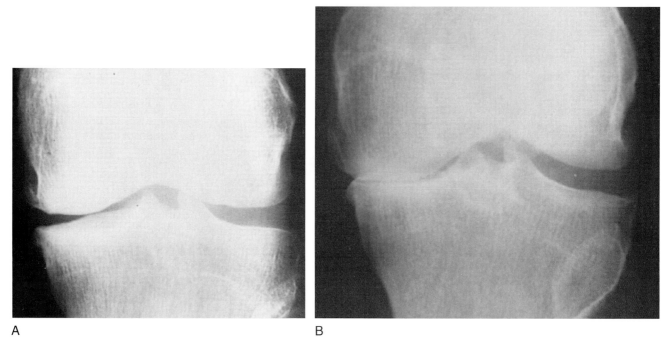

A   B

Figure 14-32 A, A standard non–weight-bearing anteroposterior radiograph. **B,** A weight-bearing radiograph of the knee in a patient with osteoarthritis; note the joint space narrowing. (From Resnick D: *Diagnosis of bone and joint disorders,* ed 4, Philadelphia, 2002, WB Saunders, p 1348.)

Table 14-3   Nonsurgical Treatment Options for Osteoarthritis

Treatment	Benefits and Possible Adverse Effects	Duration of Effects/Frequency of Use
Exercise	Decreased pain and stiffness; improved daily function and activity level; some types of exercise will aggravate some people	Indefinite
Oral Medications		
Tylenol	Pain relief	Indefinite
COX-2 selective antiinflammatory celecoxib (Celebrex)	Pain relief; decreased inflammation; potential risk for stomach upset and possible aggravation of high blood pressure	Indefinite as long as symptoms are improved and no adverse effects occur
Non–COX-2 selective anti-inflammatories: ibuprofen, diclofenac, naproxen, others	Pain relief; decreased inflammation; potentially higher adverse effect profile with increased risk of gastrointestinal ulceration and bleeding	Indefinite as long as symptoms are improved and no adverse effects noted
Glucosamine, chondroitin sulfate	Potential benefit in preventing breakdown of articular cartilage	Indefinite as long as symptoms are improved
Narcotics	Short-term use for acute pain	Short term
Injections		
Corticosteroids: betamethasone (Celestone), triamcinolone (Kenalog), dexamethasone	For acute flare-ups; give pain relief by decreasing inflammation	Short term: 1-6 mo (per injection); long term: may be repeated every 3-4 mo
Visco-supplementation (series of 3-5 injections given weekly): sodium hyaluronate (Hyalgan, Supartz), Hylan G-F 20 (Synvisc), high-molecular-weight hyaluronan (Orthovisc)	Thick, viscous fluid injected into the joint that coats the cartilage surface, decreases inflammatory mediators, and promotes the production of normal joint fluid	Long term: up to 6-12 mo; may be repeated if good response
Braces		
Elastic or neoprene knee sleeve	Offers added knee support during daily activities	Long term: worn as long as needed and symptoms are improved
Unloader brace	Reduces the stress placed on the affected compartment of the knee	Long term: worn as long as needed and symptoms are improved

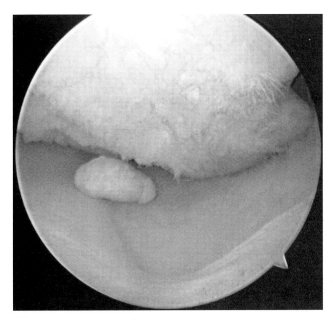

Figure 14-33 Arthroscopic débridement of joint to remove loose bodies caused by osteoarthritis may decrease the patient's symptom.

Treatment

No treatments are available that reverse OA, but many modalities, including pharmacological and surgical interventions, can be helpful in decreasing joint pain and preserving joint mobility and function (Table 14-3). Exercise and lifestyle changes to maintain and improve joint range of motion and muscular strength should be initiated. At the same time limiting impact-loading activities can decrease stress on the affected joints.

Pharmacological treatment follows a path from least invasive to most invasive by beginning with acetaminophen, progressing to nonsteroidal antiinflammatory medications, then to corticosteroid injections. Other over-the-counter treatments, such as topical ointments, may provide superficial pain relief. Supplements such as glucosamine and chondroitin sulfate have shown some promise in treating the symptoms of OA in some individuals. In addition, analgesics are used for pain in patients whose symptoms are not controlled with other means.

More invasive treatments such as corticosteroid injections have a beneficial effect on most arthritic joints, especially during flare-up of symptoms. Corticosteroid injections may safely be performed two or three times per year in any joint. More recently, injectable hyaluronic acid has been used as a series of weekly injections that may help decrease symptoms for as long as 6 to 12 months. When conservative measures are not successful in alleviating a patient's symptoms, more aggressive interventions are appropriate. These may include arthroscopic débridement (Figure 14-33) and **lavage** for intraarticular pathology, such as meniscal tears, loose bodies, and articular cartilage flaps.

Simply lavaging the joint and removing degenerative particles may also have a temporary benefit.

Other more aggressive procedures, such as osteotomy to correct joint alignment (Figure 14-34) or arthroplasty to replace or resurface the joint (Figure 14-35), may provide a better chance of long-term relief from symptoms. More recently a less invasive procedure that involves placing a small metal disk in the affected joint space of the knee has shown some promise in younger patients or patients with OA isolated to one side of the joint (Figure 14-36).

Prognosis and Return to Participation

As with all the degenerative arthropathies, the long-term prognosis for OA is not good. However, most patients do very well with some combination of therapies and are able to lead a healthy and active, if somewhat restricted, lifestyle. Specific restrictions are based on a patient's pain and progression of the disease.

Osteomyelitis

Osteomyelitis is an infection caused by a bacterium or fungus that affects the bone. Osteomyelitis can occur in any age group but is most commonly seen in young children, older adults, and individuals with underlying disease that leaves them immunocompromised.

When a bone becomes infected, the marrow may swell and press against cortical bone, causing the blood vessels in the marrow to be compromised, therefore cutting off the blood supply to the bone. Bone requires this blood supply to survive and will break down without it. The infection may also break through the cortical bone, forming abscesses in surrounding muscle or other soft tissues.

Osteomyelitis is typically caused by one of several routes: hematogenous that carries the infection through the blood stream; direct invasion from a penetrating trauma or retained metal implants; or infections in adjacent bone or soft tissues, such as soft tissue ulcerations.[32]

Signs and Symptoms

Osteomyelitis can present in many ways, but typically an individual has pain in the infected bone and may experience fevers. The area around the infection may be painful to touch, erythematous, edematous, warm, and painful with movement. General signs of infection, such as malaise and fatigue, are common.

Chronic osteomyelitis may develop if the initial bone infection is not treated adequately. This persistent infection can be very difficult to eliminate. It may be dormant for extended periods or, more commonly, cause recurrent infections in the soft tissue surrounding the bone with recurrent drainage of **purulent** fluid through a sinus tract in the skin.

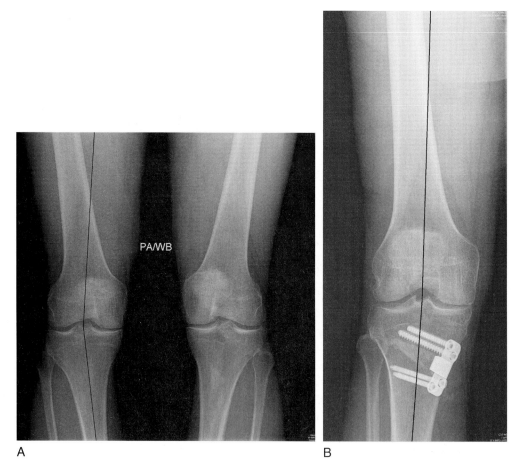

A

B

Figure 14-34 Radiographs show **(A)** malalignment of the femur and tibia and **(B)** "opening-wedge" osteotomy to correct the malalignment.

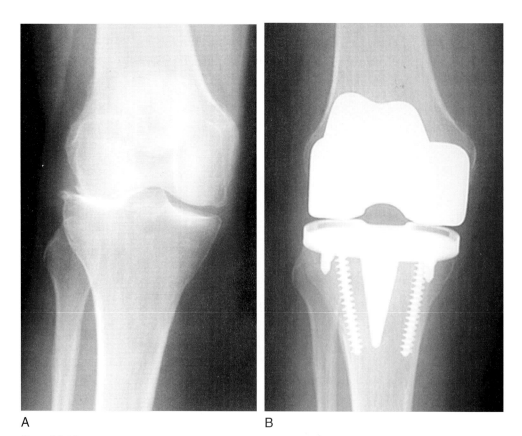

A

B

Figure 14-35 Radiographs show, **A,** an osteoarthritic knee and, **B,** following total knee replacement (arthroplasty). (Courtesy Zimmer, Inc.)

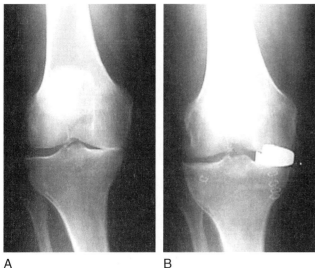

A   B

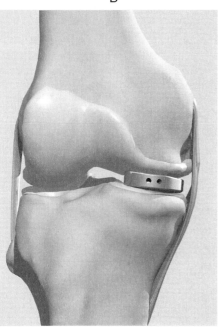

C

Figure 14-36 Surgical technique to correct alignment and unload osteoarthritic medial compartment using a small metal disk placed in the knee. A, Radiograph before procedure. B, Radiograph after procedure. C, A schematic representation of the procedure. (Courtesy Zimmer, Inc.)

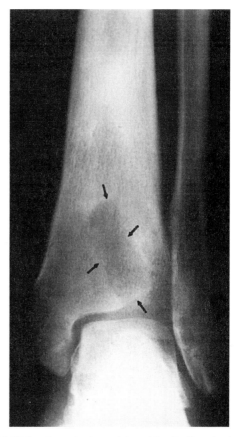

Figure 14-37 A radiograph of an epiphyseal localization of osteomyelitis in an adult ankle. (From Resnick D: *Diagnosis of bone and joint disorders*, ed 4, Philadelphia, 2002, WB Saunders, p 2389.)

An aspiration of the affected area is usually required to confirm the diagnosis. This is typically done in the operating room with preparations made for possibly surgically opening the area for thorough cleaning and débridement.[3,32]

Differential Diagnosis
Other orthopedic conditions, such as gout and stress fracture, need to be ruled out. Systemic conditions also must be considered, such as reactive bone marrow edema, cellulitis, or tumor.

Treatment
Appropriate antibiotic therapy based on the organism suspected is the basis for treatment. *Staphylococcus aureus* is the most commonly seen organism, but others may include mycobacteria, fungal infections, and even viruses. Empirical treatment is often initiated before a specific organism is identified. Intravenous antibiotics are usually begun and subsequently switched to oral medications after a period of time depending on the organism, the patient's response to antibiotics, and the patient's overall health. Antibiotics are typically continued for 4 to 8 weeks, although in some cases they may be continued for several months (see Chapter 3).

Diagnostic Tests
Blood tests usually reveal an elevated level of white blood cells (WBCs), erythrocyte sedimentation rate (ESR or sed rate), and C-reactive protein (CRP). WBCs are elevated as a response to infection, whereas ESR and CRP are elevated as a response to inflammation. Radiographs may not register any bone changes until the infection has progressed for several weeks (Figure 14-37). Bone scans, MRI, and CT scans are sensitive in detecting early osteomyelitis but limited in the specificity of the abnormality.

Prognosis and Return to Participation

If osteomyelitis is detected early and treated appropriately, the prognosis is usually very good. When chronic osteomyelitis occurs, treatment may have to be cycled intermittently for several years.

Prevention

Individuals with artificial joints or metal attached to bone in their body should use prophylactic antibiotics before any type of dental work and most surgeries because these procedures have the potential to release bacteria into the blood stream.

Inflammatory Myopathies

The inflammatory myopathies are a group of diseases characterized by inflammation of muscle and other connective tissues (i.e., skin). Inflammatory myopathies may occur as a result of bacterial, fungal, or parasitic infections; toxic exposures; or other known causes of muscle damage, such as myositis ossificans. The most common inflammatory myopathies are polymyositis and dermatomyositis.[2,4,27,30]

Polymyositis/Dermatomyositis

Signs and Symptoms

Polymyositis may present acutely or over the course of weeks to months. It is characterized by the insidious onset of proximal muscle weakness in which individuals notice the inability to rise from a chair, climb stairs, and reach overhead. It later may involve distal or pharyngeal muscles. Polymyositis is usually painless, but those affected often describe fatigue, general soreness, and cramping.

Dermatomyositis is similar to polymyositis, with insidious onset of muscle weakness, often accompanied by other systemic symptoms, including fever, malaise, arthralgias, stomach ulcerations, and cutaneous lesions that result from inflammatory changes in the skin. Additional signs and symptoms of dermatomyositis are the characteristic scaling of the skin on the face and dorsal IP joints.[33] Gottron's papules, which are erythematous plaques usually seen over extensor surfaces of the MCP joints (Figure 14-38), and the **heliotrope rash,** a purplish discoloration around the upper eyelids (Figure 14-39), are pathognomonic for the disease. Other cutaneous manifestations may include scaly rashes on other areas of the body, cuticle overgrowth, drying and cracking of the palmar surfaces of the fingers, and erythema in the V of the neck.[30]

Referral and Diagnostic Tests

Screening for creatine kinase (CK), aspartate aminotransferase (AST), alanine aminotransferase (ALT),

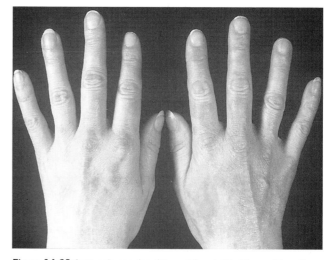

Figure 14-38 Gottron's papules. (From Klippel JH, Dieppe PA, editors: *Rheumatology,* ed 2, St Louis, 1998, Mosby, p 7.13.5.)

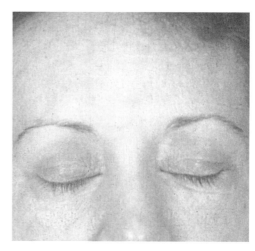

Figure 14-39 Heliotrope rash. (From Klippel JH, Dieppe PA, editors: *Rheumatology,* ed 2, St Louis, 1998, Mosby, p 7.13.5.)

lactate dehydrogenase (LD), and aldolase levels is useful to help define the severity of the disease.

Electromyography (EMG) analysis is helpful to distinguish myopathy from neuropathy and is usually abnormal with various motor unit potential changes and evidence of denervation or reinnervation in chronic cases.

Muscle biopsy is usually performed to confirm the diagnosis and rule out other potential causes of muscle inflammation. Radiographs are generally not helpful, but MRI and ultrasound may show signs of local muscle inflammation.[1,4,27,30]

Differential Diagnosis

Other conditions which may present in a similar fashion to polymyositis include Cushing's syndrome, fibromyalgia, thyroid disease, polymyalgia rheumatica, sarcoidosis, systemic lupus erythematosus, amyotrophic lateral sclerosis, infectious myositis, limb-girdle muscular dystrophy, and myasthenia gravis.

Treatment

Initial treatment includes rest until muscle inflammation subsides, with progression to passive range of motion, stretching, and flexibility exercises to prevent joint contractures. As the course of the disease subsides, a gradual increase to low impact exercise may be initiated.

Oral corticosteroids are helpful to decrease muscle inflammation. Immunosuppressive drugs are sometimes used in patients who do not respond to conventional treatments.

Prognosis and Return to Participation

Prognosis for polymyositis/dermatomyositis is extremely variable. Most patients have a good response to therapies and are able to return to moderate levels of activity, although some patients do not respond at all to therapies and are left with significant disability. Mortality is rare but may occur in patients with severe disease who develop progressive muscle weakness and eventually dysphagia, malnutrition, pneumonia, or respiratory failure.

Rhabdomyolysis

Rhabdomyolysis is a condition that ultimately leads to muscle necrosis and the release of muscle breakdown products into the blood stream, potentially leading to renal failure, cardiac arrest, and death. Rhabdomyolysis may occur as a result of genetic enzyme defects or a number of outside conditions. These outside conditions may include excessive exercise, muscle trauma, muscle ischemia, or prolonged immobilization. Other conditions include toxin exposure, acute alcohol intoxication, infection, inflammatory myopathies, and other metabolic or blood disorders.

Exertion, heat stroke, and sickle cell anemia, when exacerbated by dehydration, are the most common causes of rhabdomyolysis seen in athletes. Direct trauma or crush injuries may also lead to rhabdomyolysis in the athletic population.

The result of the acute trauma to muscle tissue or extreme eccentric loading of muscle tissue may lead to the release of extracellular calcium into muscle cells. This increased intracellular concentration of calcium activates several enzymes that induce the breakdown of muscle fibers. These breakdown products include myoglobin, potassium, and creatine kinase among others and are subsequently released into the extracellular fluid and circulatory system. An increased circulatory concentration of myoglobin is filtered by the kidneys and in sufficient quantities may lead to kidney damage. Locally, increased concentrations of these products may lead to microvascular damage,

capillary leak, increased compartment pressures, reduced tissue perfusion, and ischemia, which may in turn lead to further muscle damage.[34-36]

Signs and Symptoms

Presentation of an athlete with rhabdomyolysis can often be very subtle. Common complaints may include dark coca-cola–colored urine, muscle soreness, bruising, fatigue, fever, confusion, nausea, and vomiting. These complaints can be very mild or debilitating.

Referral and Diagnostic Tests

A high level of suspicion is needed to make a correct diagnosis. Early referral for evaluation is essential for appropriate treatment to prevent complications. Urinalysis will usually show the presence of myoglobin. A comprehensive metabolic profile (CMP) will reveal elevated levels of creatine phosphokinase (CPK), potassium, blood urea nitrogen (BUN), creatinine, uric acid, aldolase, lactate dehydrogenase (LDH), and decreased serum calcium. Electrocardiography (ECG) is performed to evaluate for cardiac arrhythmias resulting from hyperkalemia. Other diagnostic imaging tests are not really useful.[34-36]

Differential Diagnosis

Other conditions that may present in a similar manner to rhabdomyolysis include delayed-onset muscle soreness, compartment syndrome, viral infection, sickle cell crisis, heat exhaustion, heat stroke, and drug overdose.

Treatment

Intravenous hydration is begun as soon as the diagnosis of rhabdomyolysis is suspected. Dialysis is used in severe cases and when renal damage is suspected.[36] Left untreated, rhabdomyolosis may result in death.

Prognosis and Return to Participation

If rhabdomyolysis is diagnosed early and treated appropriately a full recovery is expected; however, in rare cases, or when a diagnosis is delayed, serious complications may arise. The most serious complication arising from rhabdomyolysis is acute renal failure (ARF). ARF may occur in as many as 30% of cases.[34] Other complications include disseminated intravascular coagulation (a disorder of the clotting cascade as a result of the muscle breakdown products), hypovolemia, cardiac arrhythmias, and cardiac arrest caused by hyperkalemia.

Prevention

Prevention ideally involves the elimination of precipitating factors, such as drug interactions, and recognizing underlying metabolic abnormalities. Special attention needs to be given to the hydration levels of athletes with sickle cell anemia and those most susceptible to heat illness.

Focal Conditions

Tendinopathy: Tendinitis, Tendinosis, and Peritendinitis

Tendinitis is defined as inflammation of a tendon, whereas tendinosis is defined as chronic degeneration of a tendon or inflammation of a tendon sheath. Tendinopathy is a more general term that refers to tendinitis, tendinosis, and peritendinitis. Most cases of tendinopathy caused by overuse that are encountered in athletics are tendinosis and not tendinitis. Several studies have shown that tendinosis, not inflammatory tendinitis, is the predominant pathological feature in painful overuse conditions seen at various body sites.[15,37,38]

Repeated overload of a tendon leads to collagen breakdown and eventually degeneration (Figure 14-40). This degeneration, if not relieved, eventually causes symptoms such as pain, weakness, and joint dysfunction. Repeated overload is usually due to increased demand, altered mechanics, or muscular imbalance. Treatment should be geared toward correction of the underlying abnormal stress.[39]

Signs and Symptoms

Complaints range from dull, chronic aching to more acute and sometimes debilitating pain. Weakness and pain are often associated with more acute symptoms. The affected tendon is usually tender to palpation, either diffusely or often only localized to a specific area of the tendon involved. Nodules within the tendon may be palpable, especially in chronic cases. If tenosynovitis is present, crepitus will usually be felt with motion of the tendon. Passive stretch of the tendon will often cause discomfort.

Referral and Diagnostic Tests

MRI and ultrasound are used primarily to rule out other conditions, such as tendon rupture, ganglion cyst, or deep vein thrombosis. MRI may reveal chronic degeneration and partial tearing of the tendon that often occurs in chronic cases. Radiographs may show calcifications in the tendon if present.

Differential Diagnosis

Other conditions mimicking tendinopathy include partial or complete tendon rupture, OA, ganglion cyst, cellulitis, muscle strain, delayed onset muscle soreness, and deep vein thrombosis.

Treatment

Treatment is based on the pathology; therefore many classic treatments are being phased out. First, the athletic trainer must determine any mechanical deficits that may be causing the tendon overload. This may involve equipment, such as shoes or racket; running surface; or mechanics, including throwing motion or gait. Attention is also paid to muscular imbalance, such as strength of internal versus external shoulder rotators or quads versus hamstrings.

Ice and other infrared therapies continue to have clinical relevance through their vasoconstrictive properties, even though inflammation is not the underlying pathology. Electrical and radiation therapies using galvanic stimulation or anodyne continue to have beneficial effects in clinical trials and have been shown to stimulate collagen synthesis in laboratory settings.

NSAIDs and corticosteroids have a controversial role because their primary benefit is antiinflammatory. Both probably provide some benefit as a result of

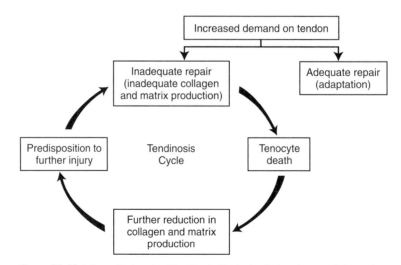

Figure 14-40 A theoretical cycle of tendinosis illustrates that an increased demand on the tendon leads to inadequate collagen and matrix production; this leads to tenocyte death, which further reduces the repair, and the process finally leads to a predisposition to further injury. (From Leadbetter WB: Cell-matrix response in tendon injury, *Clin Sports Med* 11[3]:533-578, 1992.)

their analgesic qualities; however, other benefits are questionable.[37,39,40]

Prognosis and Return to Participation

Acute cases tend to respond well to aggressive treatment as long as the underlying issues are addressed. Chronic cases are much more difficult to cure.

Prevention

Prevention is based on minimizing the overload process. Proper mechanics, techniques, muscular strength, and flexibility have all been shown to prevent the onset of chronic tendinopathy from overuse. Emphasizing eccentric strengthening and a progressive increase in activities will lead to lower instances of tendon irritation.

Bursitis

Bursitis is an acute or chronic inflammation of a bursa. Bursae are fluid-filled, saclike structures lined with synovial cells that are located around the body in areas where friction may develop between a bony prominence and overlying muscles or tendons.

Bursae allow normal movement and help minimize friction between moving parts, which may or may not communicate with the adjacent joint space. There are more than 150 bursae around the body, and inflammation can occur at any location but is commonly seen in the subacromial bursa, olecranon (student or executive elbow), prepatellar (housemaid or carpet layer knee), retrocalcaneal or Achilles, and greater trochanteric bursa.

Bursitis is most commonly caused by chronic overuse but may also be caused by direct trauma, infection, or inflammatory arthritis such as gout. When inflamed, the synovial cells that line the bursa increase in thickness and number and increase their secretion of fibrin-rich synovial fluid. Hemorrhage often occurs in acute bursitis. In chronic cases, the synovial cells may be replaced by granulation tissue as a prelude to eventual fibrous tissue formation.[41,42]

Signs and Symptoms

Symptoms of bursitis may include localized inflammation, tenderness, warmth, erythema, and edema (Figure 14-41). In acute bursitis the individual usually experiences pain and localized tenderness. Occasionally limited motion is also seen. Swelling, erythema, and warmth are common if the bursa is superficial (i.e., olecranon). Signs that may indicate an infectious etiology include fever, increased warmth, tenderness, and cellulitis.

Chronic bursitis may develop following recurrent episodes of acute bursitis or as a result of overuse. Symptoms may be intermittent or prolonged

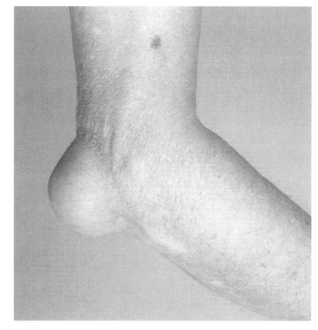

Figure 14-41 Symptoms of bursitis may include inflammation, localized tenderness, warmth, erythema, and edema as seen in this olecranon bursitis. (From Jarvis C: *Physical examination & health assessment*, ed 4, Philadelphia, 2004, WB Saunders, p 650.)

over several days to several weeks and often tend to wax and wane, but they may gradually worsen if treatment or activity modifications are not made. Eventually decreased range of motion and muscle atrophy may occur.

Referral and Diagnostic Tests

Radiographs are helpful in ruling out acute trauma causing swelling but are usually not helpful in making a diagnosis. In chronic bursitis, especially associated with gout, calcifications in the bursa may be seen. The athlete is referred to a physician for aspiration of the synovial fluid if infection or gout is suspected. Aspiration is also useful in decreasing symptoms in recalcitrant cases.

Differential Diagnosis

Differential diagnoses include other inflammatory processes such as RA, tendinitis, cellulitis, acute trauma, or a septic joint.

Treatment

Treatment for bursitis consists of controlling the inflammation and modifying activities that may be contributing to overuse. This may include mechanical corrections in activities, equipment changes, or changes in exercise routines.

In cases of trauma-induced bursitis, such as olecra non bursitis, avoidance of further trauma and direct pressure (e.g., leaning on elbow) is of paramount importance.

Continued irritation of the bursa or trauma to it may lead to chronic fibrotic changes.

Inflammation can be controlled with cryotherapy, in which ice massage has shown clinical benefits for superficial cases; NSAIDs; and corticosteroids. An injection of a corticosteroid often will completely alleviate symptoms, and together with proper activity restrictions and modifications, an injection may allow a more rapid return to activity. Rarely, surgical excision of the chronically inflamed bursal tissue may be necessary.[41,42]

Prognosis and Return to Participation

Most cases of bursitis will respond well to conservative therapy, and athletes may be allowed to continue participation as symptoms allow. Protective padding may help prevent exacerbation of the condition.

Prevention

Prevention is based on recognizing inciting factors or biomechanical conditions that may be predisposing the athlete to aggravate the bursa. Avoidance of trauma to the bursa is important after the initial trauma has occurred.

WEB RESOURCES

Medline Plus
http://www.nlm.nih.gov/medlineplus/osteoarthritis.html
Sponsored by the National Library of Medicine; has extensive information from the National Institutes of Health and other trusted sources on more than 650 diseases and conditions

Arthritis Center
http://www.arthritis.org/
Provided mainly for patients but gives information on arthritic conditions as well as lupus; has several good links to other websites on arthritis

National Institute of Arthritis and Musculoskeletal Disease
http://www.niams.nih.gov/
Sponsored by the National Institutes of Health; provides information for the practitioner as well as the patient

American College of Rheumatology
http://www.rheumatology.org/
Provides information to the practitioner on more than 100 types of arthritis and related disabling disorders of the joints, muscles, and bones

American College of Foot and Ankle Surgeons
http://www.footphysicians.com/
Provides information on foot and ankle conditions, including some of the conditions discussed in this chapter, such as gout

American College of Orthopaedic Surgeons
http://orthoinfo.aaos.org/
A searchable website, including a special section on myositis as well as other musculoskeletal conditions, such as osteoarthritis and rheumatoid arthritis

American Myositis Association
http://www.myositis.org/
Devoted to myositis, including polymyositis and dermatomyositis

---

SUMMARY

The athletic trainer is well educated and skilled in the evaluation and recognition of orthopedic injuries associated with athletic trauma and overuse. This chapter provided an introduction to nontraumatic disorders of the musculoskeletal system that will also be encountered in practice.

Extreme muscle weakness may be a sign of inflammatory myopathies and should be evaluated further. In addition, the athletic trainer should be especially suspicious of symptoms normally associated with traumatic injuries that did not arise from traumatic events. These symptoms include unexpected muscular atrophy, insidious onset of swelling, or warm, red joints. Other suspect signs and symptoms include either oligoarticular or polyarticular symmetrical swelling in the joint(s) and loss of function or range of motion.

REFERENCES

1. Koopman WJ, Boulware DW, Heudebert GR: *Clinical primer of rheumatology*, Philadelphia, 2003, Lippincott Williams & Wilkins.
2. Koopman WJ: *Arthritis and allied health conditions*, ed 1, Philadelphia, 2001, Lippincott Williams & Wilkins.
3. Turek SL, Buckwalter JA: *Turek's orthopaedics: principles & their application*, ed 5, Philadelphia, 1994, Lippincott Williams & Wilkins.
4. Resnick D: *Diagnosis of bone and joint disorders*, ed 4, Philadelphia, 2002, WB Saunders.
5. Peck DM: Apophyseal injuries in the young athlete, *American Family Physician* 51(8):1891-1895, 1997.
6. Klingele KE, Kocher MS: Little league elbow: valgus overload injury in the paediatric athlete, *Sports Medicine* 32(15):1005-1015, 2002.
7. Carson WG, Gasser SI: Little leaguer's shoulder: a report of 23 cases, *American Journal of Sports Medicine* 26:575-580, 1998.
8. Gunn VL, Nechyba C, Barone MA, Johns Hopkins Children's Medical and Surgical Center: *The Harriet Lane handbook: a manual for pediatric house officers*, ed 16, Philadelphia, 2002, Mosby.
9. Woodward TW, Best TM: The painful shoulder. I. Clinical evaluation, *American Family Physician* 61:3079-3088, 2000.
10. Morisawa K, Umemura A, Kitamura T, et al: Apophysitis of the acromion, *Journal of Shoulder & Elbow Surgery* 5(2 Pt 1):153-156, 1996.
11. Adirim TA, Cheng TL: Overview of injuries in the young athlete, *Sports Medicine* 33(1):75-81, 2003.
12. Ove P, McDevitt E: Throwing injuries and other athletic injuries of the elbow. In Brown D, Neumann R, editors: *Orthopedic secrets*, ed 3, Philadelphia, 2004, Hanley & Belfus, pp 142-150.
13. Nicholas JA, Hershman ED, Posner MA: *The upper extremity in sports medicine*, ed 2, St Louis, 1995, Mosby.
14. Cain EL, Dugas JR, Wolf RS, Andrews JR: Elbow injuries in throwing athletes: a current concepts review, *American Journal of Sports Medicine* 31(4):621-635, 2003.

15. Schenck RC, editor: *Athletic training and sports medicine,* ed 3, Rosemont, Ill, 1999, American Academy of Orthopaedic Surgeons.

16. Bloom OJ, Mackler L, Barbee J: What is the best treatment for Osgood-Schlatter disease? *Journal of Family Practice* 53(2):153-156; discussion 156, 2004.

17. Calmbach WL, Hutchens M: Evaluation of patients presenting with knee pain. II. Differential diagnosis, *American Family Physician* 68(5):917-922, 2003.

18. Gigante A, Bevilacqua C, Bonetti MG, Greco F: Increased external tibial torsion in Osgood-Schlatter disease, *Acta Orthopaedica Scandinavica* 74(4):431-436, 2003.

19. Duri ZA, Patel DV, Aichroth PM: The immature athlete, *Clinics in Sports Medicine* 21(3):461-482, 2002.

20. Tyler W, McCarthy EF: Osteochondrosis of the superior pole of the patella: two cases with histologic correlation, *Iowa Orthopaedic Journal* 22:86-89, 2002.

21. Hirano A, Fukubayashi T, Ishii T, Ochiai N: Magnetic resonance imaging of Osgood-Schlatter disease: the course of the disease, *Skeletal Radiology* 31(6):334-342, 2002.

22. Orava S, Malinen L, Karpakka J, et al: Results of surgical treatment of unresolved Osgood-Schlatter lesion, *Annales Chirurgiae et Gynaecologiae* 89(4):298-302, 2000.

23. Duri ZA, Aichroth PM, Wilkins R, Jones J: Patellar tendonitis and anterior knee pain, *American Journal of Knee Surgery* 12(2):99-108, 1999.

24. Manusov EG, Lillegard WA, Raspa RF, Epperly TD: Evaluation of pediatric foot problems. II. The hindfoot and the ankle, *American Family Physician* 54(3):1012-1026, 1996.

25. Wenger DR, Frick SL: Scheuermann kyphosis, *Spine* 24(24):2630-2639, 1999.

26. Lowe TG: Scheuermann disease, *Journal of Bone and Joint Surgery America* 72(6):940-945, 1990.

27. Ruddy S, Harris ED, Sledge CB: *Kelly's textbook of rheumatology,* ed 6, Philadelphia, 2001, WB Saunders.

28. Schumacher HR: Crystal-induced arthritis: an overview, *American Journal of Medicine* 100(2A):46S-52S, 1996.

29. O'Dell JR: Therapeutic strategies for rheumatoid arthritis, *New England Journal of Medicine* 350(25):2591-2602, 2004.

30. Klippel JH, Dieppe PA, editors: *Rheumatology,* ed 2, St Louis, 1998, Mosby.

31. McAlindon TE, Formica MK, Fletcher J, Schmid C: Barometric pressure and ambient temperature influence osteoarthritis (OA) pain. Results of a national web-based prospective study, Presentation no. 596, American College of Rheumatology, Scientific Meeting, Monday, October 18, 2004, San Antonio, TX.

32. Lew DP, Waldvogel FA: Osteomyelitis, *Lancet* 364(9431):369-379, 2004.

33. Habif T: *Clinical dermatology: a color guide to diagnosis and therapy,* ed 4, St Louis, 2004, Mosby.

34. Knochel JP: Mechanisms of rhabdomyolysis, *Current Opinion in Rheumatology* 5:725-731, 1993.

35. Poels PJ, Gabreels FJ: Rhabdomyolysis: a review of the literature, *Clinical Neurology and Neurosurgery* 95:175-192, 1993.

36. Sauret JM, Marinides G, Wang GK: Rhabdomyolysis, *American Family Physician* 65(5):907-912, 2002.

37. Khan KM, Cook JL, Bonar F, et al: Histopathology of common tendonopathies: update and implications for clinical management, *Sports Medicine* 27(6):393-408, 1999.

38. Arndt EA, editor: *Orthopaedic knowledge update. Sports medicine 2.* Rosemont, Ill, 1999, American Academy of Orthopaedic Surgeons.

39. Khan KM, Cook JL, Taunton JE, Bonar F: Overuse tendinosis, not tendinitis. I. A new paradigm for a difficult clinical problem, *Physician and Sportsmedicine* 28(5):38-48, 2000.

40. Mafulli N, Khan KM, Puddu G: Overuse tendon conditions: time to change a confusing terminology, *Arthroscopy* 14(8):840-843, 1998.

41. Butcher JD, Salzman KL, Lillegard WA: Lower extremity bursitis, *American Family Physician* 53(7):2317-2324, 1996.

42. Salzman KL, Lillegard WA, Butcher JD: Upper extremity bursitis, *American Family Physician* 56(7):1797-1806, 1997.

CHAPTER
15

Mental Health Conditions in the Athlete

Layne Prest

OBJECTIVES

At the completion of this chapter, the reader should be able to do the following:

1. Recognize emotional and behavioral signs of common mental health issues, including mood, anxiety, eating, attention deficit hyperactivity, and substance use disorders.
2. Intervene appropriately with the affected athlete through discussion, supportive confrontation, education, and referral.
3. Be aware of and establish collaborative relationships with qualified physical and mental health professionals in the recognition and treatment process.
4. Identify a variety of educational and supportive resources (printed material, web based, organizational) that are available to both professionals, and patients affected by these disorders.

INTRODUCTION

The twenty-first century is supposed to be the era of healthier people; and, of course, athletes are by definition among the healthiest. Therein lies the main dilemma when assessing and intervening in potential mental health concerns of athletes. Many people, perhaps athletes more than average people, have been conditioned to minimize or even deny physical health problems, and they are even more inclined to do so with mental health issues. Being sick or disabled physically is one thing; being crazy or weak mentally or emotionally is quite another! Professionals working with athletes are increasingly likely to have been educated about mental health issues, however, or know of someone in their personal or professional circle who has struggled with emotional or behavioral problems in the past. It is hoped that more exposure will erase stereotypes and increase the likelihood of early detection and appropriate intervention. This chapter is designed to educate the athletic trainer about the signs, symptoms, and prognosis of the most common mental health disorders. It is not intended that the athletic trainer actually counsel the athlete as this is beyond the scope of practice but rather that the athletic trainer know the appropriate situations to refer the athlete. Toward that end, this chapter outlines the mental health problems most commonly experienced by athletes, suggests red flags for earlier detection, and describes strategies for intervention.

The World Health Organization (WHO) identifies mental and behavioral health conditions as four of the ten leading causes of disability worldwide and as affecting 25% of all people at some time in their lives.[1] These four causes of disability are depression, anxiety disorders, suicide, and alcohol use. Other serious disorders include schizophrenia, bipolar disorder, dementia, obsessive-compulsive disorder, posttraumatic stress disorder, and panic disorder. Problems with attention and concentration, disordered eating, personality issues, and other forms of substance abuse also contribute greatly to the disease burden throughout the world.[2] Some of these difficulties, chiefly depression, anxiety, and substance abuse problems, are ubiquitous in American society. The others, including attention deficit hyperactivity disorder (ADHD), personality disorders, and disordered eating, are not as common. All can impair athletic performance and overall life adjustment. These conditions also can be difficult to treat, especially if allowed to escalate out of control. Therefore athletic trainers working with physically active people must be able to identify these potentially serious problems as early as possible.

Following a description of typical physical and emotional symptoms, diagnostic criteria, and potential red flags, suggestions are made for initial intervention, referral, and treatment recommendations. The diagnostic criteria are taken from the *Diagnostic and Statistical Manual of Mental Disorders,* 4th edition (DSM-IV).[3]

UNDERSTANDING THE ROLE OF MENTAL HEALTH PROFESSIONALS

At the outset, a full and comprehensive treatment plan needs to be developed in the context of the athlete's relationship with a trusted licensed professional operating within the scope of professional practice. The athletic trainer who may be among the first to detect a problem can be instrumental in getting the athlete needed help. Athletic trainers need to be familiar with the various mental health professionals to whom they may refer an athlete for professional services. A reasonable professional to start with is the athlete's primary care physician.

The U.S. federal government has designated five disciplines with competency to provide mental health services to the population: psychiatry, psychology, marriage and family therapy, social work, and psychiatric nursing (Table 15-1). Other professionals who provide mental health services include professional counselors and clergy members. Licensure and certification for most of these professionals are becoming standardized within each discipline, and the boundaries are better delineated among disciplines. A fair amount of overlap remains, however, and providers in any of these categories can potentially help with any of the clinical problems this chapter addresses. Referrals may be guided somewhat by the discipline of the professional but more importantly by the person's clinical specialty.

The training of psychiatrists and psychiatric nurse practitioners enables them to assess the patient from a medical point of view and prescribe medicine to address the underlying physiological or chemical components of the problem. They may also provide

supportive counseling, psychoeducation, or assistance in problem solving. If a major mental disorder is suspected and medical intervention is needed, a referral to one of these professionals would be appropriate.

The various types of psychologists—clinical, educational, counseling—have different but overlapping training, experience, and areas of expertise. They can be trained at either the master's or doctoral level. Typically psychologists are the professionals to contact if psychological or educational testing is needed. Psychologists also provide counseling services.

Marriage and family therapy, especially medical family therapists, views problems from the biopsychosocial point of view. Consequently their clinical approach considers various aspects of the person's life. Marriage and family therapists work with typical mental health issues, such as depression, anxiety, eating disorders, ADHD, but will often do so by including part or all of the family and in collaboration with a primary care provider.

Social workers usually specialize in addressing macro issues, such as housing, income, or food deficiencies and insurance needs, or micro issues, such as psychotherapy. Social work as a discipline also uses a holistic perspective of the client. A number of social workers also provide counseling services similar to other mental health providers.

Mental health professionals (MHPs) increasingly are being called on to demonstrate the effectiveness of their work with clients. As a result, more attention is being focused on the development of evidence-based protocols. Therapy typically begins with an intake session during which the professional gathers background information (e.g., family of origin details), a description of the problem and previous attempts to address it, and the client's goals. A contract governing frequency and duration of sessions is negotiated, and parameters of confidentiality are discussed. MHPs will obtain a signed consent for release of information, allowing them to contact other professionals including the athletic trainer or family members working with the client.

OVERVIEW OF MENTAL HEALTH ISSUES IN THE ATHLETE

Everyone has symptoms of some type of mental health issue at some time in life when one or several stressors overwhelm the body's ability to self-regulate or repair. The symptoms are usually, and arbitrarily, divided into the physical and mental categories. However, this artificial dichotomy does not match the affected person's reality. In other words, rarely is an athlete with a strained hamstring not also worried about the injury or distressed by the pain. Similarly, the most common initial warning signs of emotional or mental

Table 15-1	Disciplines Providing Mental Health Services
Discipline	**Approach**
Psychiatry	Medical approach, including medication
Psychology	Psychological testing and counseling
Marriage and family therapy	Biopsychosocial assessment and therapy
Social work	Holistic approach; social services and programs
Psychiatric nursing	Medical approach, including medication

depression are the physical symptoms of sleep, energy, and appetite disturbance. This is because humans are made up of overlapping systems of mind, body, spirit, and relationships, each integrally connected to the others. When the homeostasis of one or more systems is disrupted, people instinctively attempt to correct the problem regardless of physiological, mental, or behavioral origin. In the mental health domain, signs of distress manifesting this state of disequilibrium are emotional, mental, behavioral, and physical.

Framework for Understanding Mental Health

In virtually all situations, a variety of overlapping factors are at play and contribute to symptom development. The **biopsychosocial-spiritual model (BPSS)** is a framework for understanding the individual's responses in a given situation and development of symptoms. Symptom etiology may be conceptualized in terms of a pie metaphor (Figure 15-1). Figure 15-1 shows how these various factors overlap and contribute to overall well-being. In a given individual, the various pieces of the BPSS pie may be larger or smaller at any one time. The relative sizes of the pieces greatly influence the individual's overall adaptation and symptom development.

For example, two runners may have identical injuries, but the impact of the injury and the course of rehabilitation in these two athletes will usually differ. The amount of pain they have, as well as the length of time until they are ready to compete again, will be influenced not only by the difference in their respective levels of physical conditioning and injury history but also by other physical and emotional conditions they may be experiencing, such as pain tolerance, attitude, perception of the problem, and its implications for their lives. The situation may also be impacted by personality and temperament issues, variable resources

for coping, and so on. Another example involves two wrestlers who seem to be equally competitive, but wrestler A, in a struggle to make or maintain weight, develops more obviously disordered eating patterns than wrestler B. Perhaps wrestler A has a family history of obesity and is genetically predisposed toward weight gain more than the other; and temperamentally, wrestler A may tend to think more negatively about life challenges, become somewhat self-defeating in the face of adversity, and find emotional comfort in food and the process of eating. Often a variety of factors will help to explain the development of clinically significant problems.

This interplay of variables is the same for athletes as it is for others who are physically active regardless of whether the symptoms of an injury or condition are physical or emotional. Whereas one athlete may become depressed, another's symptoms may include anxiety or outbursts of anger and physical aggression. Sometimes one piece of the BPSS pie is so big that it seems to account for virtually the whole reason that someone is symptomatic (e.g., the chemical disequilibrium that comes with bipolar disorder). For this reason, it is a good practice to regularly consider the possibility that an organic cause may be the culprit and refer the person for a medical evaluation.

The treatment approaches that have been found to be effective for the problems discussed in this chapter are based on the same BPSS approach as in assessment and diagnosis. Different strategies are useful, depending on the biopsychosocial-spiritual components that are implicated in the assessment process. Treatment plans are often recommended by the practitioner on the basis of assessment and experience, and then negotiated with the individual or family members according to their preferences. The treatment may be offered on either an inpatient or, more commonly, outpatient basis.

Treatment may also involve the collaboration of a variety of treatment professionals. For example, eating

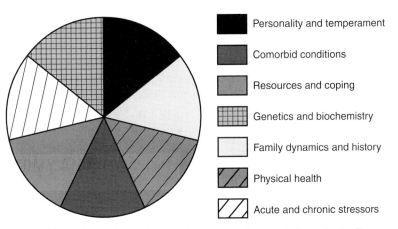

Figure 15-1 The biopsychosocial-spiritual model is a framework for understanding an individual's responses in a given situation and development of symptoms.

disorder treatment often involves a physician, registered dietitian, and psychotherapist. This determination is made on the basis of the severity of symptoms, the difficulty the athlete has in making changes, the amount of support the athlete has, and other resources that impact care, including financial concerns or insurance benefits. The important first step in treatment is accurate assessment followed by clear and well-timed communication and education with the person and family. The athletic trainer can play a valuable role here, since people are much more likely to engage in treatment or some type of change process if they become convinced that there is a problem, what it is, and that something can be done about it. This is because most people will want to know what is going on with themselves, how they "got it," and what they can do to "get rid of it" or at least cope more effectively. Additional treatment recommendations specific to various clinical problems are listed in subsequent sections.

Implications for Participation in Athletics

Early identification and treatment are very helpful in preventing problems from worsening, but sometimes the stigma still associated with mental health conditions prevents people from recognizing these problems in themselves or others. In that case, functioning in one or more areas of life can be affected, sometimes severely. Whether restricting an athlete's participation in a sport is necessary will depend on the athlete, coach, and athletic trainer's assessment of the individual's level of functioning. The treatment plan, even when it includes appropriate medication, should not affect the athlete's ability to participate. Initially, while the medication dose is being adjusted, the athlete could experience problematic adverse effects, such as nausea, headache, sedation, balance, or stimulation that could affect participation or performance. The National Collegiate Athletic Association (NCAA) has no restrictions on the medications typically used to treat these conditions except for pemoline, a medication prescribed to treat ADHD.[4]

The last general point to be made is that some people experiencing the problems described in this chapter may consider suicide or become homicidal. Most health care or other professionals are required by state law and/or their professional code of ethics to report to the authorities if someone with whom they are working is a danger to self or others. Athletic trainers, too, may encounter an individual with depression, panic disorder, or substance abuse who is considering suicide or harming someone else. The athletic trainer must seek immediate consultation if in doubt about the need for such a report. An assessment of suicidality or homicidality includes a determination that the person has a specific plan, the means to carry it out, the intention to carry it out, and a measure of how lethal the plan is. Those who have a personal or family history of this type of ideation or action, or whose judgment is impaired, perhaps through the use of substance abuse, are more at risk to follow through.

ANXIETY DISORDERS

Anxiety is one of the most common human experiences. For example, most people have experienced a momentary sensation of "butterflies" in the stomach. In fact, the ability to respond with anxiety is considered normal and even desirable; and anxiety is what helps us "get our game face on" (Figure 15-2). However, given the right set of factors—physiology, central nervous system sensitivity, perceptual filters,

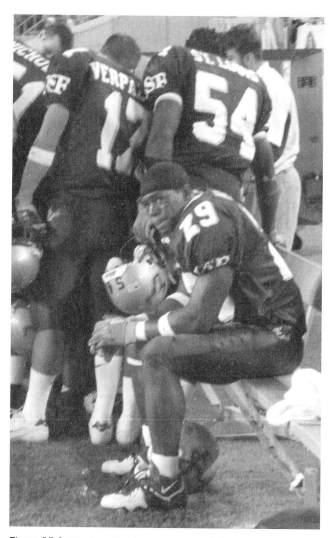

Figure 15-2 Athletes often become anxious during competitive events and may be able to use that anxiety to good advantage.

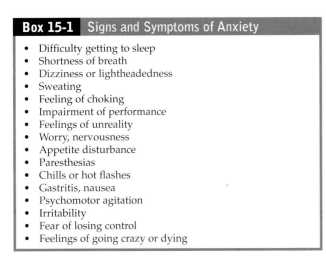

Box 15-1   Signs and Symptoms of Anxiety

- Difficulty getting to sleep
- Shortness of breath
- Dizziness or lightheadedness
- Sweating
- Feeling of choking
- Impairment of performance
- Feelings of unreality
- Worry, nervousness
- Appetite disturbance
- Paresthesias
- Chills or hot flashes
- Gastritis, nausea
- Psychomotor agitation
- Irritability
- Fear of losing control
- Feelings of going crazy or dying

Box 15-2   Criteria for Diagnosing Generalized Anxiety Disorder

- Excessive daily anxiety or worry for 6 months
- Difficulty controlling the worry
- Three or more anxiety symptoms
- Impairment in social, academic or occupational, or relational functioning because of the anxiety

belief system, coping and support system—people may respond to one or more acute or chronic stressors by developing anxiety serious enough to be considered a disorder. This is a case of too much of a good or necessary thing. The individual is wracked with very serious and debilitating apprehension, excessive and ongoing worry, overwhelming fears, or compulsive behaviors. Some 19.1 million Americans (13.3% of the population) experience one of the more debilitating forms of anxiety and have been diagnosed with an anxiety disorder.[5]

Red flags for problems with anxiety include outbursts of irritability or anger, substance abuse, changes in athletic performance, or other behaviors that are uncharacteristic for the athlete. Anxiety symptoms include both somatic-behavioral and emotional-cognitive disturbances.[6] The presence of some or all of these symptoms may signal an anxiety problem or even an anxiety disorder (Box 15-1). People can be screened for anxiety disorders using a variety of standardized measures, such as the **Hamilton Anxiety Scale (HAMA).**

Generalized Anxiety Disorder

Generalized anxiety disorder (GAD) is a condition in which the individual is worried or nervous about many or most things in life. The person may complain on a regular basis of one or more of the anxiety symptoms listed previously. Box 15-2 summarizes criteria for diagnosing generalized anxiety. It has been estimated that 4 million people, or 2.8% of the American population, have this disorder. Women are twice as likely as men to report generalized anxiety.[5] Consistent with the BPSS model described previously, the causes of GAD and other anxiety problems are varied. Fortunately, a number of effective treatment approaches and self-help measures are available.[7]

Panic Attacks

Among the 2.4 million people (1.7% of the population) who experience panic attacks, some say that these episodes seem to come out of nowhere when in fact they are probably in response to an accumulation of stressors. At other times the attacks may be stimulated by an identifiable, acutely stressful event.[5] Symptoms that seem cardiovascular in nature are particularly striking during these episodes, for example, chest pain or shortness of breath. The attacks can be so overwhelming and produce such fear and intense anxiety that the affected person may begin avoiding stressful situations and other stimuli perceived as being triggers.[8] As a result, the panic attacks may become **panic disorder** that can be accompanied by agoraphobia or avoiding going out into open spaces or public places. Panic disorder can be so severe and distressing that someone affected might consider suicide as the only way out; in fact, up to 20% of those affected consider this step. Women experience panic attacks at twice the rate of men.

Posttraumatic Stress Reactions

Similar to the intense responses involved in panic attacks are varying degrees of posttraumatic stress reactions **(posttraumatic stress disorder [PTSD])** experienced by approximately 5.2 million Americans.[5] These reactions are in response to exposure to life-threatening events or other situations outside the normal range of human experience (e.g., war, serious physical or sexual assault, motor vehicle accident). People are so overwhelmed by the event or series of events that they will go to great lengths to avoid similar situations, as well as the feelings associated with the original experience because their responses involved intense fear, helplessness, or horror.

Fairly often people will replay or reexperience the traumatic event in the form of recurrent or intrusive and distressing recollections, images, thoughts, perceptions, recurrent dreams, illusions, or hallucinations. They often experience great physiological reactivity and therefore engage in persistent avoidance of stimuli and numbing of general responsiveness. This involves avoiding associated thoughts, feelings, conversations, activities, places, and people. At times this process of compartmentalization can be so severe as to lead to an inability to recall important aspects of the event, marked **anhedonia,** detachment or estrangement, restricted range of affect, and a sense of a foreshortened future.

Obsessive-Compulsive Disorder

Approximately 11.5 million individuals, or 8% of the U.S. population, display characteristics of anxiety in a more circumscribed manner by developing phobias to specific triggers or fears about specific issues. These include abnormal anxiety regarding being in social situations, public speaking, fear of flying, or preoccupations with germs or disease.[5] These manifestations of anxiety can be less incapacitating if the person is successfully able to avoid the stimuli without compromising life and activities, but otherwise they can be quite disruptive. Attention to detail and the ability to be thorough in a task can be very valuable attributes; taken or driven to the extreme by anxiety, they can be debilitating. **Obsessive-compulsive disorder (OCD)** is a condition in which the person becomes fixated on one or more issues (i.e., obsessions) that cause anxiety. OCD affects approximately 3.3 million people in the United States and is equally common among men and women. The basis for OCD consists of persistent thoughts, impulses, or images about exaggerated or imaginary circumstances. The thoughts the person has are experienced as intrusive or inappropriate to the situation. Compulsive or repetitive behaviors are paired with the obsessions, with the goal of eliminating, reducing, or ignoring the resultant anxiety. As with the obsessions, the person frequently recognizes that the compulsive behaviors are, to some degree, excessive or unreasonable, especially if they impede the person's performance, routine, or social activities. The most common obsessive thoughts are those concerning contamination, doubts, loss of order, horrible trauma, and sexuality. Table 15-2 summarizes common compulsive behaviors, and Box 15-3 lists diagnostic criteria for OCD.

Treatment of Anxiety Disorders

Treatment plans for anxiety disorders are often recommended by the practitioner on the basis of assessment and experience, and then negotiated with the individual or family members according to their preferences. The treatment plan for addressing anxiety can include one or all of a group of evidence-based interventions.

When there is a strong family history of anxiety problems, there is likely a biological or physiological

Table 15-2   Common Compulsive Thoughts and Behaviors Associated with Obsessive-Compulsive Disorder

Worrisome Thoughts	Compensatory Behaviors
Contamination or infection	Washing of hands Excessive cleaning
Doubts	Requesting or demanding assurance
Loss of order	Ritualized behaviors Certain order to getting dressed
Personal safety	Making sure doors are locked Checking to make sure appliances are turned off (e.g., stove and coffee maker)
Sexuality	Religious or psychological correction Self-flagellation Defense

Box 15-3   Diagnostic Criteria for Obsessive-Compulsive Disorder

- Obsessions or recurrent and persistent thoughts, impulses, or images that are not simply about life problems
- Attempts to suppress or neutralize such thoughts with other thoughts or actions while recognizing they are a product of the person's own mind
- Compulsive thoughts or actions engaged in according to rigid rules even though they may not be rationally connected to the intrusive thoughts

predisposition that can be ameliorated through psychopharmacological measures. One class of **psychotropic medications** often used includes those that act on the serotonin system. These include selective serotonin reuptake inhibitors such as fluoxetine (Prozac), paroxetine (Paxil), and escitalopram (Lexapro). When anxiety coexists with depression, medications that affect dopamine or norepinephrine, as well as serotonin, can be useful. These include venlafaxine (Effexor), and mirtazapine (Remeron). **Benzodiazepines** have been used for many years to treat anxiety and consequently are fairly well known. These medications include diazepam (Valium), lorazepam (Ativan), and alprazolam (Xanax).

The anti-anxiety drugs are prescribed according to their rate of onset, effects, and adverse effect profiles. Medication can be used from the outset or added after treatment begins. It is usually recommended that the person stay on the medication for 9 to 12 months or until symptoms are fully resolved. The medication dosage may need to be adjusted, or a different type or class of medication altogether may be needed. In the case of first or second episodes of anxiety, medication can be discontinued after the person has developed healthy, alternative coping strategies. If the anxiety recurs, then the individual may need to take the medication for the duration.

Other important steps to take to reduce anxiety on a physical level are getting regular exercise and regulating sleep. Exercise, particularly at aerobic levels, has been shown to significantly reduce levels of anxiety. This may be a moot point for those who are already physically active, but at times people will discontinue exercise if they are sufficiently distressed. For the injured athlete, the importance of maintaining aerobic conditioning during rehabilitation is equally important for mental as well as physical well-being. Most people should be encouraged to slowly reestablish healthy patterns of physical activity. Similarly, good sleep hygiene addresses the basic human need for restful sleep, which in turn supports well-being and stable functioning (Key Points—Good Sleep Hygiene).

> ## KEY POINTS
> ### Good Sleep Hygiene
>
> - Establish regular times for going to bed and awakening.
> - Minimize distractions and noises.
> - Avoid stimulating activity or substances before bedtime (e.g., exercise, caffeine).

In addition, self-defeating or negative patterns of thought or behavior can exacerbate anxiety. Consequently, cognitive-behavioral psychotherapy is used to help people recognize automatic thoughts and reflexive behaviors and replace them with more constructive and positive alternatives. On a related note, minimizing stress and distinguishing those things over which individuals have control versus no control are important steps in addressing anxiety problems. Stress management strategies include breathing exercises, progressive muscle relaxation, guided imagery, meditation, and prayer. Problem solving and conflict resolution skills can be learned. Developing social support systems is also helpful.

Generalized anxiety disorder (GAD), obsessive-compulsive disorder (OCD), and panic attacks are often treated through a combination of medication and support techniques. These include stress management, conflict resolution, problem solving, supportive relationships with others, exercise, and good sleep hygiene. In addition, psychotherapy emphasizing cognitive behavioral and interpersonal therapy is important. Acute or posttraumatic stress disorders often benefit from the addition of group therapy because this process helps to normalize the sense of unreality or disconnection that victims of trauma often experience. People with phobias do not usually respond to the use of medication; instead, a process of systematic desensitization helps to lessen or even eliminate their phobic responses.

MOOD DISORDERS

Transient feelings of sadness or depressed mood are normal in response to life's ups and downs. At the other end of the spectrum, however, depression can be so severe that people experience psychotic symptoms. Like anxiety, depression can manifest its effects in changes in physical, mental, emotional, relational, or spiritual well-being. Depression can be mild, moderate, or severe, and it can be situational or global. The incidence of depression is highest in middle age[1]; however, it can affect people at any time of life. Up to 2.5% of children, 8.3% of adolescents,[9] 5.8% of men, and 9.5% of women are affected within a 1-year period.[1] In addition, comorbidity between anxiety and mood disorders is high.[10] Some people become depressed in response to situational stressors (e.g., a change in playing status, a move, illness in a family member) (Figure 15-3) or developmental stressors (e.g., the transition from high school to college, birth of a baby in the family). Most often the experience of depression, with its multisystem symptoms, will come and go within a limited time (Key Points—Stressors That Sometimes Lead to Depression in Athletes).

> ## KEY POINTS
> ### Stressors That Sometimes Lead to Depression in Athletes
>
> **Situational Stressors**
> - Change in playing status, coaches, teams, partners
> - Death or serious illness in a family member
> - Relationship breakup
>
> **Developmental Stressors**
> - Major life transitions (e.g., move, change of schools)
> - Birth of a baby in the family

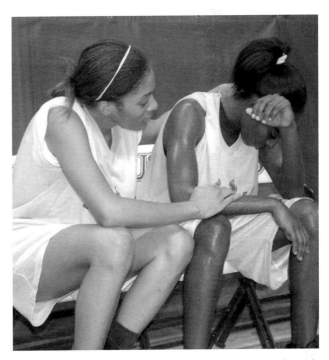

Figure 15-3 An athlete may become depressed in response to a change in playing status caused by either performance or injury.

Persistent symptoms, however, may be a sign of a more serious problem developing (Red Flags—Depression). For those people who develop more serious forms of depression and are not adequately treated, 35% will relapse within 2 years and 60% will relapse within 12 years.[1] As with the other conditions discussed in this chapter, the development, progression, and recovery or relapse of depression are affected by multiple factors, which again reflect the pieces of the BPSS pie.[11,12] In more serious forms of depression, the individual experiences depressed mood and also diminished interest in usual activities. Accordingly, red flags for depression include uncharacteristic outbursts of irritability or anger, diminished performance, substance abuse, social withdrawal or isolation, and other behaviors that are not the norm for the athlete.

> **Red Flags for Depression**
> - Depressed mood
> - Diminished interest in usual activities
> - Irritability or anger
> - Diminished performance
> - Substance abuse
> - Social withdrawal or isolation
> - Preoccupation with escape or death

Typical physical symptoms include both somatic-behavioral and emotional-cognitive disturbances. On an organic level, the athlete may experience changes in sleeping patterns, usually waking in the early hours of the morning and then being unable to return to a restful sleep or, alternatively, wanting to sleep all the time. Other symptoms include a loss of appetite with no interest in eating or eating more than usual; loss of energy or fatigue; and problems concentrating (Key Points—Depression in Daily Activities). A depressed

KEY POINTS
Depression in Daily Activities

The athlete with depression may exhibit changes in the following:
- Sleep patterns
- Appetite
- Energy
- Concentration

athlete is also very likely to complain of various somatic pains or irregularities, such as muscle aches, bowel problems, or headaches.[13] Emotionally, a depressed person is often sad, can become self-critical, and feels out of control of life, despairing, and hopeless, even to the point of being suicidal.

The minor form of a mood disorder is called an adjustment disorder. The DSM-IV guidelines, although somewhat arbitrary, suggest that an adjustment disorder is two to four symptoms with onset within 3 months

and resolution within 6 months of termination of the stressor.[3] If the symptoms are more severe in number or quality, an even more significant problem may have developed. This more serious form, major depressive episode, involves a greater number and more severe depressive symptoms for at least 2 weeks.[3] Box 15-4 summarizes the criteria for a major depressive episode. Mood disorders such as major depressive disorder can be assessed according to diagnostic criteria such as those listed previously; but the busy practitioner or athletic trainer who is not an expert in this area can use one or more screening instruments to measure the level of impairment. One example is the **Zung Self-Rating Depression Scale.**[14]

Even depressed people can have periods from days to weeks or even months during which they do not feel so bad and can rally to perform well. Some people have cyclical fluctuations in mood, energy, and appetite. Not surprisingly, one mood disorder variation is termed **cyclothymia.** In this case, the athlete may perform well in practice or competitions for several days or weeks but inexplicably hit a slump. Another form of fluctuating depression, **seasonal affective disorder (SAD),** is tied to exposure to changing amounts of sunlight. The prevailing theory is that sunlight, by way of the optic nerve, stimulates the brain to produce melatonin, a chemical related to serotonin. The hormone serotonin helps to regulate mood, appetite, activity level, and the wake-sleep cycle. When there is relatively less exposure to sunlight, less of this chemical is being produced, which in turn leads to depression.[5] These cycles are often tied to the changing of the seasons. Therefore the changes in mood, energy, and performance may take place over longer periods.

The most debilitating mood disorder, manic-depressive illness or **bipolar disorder,** is associated with significant fluctuations of symptoms. In this condition, people may experience periods of depression (i.e., hypodepression), mania (i.e., hypomania), or both. Mania and hypomania are on a continuum with a normal sense of well-being and the depression

Box 15-4   Criteria for a Major Depressive Episode

At least 2 weeks of the following:
- Lack of interest in usual activities
- Depressed mood

Plus four or more of the following:
- Appetite change along with weight gain or loss
- Insomnia or hypersomnia
- Psychomotor agitation or retardation
- Fatigue
- Worthlessness or guilt
- Difficulty concentrating or indecisiveness
- Recurrent thoughts of death or suicide

previously described. Mania is characterized by extremes of energy, euphoria, irritability, frustration, and rapid or grandiose thinking, speaking, and acting. In more moderated circumstances, people can be very productive and creative; but in extreme situations they can be driven to put themselves and others at risk because of impulsivity, poor judgment, and lack of focus and concentration. Mania is also characterized by and thrill seeking, such as risky sexual behavior, substance use, impulsive travel, or buying sprees.

Treatment of depression is actually fairly similar to treatment of anxiety problems because the biopsychosocial-spiritual issues underlying these disorders overlap to a great degree. As a result, the interventions that are evidenced based or have been used extensively on a clinical level are those mentioned previously: medication, psychotherapy, sleep hygiene, exercise, skill building, stress management, and social-spiritual support (Figure 15-4).

Research has shown that in cases of mild depression or adjustment disorders, medication is usually not necessary.[11,13] People tend to heal with time, reassurance, supportive relationships with others, exercise, good sleep hygiene, and sometimes a short course of psychotherapy, either cognitive-behavioral or interpersonal therapy. When the depression is more serious, research-based practice indicates that psychotherapy and medication can both be helpful.[13]

Whereas medication is more effective in the short term, therapy tends to be more helpful over longer periods. Severe depression requires aggressive treatment with both medication and psychotherapy. The other strategies are helpful additions to the treatment plan in both moderate and severe depression.

EATING DISORDERS

It is estimated that 5 million Americans are affected by eating disorders each year, but many more experience disordered eating.[15] Perhaps this is because members of modern American society have a love-hate relationship with food and their bodies. A wide and tempting variety of high-calorie foods with high fat and sugar content is increasingly cheaper and easily available. As a result, an increasing focus on fitness and healthy lifestyles is paired incongruously against record levels of obesity and related health problems, such as diabetes, coronary artery disease, and stroke.[16] Resulting disordered patterns of eating often have their onset in childhood and early adolescence,[17] a time when the individual is becoming increasingly aware of self and attuned to peer group messages regarding acceptability, attraction, and competence.

Even though athletes are usually more physically active and fit than the average person, the demands related to performance, such as maintaining a certain body weight or proportions, can exacerbate an individual's attitude toward and behaviors regarding food. Wrestlers, gymnasts, dancers, and swimmers are among the athletes stereotyped as people who are prone to developing problems with food and weight. One recent estimate is that up to one third of female athletes display disordered eating patterns.[18]

Like the other issues discussed in this chapter, disordered eating can be conceptualized according to a spectrum of severity. People with these problems do not often fit into clear-cut categories (Red Flags—Eating Disorders).

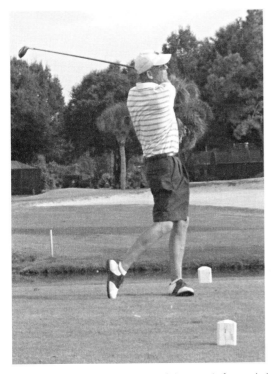

Figure 15-4 Exercise is both preventive and therapeutic for psychological health at all ages.

> ### 🏳 Red Flags for Eating Disorders
> - Frequent comments about feeling fat or overweight
> - Fluctuations or other changes in weight
> - Secretive, peculiar, or ritualized eating habits
> - Avoidance of social situations involving food
> - Mood changes
> - A history of weight problems
> - Excessive training regimen
> - Gastrointestinal problems
> - Dizziness
> - Dental or oral problems
> - Recall specificity about food portions
> - Wearing baggy clothing

- Refusal to maintain weight at a minimum of 85% of expected
- Intense fear of gaining weight or being fat
- Disturbance in perception of body weight or body image
- Absence of at least three consecutive menstrual cycles

Anorexia Nervosa

Anorexia nervosa is a potentially life-threatening condition with long-term mortality rates approaching 20%.[18] Anorexia develops when the person restricts or otherwise compensates for eating to the point that the person drops below 85% of ideal body weight (Box 15-5). An important point for athletic trainers to consider is that overtraining is a common compensatory behavior.

Anorexia is a relatively rare condition, with about 5 to 10 new cases per 100,000 persons each year and a prevalence of 0.5%.[19] The vast majority of cases of anorexia are found in females (Figure 15-5), but approximately 10% to 15% of cases occur in boys and men.[15] It is found more frequently in industrialized than nonindustrialized societies. The two subtypes of anorexics are the restricting type and the binge eating–purging type. Individual patients' behaviors may vary from time to time.

The possible physical sequelae include gastrointestinal problems (stomachache, diarrhea, constipation, heartburn), amenorrhea or other menstrual irregularities, dehydration, electrolyte imbalance, bradycardia, hypotension, decreased muscle mass and body fat, musculoskeletal injuries, lowered core body temperature, development of **lanugo** hair on the body, and fatigue and weakness.[18] Emotionally and mentally, people develop a distorted body image, emotional lability, cognitive rigidity, perfectionist attitudes, social isolation, an intense fear of becoming fat, and eventual impairment in mental functioning.[3]

Bulimia

Bulimia is another type of eating disorder that affects athletes and is more common than anorexia. Even though the individual is often at or slightly above normal weight, bulimia can also be life threatening. It is characterized by binge eating followed by an inappropriate compensatory mechanism designed to prevent weight gain and, perhaps more importantly, combat the person's sense of being out of control.[19] These compensatory mechanisms include restricting food (dieting or fasting), vomiting, laxative or diuretic use, and exercise. Binges stereotypically involve the secretive ingestion of large amounts of food in a short period of time. In reality, people may or may not be particularly secretive, and the amount of food constituting a binge is a matter of perception. People with bulimia who believe they have eaten too much may see even one too many cookies or slices of pizza as a binge. In response, they engage in one or more compensatory behaviors.

The repercussions for this pattern include fluid and electrolyte imbalance, gastrointestinal difficulties, inflammation of the esophagus and parotid glands, dental conditions, visual disturbances, muscle weakness, and menstrual irregularities. Vomiting, laxatives, or diuretics usually are what cause these difficulties. From psychological and behavioral points of view, people with bulimia often exhibit a great concern regarding body weight and shape, irritability, social withdrawal, depression, and impulsive behavior.[3] Box 15-6 summarizes the criteria for diagnosing bulimia.

Eating disorders of all types require a thorough assessment and multidisciplinary treatment. This treatment can be on an outpatient basis or, for more serious problems that create life-threatening electrolyte imbalances or starvation, inpatient stabilization. The most effective treatment teams include medical, nutritional, and mental health practitioners. The antianxiety and

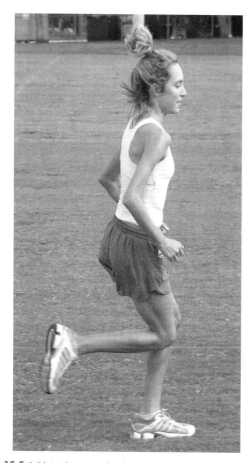

Figure 15-5 Athletes in sports that have weight or appearance standards are at higher risk for eating disorders.

> **Box 15-6** Criteria for Diagnosing Bulimia
>
> - Recurrent eating of a larger amount of food than normal in a discrete amount of time and in an out-of-control manner
> - Recurrent, inappropriate compensatory behavior, such as vomiting or laxative or diuretic abuse
> - Compensatory excessive exercise
> - Behavior happens regularly over at least 3 months
> - Behavior influenced by perceptions of body weight or image
> - Excessive dental caries resulting from frequent vomiting or malnutrition

depression medications described previously are used to treat underlying or comorbid conditions and symptoms. These medications are especially useful in treating the dysphoria associated with low self-esteem and disturbed identity, anxiety that comes with changing eating-related behaviors (e.g., eating but not purging; fear of gaining weight), and the obsessive-compulsive nature of the disorder.

Group therapy, or more generally milieu therapy, has been found to be helpful in assisting the patient to confront unrealistic expectations, maladaptive behaviors, and distorted thinking. Nutritionists work with eating-disordered patients to achieve a more realistic understanding of the body's physiology and nutritional needs, as well as expectations about diet and exercise. Individual and family therapy is especially helpful with children and adolescents and address the dysfunctional social, cultural, and family dynamics within which eating behaviors are embedded.

SUBSTANCE ABUSE AND DEPENDENCE

As with eating and weight issues, the social messages around drug and alcohol use seem to conflict and exacerbate the associated problems. On one hand, alcohol use in the United States is legal and normative for those over the ages of 18 to 21 years old, depending on state laws. On the other hand, millions of dollars are spent on alcohol and drug awareness programs delivered to children throughout their school years. However, peer pressure among younger adolescents often encourages alcohol use. At any rate, the use of mind- or mood-altering substances takes many forms, including use, misuse, abuse, and addiction.

Delineating the boundaries among appropriate use, misuse, abuse, and addiction is fraught with many legal, ethical, and moral difficulties; but from a health care professional's point of view, and perhaps that of an athletic trainer, the categories might be defined by the impact the degree of use is having on the person's overall health and well-being, including performance.

Drug or alcohol use involves the person using the substance without meaningful impairment. Substance misuse includes an individual who occasionally uses an illegal substance or uses a legal substance to excess and who experiences a resulting impairment in ability to function. Substance abuse is a maladaptive pattern of substance use occurring within a 12-month period that causes impairment in social or occupational functioning (e.g., job, legal, and interpersonal problems). In this case, the abuser continues use despite ongoing or increasing consequences. Substance dependence or addiction is a maladaptive pattern of substance abuse occurring within a 12-month period that leads to significant impairment or distress and is characterized by either tolerance—the need for markedly increased amounts of the substance or marked diminished effect with continued use of the same amount of substance—or withdrawal, even if withdrawal does not happen because the patient uses a substance to relieve or avoid withdrawal symptoms.

Alcohol, prescription drugs, illegal drugs (e.g., cocaine, methamphetamine, ecstasy), and other substances (e.g., inhalants such as glue, gasoline, propellants) can be used for their intoxicating effects. The highest rates of inhalant use are found among younger children aged 8 to 12 years. The highest rates of illicit drug use, at 36%, are found in 16 to 20 year olds, with marijuana and alcohol as the most commonly used drugs.[20] The 18- to 29-year-old age group includes the highest prevalence of problem drinkers.[21] Alcohol is the third leading cause of preventable mortality, contributing to 100,000 deaths annually.[22]

The misuse of substances can be found in families of all socioeconomic, racial, and ethnic backgrounds and negatively affects the lives of family members at many levels because of associated relational, social, and legal difficulties. Paradoxically, substance abusers are often enabled by family members who may rationalize or cover for their compulsive or addictive behavior patterns. The impact of substance abuse on the individual and the family depends on the type of drug, length of use, amount being used, and any comorbid conditions. In situations in which athletes are experiencing training- or performance-related difficulties, the athletic trainer should be aware of the possibility of substance abuse as a contributor to performance-related difficulties. Denial is often a complicating factor, however, when working with these individuals and families. For this reason, they will not usually want to acknowledge or discuss substance abuse problems. Because of these denial issues, the athletic trainer needs to be alert for simple clues such as performance problems, work absenteeism, marital discord, or vehicular and everyday accidents. It also helps if the athletic trainer can provide a safe, nonjudgmental environment within which athletes can share their struggles. Successful intervention is based on the individual's desire to stop, willingness to find alternative coping strategies, and, when indicated, effective detoxification, treatment of dual diagnoses, or relapse prevention through individual or family treatment or participation with groups such as Alcoholics Anonymous.

Substance abuse is associated with a variety of possible comorbid conditions that either contribute to or result from the substance abuse itself. Many individuals with comorbid problems self-medicate with alcohol or other drugs, apparently to correct or compensate for the difficulty with mood, anxiety, or concentration (Box 15-7).

The first step in substance abuse intervention is usually assessment by a qualified professional such as a certified drug and alcohol abuse counselor, mental health practitioner, or physician trained in addictions. If the person is determined to be dependent on alcohol or other drugs, inpatient or outpatient detoxification may be necessary. This individual needs to be educated and even confronted about the deleterious effects of the substance use and abuse. Treatment options include a referral to a 12-step group (e.g., Alcoholics Anonymous, Narcotics Anonymous), an alternative treatment method (e.g., Rational Recovery [RR], Moderation Management), outpatient individual or group psychotherapy, or inpatient treatment and aftercare follow-up. (Box 15-8). The RR is an alternative

to the 12-step disease model and is based on a perspective that considers substance use a pattern of problematical behavior and thinking as opposed to a lifelong addictive disease. RR is not a group-based approach to substance use and abuse; rather, the organization provides information and training on their alternative to AA.

Relapse is considered a normative part of the change process with most lifestyle, behavioral, or addiction problems. This is obviously the case with substance abuse as well. In addition to education and referral, the athletic trainer can play an important role in offering ongoing support and encouragement for the person to stay with the behavior change and recovery process.

ATTENTION DEFICIT HYPERACTIVITY DISORDER

Attention deficit hyperactivity disorder (ADHD) is a neurobehavioral condition that impairs a person's ability to sustain attention or control activity and impulses in at least two settings (e.g., home and school or work). As with the other conditions discussed in this chapter, ADHD can be mild, moderate, or severe in its impact on the individual's ability to function. It is often first detected in childhood, especially when children enter classroom settings; however, adult ADHD is increasingly becoming a focus of clinical concern. It has been estimated that 4% to 12% of children are affected by ADHD[23]; it appears to affect boys more than girls by a ratio of 3:1. Girls are more likely to manifest the inattentive type, and boys generally display the hyperactive or combined type.[24] Differences in socialization may account for some of this discrepancy.

Increasing attention is being given to this disorder among adults because of its long-term consequences if unrecognized and untreated.[23] Initially, the athlete with ADHD is much less likely than the student with ADHD to come to the attention of school personnel or other concerned adults. This is because the athlete may just seem to have more energy than peers, but eventually coaches and even teammates may become irritated or frustrated with the athlete's difficulty sitting still, listening to directions, and following through on plans.

ADHD is seen in several forms: primarily hyperactive, primarily inattentive, or mixed.[3] People with primarily hyperactive ADHD can be very easy to detect because they are "wound up like a top." Those with primarily inattentive disorder may be more difficult to detect because they fade into the academic woodwork. Most people with ADHD have elements of hyperactivity, impulsivity, and inattention (Box 15-9).

Box 15-7   Comorbid Conditions Associated with Substance Abuse

- Mood and anxiety disorders
- Marital or family dysfunction
- Partner or child abuse
- Physical injury to self
- Engaging in dangerous behaviors
  - Driving while intoxicated
  - Falls (especially in older adults, elderly)
  - Overdosing
- Physical complaints
  - Gastrointestinal problems
  - Malnutrition
  - Numbness
  - Weakness and fatigue
  - Hypertension
  - Palpitations

Box 15-8   Support Groups for Individuals with Substance Abuse Problems

- Alcoholics Anonymous (AA)
  http://www.alcoholics-anonymous.org
  Numbers of local support groups may be found on their website or in the phone book under AA
- Narcotics Anonymous (NA)
  http://www.na.org
  1-888-773-9999
  Numbers of local support groups may be found at the NA website or in the phone book under NA
- Rational Recovery
  http://www.rational.org

Generally, people with ADHD do not perform academically as well as they should according to standardized test scores. Thus, if ADHD is suspected in an athlete, questions about classroom performance and standardized tests can be helpful. It is also useful to understand the diagnostic criteria for ADHD (Box 15-10). Diagnosis with ADHD is based on an individual experiencing inattention for at least 6 months, including the following:

- Problems attending to detail or makes careless mistakes
- Difficulty sustaining attention
- Appearance of not listening
- Difficulty with follow through on tasks or instructions
- Difficulty with organization
- Avoidance or dislike of tasks requiring sustained mental effort
- Problems losing things
- Easily distracted
- Forgetful

There is a high comorbidity among ADHD, substance abuse, mood and anxiety disorders, and other mental health and behavioral problems.[23] In fact, people with untreated ADHD are almost twice as likely as those who are treated with medication to develop substance abuse problems.[24] In addition, many professionals believe that people with ADHD who also use or abuse substances are, at least in part, self-medicating the underlying problem. As a result, treatment needs to address the medical, behavioral, family, and psychoeducational needs of the patient with respect to ADHD and these comorbid conditions (Box 15-11).

The clinical practice guidelines developed by the American Academy of Pediatrics suggest that assessment begin with an interview, medical checkup, and administration of checklists.[25] From a medical standpoint, first-line ADHD treatment includes the use of stimulant medication (e.g., methylphenidate in its various forms). Older tricyclic antidepressants such as imipramine, newer dopaminergic agents such as bupropion (Wellbutrin), or drugs that block norepinephrine reuptake such as atomoxetine (Straterra) are also being used. Bupropion is indicated for the treatment of ADHD in adults, and atomoxetine is useful for people with comorbid ADHD and depression because of its norepinephrine effects.

Children, adolescents, and adults with ADHD all benefit from education about the nature of the disorder. Those with ADHD also benefit from coaching to reinforce constructive coping strategies that address the problematic behavior and thought processes, such as eliminating distraction, setting short-term goals, and seeking frequent feedback on performance. Family sessions can help others develop realistic expectations for the individual and open up communication about what may have been a very painful and disruptive set of behaviors. Similar communication with teachers, coaches, or work supervisors can be valuable as well.

STAGES OF READINESS

The concerned athletic trainer will routinely screen troubled athletes for one or more of the problems described in this chapter. The athletic trainer who

---

Box 15-9 Typical Symptoms of Hyperactivity, Impulsivity, and Inattention

Hyperactivity and Impulsivity
- Difficulty unwinding
- Restless, fidgety, or always "on the go"
- Talking excessively or interrupting
- Difficulty remaining still when required (e.g., waiting turns)
- Difficulty engaging in quiet activities
- Irritability
- Impulsive behavior (e.g., clowning around, unnecessarily touching others)

Inattention
- Difficulty paying attention, especially to details
- Problems concentrating on instructions
- Failure to follow directions
- Difficulty following through to a goal
- Making careless mistakes
- Distractibility
- Memory problems (e.g., appointments, deadlines)

Box 15-10 ADHD Diagnosis

In order to be diagnosed with ADHD, an individual must, for at least 6 months, experience inattention including the following:
- Problems attending to details or makes careless mistakes
- Difficulty sustaining attention
- Appears to not be listening
- Difficulty with follow through on tasks or instructions
- Difficulty with organization
- Avoids or dislikes tasks requiring sustained mental effort
- Often loses things
- Easily distracted
- Forgetfulness

ADHD, Attention deficit hyperactivity disorder.

Box 15-11 Treatment of ADHD

Mild
- Educate patient and family about the disorder.
- Initiate development of adaptive strategies that increase organizational skills and concentration.

Moderate-Severe
- Add medication.
- Use individual therapy to problem solve.
- Add family therapy.
- Reinforce development strategies.
- Address problematical interpersonal dynamics.

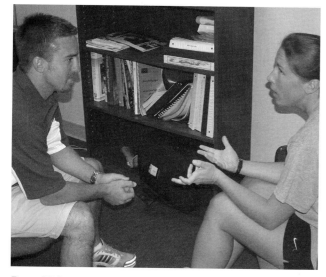

Figure 15-6 The athletic trainer is often in a position to recognize potential psychological disorders in the athlete. It is imperative that the athletic trainer has a referral and support system in place for those athletes in need of further counseling or treatment.

finds that the athlete does indeed have a problem that needs to be addressed will be in the position of educating the person about the problem and contributing factors, as well as discussing options (Figure 15-6). Part of the screening process, however, should first include an assessment of the athlete's readiness to recognize that a problem exists and desire to do something about it. Prochaska and DiClementi[26] developed a useful framework for this step. It involves assessing the athlete's readiness for change. People in need of change can be in one of five different stages of the change process:

1. Precontemplation stage—the athlete has not considered that there is a problem with substance use, eating habits, or mood. This person needs to be educated and encouraged to consider the presence of a problem.

2. Contemplation stage—the athlete has begun to think about the problem and has wondered whether it is time to change, that is, to stop using the substance or seek medical treatment. This needs to be encouraged, and an athletic trainer can be the facilitator by helping the athlete look honestly at the impact of the condition on performance, satisfaction, or general life circumstances.

3. Preparation stage—once the athlete has made the decision to change or seek help, a plan needs to be formulated. The athletic trainer can help by brainstorming possible components of an effective plan for change.

4. Action stage—the athlete has begun making behavioral, situational, or attitudinal changes, including seeking professional help. Referrals from the athletic trainer can be very important now.

5. Follow-up or relapse prevention stage—involves continued implementation or alteration of the plan despite possible setbacks. The athletic trainer can use contacts with the athlete on the field or in the office to support the athlete's decision to address the problem, support progress, or confront relapse.

It will not be a productive use of time or relationship capital for the athletic trainer to attempt getting the athlete to do something that is not congruent with the athlete's current stage of readiness. In other words, it will not work to try to get someone to develop a plan of action or even take steps to correct the problem, such as going to Alcoholics Anonymous, seeing a physician, or being more reasonable with the workout schedule, when still in denial about the problem. The athletic trainer who tries to get the athlete to move from one stage to the next by first assessing and asking good questions, providing support, and offering educational input will be more effective. When the person moves from precontemplation to contemplation and preparation, then it is time for the person and the athletic trainer to partner in developing a plan.

SUMMARY

The certified athletic trainer attends to the athlete as a whole person, not just to physical health and performance. This is because performance, physical health, mental health, behaviors, and life situation affect each other. Accordingly, this chapter has highlighted the most common mental health conditions experienced by athletes that athletic trainers need to recognize. Based on this information and continuing education, athletic trainers should be able to identify emotional and behavioral signs of common mental health issues, including mood, anxiety, eating, attention deficit hyperactivity, and substance use disorders.

Subsequently, the athletic trainer will be equipped to appropriately intervene with the affected athlete through discussion, supportive confrontation, education, and referral. This part of the process involves being aware of and establishing collaborative relationships with qualified physical and mental health professionals and knowing when to refer. Last, various educational and supportive resources, such as organizational procedure, printed materials, and web-based resources, have been identified and are available to both professionals and patients affected by these disorders.

REFERENCES

1. World Health Organization: *World health report 2001—mental health: new understanding*, World Health Organization. Available at http://www.who.int/whr2001. Accessed December 2003.
2. Murray C, Lopez A, editors: *A comprehensive assessment of mortality and disability from diseases, injuries, and risk factors in 1990 and projected to 2020*, Cambridge, Mass, 1996, Harvard University Press.
3. American Psychiatric Association: *Diagnostic and statistical manual of mental disorders*, ed 4, Washington, DC, 1994, APA.
4. National Collegiate Athletic Association (NCAA): Banned drug classes. Available at www1.ncaa.org/membership/ed_outreach/health-safety/drug_testing/banned_drug_classes.pdf. Accessed December 2003.
5. Anxiety Disorders Association of America: Anxiety disorders. Available at www.adaa.org. Accessed November, 2003.
6. Antony M, Swinson R: *Phobic disorders and panic in adults: a guide to assessment and treatment*, Washington, DC, 2000, American Psychological Association.
7. Gorman J: Treatment of generalized anxiety disorder, *Journal of Clinical Psychiatry* 63(suppl 8):17-23, 2002.
8. Roy-Byrne P, Russo J, Dugdale DC, et al: Under-treatment of panic disorder in primary care: role of patient and physician characteristics, *Journal of the American Board of Family Practice* 15(6):443-450, 2002.
9. Birmaher B, Ryan N, Williamson D: The NIMH diagnostic interview schedule for children, version 2.3 (disc 2.3): description, acceptability, prevalence rates, and performance in the MECA study, *Journal of the American Academy of Child and Adolescent Psychiatry* 35(7):865-877, 1996.
10. Levine J, Cole DP, Chengpappa KN, Gershon S: Anxiety disorders and major depression, together or apart, *Depression and Anxiety* 14:94-104, 2001.
11. Manber R, Allen JB, Morris MM: Alternative treatments for depression: empirical support and relevance to women, *Journal of Clinical Psychiatry* 63:628-640, 2002.
12. Wang JL, Patten SB: The moderating effects of coping strategies on major depression in the general population, *Canadian Journal of Psychiatry* 47:167-173, 2002.
13. Culpepper L: The active management of depression, *Journal of Family Practice* 51(9):769-776, 2002.
14. Zung WW: A self-rating depression scale, *Archives of General Psychiatry* 12:63-70, 1965.
15. Becker AE, Grinspoon SK, Klibanski A, Herzog DB: Current concepts: eating disorders, *New England Journal of Medicine* 340:1092-1098, 1999.
16. Maddox RW: Eating disorders: current concepts, *Journal of the American Pharmaceutical Association* 39:378-387, 1999.
17. Mitan LA: Eating disorders in adolescent girls, *Current Women's Health Report* 2:464-467, 2002.
18. Tamburrino MB, McGinnis RA: Anorexia nervosa. A review, *Panminerva Medica* 44:301-311, 2002.
19. Lock J, Le Grange D, Agras, WS. Treatment manual for anorexia nervosa: A family-based approach. *Behavior Research & Therapy* 40(11):1364-1365, Nov 2002.
20. National Institute on Drug Abuse (NIDA): *National household survey on drug abuse*. Bethesda MD, 1997, NIDA.
21. National Institute on Drug Abuse (NIDA): Guide to assessing drug abuse within and across communities. *Alcohol Health & Research World* 18(3):243, 1994.
22. McGinnis J, Foege W: Actual causes of death in the United States, *JAMA* 270(18):2208, 1993.
23. Brown R, Freeman W, Perrin J, et al: Prevalence and assessment of attention-deficit/hyperactivity disorder in primary care settings, *Pediatrics* 107(3):1-11, 2001.
24. Giedd J: ADHD & substance abuse, *Medscape Psychiatry & Mental Health* 8(1), 2003.
25. Homer CJ et al: Clinical practice guideline: diagnosis and evaluation of the child with attention deficit/hyperactivity disorder, *Pediatrics* 105(5):1158-1169, 2000.
26. Prochaska J, DiClementi C: Stages and processes of self-change of smoking: towards an integrative model of change, *Journal of Consulting and Clinical Psychology* 51:390, 395, 1983.

CHAPTER 16

Special Populations

Monique Butcher-Mokha

OBJECTIVES

At the completion of this chapter, the reader should be able to do the following:

1. Determine components of the general medical history necessary when assessing persons with selected disabilities.
2. Recognize the importance of the preparticipation physical examination in identifying baseline norms in the athlete with a disability.
3. Identify typical symptoms and clinical signs of pathological conditions seen in athletes with selected disabilities.
4. Appreciate typical treatment and prevention measures of pathological conditions seen in persons with selected disabilities.
5. Understand the interaction of disability-related attributes with illness-related characteristics.
6. Describe manners of effective communication with athletes with selected disabilities.

INTRODUCTION

Participation in organized sports and recreation by athletes with disabilities has increased significantly, with over three million individuals participating in the United States alone. This has created a deeper field of competition, requiring athletes to train and compete at higher levels to attain success. Athletes in wheelchairs have broken the 4-minute mile and have completed 26-mile marathons in less than 90 minutes. Marlon Shirley from the United States has run the 100 m on a prosthetic leg with a time of 11.08 seconds.

The need for quality sports medicine care in special populations is as important as it is in the able-bodied population. Although risks of injury and illness are inherent in all physical activity and injury rates for athletes with disabilities have generally been found to be within the same range as for athletes without disabilities, athletes with disabilities do pose some unique concerns related to the general medical assessment. Musculoskeletal injuries accounted for 79.7% of the reported injuries to athletes with disabilities, and general medical problems (i.e., illness or disability-related) accounted for 20.3% of those athletes who were unable to participate.[1]

Person-first terminology should be used to refer to athletes with disabilities. Person-first terminology recognizes the individual before the disability. For example, the athletic trainer identifies the athlete as a person with spina bifida or an athlete with a visual impairment, rather than a disabled or blind athlete. Using appropriate terminology reflects an overall philosophy of the person being first to the athletic trainer, and the disability being second.

This chapter focuses on issues related to the general medical concerns for the athlete with a disability. The specific disabilities covered are traumatic tetraplegia and paraplegia, spina bifida, poliomyelitis, cerebral palsy, amputations, sensory disabilities, and intellectual disabilities.

PREPARTICIPATION EXAMINATION FOR ATHLETES WITH DISABILITIES

Athletes must complete a thorough preparticipation physical examination (PPE) so that baseline norms can be established. The general approach of the PPE for athletes with disabilities is similar to that of athletes without disabilities (see Appendix A). However, often the focus is on the primary condition or disability, and the athletic trainer and other members of the sports medicine team may overlook medical issues that exist other than the primary disability. This is known as diagnostic overshadowing.[2,3] Patel and Greydanus[2,3] stress the importance of a detailed history and suggest that the PPE be completed by a sports medicine team that is involved in the athlete's long-term care and who know the athlete's baseline functioning. It is also suggested that the mass or station method of the PPE be avoided with these athletes. Specific recommendations are that medical personnel talk at eye level with an athlete in a wheelchair, ask the athlete what movement patterns are possible and which parts of the body have normal sensation, and be cognizant of skin conditions and pressure sores.[4]

Many athletes with spinal cord disabilities have constant or residual pain from their disability and may not be able to distinguish pain due to a sport injury from pain due to a disability. Having a baseline appreciation for the athlete's unique condition will help the assessment process should a general medical condition arise later. An additional component of the examination includes careful evaluation to ensure proper fit and adequacy of any prostheses, orthoses, sports wheelchairs, or other assistive devices being used by the athletes. Athletic trainers seek assistance from professionals with expertise in the specific area of disability. Other aspects to consider during the PPE for an athlete with a disability are listed in Box 16-1.

To identify medical problems, provide baseline data, and identify training goals, Jacob and Hutzler[5]

developed the Sports-Medical Assessment Protocol (SMAP), a tool for the evaluation of athletes with neurological disabilities. The SMAP includes a clinical interview, cardiopulmonary testing, and physical and functional assessments. In regard to participation guidelines, the American Academy of Orthopaedic Surgeons developed a sport participation possibility chart designed to provide initial guidance for the athlete and sports medicine team regarding which sports are appropriate. Factors influencing how to match an athlete to a particular sport include the psychological maturity of the athlete, adaptive and protective equipment, modification of the sport, the athlete's and parents' understanding of the inherent risks of injury, current health condition of the athlete, and level of competition and position played.[2]

OVERVIEW OF ANATOMY AND PHYSIOLOGY

The anatomy and physiology pertinent to traumatic spinal cord injury is also pertinent to spina bifida, poliomyelitis, and cerebral palsy. The reader is referred to Chapters 8, 9, 10, and 14 to review the anatomy and physiology related to intellectual and sensory disabilities and amputation. Recall from Chapter 8 that the spinal cord is a cylindrical mass of nerve tissue that consists of 31 pairs of spinal nerves and extends from the medulla to the first or second lumbar vertebra. It is protected by the vertebral column that consists of 7 cervical, 12 thoracic, 5 lumbar, 5 fused sacral, and 4 or more fused coccygeal bones (Figure 16-1). The lumbar and sacral roots of the spinal cord fan out like a horse's tail at L1-2, giving rise to the term **cauda equina.**

Nerve impulses are conducted via the spinal cord and nerves between the brain and other parts of the body, and trauma to the spine can severely affect these intricate processes. In addition, the nervous system has other nonmotor functions. The autonomic nervous system consists of the sympathetic and parasympathetic systems (Key Points—Autonomic Nervous System).

Box 16-1 | **Special Considerations During the Preparticipation Exam**

Follow these special considerations when examining and recording the health history for athletes with disabilities:
- Inspect all braces, orthoses, wheelchairs and assistive devices
  - Make sure they are clean and free of rough areas
  - Ensure a proper fit for the specific athlete
- Obtain a resting blood pressure in at least two positions: supine and sitting or standing
- Inquire about bladder and bowel habits
  - Ask about the management plan
  - Determine the method of voiding and evacuating (i.e., catheter, bag)
- Inquire about autonomic dysreflexia and the offending agent
- Inquire about history of heat-related illnesses
- Inquire about experiences with stimuli that cause spasms
- Note history and frequency of urinary track or bladder infections
- Note history of spina bifida
- Note presence of a cerebral shunt
- Note history of latex allergy
- Note history of poliomyelitis
- Note history of seizures and management plan (i.e., medications, last seizure, type of seizure)
- Note history of visual impairment (i.e., age at onset, cause, protective lenses)

KEY POINTS
Autonomic Nervous System

The autonomic nervous system consists of the "fight or flight" physiological responses necessary to protect against perceived danger. Specifically, this system and their actions have two components:
Sympathetic system
- Increases heart rate
- Increases blood pressure
- Increases core temperature
Parasympathetic system
- Decreases heart rate
- Decreases blood pressure
- Decreases core temperature

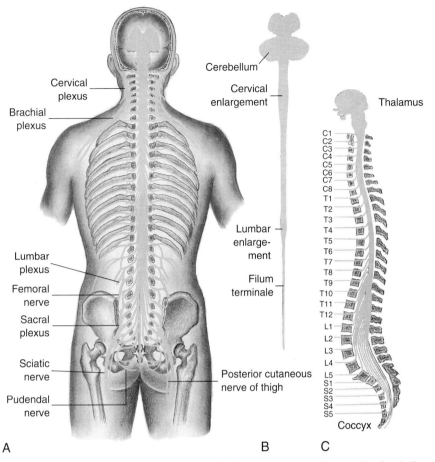

Figure 16-1 The spinal cord has 31 pairs of nerves that interpret sensory and motor stimuli and allow movement to occur. The level of a lesion to the cord is associated with type of disability, typically sensory and motor, and will affect all areas distal to the lesion. (From Rudy EB: *Advanced neurological and neurosurgical nursing,* St. Louis, 1984, Mosby.)

The sympathetic system controls increases in heart rate, blood pressure, and temperature, whereas the parasympathetic system controls decreases in heart rate, blood pressure, and temperature.

PATHOLOGICAL CONDITIONS

Spinal cord disability results from some form of injury or disease to the vertebrae and/or the nerves of the spinal column. Usually some degree of paralysis accompanies the disability. The degree of the paralysis is a function of the location of the injury on the spinal column (e.g., C5) and the number of neural fibers that are destroyed as a result of the injury. The level of function for an athlete with a spinal cord disability is dependent upon the level of the lesion. The lower the level of lesion on the spinal cord, the greater the functional ability of the athlete. Table 16-1 provides a summary of the relationship between level of lesion and functional ability. In addition, note that athletes with lesions above S2 will experience bowel and bladder concerns.

The pathological conditions associated with spinal cord injury (SCI), whether tetraplegia or paraplegia, spina bifida, or poliomyelitis, are often seen in cerebral palsy as well. Sequelae unique to specific conditions are discussed here in order to provide the athletic trainer with the knowledge base to assess each individual athlete.

Pathological conditions associated with amputation, sensory disabilities, and intellectual disabilities are also covered in this chapter.

Traumatic Tetraplegia and Paraplegia

The extent of an SCI is generally described by using a five-point grading system: complete, incomplete with sensation only, incomplete with nonfunctional motor ability, incomplete with motor function, and complete recovery. An athlete with complete **tetraplegia** (formerly called **quadriplegia**) has a lesion above T1 that involves the cervical spine and affects all four limbs, has no trunk control or sitting balance, and usually uses a high-backed sports wheelchair. The athlete will also be strapped in for safety. An athlete with complete **paraplegia** has a lesion below T-1 that affects the lower extremities, has full use of the upper extremities, and may or may not have trunk control and sitting balance. Training apparatus is available to encourage correct movement.

Athletes with incomplete spinal lesions will have varied and unpredictable responses to many neurological tests. For example, a wheelchair basketball player with a T10 incomplete lesion may respond within normal limits to dermatome testing below T10.

Athletes with SCI have higher resting heart rates and lower blood pressures than their able-bodied counterparts. The higher heart rate is primarily due to the smaller venous return from the nonworking muscles in the lower extremities. To maintain cardiac output when stroke volume is less, the heart compensates by increasing its rate. In turn, the blood pressure lowers to accommodate a decreased perfusion need in the nonworking limbs. During the general medical assessment, the athletic trainer is aware that the baseline blood pressure for adults with quadriplegia may

be as low as 90/60 mm Hg and that peak heart rates for persons with quadriplegia typically do not exceed 130 beats per minute. As part of the PPE, blood pressure should be obtained in 2 of 3 positions: supine and sitting or standing, as applicable.[6] A change of ≤10 mm Hg between positions is acceptable. Resting pulse is checked, as tachycardia (i.e., heart rate > 120 beats per minute) may be the only sign of pneumonia or pulmonary embolus in an athlete with a high-level SCI.

Autonomic Dysreflexia

Autonomic dysreflexia (AD), also known as hyperreflexia, is a clinical phenomenon unique to individuals with SCI above the major sympathetic nervous system outflow tract. It is a potentially life-threatening complication from SCI particular to those with lesions above T6. With AD, the athlete's blood pressure rises to dangerous levels and, if not treated, can lead to stroke or death.

AD is an imbalanced reflex sympathetic discharge that occurs when there is a painful, irritating, or even strong stimulus below the level of injury, such as an insect bite, bone fracture, or distended bladder (Box 16-2). Intact peripheral sensory nerves transmit impulses that stimulate sympathetic neurons in the spinal cord below the level of the lesion. The inhibitory outflow above the SCI is increased but it is unable to pass below the block of the SCI. The large sympathetic outflow causes release of various neurotransmitters such as norepinephrine and dopamine, causing a sudden rise in blood pressure. Vasomotor brainstem reflexes attempt to lower blood pressure by increasing parasympathetic stimulation to the heart through stimulation of the vagus nerve, resulting in bradycardia. Because the parasympathetic system's messages cannot pass through the SCI, the blood pressure remains elevated. The most common cause of AD is impairment

Table 16-1	Level of Spinal Cord Lesion Related to Functional Ability
Level of Lesion	**Functional Abilities**
C4	Use of neck and diaphragm Needs total assistance for transfers Limited respiratory endurance Controls electronic wheelchair by mouth-operated joystick
C7	Ability to extend elbow and flex and extend fingers Uses wheelchair independently Transfers to some extent independently Weak grasp
T1-9	Ability to use upper extremities Little or no use of lower extremities Lower level injury: some control of upper back, abdominal, and rib muscles Lower level injury: may ambulate with braces
T10-12	Complete control of upper back, abdominal, and rib muscles Ambulates mainly with use of long leg braces or crutches Use wheelchair for convenience or wheelchair sport possible
L1-3	Hip joint flexibility and ability to flex hip Ambulates independently with short leg braces, cane, or crutches
S1	Ability to flex knees and lift foot Ambulates without crutches but may require ankle braces or orthopedic shoes

Box 16-2	Common Causes of Autonomic Dysreflexia

- Bladder distention
- Urinary tract infection
- Epididymitis or scrotal compression
- Bowel distention
- Bowel impaction
- Gastric ulcers or gastritis
- Appendicitis or other abdominal trauma
- Menstruation
- Contact with hard or sharp objects
- Temperature fluctuations
- Constrictive clothing, shoes, or equipment
- Fractures or other trauma
- Ingrown toenails
- Burns or sunburns
- Blisters
- Insect bites
- Pain

in the urinary system, but others are illustrated in Key Points—Inadvertant Causes of Autonomic Dysreflexia. Everyday training and rehabilitation sessions have the potential for provoking AD.

Signs and Symptoms

AD is characterized by sudden-onset high blood pressure and slowed heart rate, profuse sweating above the lesion level, piloerection (i.e., goose bumps), flushing of the skin above the lesion level, headache, and nasal congestion. It is possible for signs or symptoms to be absent despite the elevated blood pressure. It is paramount that the athletic trainer take a blood pressure reading when AD is suspected. Special attention is paid to any BP more than 20 mm Hg to 40 mm Hg above the reference range for systole. The athletic trainer must know the athlete's normal blood pressure so that changes can be detected. The heart rate should also be monitored for atypical decreases. An athlete may present with flushed skin, particularly in the face and neck area, and piloerection (Red Flags for Autonomic Dysreflexia). The athlete may also have a headache or

> ### ⏵ Red Flags for Autonomic Dysreflexia
> Examine an athlete immediately who presents with the following signs or symptoms of autonomic dysreflexia and treat by removing the offending stimulus:
> - Sudden on-set elevated blood pressure
> - Accompanying lowered heart rate
> - Profuse sweating above the level of impairment
> - Piloerection
> - Flushing of the skin above level of impairment
> - Headache
> - Nasal congestion

nasal congestion in response to the high blood pressure. Because impacted bowels and distended bladders can lead to AD, the athletic trainer should also inquire about bowel and bladder habits.

Treatment, Prognosis, and Return to Participation

Response to AD needs to be quick and thorough. The offending stimulus must be removed and the athlete should be in a sitting position, because sitting leads to pooling of blood in the lower extremities and may aid

in reducing blood pressure. Clothing is loosened, as is protective equipment. A thorough inspection should begin with the urinary system. Indwelling catheters are checked along the entire length of the system for constrictions, obstructions, or kinks. Athletic trainers need to be aware and comfortable with the mechanism of these catheters, since they are common to many athletes with SCI. The bladder should be drained; fecal matter is evacuated. If neither bladder nor colon is full, the athletic trainer checks for other causes such as sunburn, pressure sores, ingrown toenails, and insect bites. A physician may administer sublingual nifedipine to reduce the blood pressure while the causes of AD are being examined. Caution is recommended when using antihypertensives with older adults or those with coronary artery disease.

It is essential that the underlying causal agent be found and removed. If symptoms do not seem to resolve immediately or if the cause of the AD has not been identified, emergency medical services should be summoned. Return to play should be based on a physician's clearance. The athlete's symptoms and blood pressure are monitored for at least 2 hours after resolution of the episode to ensure that AD does not recur.

Prevention

Prevention is the key with AD, and because most episodes result from forgetfulness or carelessness about urine needs,[7] athletes should inspect catheters and void the bladder before activity. Athletes must be asked what type of bowel and bladder management program they maintain. They should avoid the risk of sunburn by using sunscreen, wearing hats or visors, seeking shade during nonactivity, and covering susceptible areas. Careful inspection after training or competition by the athlete and the athletic trainer for contributors such as blisters, sunburn, pressure sores, constricting clothing or equipment will aid in preventing episodes of AD. To date, no specific relationship has been documented between AD and age. Because more males sustain SCI, AD is primarily a male phenomenon.

Boosting

Boosting is a dangerous technique used by some athletes with SCI in an attempt to gain an advantage over an opponent or to improve race times. Although this condition is potentially life threatening, many athletes have intentionally induced AD in order to gain better performance results from increased blood circulation. Athletes with SCI can induce AD by holding their urine or clamping their catheters before an event, sitting on a sharp object (e.g., tack), strapping their legs very tightly, or aggressively pinching or striking themselves. Self-induced lower leg fractures have also been reported.[2]

A 9.7% improvement in track and swimming times have been reported in athletes with disabilities who used this tactic.[8] This would be equivalent to reducing the able-bodied 26-mile marathon record by 12 minutes! However, research has reported this practice is, at the very least, unethical and must be prevented at all costs.[9] The International Paralympic Committee bans boosting as a method of doping. The athletic trainer must know that this is an extremely risky behavior and must strongly discourage it. Athletes may think they are only receiving a catecholamine response and heart rate reserve that could normally be attained if uninjured. However, the significant rise in blood pressure that occurs with AD cannot be controlled by the body's autonomic nervous system. Other factors, such as inadequate hydration, fatigue, thermal stress, illness, or anxiety, can add to the AD and push the athlete to the point of autonomic shutdown, which can lead to death.[9]

Thermoregulation Concerns

Evaporative cooling is the most effective heat loss mechanism for the body, providing more than 80% of heat loss in the able-bodied athlete. Individuals with spinal cord injury are unable to depend on the autonomic nervous system to lower their core temperature by regulating blood flow. In addition, sweating is often impaired below the level of the spinal cord lesion, requiring the athlete's body to rely upon less surface area for evaporative cooling.[6] Therefore athletes with SCI are at greater risk of heat illness than their able-bodied counterparts, and the athletic trainer needs to keep careful watch over athletes during high-energy sports that raise their core temp (Figure 16-2). Individuals with tetraplegia and those with lesions above T6 are particularly vulnerable to heat illness because they are unable to increase heart rate to sustain cardiac output when blood must flow to both the muscle and the skin.[4,10]

Likewise, in cold conditions these athletes may lack normal warming mechanisms, such as producing piloerection, shivering, and circulatory shunting. A lack of working muscle mass below the level of lesion contributes to temperature regulation problems. Even temperatures around 50° F may pose problems for an athlete with a cervical or high thoracic lesion.[11] Impaired or absent sensation intensifies the risk of hypothermia because these athletes may be unaware that damp clothing increases the loss of body heat (Box 16-3).

Heat illness and hypothermia occur in the athlete with SCI in the same manner as for able-bodied athletes. Athletes with SCI are more vulnerable because of the reasons described previously. Athletic trainers need to alert all athletes to the factors that can contribute to temperature-related illnesses (Key Points—Contributing

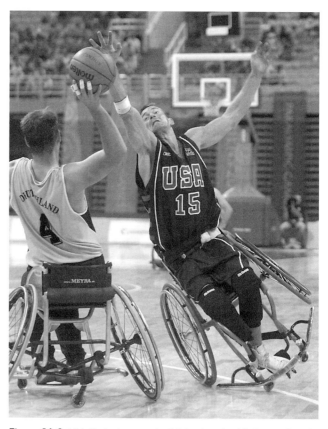

Figure 16-2 Athletic trainers and athletes in wheelchairs need to be mindful of the athletes' core body temperatures and schedule breaks so that they can cool down.

Factors to Heat-Related Illness). Athletic trainers must also be able to recognize conditions that put athletes at risk for hyperthermia and understand that these factors may occur in combination to create the risky environment for the athlete.

Signs and Symptoms
Recognizing the early warning signs and symptoms of dehydration is crucial in preventing severe complications

---

KEY POINTS
Contributing Factors to Heat-Related Illness

- Hot, humid day
- Recent illness
- Inability to sweat
- Not acclimated to temperature
- High-intensity workout
- Dehydrated
- Dark-colored clothing
- Use of medications or dietary supplements
- Out of shape; not fit
- Over-motivated
- Behavior risks (e.g., lack of sleep, alcohol intake)
- Amount and type of clothing or equipment causing impaired evaporation

Modified from Casa D, Almsquist J, Anderson S: Inter-Association task force statement on exertional heat illnesses consensus statement, *NATA News,* June 2003:24-29, 2003.

Box 16-3 **Contributory Factors for Hypothermia**

Athletes with neurological disorders such as SCI are particularly susceptible to cold. The athlete, athletic trainer, coaches, and other team members need to be mindful of the following:
- Low temperatures
- Presence of wind or chill factor
- Inadequate clothing (e.g., nonwicking fabric, inappropriate layers, no wind or rain barrier)
- Prolonged periods of inactivity during the competition or training session
- Environmental dampness or wetness
- Damp or wet clothing
- High spinal cord lesion
- Improper warm-up
- Dehydration

from heat stress. Signs and symptoms include thirst, irritability, fatigue, headache, weakness, dizziness, decreased performance, erratic wheelchair propulsion, flushed skin, head or neck heat sensations, vomiting or nausea, and general discomfort. In able-bodied athletes chills and muscle cramps are common; such signs may not be present in athletes with SCI if piloerection is impaired. Usually muscle cramps are common in the gastrocnemius and abdominal muscles, but these muscles are often nonworking in individuals with SCI.

Heat stroke, a life-threatening emergency, is characterized in the able-bodied population as having a core temperature of 104° F or higher[12]; a rapid increase in pulse is present as well (160-180 bpm). The chief symptom of heat stroke is central nervous system dysfunction. Other symptoms are similar to those associated with concussions, namely confusion, agitation, inappropriate behavior or language, apathy, vacillating emotions, stupor, and coma or death if untreated.

Dehydration can also occur in hyperthermal situations conjunction with cold weather conditions or when hypothermia exists. Dehydration causes reduced blood volume, resulting in less fluid available to cool or warm tissue. Low temperatures accentuated by wind and dampness can pose a major threat to any athlete but especially to the athlete with a spinal cord injury, who may lack the normative mechanisms for warming as mentioned previously.

Referral, Diagnostic Tests, and Differential Diagnosis

Thermoregulatory problems are often incorrectly attributed to athlete fatigue, illness, hypoglycemic reactions, concussion, or head injury.[12] To determine hyperthermia, the athletic trainer feels for hot skin of a distressed athlete.[13] Because the individual with SCI has a decreased ability to regulate blood flow beneath the lesion, rectal temperatures may not be as accurate for measuring core temperature in athletes with spinal cord injuries.[14] In addition, when the thermoregulatory system is impaired, typical signs such as shivering

might not be observable. It is critical that the athletic trainer be able to review a thorough medication and nutritional supplement history for the athlete that includes prescription and over-the-counter products. Sympathomimetics and anticholinergics affect thermoregulation, as do diuretics and excessive caffeine.[2] Emergency referral is warranted if the athlete is not responding to treatment or if heat stroke is suspected.

Treatment

Treating thermoregulatory problems in the athlete with a spinal cord disability is similar to treatment for the able-bodied athlete. For hyperthermia, the athlete is moved to a shaded or cooled area, clothing is loosened, equipment removed, oral fluids are administered, and cooling is accomplished with cold water. Intravenous fluids are administered if the athlete is not coherent. If heat stroke is suspected, emergency measures to reduce the athlete's temperature (e.g., emersion in cold water bath or sponge cool water, fanning body with a towel) are performed first; then the athlete must be transported to an advanced emergency care facility.[15] It should be stressed that while immersion in an ice bath has been recommended for able-bodied athletes, this treatment should be used with caution in the athlete with a spinal cord injury, especially one with a complete, high level of lesion because the thermoregulatory system is impaired. Cooling may occur too rapidly. To date, research is this area for athletes with spinal cord injury is incomplete. Therefore, indications and contraindications should be discussed with the physician who is most familiar with the individual athlete.

Treating hypothermia involves administering warm fluids, transporting the athlete to a warm environment, removing wet clothing immediately, and replacing them with warm, dry clothing. The use of heating pads or hot water bottles on paralyzed areas should be avoided because using heat on areas without sensation is contraindicated.

Prognosis and Return to Participation

The National Athletic Trainers' Association established an Inter-Association Task Force that created a statement on exertional heat illness contain return-to-activity guidelines for able-bodied athletes.[15,16] In general, these guidelines include clearance from a physician and a gradual and monitored return to activity and may be used for the athlete with SCI.

Prevention

Heat-related illnesses are entirely preventable (Box 16-4). Wheelchair athletes should attach a water bottle to the wheelchair. A tented area adjacent to the competition for ready access to shade needs to be provided. The medications that athletes are taking

Box 16-4 | Prevention of Hyperthermia

Hyperthermia is always preventable. Athletic trainers need to educate coaches and athletes about heat-related illnesses and the steps to prevention.

- Ensure proper acclimatization and hydration
- Advise the athlete to drink plenty of fluids
- Provide readily accessible fluids
- Rehydrate after activity
- Use electrolyte drinks as available
- Seek shelter from the sun frequently
- Spray externally with cool water using a spray bottle or hose

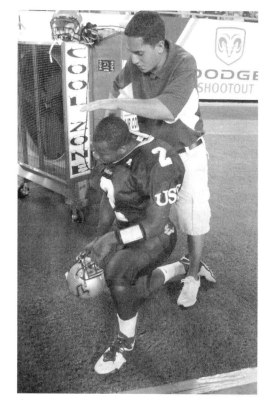

- Wear appropriate clothing made of breathable fabric with wicking properties
- Adapt activities to the environment as necessary
- Screen participants for a past history of heat illness

should be monitored. Some prescription, over-the-counter, and recreational drugs, as well as nutritional supplements, can adversely influence heat production and heat loss. The risk of heat illness in able-bodied athletes is much greater for individuals who consume these drugs. It stands to reason that some medications could influence similar mechanisms in athletes with SCI. Certain medications may also predispose the athletes to temperature regulation problems in the cold.

Preventing hypothermia includes encouraging the athlete to: drink plenty of fluids, warm-up properly, wear adequate clothing (i.e., layers), change wet clothing immediately after exercise, and wear a hat. Athletic trainers should screen participants for a past history of hypothermia.

Special Concerns for Youth and Older Adults

Just as with the able-bodied athletic population, athletic trainers should exercise caution with youth or master's level athletes in terms of thermoregulatory conditions.[15] Children tend to absorb more heat from their surroundings, have a lower sweating capacity, and produce more metabolic heat per mass unit than adults. Therefore, exercise time and intensity is reduced when environmental conditions are extreme. In addition, athletic trainers should ensure that children have 10 to 14 days of acclimatization. Older adults may have decreased fitness levels and lean body mass, chronic diseases, or prescription medications, all of which may affect the athlete's reaction to the environment. It is important for the athletic trainer to check for fitness, acclimatization, and frequent intake of fluids, as well as consult with the athlete's physician regarding medications.

Skin Breakdown and Pressure Sores

The inability of athletes with complete SCI to feel sensation makes them susceptible to skin breakdown. Wrinkles in socks, poorly fitted shoes, or orthoses can cause blisters that become infected. Inattention to personal hygiene may also cause skin breakdown.[7] Circulatory problems related to paralysis increase the risk of infection and slow healing. Pressure sores, or **decubitus ulcers,** result in loss of training and competition time and could lead to bed rest, hospitalization, or, in extreme cases such as Christopher Reeve, death. Skin over bony prominences is at the greatest risk (e.g., pelvis, buttocks, and ankles). Athletes with pressure sores should not be allowed to compete.

Wheelchair athletes who race for long periods of time in a knees-up, forward-seated position are particularly at risk for skin breakdown on the buttocks area. This is due to the weight of the body that creates shear and compressive forces when engaged in sport. Chairs designed with the knees higher than the buttocks contribute to increased pressure over the sacrum and ischial tuberosities.[17] Impaired circulation is exacerbated by friction with the chair and perspiration. Wheelchair athletes such as tennis and basketball players who may train without shirts or in perspiration-soaked shirts can develop skin breakdown on their upper backs from contact with the back of their chairs.

Signs and Symptoms

Skin appearance will vary with the severity of the breakdown (Figure 16-3). A Stage I sore is red or discolored, but the skin is not broken. The discoloration or redness does not disappear within 30 minutes of pressure being removed from the site. In a Stage II sore, the epidermis or top layer is broken, creating a

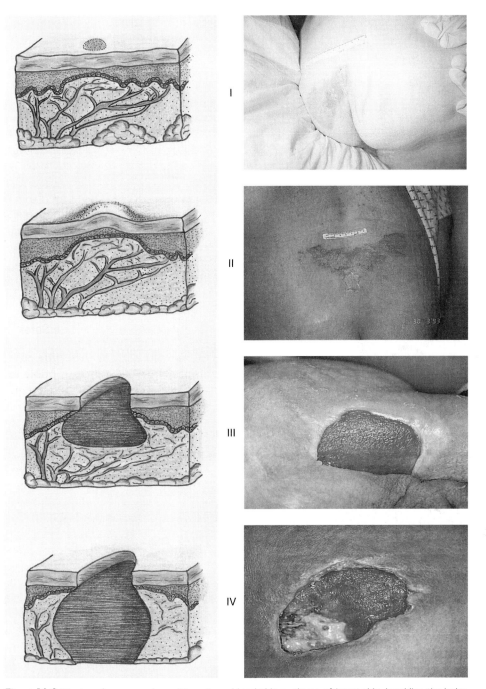

Figure 16-3 Staging of pressure ulcers: Stage I, nonblanchable erythema of intact skin, heralding the lesion of skin ulceration; Stage II, partial-thickness skin loss involving epidermis or dermis; Stage III, full-thickness skin loss involving damage or necrosis of subcutaneous tissue that extends down to but not through underlying fascia; Stage IV, full-thickness skin loss with extensive destruction, tissue necrosis, or damage to muscle, bone, or supporting structures. (From Potter PA, Perry AG: *Fundamentals of nursing concepts, process and practice,* ed 4, St. Louis, 1997, Mosby.)

shallow, open sore, but drainage may or not be present. In a Stage III sore, the break in the skin has extended deep through the dermis or second layer into the subcutaneous and fat tissue and drainage is present. Stage IV is more severe in that the breakage extends into the muscle tissue and possibly down to the bone and extensive dead tissue and drainage are

present. Signs and symptoms that indicate further complication of a pressure sore include fever, black areas around the sore, greenish drainage, and an odor.

Referral, Diagnostic Tests, and Differential Diagnosis
Sores are typically overlooked because an athletic trainer or other health care provider may not inspect for them,

or they are dismissed as abrasions or contusions from equipment. A thorough visual inspection of the skin over at-risk body parts is necessary by the athletic trainer and athlete. Young athletes need special reminders to make this inspection a habit. When a pressure sore is discovered, the offending pressure needs to be removed (e.g., the athlete transfers from the wheelchair to a treatment table or the athlete stops lying or sitting on that particular skin area). If the discoloration or redness does not disappear within 30 minutes, the location and color should be noted, along with any drainage, in the athlete's medical file. If there is drainage, the athletic trainer inspects, monitors, and notes the color and odor and refer the athlete to a physician.

Treatment

Keeping pressure off of the sore is the first and foremost treatment. If this is not possible during athletic activity and the sore is not severe enough to warrant the athlete's restriction from activity, the athlete must relieve pressure from the area when not participating in athletics. These sores must be cleaned and treated as a potential infection. Appropriate hygiene and sanitation must be maintained, and medicated dressing applied if necessary (Box 16-5).

Prognosis and Return to Participation

Only when a pressure sore is completely healed will the area be able to receive pressure. The epidermis should not be broken nor should there be any redness or discoloration. One recommendation for determining whether a sore is completely healed is to gradually allow pressure to be accepted by the area again.

Box 16-5   Care Associated with Pressure Sore Stages

Stage I
- Remove pressure
- Practice proper hygiene (avoid vigorous scrubbing; pat dry)
- Evaluate diet for nutritional deficits
- Evaluate mattress, wheelchair cushions, transfer techniques
- Apply Tegaderm or similar dressing to prevent friction
- Refer if sore persists 3-5 days

Stage II
- Continue Stage I plan
- Cleanse with saline and pat dry
- Apply dressing such as Tegaderm or Duoderm
- Refer if sign of infection

Stage III
- Continue Stage I and II plans except for dressing
- Use pressure-relieving mattress (physician can authorize)
- Apply advanced wound care for cleansing, debriding and packing; most likely will need referral
- Administer oral or topical antibiotics

Stage IV
- Consult with physician immediately
- Most often surgery is required

For example, 15 minutes of pressure could be allowed, followed by 15 minutes of waiting for the redness to subside. If the discolorization does not subside, the area is not ready to accept pressure. If the redness does subside, the procedure can be repeated in an hour. After three successful and consecutive 30-minute trials, the area is usually ready to accept pressure. Athletes with pressure sores should not be allowed to compete.

Prevention

Prevention of pressure sores and skin breakdown includes regular inspection of the skin, the use of seat cushions in the everyday wheelchair, changing position frequently, proper transferring mechanics (i.e., avoidance of shear), good hygiene, adequate nutrition, and keeping the skin dry. Athletes should promptly towel dry to remove perspiration after heavy exercise, swimming, and bathing or showering.

Special Concerns for Youth and Older Adults

Children especially need to be reminded of the preventive measures that can be taken to avoid skin breakdown, such as proper hygiene, adequate nutrition, and routine visual inspections.[18] Because the skin of older adults who are physically active will be more inclined to break down, it is paramount that preventive measures be stressed with this group of participants as well.

Spasms

Spasms can occur in athletes with spinal cord lesions above L1. Spasms are caused by excessive reflex activity below the lesion level and appear as the sudden, involuntary jerk of a body part. In an able-bodied person the brain coordinates reflex activity, but in spinal paralysis impulse transmission is impaired. A spasm in a muscle group can be of sufficient force to launch an athlete out of a wheelchair. Spasms are frustrating for the athlete but have been considered good for circulation, especially for those who use wheelchairs.[7] Most people in wheelchairs get spasms, although ambulatory people with incomplete SCI can get them, too.

The stimuli that provoke spasms differ from one person to another. Three main stimuli are responsible: (1) sensory input, generally from touching hot or cold items, (2) pathology (e.g., bladder infections, skin breakdowns), and (3) menstrual period.

Signs and Symptoms

A spasm may vary in its duration and intensity but is most often a sudden, rapid, and involuntary jerking of the paralyzed limb. The strength, frequency, and duration of the spasms should be noted and compared with the athlete's norm, since this information will vary from athlete to athlete.

Referral, Diagnostic Tests, and Differential Diagnosis
Athletic trainers obtain a history regarding spasms in the PPE in order to have comparison data. During the general medical assessment, questions regarding stimuli that can cause spasms are also noted. Having a record of the athlete's baseline when problems arise is the reason a complete history is essential. For example, an athlete who reports severe or more frequent spasms might be asked about a possible bladder infection. The athlete is referred to a physician for a complete urinalysis when bladder infection is suspected. In addition, the athlete is always referred to a physician if conservative measures do not alleviate the spasms and improve the condition. Spasms can be confused with seizure disorders or spasticity.

Treatment, Prognosis, and Return to Participation
Typically no treatment is necessary for spasms, especially once the cause is addressed. However, when spasms are too severe, treatments such as stretching, drug therapy (e.g., baclofen, dantrolene, valium, diazepam), nerve blocks, and surgery are options.

Athletes usually do not need to be restricted from activity because of spasms. If the spasms are excessive for the particular athlete, then the underlying cause (e.g., bladder infection) needs to be addressed. Otherwise, spasms usually pose no medical threat to participation.

Prevention
Spasms are not inherently a negative occurrence and may not be preventable since they are associated with the reflex activity in spinal cord lesions above L1. However, because bladder infections may contribute to the intensity and frequency of spasms, avoiding such infections is critical.

Bladder Dysfunction

Athletes with SCI have a neurogenic bladder, meaning that the bladder does not always empty properly or completely, causing infections, kidney stones, and obstructions.

The athletic trainer must ask the athlete about his bladder management plan. Ideally, this is done during the PPE. Perhaps the athlete uses an indwelling catheter to drain the bladder. Athletes who use indwelling catheters usually have frequent if not constant bacteria in their urine.[11] Bacteria in the bladder can spread to the kidneys and bloodstream to cause further illness and even fatality. Athletes who use intermittent catheterization, such as self-catheterization only when the urge to urinate is sensed, are also at risk for bladder infections, although to a lesser degree than those who use indwelling catheters. The athletic trainer should be aware if timely access to appropriate facilities is a problem. These factors, as well as inadequate hydration, lead to an increased risk for urinary tract infections athletes with SCI.

Athletes with SCI also have problems with constipation and stool retention that require that they regularly follow a bowel regimen.

Signs and Symptoms
The athlete with a spinal cord injury will not sense symptoms of pain and burning as an able-bodied athlete does. Other signs and symptoms include bacteria in the urine, discolored urine (i.e., cloudy, dark), and fever. As stated previously, a bladder problem is the most common cause of autonomic dysreflexia, which can cause death (Red Flags for Bladder Dysfunction in Athletes with SCI).

> **Red Flags for Bladder Dysfunction in Athletes with SCI**
> Identify and immediately treat athletes with SCI who have bladder dysfunction because this condition can lead to autonomic dysreflexia; AD, when untreated, can cause death because of the combination of raised blood pressure and lowered heart rate.

A proper assessment includes in-depth questions regarding the bowel and bladder routine (e.g., type, frequency, hygiene), an inspection of the catheter, urinalysis, body temperature assessment, and hydration history. The athletic trainer should be aware that, while on road trips, athletes have often been known to withhold hydration, thereby avoiding the perceived hassle of bladder voiding, but arriving at the competition in a less than hydrated condition.

Referral, Diagnostic Tests, and Differential Diagnosis
As mentioned previously, urinalysis and body temperature assessment is necessary. Chapter 2 provides a description of how to take a dip-stick reading for an on-site evaluation for many properties of the urine; Table 2-4 lists the normal values for urine.

Kidney infection, kidney stones, bladder infection, urinary tract infection, contusion to ureter, bladder, and urethra, urethritis, cystitis are the differential diagnoses for bladder dysfunction.

Treatment and Return to Participation
Antibiotics are the typical treatment for bladder infections. Athletes refrain from training and competition for at least 8 hours after initiating antibiotic treatment, in addition to being free from fever for at least 24 hours.

Prevention
Athletes need to drink at least 2 liters of water a day in order to regularly flush the bladder. They should be advised to use sterile voiding techniques in order to avoid contamination during catheterization and urinary drainage. In addition, the athletic trainer creates and promotes an environment in which athletes do not feel

self-conscious about taking care of their bowel and bladder needs.

Special Concerns for Youth

Children need education and encouragement about independent care of bowel and bladder habits. Different routines (e.g., new environment, school), accidents, and odor may cause embarrassment in the young athlete.[18] In addition, this athlete may be too preoccupied with the sporting activity to adhere to a prescribed routine. This behavior adds to the risk of infection as well as embarrassment should an accident occur.

Spina Bifida

Spina bifida is a congenital spinal cord disability in which the neural tube fails to close completely during the first four to six weeks of fetal development. Subsequently, the posterior arch of one or more vertebrae does not develop properly, leaving an opening in the spinal column. It occurs most often in the low back and is more prevalent in females than males. It causes muscular weakness or paralysis below the deficit. From least to most severe, the types of spina bifida are (1) occulta, (2) meningocele, and (3) meningomyelocele. Spina bifida occulta is given its name because the defect is hidden under the skin, **occult** meaning hidden or secret. This mild form of spina bifida does not cause paralysis or muscle weakness. However, it is associated with low back pain in adults. In some people with spina bifida occulta, a birthmark, dimple, or a tuft of hair (i.e., **Faun's Beard**) will mark the occulta. Usually diagnosis is obtained incidentally by radiographs for other problems.

Meningocele is characterized by the protruding of the meninges, the spinal cord covering, through a vertebral cleft into a sac, resulting in weakness in the lower extremities (Figure 16-4).

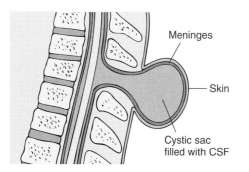

Figure 16-4 Meningocele is a form of spina bifida in which the meninges herniate through the skin between an incomplete closure in the spinal column. The resulting cyst is filled with cerebrospinal fluid but no neural tissue. (From Huether SE, McCance KL: *Understanding pathophysiology,* ed 2, St. Louis, 2000, Mosby.)

Labels in figure: Meninges; Skin; Cystic sac filled with CSF

The most common type of spina bifida is **meningo-myelocele**, also termed **myelomeningocele** (Figure 16-5, *A*). In this condition, the spinal cord and nerve roots exit through a vertebral cleft and fill a tumorous sac, causing a significant deficit below the lesion (Figure 16-5, *B*). The latter two conditions require surgical correction for spinal cord fluid leakage into the sac. Spina bifida is nonprogressive; the defect at the spine will not become worse with time.

Athletes with spina bifida experience many problems common to all forms of spinal paralysis, including bladder and bowel dysfunction, spasms, and skin lesions. However, problems are greater for children.[7] Without sensation to the lower extremities, children with meningomyelocele might not notice and report skin lesions until serious infection occurs. This is due to children's proclivity to play with abandon, disregarding seemingly mild contusions and abrasions. Children are also more likely to be wearing splints and braces than adults. The athletic trainer needs to be diligent in the visual inspection of areas covered by assistive devices. Proper fitting of assistive devices must be assured to avoid skin problems.

In addition, individuals with spina bifida often have a heightened gag reflex, which is related to the vagus nerve.[19] The exaggerated gag reflex may make swallowing pills, having the throat examined, or having a complete cranial nerve assessment more difficult for this athlete.

Cerebral Shunts

The athlete with spina bifida may have an implanted cerebral shunt to control cerebral spinal fluid that backs up into the ventricles of the brain. The shunt relieves **hydrocephalus,** the increased cerebrospinal fluid in the ventricles of the brain. One end of a tube, which has a one-way valve for outflow of fluid, is inserted into the ventricles; the other end is threaded just under the skin down to the abdomen, where fluid is then reabsorbed by blood vessels in the membranes surrounding internal organs.[7] Athletic trainers should be sure to inquire about a shunt in the PPE. Shunts typically pose no restrictions on activity except avoidance of trauma to the head such as experienced in soccer heading. Some athletes will wear an appropriate helmet or headgear for protection. A small scar may be noticed behind the ear of an athlete with spina bifida who has a shunt.

Shunts can sometimes become clogged or may malfunction. Signs and symptoms of shunt problems include headaches, vomiting, seizures, lethargy, irritability, redness along the shunt tract, and changes in personality or sport performance. The athlete with suspected shunt problems should be referred to a physician. If this athlete sustains sufficient impact to

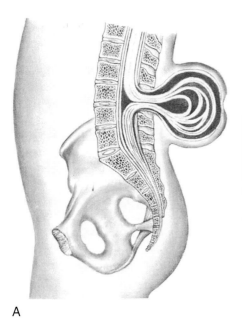

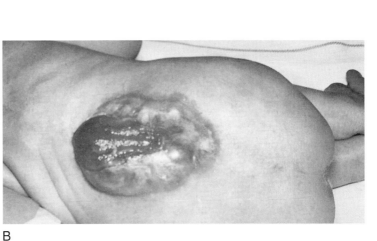

A   B

Figure 16-5 Meningomyelocele, or myelomeningocele, is a form of spina bifida that is apparent at birth. **A,** The herniation contains cerebrospinal fluid and a portion of the spinal cord. **B,** Because a portion of the spinal cord is outside the protection of the body and vertebral column, it is susceptible to continuous damage and immediate surgery is required to repair the defect. There are typically profound neurological repercussions associated with this defect. (From Seidel HM, Ball JW, Dains JE, Bendeict GW: *Mosby's guide to physical examination*, ed 5, St. Louis, 2003, Mosby, Figure 20-73, p 761.)

cause a laceration to the skin overlying the shunt, referral to a neurosurgeon should occur immediately. [2]

Latex Allergy

Athletes with spina bifida have a higher incidence of latex allergy (Red Flags for Latex Allergies). Latex

> **⚑ Red Flags for Latex Allergies**
>
> Signs and symptoms of latex allergies include the following:
> - Sneezing or runny nose
> - Itchy, red, watery eyes
> - Coughing
> - Rash or hives
> - Shock
> - Chest tightness and shortness of breath
> - Change in voice or hoarseness
> - Difficulty breathing

products such as gloves, stretch bands or rubber tubing, adhesive bandages and tape, and rescue breathing masks should never come into contact with athletes with spina bifida. The athletic trainer needs to have nonlatex substitutes available when working with athletes with spina bifida. It is wise to have substitutes on-hand for the general athlete population since latex allergies can exist in any athlete. While most reactions are mild, some persons may have a life-threatening reaction to latex.

Treatment for severe reactions includes use of a prescription epinephrine-injecting pen (Epi-pen). The method for administration of the Epi-pen is discussed in Chapter 3. Because the best method is prevention,

the use of nonlatex products on athletes known to have this allergen is crucial. An allergist can conduct testing to confirm the allergy.

Poliomyelitis

Poliomyelitis, or polio, is a form of paralysis caused by a viral infection that affects motor cells of the spinal cord. Sensation, as well as bowel and bladder control, is not affected in the athlete with polio. The severity and degree of paralysis depends on the number and location of the motor cells destroyed by the virus. Because of the widespread use of the Salk vaccine developed in the 1950s, occurrence of polio is rare in school-aged athletes. However, in third world countries, polio continues to cause paralysis. Worldwide, about 5 million new cases appear each year.[7]

Many people who have previously had polio have experienced a recurrence of many of the symptoms of polio later in life. These symptoms include new muscle and joint pain, muscle weakness at old and new sites, severe fatigue, profound sensitivity to cold, and new respiratory problems.[7] This combination of symptoms, known as **post-polio syndrome,** affects 23% of persons who have previously had polio, usually 35 to 40 years after the original onset.[20]

Polio is similar to SCI and spina bifida in that muscles are paralyzed. However, because the virus does not attack sensory nerve fibers, sensation is intact. The paralysis is often incomplete, which makes judging the level of lesion difficult.[7] Therefore, a complete assessment of functional abilities should be conducted during the PPE.

Other than the possible presence of post-polio syndrome, few general medical conditions are unique to these athletes. The overall general medical assessment process is facilitated in this group of athletes since they have sensation and can detect pain.

Cerebral Palsy

Cerebral palsy (CP) is a chronic neurological disorder caused by a lesion in the brain that affects movement and posture. CP occurs before, at, or soon after birth and is not hereditary or progressive. CP affects the ability to move and maintain balance and posture because of the damage to the areas of the brain that control muscle tone and spinal reflexes. The disorder varies from mild, evidenced by general clumsiness and a slight limp, to severe, in which the affected individual is dominated by reflexes, unable to ambulate without a motorized chair, and nonverbal.

The United States Cerebral Palsy Athletic Association uses a classification system based on an individual athlete's functional ability. This system also includes athletes with other conditions characterized by nonprogressive brain lesions. Neurotrauma such as stroke and traumatic brain injury are included in the classification, since many paralympic sports use a functional classification system across disabilities rather than isolated competition within disabilities. The system is controversial but was designed to allow for the grouping of athletes with similar abilities to compete within specific categories.

Some individuals with CP will have associated conditions such as deafness, vision disturbances, impaired hand-eye coordination, and mental retardation. These factors influence the risk of injury but not necessarily illness in the athlete with CP. Because the affliction can be complicated by other impairments, communication with the athlete with CP is critical (Key Points—Communication Considerations).

KEY POINTS
Communication Considerations

Communication considerations with an athlete who has Cerebral Palsy include the following:
- Be patient and allow the athlete enough time to communicate; speech may be very slow or difficult to understand.
- Position the athlete carefully during assessment because incorrect positioning on a treatment table can elicit abnormal reflexes that will interfere with movement.
- Use word boards or other visual aids related to the general medical condition.
- Avoid ballistic movements during assessment; move the athlete's body parts slowly to avoid increased muscle tone or abnormal reflexive responses.

CP is characterized by spasticity, athetosis, or ataxia. Athletes may present with decreased musculotendinous flexibility, decreased strength, and considerable muscle imbalance. Flexibility is the most important fitness goal in the athlete with CP.

Spasticity

Spasticity, the most common type of CP, is characterized by hypertonic muscle tone during voluntary movement. Typically, the flexor muscles are stronger than extensor muscles. Associated with spasticity is an exaggerated myotatic reflex. This reflex normally serves as a protective mechanism, but in athletes with an exaggerated myotatic reflex, mild stretching may evoke a heightened response varying from a mild recoil to a violent withdrawal of the limb. In some athletes, this reflex is so disruptive that they strap their limbs down. It is important for athletes with CP to start stretching after a period of warm-up. This stretching is slow and sustained to prevent activation of the myotatic reflex.

Athletes who are ambulatory may walk with a scissors gait which is characterized by a pigeon-toed walk caused by extreme tightness of the hip flexors, adductors, and internal rotators. The knee flexors and ankle plantar flexors are also abnormally tight causing the knees to be bent when walking, and the athlete to walk on his or her toes. The athletic trainer needs to be aware that spasticity increases with stress and fatigue.

Athetoid Cerebral Palsy

Athetosis, the second most common type of motor disorder, is characterized by constant, purposeless, and unpredictable movement that is caused by fluctuating muscle tone. Fluctuating muscle tone occurs when muscles are hypertonic and are periodically hypotonic. This causes characteristics of drooling, lack of head control (i.e., rolling from side to side), and troubles with speaking, eating, and writing. Most individuals with athetosis are tetraplegic; some use wheelchairs and others walk with an unsteady gait. Signs and symptoms of athetosis increase with stress and fatigue.

Ataxic Cerebral Palsy

Ataxia can result from disorders to the spinal cord as well as the brain. It varies from mild to severe and occurs in approximately 10% of persons who have CP. It is diagnosed only in individuals who can walk unaided. Athletes with ataxia have balance and coordination disturbances. This athlete can usually maintain balance when eyes are open but not when they are closed. Walking on uneven ground, managing stairs, and stepping over objects pose problems for athletes with CP.

Seizures

Seizure control is a common medical issue in athletes with CP. Seizures should be identified at the PPE and then carefully monitored on an ongoing basis. The sports medicine team should be especially familiar with the different options available for anti-seizure medication as well as the potential side effects. Side effects include impaired attention span, ataxia, nystagmus, strabismus, and cognitive impairment. Seizure medications are chosen for an individual based on type of seizures. Because no one drug controls all types of seizures, athletes with CP may be on different medications, and some may require a combination of seizure medications to achieve good seizure control. Carbamazepine is recommended for this athletic population because its side effects are believed to have less likelihood of affecting athletic performance.[21] Seizures during aerobic activity are rare, but that does not preclude caution. Compliance with medication is extremely important. Therefore, medications are kept on the athlete's person so that doses are not missed. During competition that involves travel, athletic trainers need to prompt athletes to take medications at the correct times, because travel often disrupts routines, making many athletes more likely to forget doses. Also, the athletic trainer should be aware when athletes have had their anti-seizure medications adjusted. The athlete, physician, and athletic trainer work together to set up the most appropriate seizure control plan.

Pathological Reflexes

In infants, the involuntary, predictable muscle and postural tone shifts that occur are normal and considered important for development. However, reflexes that are not integrated at the developmentally appropriate times become pathological and affect the smoothness and coordination of movement. These reflexes can be elicited spontaneously or by an external stimulus.

CP patients have a high incidence of exhibiting these pathological reflexes. During an assessment the athletic trainer should be aware of what reflexes the athlete has not integrated so that the athlete can be positioned in a manner so as not to elicit the reflex which may interfere with the examination. Although a comprehensive discussion of the over 25 primitive reflexes that might be present in this population is beyond the scope of this chapter, a few are presented in Box 16-6.

Athletic trainers need to remember that these reflexes are involuntary motions or postures, and although they are not painful, they can compromise certain body positions. Communication with the athlete can be enhanced by understanding the reflexes and working around the stimuli that elicit them.

Box 16-6   Problematic Reflexes in the Athlete with Cerebral Palsy

Four reflexes are considered troublesome because they are initiated by head movements:

- *TLR-prone* (tonic labyrinthine reflex–prone): This reflex is characterized by an increased flexor tone elicited by a change in position of the head. When gravity acts to pull the head downward and the total body responds by assuming a flexion posture, this is evidence of the TLR-prone.
- *TLR-supine* (tonic labyrinthine reflex–supine): In contrast to the TLR-prone, this reflex is characterized by an increased extensor tone in response to any change in head position. If the head is thrown backward and the total body responds in an extension posture, this is evidence of the TLR-supine.
- *ATNR* (asymmetrical tonic neck reflex): This reflex is also known as the fencing reflex since when activated, the upper extremity assumes an "on-guard" position. Rotation or lateral flexion of the neck cause obligatory extension of the arm on the face side and simultaneous flexion on the non-face side. Positioning in front of the athlete prior to addressing him (to avoid head turning) will reduce the chance of eliciting this reflex.
- *STNR* (symmetrical tonic neck reflex): This reflex is characterized by bilateral arm and leg responses to up and down head movements. Head flexion causes flexor tone of the upper body and extensor tone of the lower body; head extension elicits the opposite. Positioning at eye level with the athlete will aid in reducing the chance of eliciting this reflex.

Amputations

Prostheses and orthoses are typically used by individuals with limb amputations. Sports governing bodies have rules that allow or disallow athletes to participate with prosthetic devices. Currently, the National Federation of State High School Associations allows athletes to wear these devices in many sports, including football, wrestling, soccer, and baseball. Factors considered in their use include the type of amputation and prosthesis, the potential harm to other players, and the question of an unfair advantage for the athlete because of the prosthetic device. Extremity prostheses can allow an athlete full range of motion for competitive success in a variety of sports, including basketball and throwing sports (Figure 16-6, *A* and *B*).

Track and field and swimming events are the most popular for athletes with amputations. The rules for individual events are the same as for able-bodied competition. The athletes may use prostheses, but no other assistive device is allowed. Prosthesis use is optional in most events but is not permitted in the high jump. The athletic trainer is aware that balance may be adversely affected in athletes with amputations because of the alterations in their center of gravity. Athletes with double amputations compete in wheelchair tennis or basketball events.

Congenital or acquired disorders may necessitate limb amputation. Common indications for amputation include a necrotic extremity associated with peripheral

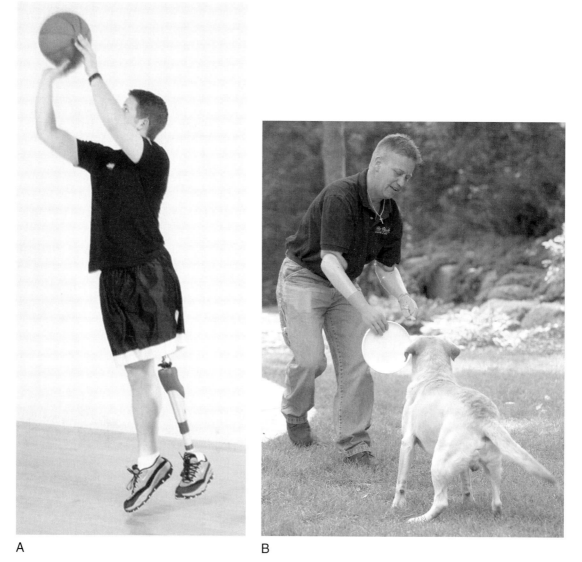

A   B

Figure 16-6 Examples of extremity prostheses. **A,** The C-leg in Action provides stability and ease of motion to the athlete during basketball practice. **B,** Using both body-powered and myoelectric technology support effective upper extremity function. (Courtesy Otto Bock HealthCare, Minneapolis, MN.)

vascular diseases or diabetes; life-threatening emergency conditions related to cancer or infection; and congenital deformity or injuries to the brachial plexus, which cause the arm to be insensate and are sometimes deemed a "nuisance extremity."[22]

Individuals who have had amputations can continue to participate in sporting events despite loss of one or both of the upper or lower extremities. Amputations are categorized by location and number for identification in sport classifications (Box 16-7). The primary medical problems seen in athletes who have had amputations are skin breakdown and phantom leg pain.

Skin Breakdown

This athlete is generally aware of skin irritation or breakdown when it begins. Prevention includes ensuring

that the prosthesis fits properly. An excessively loose or tight fit will increase stress at the junction. Prostheses can increase local skin pressure and contribute to abrasions, blisters, and rashes. Various materials, such as gels, soft materials, and foam padding, have been used

Box 16-7   Amputation Categories
Amputation categories describe location and number when used for sporting event classifications: <ul><li>(A1) AK (above-the-knee) double</li><li>(A2) AK single</li><li>(A3) BK (below-the-knee) double</li><li>(A4) BK single</li><li>(A5) AE (above-the-elbow) double</li><li>(A6) AE single</li><li>(A7) BE (below-the-elbow) double</li><li>(A8) BE single</li><li>(A9) Combined lower and upper limb</li></ul>

Chapter 16   Special Populations   407

between the skin and the socket to reduce the stress from vigorous athletic activity. Cleaning and thoroughly drying the stump and changing the padding that has become moist because of perspiration is warranted. If skin breakdown is in an advanced state, the athlete may have to temporarily discontinue use of the prosthesis and reduce athletic participation. An athlete participating in wheelchair sports does not have to discontinue play.

Younger athletes with amputations have special needs because their appliances are small and require frequent adjustments to accommodate for growth. However, skin breakdown is less frequent at younger ages.

Phantom Pain Syndrome

Phantom pain syndrome, or pain that seems to come from the amputated body part, is more common in adults than children. It can range from mild to severe. For severe pain, antidepressants have be used to provide relief. In the nonathletic population, narcotics have also been prescribed. Any person using narcotics for phantom pain needs to consult a physician before entering an exercise program.[23]

Sensory Disabilities

Athletes with sensory disabilities make up a unique segment of the athletic population. The general treatment of illness and sport-related injuries in athletes with sensory disabilities is similar to treatment for other athletes. The only special concern is in regard to communication.[22] The medical team should be prepared to find alternative methods of delivering and obtaining information. In each of the following sections, recommendations for communication will be presented. Sensory disability in this chapter refers to visual impairments and blindness, as well as deafness and hardness of hearing.

Visual Impairments and Blindness

Athletes with visual impairments have a range of visual acuity from legal blindness with partial sight to total blindness. Athletes with visual impairments compete and excel in a variety of sports, such as track and field events (Figure 16-7), wrestling, swimming, tandem cycling, power lifting, goal ball, judo, gymnastics, skiing, baseball, and golf. Participation may be facilitated by the use of assistive technology such as Joint Optical Reflective Display (Jordy 2), sighted guides (Figure 16-8), step or stroke counting, a tether or guide wire, or a sound source, depending on the degree of visual impairment. Table 16-2 lists the classification system for sport competition utilized by the United States Association of Blind Athletes.

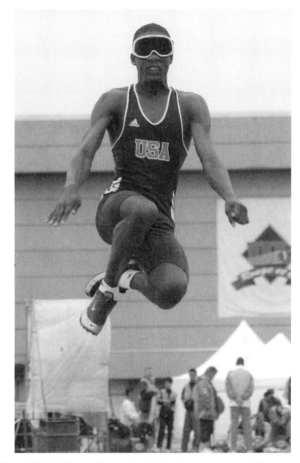

Figure 16-9 Athletes who are visually impaired can successfully compete in a wide range of high-level athletic events, as evidenced by this college-age high jumper. (Courtesy U.S. Association of Blind Athletes and photographer, Yverick Rangom.)

The cause of the athlete's blindness should be noted. Blindness can be caused by birth defects, including congenital cataracts and optic nerve disease. Excessive oxygen in incubation in babies born in the 1950s was a common cause but has decreased. Other causes include tumors, albinism, injuries, and infectious diseases. In older participants, common causes of blindness are diabetes, macular degeneration, glaucoma, and cataracts.

During the PPE the useful vision of the athlete is determined. About 80% to 90% of people who are blind have some residual vision.[7,23] Residual vision can be ascertained by questioning the athlete in-depth about what he or she sees, in addition to conducting a visual acuity examination. The athletic trainer must also be sensitive to the fact that lighting in the clinic or athletic training room may affect the athlete's ability to see. The athletic trainer should determine at what age this athlete became visually impaired and if loss of sight was congenital or occurred later in life.

Overall, there are few special concerns in sports medicine regarding the athlete with a visual impairment. First and foremost is the issue of communication. It is up to the athletic trainer to effectively

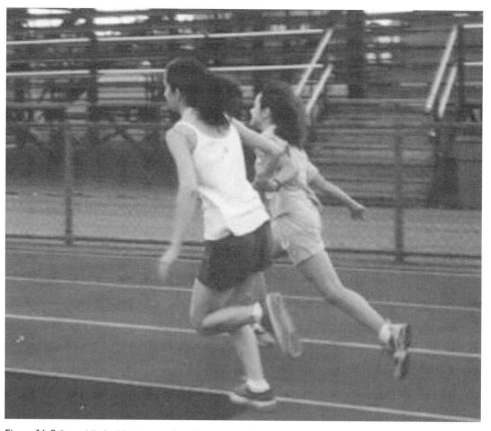

Figure 16-8 Some blind athletes appreciate the support of a sighted guide during practice workouts.

Table 16-2	USABA Visual Classification System for Sport Competition

Level	Characteristics
B1	No light perception in either eye up to light perception but inability to recognize the shape of a hand at any distance or in any direction
B2	From ability to recognize the shape of a hand up to visual acuity of 20/600 and/or a visual field of less than 5 degrees in the best eye with the best practical eye correction
B3	From visual acuity above 20/600 and up to visual acuity of 20/200 and/or a visual field of less than 20 degrees and more than 5 degrees in the best eye with the best practical eye correction
B4	From visual acuity above 20/200 and up to visual acuity of 20/70 and a visual field larger than 20 degrees in the best eye with the best practical eye correction.

From U.S. Association of Blind Athletes: U.S. Association of Blind Athletes (USABA) visual classification. Available at http://www.usaba.org/.

KEY POINTS
Communication Considerations

Communication considerations with an athlete who is visually-impaired include the following:
- Always start an interaction by stating your name, "James, hi. It's Jessica and I'm going to discuss your symptoms with you." Do not expect the athlete to recognize you by the sound of your voice.
- Ask the athlete if assistance is needed with mobility. Do not grab the athlete's arm but rather offer an upper arm; allow the athlete to grasp it.
- Provide the athlete with verbal cues that indicate changes in surface, location of the examining table, doors to be opened in or out, stepping up or down.
- Use tactile sense when performing an assessment; allow the athlete to follow the examiner's hands through the evaluation.
- Demonstrate a maneuver within the athlete's field of vision.
- Enhance visual cues: conduct assessment in a brightly lit area and use colored instruments or materials that contrast with the background (e.g., brightly colored stethoscopes and reflex hammers, colored tape around edges of furniture or doorways).
- Understand that athletes who have albinism and glaucoma can better distinguish solid-colored objects under nonglare lights and away from glare from sunlight.
- Ask the athlete's preference when providing material that is usually in a written format, such as treatment instructions or medical staff contact information; ask what works best—large print, Braille, audio tapes, or computer software–based files.
- Keep the examination and treatment areas free of clutter and low-hanging objects.

communicate information to the athlete, especially since so much of the general assessment is gained through the preparticipation history. Good documentation will help the athletic trainer and coaches provide a positive athletic experience and can be obtained through a variety of communication modes (Key Points—Communication Considerations).

Some individuals who are blind often exhibit blindisms, repetitive movements such as rocking, hand waving, finger flicking, or digging the fingers into the eyes. There is no inherent harm in displaying blindisms other than social stigma. Many parents, teachers, and coaches have worked with children who are blind to stop these movements in certain situations. Postural deviations, such as the forward head and slumping, may also be prevalent, especially in those athletes who are congenitally blind and have never seen others sit, stand, and move. Most experienced adult athletes develop proper posture through cueing and physical activity. Some novice athletes with visual impairments may exhibit poor balance, fewer social skills, and low cardiovascular fitness.

Documentation of illness and other general medical conditions in athletes who are visually impaired is extremely limited. Musculoskeletal injury data show that these athletes have a high proportion of lower extremity injuries. Athletes with visual impairments expend more energy than matched sighted athletes and therefore are more likely to fatigue quickly. This could be an important consideration when determining return-to-play guidelines after illness.

Albinism

Albinism is characterized by a lack of pigment in the iris and throughout the body. Eyes are sensitive to light. Therefore, the athlete with albinism may need to wear tinted glasses inside and outside to help reduce glare. **Nystagmus** may also be present and should be noted in the PPE. Because athletes with albinism are more susceptible to sunburn, the athlete who exercises outdoors, even in overcast or cool weather, should generously and repetitively use sunscreen. Hats or visors and long-sleeved shirts are also advised.

Glaucoma

Glaucoma is an increase in pressure in the globe of the eye caused by inability of the intraocular fluid to properly drain. This excess pressure damages the optic nerve. Visual loss may be gradual, sudden, or present at birth. An early sign of glaucoma is reports of lights that appear to have halos around them. Athletes with glaucoma must avoid isometric activities, swimming under water, inverted body positions, excess fluid intake, use of antihistamines, and other practices that could increase eye pressure.[7] Athletes with glaucoma may also need to use moistening eye drops.

Deafness and Hard of Hearing

In the United States, deaf persons do not consider themselves disabled but rather members of a subculture of American society. Person-first terminology, discussed at the beginning of this chapter, is not supported by these athletes. The preferred terminology is "Deaf," with an uppercase D. Hearing loss is a general term that describes people who are hard of hearing or deaf. Hard of hearing is defined as a condition that makes understanding speech difficult through use of the ears alone, with or without a hearing aid. The term previously used for hard of hearing was hearing impaired. Deaf is a condition in which a person is unable to understand speech through the use of the ears alone, with or without a hearing aid.[23] Hearing loss can range from mild to profound and is classified as one of three types: conductive, sensorineural, and mixed.

In conductive hearing loss, sound does not pass through the external and middle ear to reach the inner ear. Buildup of impacted wax, injury, or infection in the external ear can cause conductive loss. See Chapter 10 for other conditions related to temporary hearing loss.

Sensorineural loss is more serious and involves the inner ear, where sensory receptors convert sound waves into neural impulses that are transmitted to the brain for translation. Most people who are born deaf have this type of loss. Causes of this type of loss are generally idiopathic. Others identified include hereditary factors, meningitis, measles, scarlet fever, mumps, and encephalitis. Balance problems sometimes accompany this type of loss.

The mixed type of loss is a combination of conductive and sensorineural losses. It is more common in seniors, and thus might not be seen as frequently in the athletic population as the other types of losses.

Communication is the primary factor related to the care of Deaf athletes and needs to be addressed during the PPE (Box 16-8). It is up to the practitioner to find alternative techniques for communication (Key Points—Communication Considerations). One method of communication relatively easy for medical personnel

---

Box 16-8 | Special Considerations During the Preparticipation Exams of Athletes Who are Hearing Impaired or Deaf

In addition to the standard preparticipation exam, ask the following questions of athletes who are hearing-impaired or Deaf:
- Has the hearing loss progressed? Has it worsened, stayed the same, improved with aids?
- At what age did the loss occur?
- What method of communication does the athlete prefer (e.g., sign language, speech reading)?
- Does the athlete use hearing aids or have cochlear implants?
- Does the athlete use ear plugs during swimming and water activities?
- Does the athlete have a history of ear infections?
- Is the hearing loss related to or accompanied by balance problems or vertigo?

KEY POINTS
Communication Considerations

Communication considerations with a Deaf athlete include the following:
- Maintain eye contact and face the athlete in order to facilitate speech or lip reading; even the best speech readers will understand only about 30% of what is said.
- Speak normally if the athlete uses a hearing aid.
- Use facial expressions, body language, gestures, and common signs such as thumbs up or down for OK and not OK.
- Demonstrate any technique before performing it on an athlete.
- Use video, computer movie files, or other visual media as another form of demonstration.
- Use visual and tactile cues.
- Learn basic American Sign Language.
- Orient the athlete to all aspects of the facility, with special attention to exits and fire evacuation procedures.
- Do not pretend to understand the athlete if speech is unclear to you; instead, ask for repeats.
- Use strobe fire alarms or other visual alerting devices in the facility so that the athlete has notification in the case of an emergency; point out these systems to the athlete.
- Loud or constant music or background noise, even at low levels, reduces hearing aid effectiveness and may even cause the athlete to develop headaches.
- Avoid "visual noise" such as extra physical or visual movements behind a person who is speaking.

to learn is American Sign Language. Although there are shortcuts to certain words and phrases, the simple alphabet can be articulated by hand signs, and is depicted in Figure 16-9.

Hearing Aids and Implants

A variety of hearing aids exist for the Deaf. Hearing aids do not clarify or make speech sound clearer; they simply amplify sound. The four basic types of hearing aids worn are as follows: (1) on the chest or body, (2) behind the ear, (3) in the ear, and (4) on the eyeglasses.

Cochlear implants are recommended for those individuals for whom a hearing aid is not helpful. The implants are surgically placed in the inner ear and are activated by an external speech processor worn on a belt or in a pocket. A microphone is worn as a headpiece externally behind the ear. Sound is translated by the speech processor into distinctive electrical signals that travel up a thin cable to the headpiece and are transmitted across the skin via radio waves to the implanted electrodes in the cochlea. The auditory nerve is stimulated, and information is transmitted to the brain where it is interpreted (Figure 16-10). Some newer models do not have external wires. The external apparatus should be removed during exercise to reduce the chance of electrostatic discharge.[23] Athletes with cochlear implants must also stay away from plastic mats, balls, and equipment to prevent electrostatic discharge that can damage the electrodes.

Once communication barriers, type and care of hearing aids or implants, and any related conditions (e.g., balance problems, ear infections) have been addressed, the general medical assessment will not be any different than for an athlete who is not deaf or hard-of-hearing.

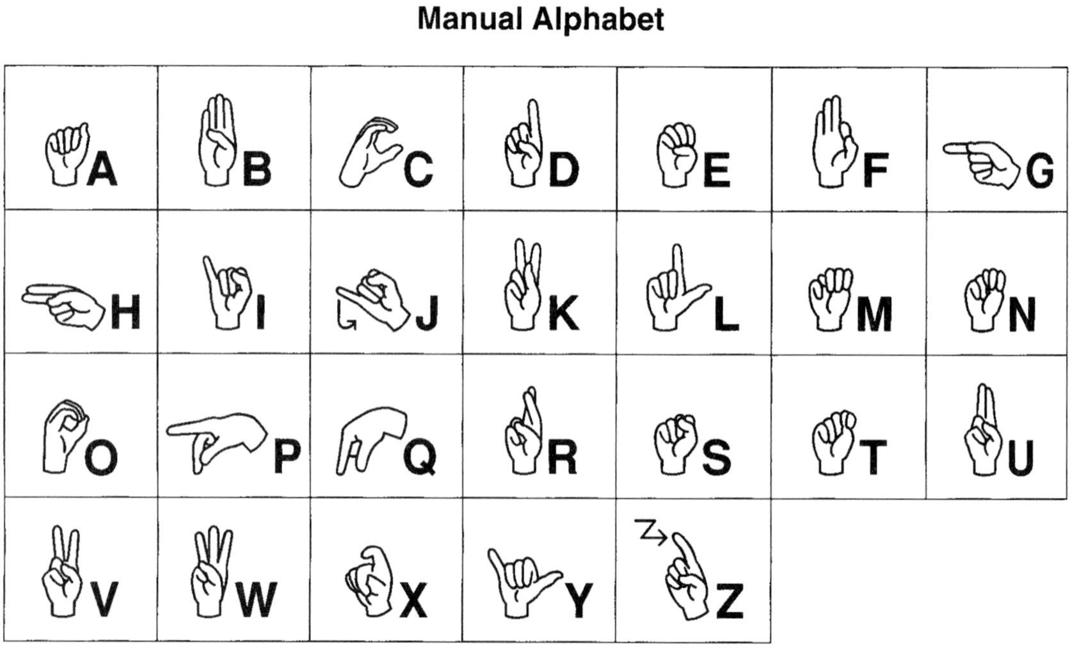

Manual Alphabet

Figure 16-9 The ASL alphabet can be used to communicate effectively with Deaf athletes. ASL has short cuts and abbreviations for words or phrases that facilitate communication, but this alphabet shows the basis for the language. *ASL,* American Sign Language. (From *Mosby's medical, nursing, and allied health dictionary,* ed 6, St. Louis, 2002, Mosby.)

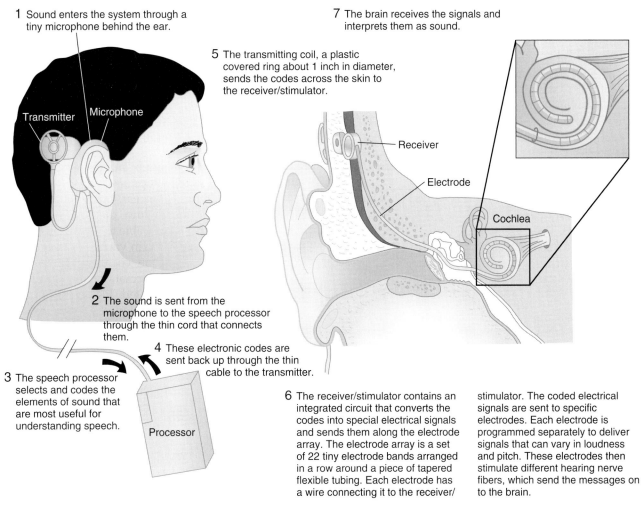

1 Sound enters the system through a tiny microphone behind the ear.

7 The brain receives the signals and interprets them as sound.

5 The transmitting coil, a plastic covered ring about 1 inch in diameter, sends the codes across the skin to the receiver/stimulator.

Transmitter   Microphone

Receiver

Electrode

Cochlea

2 The sound is sent from the microphone to the speech processor through the thin cord that connects them.

4 These electronic codes are sent back up through the thin cable to the transmitter.

3 The speech processor selects and codes the elements of sound that are most useful for understanding speech.

Processor

6 The receiver/stimulator contains an integrated circuit that converts the codes into special electrical signals and sends them along the electrode array. The electrode array is a set of 22 tiny electrode bands arranged in a row around a piece of tapered flexible tubing. Each electrode has a wire connecting it to the receiver/ stimulator. The coded electrical signals are sent to specific electrodes. Each electrode is programmed separately to deliver signals that can vary in loudness and pitch. These electrodes then stimulate different hearing nerve fibers, which send the messages on to the brain.

Figure 16-10 A cochlear implant can restore hearing through electronic assistive devices, which include an external processor, transmitter, and microphone that transmits sound to an implanted receiver/stimulator and electrode to stimulate various hearing nerve fibers in the cochlea. (From Black JM, Hawks JH: *Medical-surgical nursing: clinical management for positive outcomes*, ed 7, St. Louis, 2005, Saunders.)

Intellectual Disabilities

Intellectual disabilities were formerly called mental retardation in the United States. Intellectual disabilities have become one of the best known disabilities because the Special Olympics gives it extensive visibility.[7] Athletes with intellectual disabilities compete in over 15 different sports, such as aquatics, basketball, gymnastics, figure skating, and alpine skiing. Special Olympics competition was begun in 1968 by Eunice Kennedy Shriver as a means for awareness, attitude change, and equal opportunity. It is the premier sports event for persons with intellectual disabilities.

The American Association on Mental Retardation in 2002 defined an **intellectual disability** as "a disability characterized by significant limitations both in intellectual functioning and in adaptive behavior as expressed in conceptual, social, and practical skills. This disability originates before age 18." Intellectual disabilities can be subdivided into the following levels

of severity according to the intelligent quotient (IQ) scale: mild (IQ 52-70), moderate (IQ 36-51), severe (IQ 20-35), and profound (19 and lower). Note that the average IQ is 100. Approximately 90% of all individuals classified with intellectual disabilities fall into the mild classification, 5% into the moderate, 3.5% severe, and 1.5% profound.[24]

Clearly, athletic trainers will most likely be serving athletes who fall into the mild category. In general, these individuals will function academically between the third and sixth grades.[7] Terminology and directions used in the assessment of athletes with intellectual disabilities need to be very clear and concise. Athletic trainers should provide ample time for athletes to familiarize with the treatment or athletic training facility. Demonstrating the task first is best accompanied by simple, one-step instructions reinforced to the athlete verbally and continually. Athletes should be asked to repeat instructions to ensure that they understand.

Down syndrome is the most common chromosomal abnormality that causes intellectual disability. It is an autosomal chromosomal condition that results in a whole host of medical concerns in addition to those seen in other athletes with intellectual disabilities (Box 16-9).

Individuals with intellectual disabilities vary so widely on abilities and medical issues that generalizations are difficult. Assessment during the PPE is the best method of determining normative values per athlete. Maximal heart rates of persons with intellectual disabilities are 8% to 20% lower than expected. They exhibit maximal heart rates of 10 to 15 contractions/min below expected levels, and people with Down syndrome have even lower maximal heart rates (e.g., approximately 30-35 contractions/min below expected levels). In the general population, individuals with cognitive disorders have lower fitness levels than those without intellectual disabilities.

Associated Medical Concerns

Documented medical concerns that are associated with intellectual disabilities include seizures, pain insensitivity, and medication use. Seizures occur in approximately 20% of individuals with mild intellectual disabilities. The PPE should include inquiries about seizure control methods and medications. Approximately 25% of individuals with intellectual disabilities show signs of pain insensitivity or indifference that place them at serious medical risk.[25] Reports have documented individuals with intellectual disabilities who have died from appendicitis and bowel obstruction that went undiagnosed because no indication of pain was given.[7] The athletic trainer needs to carefully check for signs of trauma and not rely exclusively on what the athlete reports (Red Flags for Pain).

Red Flags for Pain

Athletes who are intellectually disabled may have insensitivity or indifference to pain or may not be able to articulate the severity of pain they are experiencing. It is essential that the athletic trainer thoroughly evaluate for signs of trauma or illness if there is cause to believe something is wrong.

Box 16-9   Medical Conditions Associated with Down Syndrome

The following medical conditions are associated with Down syndrome:
- Atlantoaxial instability
- Balance deficits
- Obesity
- Poor hand-eye coordination
- Postural or orthopedic posture problems (e.g., kyphosis, club foot, lordosis)
- Vision concerns (e.g., strabismus, nystagmus, cataracts)
- Cardiac concerns (e.g., ventricular septal defect, atrioventricular canal defect, mitral valve prolapse)

Anticonvulsive, hypnotic, neuroleptic, and antidepressant medications are commonly used in this population. Hypothyroidism is common in persons with Down syndrome, and many of these athletes may be on thyroxine replacement therapy. Side effects of some of these hypothyroidism medications can cause angina until a stable dose has been determined.[23]

Atlantoaxial Instability

Atlantoaxial instability is laxity in the ligaments and muscles that surround the first and second cervical vertebrae. Because approximately 17% of persons with Down syndrome have atlantoaxial instability,[23] the Special Olympics requires radiographic results to confirm the condition.

The full participation of the medical team in completing a thorough PPE that screens for the above health problems is paramount. An athlete with Down syndrome should have the presence of atlantoaxial instability ruled out before unrestricted participation in sport is approved. Without medical clearance

---

WEB RESOURCES

United States Association of Blind Athletes (USABA)
   http://www.usaba.org/

International Blind Sports Federation
   http://www.ibsa.es/

Wheelchair Sports USA (WSUSA)
   http://www.wsusa.org/wsusa/

American Athletic Association for the Deaf (AAAD)
   http://www.usadsf.org/

United States Cerebral Palsy Athletic Association (USCPAA)
   http://www.cpalsy.baikal.ru/lifestyle/sport/uscpaa.html

Special Olympics (SO)
   http://www.specialolympics.org/Special+Olympics+Public+Website/default.htm

Disabled Sports USA (DSUSA)
   http://www.dsusa.org/

Paralympics
   http://www.usparalympics.org/

National Wheelchair Basketball Association (NWBA)
   http://www.nwba.org/index.php

International Tennis Federation (wheelchair division)
   http://www.itfwheelchairtennis.com/

Amputee Online Magazine
   http://www.amputee-online.com/

Amputees in Motion
   http://www.amputeesinmotion.com/

Sports n' Spokes Magazine
   http://www.pvamagazines.com/sns/

Cerebral Palsy–International Sport and Recreation Association
   http://www.cpisra.org/

National Federation of High Schools Association
   http://www.nfhs.org

American Association on Mental Retardation
   http://www.aamr.org

on file, athletes with Down syndrome are restricted from participating in gymnastics, diving, butterfly stroke and diving starts in swimming, high jump, penthathalon, soccer, and warm-up exercises, which place pressure on the head and neck muscles.[7]

SUMMARY

Although athletes with disabilities do not have a higher incidence of general medical conditions than their able-bodied counterparts, they do present with some unique conditions that the athletic trainer must be prepared to recognize through assessment. Athletes with spinal cord injury are susceptible to autonomic dysreflexia, thermoregulatory problems, bowel and bladder complications, spasms, and skin breakdown. In addition, athletes with spina bifida may have latex allergies.

The athletic and medical teams need to be creative and committed when communicating with athletes who are sensory impaired whether they are Deaf, hard of hearing, visually impaired, or blind. Knowing the common limitations associated with each disability can enable the athletic trainer to be prepared to provide quality care to these athletes.

Appreciating the critical importance of a thorough PPE enables the athletic trainer to discover possible future problems and address them before they arise. The PPE is the most powerful tool team members have in managing the sports health care of the athlete with a disability. Each athlete presents with unique characteristics, and baseline measurements are imperative.

REFERENCES

1. Ferrara M, Buckley W: Athletes with disabilities injury registrar. *Adapted Physical Activity Quarterly,* 13:50-60, 1996.
2. Patel D, Greydanus D: The pediatric athlete with disabilities. *Pediatric Clinics of North America* 49:803-827, 2002.
3. Boyajian-O'Neill L, Cardone D, Dexter W, et al: The prepartcipation examination for the athlete with special needs. *The Physician and Sportsmedicine* 32(9):13-19, 42, 2004.
4. Ferrara M, Buckley W: Epidemiology of sports related injuries for athletes with disability. *Athletic Therapy Today* 2(1):30-33, 1997.
5. Jacob T, Hurtzler Y: Sports-medical assessment for athletes with a disability. *Disability rehabilitation* 20:116-119, 1998.
6. Dec K, Sparrow K, McKeag D: The physically-challenged athlete: medical issues and assessment. *Sports Medicine* 29(4):245-258, 2000.
7. Sherrill C: *Adapted physical activity, recreation and sport: cross disciplinary and lifespan,* ed 5. Dubuque, 1998, McGraw-Hill.
8. Peck D, McKeag D: Athletes with disabilities: removing the barriers. *Physician and sportsmedicine* 2(4):59-62, 1994.
9. Stopka C: Sports medical concerns for conditioning athletes with disabilities. *Strength and conditioning* 20(1): 24-31, 1998.
10. Hopman M, Binkhourst R: Spinal cord injury and exercise in the heat. *Sports Science Exercise* 10:1-4, 1997.
11. Curtis K: Prevention and treatment of wheelchair athletic injuries. *Athletic Therapy Today* 2(1):19-25, 1997.
12. Prentice W: *Arnheim's Principles of Athletic Training,* ed 11, Boston, 2002, McGraw-Hill.
13. Bloomquist L: Injuries to athletes with physical disabilities: prevention implications. *The Physician and Sports Medicine* 14(9):97-105, 1986.
14. Armstrong L, Maresh C, Riebe D, et al: Local cooling in wheelchair athletes during exercise-heat stress. *Medicine and Science in Sports and Exercise* 27:211-216, 1995.
15. Casa D, Almsquist J, Anderson S: Inter-Association task force statement on exertional heat illnesses consensus statement. *NATA News* June 2003:24-29, 2003.
16. Binkley H, Beckett J, Casa D, et al: National Athletic Trainers' Association position statement: exertional heat illness. *Journal of Athletic Training* 37(3):329-343, 2002.
17. Madorsky J, Curtis K: Wheelchair sports medicine. *American Journal of Sports Medicine* 12(2):128-132, 1984.
18. Patel D, Roth A: Pediatric athletes with physical disabilities. *Athletic Therapy Today* 9(2):16-19, 2004.
19. Coutts K, McKenzie D, Loock C, et al: Upper body exercise capacity in youth with spina bifida. *Adapted Physical Activity Quarterly* 10:22-28, 1993.
20. Winnick J: *Adapted Physical Education and Sport,* ed 3, Champaign, IL, 200, Human Kinetics.
21. Ferrara M, Richter K, Kaschalk S: Sport for the athlete with a physical disability. In Scuderi G, McCann B, Bruno P, eds, *Sports medicine: principles of primary care.* Saint Louis, 1997, Mosby. pp. 598-608.
22. Lai A, Standish W, Standish H: The young athlete with physical challenges. *Clinics in sports medicine* 19(4): 793-819, 2000.
23. ACSM: *American College of Sports Medicine's Exercise Management for persons with chronic diseases and disabilities.* Champaign, 1977, Human Kinetics.
24. American Association on Mental Retardation: Guidelines to qualify as developmentally disabled. Available at www.aamr.org. Accessed November, 2004.
25. Biersdorff K: Incidence of significantly altered pain experience among individuals with developmental disabilities. *American Journal on Mental Retardation* 98(5):619-631, 1994.
26. Davis R, Ferrara M: Sports medicine and athletes with disabilities. In PePauw K, Gayron S, eds, *Disability and sport,* Champaign, 1995, Human Kinetics.

APPENDIX
A

Preparticipation Physical Evaluation

HISTORY FORM

DATE OF EXAM _____

Name _____ Sex _____ Age _____ Date of birth _____

Grade ____ School _____ Sport(s) _____

Address _____ Phone _____

Personal physician _____

In case of emergency, contact

Name _____ Relationship _____ Phone (H) _____ (W) _____

Explain "Yes" answers below.
Circle questions you don't know the answers to.

Yes No

1. Has a doctor ever denied or restricted your participation in sports for any reason? ☐ ☐
2. Do you have an ongoing medical condition (like diabetes or asthma)? ☐ ☐
3. Are you currently taking any prescription or nonprescription (over-the-counter) medicines or pills? ☐ ☐
4. Do you have allergies to medicines, pollens, foods, or stinging insects? ☐ ☐
5. Have you ever passed out or nearly passed out DURING exercise? ☐ ☐
6. Have you ever passed out or nearly passed out AFTER exercise? ☐ ☐
7. Have you ever had discomfort, pain, or pressure in your chest during exercise? ☐ ☐
8. Does your heart race or skip beats during exercise? ☐ ☐
9. Has a doctor ever told you that you have (check all that apply):
   ☐ High blood pressure ☐ A heart murmur
   ☐ High cholesterol ☐ A heart infection
10. Has a doctor ever ordered a test for your heart? (for example, ECG, echocardiogram) ☐ ☐
11. Has anyone in your family died for no apparent reason? ☐ ☐
12. Does anyone in your family have a heart problem? ☐ ☐
13. Has any family member or relative died of heart problems or of sudden death before age 50? ☐ ☐
14. Does anyone in your family have Marfan syndrome? ☐ ☐
15. Have you ever spent the night in a hospital? ☐ ☐
16. Have you ever had surgery? ☐ ☐
17. Have you ever had an injury, like a sprain, muscle or ligament tear, or tendinitis, that caused you to miss a practice or game? If yes, circle affected area below: ☐ ☐
18. Have you had any broken or fractured bones or dislocated joints? If yes, circle below: ☐ ☐
19. Have you had a bone or joint injury that required x-rays, MRI, CT, surgery, injections, rehabilitation, physical therapy, a brace, a cast, or crutches? If yes, circle below: ☐ ☐

Head	Neck	Shoulder	Upper arm	Elbow	Forearm	Hand/ fingers	Chest
Upper back	Lower back	Hip	Thigh	Knee	Calf/shin	Ankle	Foot/toes

20. Have you ever had a stress fracture? ☐ ☐
21. Have you ever been told that you have or have you had an x-ray for atlantoaxial (neck) instability? ☐ ☐
22. Do you regularly use a brace or assistive device? ☐ ☐
23. Has a doctor ever told you that you have asthma or allergies? ☐ ☐

Yes No

24. Do you cough, wheeze, or have difficulty breathing during or after exercise? ☐ ☐
25. Is there anyone in your family who has asthma? ☐ ☐
26. Have you ever used an inhaler or taken asthma medicine? ☐ ☐
27. Were you born without or are you missing a kidney, an eye, a testicle, or any other organ? ☐ ☐
28. Have you had infectious mononucleosis (mono) within the last month? ☐ ☐
29. Do you have any rashes, pressure sores, or other skin problems? ☐ ☐
30. Have you had a herpes skin infection? ☐ ☐
31. Have you ever had a head injury or concussion? ☐ ☐
32. Have you been hit in the head and been confused or lost your memory? ☐ ☐
33. Have you ever had a seizure? ☐ ☐
34. Do you have headaches with exercise? ☐ ☐
35. Have you ever had numbness, tingling, or weakness in your arms or legs after being hit or falling? ☐ ☐
36. Have you ever been unable to move your arms or legs after being hit or falling? ☐ ☐
37. When exercising in the heat, do you have severe muscle cramps or become ill? ☐ ☐
38. Has a doctor told you that you or someone in your family has sickle cell trait or sickle cell disease? ☐ ☐
39. Have you had any problems with your eyes or vision? ☐ ☐
40. Do you wear glasses or contact lenses? ☐ ☐
41. Do you wear protective eyewear, such as goggles or a face shield? ☐ ☐
42. Are you happy with your weight? ☐ ☐
43. Are you trying to gain or lose weight? ☐ ☐
44. Has anyone recommended you change your weight or eating habits? ☐ ☐
45. Do you limit or carefully control what you eat? ☐ ☐
46. Do you have any concerns that you would like to discuss with a doctor? ☐ ☐

FEMALES ONLY
47. Have you ever had a menstrual period? ☐ ☐
48. How old were you when you had your first menstrual period? _____
49. How many periods have you had in the last 12 months? _____

Explain "Yes" answers here: _____
_____
_____
_____
_____
_____
_____
_____

I hereby state that, to the best of my knowledge, my answers to the above questions are complete and correct.

Signature of athlete _____ Signature of parent/guardian _____ Date _____

APPENDIX
B

Common Medical Abbreviations

Abbreviation/Symbol	Interpretation
A	Assessment
abd	Abduction
ac	Before meals
AIIS	Anterior inferior iliac spine
AMA	Against medical advice
amb	Ambulation, ambulating, etc.
ant	Anterior
AP	Anterior-posterior
AROM	Active range of motion
ASA	Aspirin
ASAP	As soon as possible
ASIS	Anterior superior iliac spine
bid	Twice per day
bilat	Bilaterally
BM	Bowel movement
BP	Blood pressure
bpm	Beats per minute
CA	Cancer, carcinoma
cal	Calories
CBC	Complete blood count
CC, C/C	Chief complaint
cc	Cubic centimeter
CHF	Congestive heart failure
CNS	Central nervous system
c/o	Complains of
cont.	Continue
CP	Cerebral palsy
CPR	Cardiopulmonary resuscitation
CSF	Cerebrospinal fluid
CWI	Crutch walking instructions
DM	Diabetes mellitus
DTR	Deep tendon reflex
Dx	Diagnosis
ECG, EKG	Electrocardiogram
ED/ER	Emergency department/Emergency Room
EEG	Electroencephalogram
EENT	Ear, eyes, nose, throat
EMG	Electromyogram, electromyography
eval	Evaluation
ext.	Extension
F	Fair (muscular strength)

Abbreviation/Symbol	Interpretation
FBS	Fasting blood sugar
FH	Family history
flex	Flexion
ft	Foot, feet (measurement only)
FUO	Fever, unknown origin
FWB	Full weight bearing
fx	Fracture
G	Good (muscular strength)
GB	Gallbladder
GI	Gastrointestinal
gm	Gram
GYN	Gynecology
H & H, H/H	Hematocrit and hemoglobin
H & P	History and physical
HA, H/A	Headache
Hb, Hgb	Hemoglobin
HEENT	Head, ear, eyes, nose, throat
HIV	Human immunodeficiency virus
HR	Heart rate
hr.	hour
hs	At bedtime
ht.	height
Ht.	Hematocrit
Htn	Hypertension
Hx	History
ICU	Intensive care unit
IM	Intramuscular
imp.	Impression
in.	Inches
indep	Independent
inf	Inferior
IV	Intravenous
kcal	Kilocalories
kg	Kilogram
KUB	Kidney, ureter, bladder
L, l	Liter
Ⓛ	Left
lb.	Pound
LBP	Low back pain
LE	Lower extremity
LOC	Loss of consciousness

Continued

Abbreviation/Symbol	Interpretation
LP	Lumbar puncture
m	Meter
max	Maximal
Meds	Medications
MI	Myocardial infarction
min	Minimal
min.	Minutes
mm Hg	Millimeters of mercury
MMT	Manual muscle test
mo.	Month
mod	Moderate
MS	Multiple sclerosis
N	Normal (muscular strength)
neg.	Negative
noc	Night
NSR	Normal sinus rhythm
O:	Objective
OB	Obstetrics
od	Once daily
O.P.	Outpatient
O.R.	Operating room
oz.	ounce
P	Poor (muscular strength)
P:	Plan
P.A.	Physician's assistant
PA	Posterior-anterior
para	Paraplegia
pc	After meals
PEARL	Pupils, equal and reactive to light
per	By/through
per os, p.o.	By mouth
P.H.	Past history
pos.	Positive
poss	Possible
post-op	After surgery
pre-op	Before surgery
prn	Whenever necessary
PROM	Passive range of motion
Pt., pt.	Patient
PVD	Peripheral vascular disease
q	every
qd	Every day
qh	Every hour
qid	Four times per day
qn	Every night
qt.	quart
Ⓡ	Right

Abbreviation/Symbol	Interpretation
RA	Rheumatoid arthritis
RBC	Red blood cells
re:	Regarding
resp	Respiratory, respiration
R/O, r/o	Rule out
ROM	Range of motion
ROS	Review of systems
Rx	Treatment, prescription
SCI	Spinal cord injury
sig	Directions for use
SLE	Systemic lupus erythematosus
SOB	Shortness of breath
spec	Specimen
stat.	Immediately
Sx	Symptoms
T	Trace (muscular strength)
tab	Tablet
TB	Tuberculosis
TIA	Transient ischemic attack
tid	Three times per day
TNR	Tonic neck reflex
t.o.	Telephone order
TPR	Temperature, pulse, respiration
UA	Urine analysis
UMN	Upper motor neuron
URI	Upper respiratory infection
US	Ultrasound
UTI	Urinary tract infection
VD	Venereal disease
v.o.	Verbal order
v.s.	Vital signs
WBC	White blood cells
w/c	Wheelchair
wk.	Week
WNL	Within normal limits
y/o, y.o.	Years old
yr	Year
♂	Male
♀	Female
$\bar{s}$	Without
$\bar{c}$	With
$\bar{p}$	After
$\bar{a}$	Before
/	Per
↑	Increase
↓	Decrease

Data from Kettenbach G: *Writing SOAP notes*, ed 2, Philadelphia, 1995, FA Davis; Dirckx J, editor: *Stedman's concise medical dictionary for the health professions*, ed 3, Philadelphia, 1997, Williams & Wilkins; Anderson DM, chief lexicographer: *Dorland's illustrated medical dictionary*, ed 30, Philadelphia, 2003, WB Saunders.

Centimeter to Inches Conversion Chart

Inches*	Centimeters	Centimeters	Inches
1	2.54	1	0.4
2	5.08	2	0.8
4	10.16	3	1.2
6	15.24	4	1.6
8	20.32	5	2.0
10	25.40	6	2.4
20	50.80	8	3.1
30	76.20	10	3.9
40	101.60	20	7.9
50	127.00	30	11.8
60	152.40	40	15.7
70	177.80	50	19.7
80	203.20	60	23.6
90	228.60	70	27.6
100	254.00	80	31.5
150	381.00	90	35.4
200	508.00	100	39.4

From Seidel HM, Ball JW, Dains JE, Benedict GW: *Mosby's guide to physical examination*, ed 5, St Louis, 2003, Mosby, p 942.
*1 inch (in.) = 2.54 centimeters (cm); 1 centimeter (cm) = 0.3937 inch (in.).

Pounds to Kilograms Conversion Table

Pounds*	Kilograms	Kilograms	Pounds
1	0.5	1	2.2
2	0.9	2	4.4
4	1.8	3	6.6
6	2.7	4	8.8
8	3.6	5	11.0
10	4.5	6	13.2
20	9.1	8	17.6
30	13.6	10	22
40	18.2	20	44
50	22.7	30	66
60	27.3	40	88
70	31.8	50	110
80	36.4	60	132
90	40.9	70	154
100	45.4	80	176
150	66.2	90	198
200	90.8	100	220

From Seidel HM, Ball JW, Dains JE, Benedict GW: *Mosby's guide to physical examination*, ed 5, St Louis, 2003, Mosby, p 942.
*1 pound (lb) = 0.454 kilogram (kg); 1 kilogram (kg) = 2.204 pound (lb).

Body Mass Index Table

BMI	19	20	21	22	23	24	25	26	27	28	29	30	31	32	33	34	35
Height (Inches)								**Body Weight (Pounds)**									
58	91	96	100	105	110	115	119	124	129	134	138	143	148	153	158	162	167
59	94	99	104	109	114	119	124	128	133	138	143	148	153	158	163	168	173
60	97	102	107	112	118	123	128	133	138	143	148	153	158	163	168	174	179
61	100	106	111	116	122	127	132	137	143	148	153	158	164	169	174	180	185
62	104	109	115	120	126	131	136	142	147	153	158	164	169	175	180	186	191
63	107	113	118	124	130	135	141	146	152	158	163	169	175	180	186	191	197
64	110	116	122	128	134	140	145	151	157	163	169	174	180	186	192	197	204
65	114	120	126	132	138	144	150	156	162	168	174	180	186	192	198	204	210
66	118	124	130	136	142	148	155	161	167	173	179	186	192	198	204	210	216
67	121	127	134	140	146	153	159	166	172	178	185	191	198	204	211	217	223
68	125	131	138	144	151	158	164	171	177	184	190	197	203	210	216	223	230
69	128	135	142	149	155	162	169	176	182	189	196	203	209	216	223	230	236
70	132	139	146	153	160	167	174	181	188	195	202	209	216	222	229	236	243
71	136	143	150	157	165	172	179	186	193	200	208	215	222	229	236	243	250
72	140	147	154	162	169	177	184	191	199	206	213	221	228	235	242	250	258
73	144	151	159	166	174	182	189	197	204	212	219	227	235	242	250	257	265
74	148	155	163	171	179	186	194	202	210	218	225	233	241	249	256	264	272
75	152	160	168	176	184	192	200	208	216	224	232	240	248	256	264	272	279
76	156	164	172	180	189	197	205	213	221	230	238	246	254	263	271	279	287

BMI	36	37	38	39	40	41	42	43	44	45	46	47	48	49	50	51	52	53	54
58	172	177	181	186	191	196	201	205	210	215	220	224	229	234	239	244	248	253	258
59	178	183	188	193	198	203	208	212	217	222	227	232	237	242	247	252	257	262	267
60	184	189	194	199	204	209	215	220	225	230	235	240	245	250	255	261	266	271	276
61	190	195	201	206	211	217	222	227	232	238	243	248	254	259	264	269	275	280	285
62	196	202	207	213	218	224	229	235	240	246	251	256	262	267	273	278	284	289	295
63	203	208	214	220	225	231	237	242	248	254	259	265	270	278	282	287	293	299	304
64	209	215	221	227	232	238	244	250	256	262	267	273	279	285	291	296	302	308	314
65	216	222	228	234	240	246	252	258	264	270	276	282	288	294	300	306	312	318	324
66	223	229	235	241	247	253	260	266	272	278	284	291	297	303	309	315	322	328	334
67	230	236	242	249	255	261	268	274	280	287	293	299	306	312	319	325	331	338	344
68	236	243	249	256	262	269	276	282	289	295	302	308	315	322	328	335	341	348	354
69	243	250	257	263	270	277	284	291	297	304	311	318	324	331	338	345	351	358	365
70	250	257	264	271	278	285	292	299	306	313	320	327	334	341	348	355	362	369	376
71	257	265	272	279	286	293	301	308	315	322	329	338	343	351	358	365	372	379	386
72	265	272	279	287	294	302	309	316	324	331	338	346	353	361	368	375	383	390	397
73	272	280	288	295	302	310	318	325	333	340	348	355	363	371	378	386	393	401	408
74	280	287	295	303	311	319	326	334	342	350	358	365	373	381	389	396	404	412	420
75	287	295	303	311	319	327	335	343	351	359	367	375	383	391	399	407	415	423	431
76	295	304	312	320	328	336	344	353	361	369	377	385	394	402	410	418	426	435	443

From Jarvis, C: *Physical examination & health assessment*, ed 4, Philadelphia, 2004, Saunders, p. 863; source: National Institutes of Health: *The practical guide: identification, evaluation, and treatment of overweight and obesity in adults*, Washington, DC, 2000, NHLBI Obesity Education Initiative (monograph).

APPENDIX
F

Temperature Equivalents

Celsius*	Fahrenheit	Celsius	Fahrenheit
34.0	93.2	38.6	101.4
34.2	93.6	38.8	101.8
34.4	93.9	39.0	102.2
34.6	94.3	39.2	102.5
34.8	94.6	39.4	102.9
35.0	95.0	39.6	103.2
35.2	95.4	39.8	103.6
35.4	95.7	40.0	104.0
35.6	96.1	40.2	104.3
35.8	96.4	40.4	104.7
36.0	96.8	40.6	105.1
36.2	97.1	40.8	105.4
36.4	97.5	41.0	105.8
36.6	97.8	41.2	106.1
36.8	98.2	41.4	106.5
37.0	98.6	41.6	106.8
37.2	98.9	41.8	107.2
37.4	99.3	42.0	107.6
37.6	99.6	42.2	108.0
37.8	100.0	42.4	108.3
38.0	100.4	42.6	108.7
38.2	100.7	42.8	109.0
38.4	101.1	43.0	109.4

From Hoekelman RA, Friedman SB, Seidel HM, et al: *Primary pediatric care*, ed 3, St Louis, 1997, Mosby.

*To convert Celsius to Fahrenheit: $(9/5 \times$ temperature$) + 32$; to convert Fahrenheit to Celsius: $5/9 \times ($temperature $- 32)$.

NCAA Banned Drug Classes 2004-2005

The National Collegiate Athletic Association (NCAA) in the United States lists banned-drug classes that are subject to change by the NCAA Executive Committee. The current list is available from the NCAA education services or at the organization's website: www.ncaa.org/health-safety. The term related compounds comprises substances that are included in the class by their pharmacological action or chemical structure. No substance belonging to the prohibited class may be used, regardless of whether it is specifically listed as an example.

Many nutritional or dietary supplements contain NCAA banned substances. In addition, the U.S. Food and Drug Administration (FDA) does not strictly regulate the supplement industry; therefore purity and safety of nutritional or dietary supplements cannot be guaranteed. Impure supplements may lead to a positive NCAA drug test. The use of supplements is at the student-athlete's own risk. Student-athletes should contact their institution's team physician or athletic trainer for further information.

BANNED DRUGS

The following is the list of banned-drug classes, with examples of substances under each class:

Stimulants

Amiphenazole
Amphetamine
Bemigride
Benzphetamine
Bromantan
Caffeine* (guarana)
Chlorphentermine
Cocaine
Cropropamide
Crothetamide
Diethylpropion
Dimethylamphetamine
Doxapram
Ephedrine (ephedra, ma huang)
Ethamivan
Ethylamphetamine
Fencamfamine
Meclofenoxate
Methamphetamine
Methylenedioxy-methamphetamine (MDMA; ecstasy)
Methylphenidate
Nikethamide
Pemoline
Pentetrazol
Phendimetrazine
Phenmetrazine
Phentermine
Phenylephrine
Phenylpropanolamine (ppa)
Picrotoxine
Pipradol
Prolintane
Strychnine
Synephrine (citrus aurantium, zhi shi, bitter orange) and related compounds

Anabolic Agents

Anabolic steroids
Androstenediol
Androstenedione
Boldenone

Clenbuterol
Clostebol
Dehydrochlormethyl-testosterone
Dehydroepiandrosterone (DHEA)
Dihydrotestosterone (DHT)
Dromostanolone
Fluoxymesterone
Gestrinone
Mesterolone
Methandienone
Methenolone
Methyltestosterone
Nandrolone
Norandrostenediol
Norandrostenedione
Norethandrolone
Oxandrolone
Oxymesterone
Oxymetholone
Stanozolol
Testosterone[†]
Tetrahydrogestrinone (THG)
Trenbolone and related compounds

Substances Banned for Specific Sport (i.e., rifle)

Alcohol
Atenolol
Metoprolol
Nadolol
Pindolol
Propranolol
Timolol and related compounds

Diuretics

Acetazolamide
Bendroflumethiazide
Benzthiazide
Bumetanide
Chlorothiazide
Chlorthalidone

Ethacrynic acid
Flumethiazide
Furosemide
Hydrochlorothiazide
Hydroflumethiazide
Methyclothiazide
Metolazone
Polythiazide
Quinethazone
Spironolactone
Triamterene
Trichlormethiazide and related compounds

Street Drugs

Heroin
Marijuana[‡]
THC (tetrahydrocannabinol)[‡]

Peptide Hormones and Analogs

Chorionic gonadotropin (HCG [human chorionic gonadotropin])
Corticotropin (ACTH)
Growth hormone (HGH, somatotropin)
All the respective releasing factors of the above-mentioned substances also are banned.
Darbypoietin
Erythropoietin (EPO)
Sermorelin

Medical Exceptions

The NCAA recognizes that some banned substances are used for legitimate medical purposes. Accordingly, the NCAA allows exception to be made for those student-athletes with a documented medical history demonstrating the need for regular use of such a drug. Exceptions may be granted for substances included in the following classes of banned drugs: stimulants, beta-blockers, diuretics, and peptide hormones.

From National Collegiate Athletic Association: *The NCAA drug testing program 2004-2005 handbook*, pp 6-7, www.ncaa.org/health-safety.
Definitions of positive depend on the following:
*For caffeine—if the concentration in urine exceeds 15 mcg/ml.
[†]For testosterone—if the administration of testosterone or the use of any other manipulation has the result of increasing the ratio of the total concentration of testosterone to that of epitestosterone in the urine to greater than 6:1, unless there is evidence that this ratio is due to a physiological or pathological condition.
[‡]For marijuana and THC—if the concentration in the urine of THC metabolite exceeds 15 ng/ml.

GLOSSARY

Abdominal aortic aneurysm – Common type of aneurysm involving localized dilation of the abdominal aorta

Abscess – A collection of pus appearing in acute or chronic localized infections

Absorption – The process of getting drugs into the body through a variety of routes, including oral, rectal, vaginal, intravenous, intramuscular, inhalation, and topical application to the skin

Acne – Condition of the pilosebaceous unit consisting of inflammatory (red papules, pustules, or deep cysts) or noninflammatory (open and closed comedones) lesions

Acquired coagulopathies – Acquired conditions that affect the ability of the blood to coagulate (clot)

Actinic dermatitis – Inflammation of the skin resulting from exposure to sunlight or another irritating light source

Acute myelogenous lymphoma (AML) – Malignant growth of tissue characterized by a proliferation of granular leukocytes

Acute poststreptococcal glomerulonephritis – Kidney disorder brought about by certain group A streptococci

Adenoids – Pharyngeal tonsils

Adenoma – Benign tumor composed of epithelial cells

Adenomatous polyp – Tumor that develops in glandular tissue

Adenovirus – Medium-sized virus that can cause an upper respiratory infection as well as a gastrointestinal infection

Adnexal – Pertaining to accessory organs or tissues

Adventitious breath sounds – Abnormal breath sounds superimposed over normal breath sounds: crackles, rhonchi, wheezes, pleural friction rubs

Afebrile – Without a fever; apyretic

Afferent pupillary defect – Apparent dilation of the pupil of injured eye when light source is moved from normal eye to injured eye; indicates injury to the optic nerve

Agglutination – Clumping together of cells as a result of the interaction with specific antibodies called agglutinins

Agnosia – Impaired ability to recognize familiar sensory stimuli

Agonists – Drugs that exert their effect by attaching to cellular receptors in the body, causing stimulation of the receptor

Albinism – Disorder characterized by a lack of pigment in the iris and throughout the body

Allodynia – Condition in which normally nonpainful stimuli evoke pain

Alopecia areata – A disease causing well-defined bald patches in the scalp

Amblyopia – A condition resulting from no apparent pathology in which vision is reduced or dimmed; also known as lazy eye

Ambient temperatures – Encompassing prevailing temperatures

Amyloidosis – Metabolic disorder resulting from protein fibril deposits in tissue, which may eventually lead to organ failure

Anaphylactic shock – A severe and often fatal systemic allergic reaction

Anemia – A decrease in the hemoglobin in the blood that falls below the normal ranges of 12-16 g/dl in women and 13.5-18 g/dl in men resulting from a decrease in red blood cell production, an increase in red blood cell destruction, or loss of blood (see Chapter 1 for normal values)

Anesocoria – Unequal pupil sizes commonly associated with head trauma

Aneurysm – Fluid- or coagulated blood–filled sac resulting from dilatation or stretching of the wall of an artery, vein, or heart

Angina – Pain or pressure in the chest

Angioedema – A dermal or subcutaneous painless swelling of short duration often associated with hives

Angiotensin-converting enzyme (ACE) inhibitor – Drug that promotes vasodilation and decreases sodium and water retention, blood pressure, and heart size

Anhedonia – Inability to experience pleasure in acts that are typically pleasurable

Ankylosing spondylitis – Chronic inflammatory condition that may lead to fusions of affected joints; usually originates in the spine and progresses to other areas

Anorexia nervosa – Eating disorder that results in loss of weight, emaciation, intense fear of weight gain, and distorted body image; characterized by stringent diet restrictions, refusal to eat, or purging of ingested food

Anosmia – Ability to discern only the smell of ammonia

Antagonists – Drugs that exert their effect by binding to cellular receptors but do not cause stimulation of the receptor

Antiemetic agents – Medications used to alleviate symptoms of nausea or vomiting

Antiphospholipid antibodies – A condition of hypercoagulability and high blood levels of certain antibodies against phospholipids; typically associated with certain autoimmune diseases

Antipyretic – A medication to reduce fever

Aortic regurgitation – Flow of blood during systole back into the left ventricle from the aorta

Aortic stenosis – Narrowing of the aortic valve

Aphasia – Neurological condition resulting in impaired speech

Apical systolic murmurs – Heart sound heard at the apex of the heart marked by pulsation of the left ventricle; palpable at 5th intercostals space

Aplastic anemia – Deficiency of all the formed elements of blood; may represent a failure of the cell-generating capacity of bone marrow

Apnea – Absence of spontaneous respiration

Appendicitis – Inflammation of the vermiform appendix

Apraxia – Loss of motor coordination

Arboviruses – Group of viruses largely from bats, rodents, and arthropods

Arnold-Chiari malformation – Herniation of the brain stem into the vertebral canal

Arrhythmogenic right ventricular dysplasia (ARVD) – A rare, genetic cardiomyopathy characterized by the muscles of the right ventricle being replaced by fat and fibrosis, which causes abnormal heart rhythms; a leading cause of sudden death in young athletes

Arteriography – Radiographic examination of arteries injected with a radiopaque dye

Asherman's syndrome – Secondary amenorrhea in a hormonally normal woman caused by obliteration of endometrial cavity by adhesions

Asymmetrical tonic neck reflex (ATNR) – Pathologic reflex associated with cerebral palsy marked by the upper extremity assuming an on-guard position when the neck is rotated or laterally flexed; causes obligatory extension of the arm on the face side and flexion of the arm on the nonface side

Ataxia – Lack of muscle coordination during gait

Atherosclerotic coronary artery disease – Thickening and hardening of the arterial wall marked by cholesterol-lipid-calcium deposits

Athetosis – Condition characterized by snakelike movements of the upper extremity commonly seen in cerebral palsy patients

Athlete's heart – Term used to refer to many of the physiologic and morphologic adaptations that an athlete's cardiovascular system may undergo as a result of chronic exercise training

Atrioventricular (AV) block – Prolonged, intermittent absent conductions of impulses that occur between the atria and ventricles

Attention deficit hyperactive disorder (ADHD) – Neurobehavioral condition that impairs the person's ability to maintain attention

Audiometry – The measurement of auditory acuity at various frequencies of sound waves

Auscultation – A technique used to listen to the sounds of the heart, lungs, blood vessels, and other internal organs; most commonly done using a stethoscope

Autoinoculation – Introduction of a substance into the body (inoculate) from a lesion on one's own body, causing a secondary infection

Autonomic dysreflexia (AD) – Hyperreflexia found in patients who have sustained a spinal cord injury above the major sympathetic nervous system outflow tract

Azotemia – Excess of urea or other nitrogenous bodies in the blood indicative of renal failure; characterized by fatigue, malaise, and loss of appetite

Bacterial vaginosis – Chronic inflammation of the vagina caused by a bacterium

Bactericidal – Antibiotic that causes bacterial cell death

Bacteriostatic – Antibiotic that inhibits further replication of bacteria but does not cause cell death

Bacteriuria – Presence of bacteria in the urine

Balanitis – Inflammation of the glans penis

Bell clapper deformity – Failure of normal posterior anchoring of the epididymis and testis that allows the testes to swing freely in the tunica vaginalis of the scrotum

Benzodiazepines – Psychotropic medication used to alleviate anxiety

Beta-blocker – Drug used to block the response to norepinephrine bound to alpha-adrenergic receptors to reduce the smooth muscle tone in peripheral blood vessels, causing an increase in peripheral circulation and a decrease in blood pressure

Bifed – Split into two parts

Biguanide – Oral antihyperglycemic agent that regulates control of glucose absorption and production

Biliary colic – Smooth muscle or visceral pain associated with the passing of stones in the bile ducts

Bioequivalence – When two drugs have similar effects on the body

Biopsy – The removal and examination of tissue from a living body

Biopsychosocial–spiritual model (BPSS) – Framework for understanding an individual's response in a given situation

Bipolar disorder – Mental disorder marked by episodes of mania and depression

Bisferiens pulse – Arterial pulse that has two peaks

Bleb – Accumulation of fluid under the skin

Blepharospasm – Squeezing of the eyelid

Boosting – Purposeful self-induced autonomic dysreflexia to gain an advantage over other disabled athletes; potentially life threatening

Bouchard's nodes – Bony or cartilaginous nodes that form in the proximal interphalangeal joint as a result of degenerative arthritis

Bradycardia – A resting heart rate of 60 beats/min or less

Bradypnea – Abnormally low rate of breathing

BRCA 1 – Symbol for breast cancer gene

Broca's aphasia – Condition characterized by intact comprehension with inability to express speech; also known as expressive aphasia

Bronchial breath sounds – Predominately expiratory sound that is loud and high pitched

Bronchophony – Increased intensity and clarity of vocal resonance due to increased density of lung tissue

Bronchovesicular – Pertaining to the bronchi, bronchioles, and alveoli

Brudzinksi's sign – When the neck is actively flexed, eliciting pain due to the elongation of the spinal cord; useful for detecting meningitis

Bruit – Abnormal swishing sound or murmur heard during auscultation of carotid artery

Buerger's disease – Vascular condition in which the small- and medium-sized arteries become inflamed and thrombotic, especially in the lower extremity

Bulbar conjunctiva – Conjunctiva overlying the sclera

Bulimia nervosa – Eating disorder characterized by repeated incidences of binge eating and self-induced vomiting or diarrhea, or excessive exercise

Bulla – Blister of skin greater than 1 cm containing serous fluid

Caisson's disease – Formation of nitrogen gas bubbles within the tissue of those who move too quickly from high to low atmospheric pressures (divers); these gases may accumulate in joint spaces and cause severe pain; also known as decompression sickness

Candidiasis – Infection caused by *Candida* characterized by white exudates; commonly found in the mouth, vagina, or skin folds

Carbuncle – A collection of several coalescing faruncles or boils

Cardiac dilatation – Enlargement of the heart caused by stretching of a weak blood vessel or myocardium

Cardioangiography – Technique used to produce radiographs of the heart by injecting a radiopaque contrast into the heart

Cataract – Clouding of the lens of the eye

Cauda equina – Lumbar and sacral roots of the spinal cord

Causalgia – Severe sensation of burning pain as a result of nerve injury

Cellulitis – Inflammation of the soft or connective tissue in which a thin, watery exudates spreads through the interstitial spaces; may lead to ulceration and abscesses

Cerebellar peduncles – Three large bundles of nerve fibers conducting information between the brain and spinal cord

Cerebral palsy (CP) – Chronic neurological disorder that affects movement and posture; caused by a lesion in the brain

Cerebral spinal fluid (CSF) – The fluid that protects the four ventricles of the brain, the subarachnoid space, and the spinal canal; is generated in the choroid plexus

Cerebrovascular accident (CVA) – Condition due to the lack of oxygen to the brain that may lead to reversible or irreversible paralysis often caused by interrupted blood flow to the brain; also known as a stroke

Cerumen – The waxlike substance normally found in the external canal of the ear; earwax

Chancroid – Highly contagious sexually transmitted disease caused by an infection with the bacillus *Haemophilus ducreyi*

Cheerleader's nodules – Laryngitis caused by excessive use of the voice

Chemoprophylaxis – Antimicrobial medication that prevents the spread of pathogens from one area of the body to another

Cheyne-Stokes respiration – Breathing pattern characterized by periods of apnea

Chlamydia – Bacterial infection that is one of the most common sexually transmitted diseases

Chlamydia trachomatis – Infection characterized by ulcerative genital lesions, swelling of the lymph nodes in the groin, headache, fever, and malaise

Choanae – The posterior openings in the nasal cavity that connect the nasal cavity with the nasopharynx, allowing the inhalation and expiration of air

Cholecystitis – Acute or chronic inflammation of the gallbladder

Cholelithiasis – Gallstones

Cholinergic – Agent that stimulates the elaboration of acetylcholine at the myoneural junction

Choriocapillaris – Vascular tissue between the retina and the sclera

Chronic fatigue syndrome (CFS) – Disabling illness, the primary symptom of which is persistent severe fatigue; is often accompanied by musculoskeletal, immunologic, and neurological complaints such as headache; may result from a virus, infection, or immune system malfunction

Chronic lymphocytic leukemia (CLL) – Tissue growth characterized by proliferation of lymphocytes in bone marrow, blood, and liver

Chronic myeloid leukemia (CML) – Marked by unrestrained overgrowth of granulocytes in the bone marrow and associated with chromosomal abnormality, also known as chronic granulocytic leukemia

Chronic obstructive pulmonary disease (COPD) – Condition characterized by decreased capacity of inspiratory and expiratory function of the lungs

Claudication – Cramping pains in the calves due to poor circulation of blood to the muscles in the leg

Clonic contractions/seizures – Rhythmic involuntary contraction and relaxation of muscles

Closed comedones – Lesion caused by an accumulation of keratin and sebum within the opening of a hair follicle; also known as *whiteheads*

Colchicine – A gout suppressant

Colostrum – Fluid secreted by the breast during pregnancy and shortly after birth

Commotio cordis – Trauma to the chest wall that results in a disruption of the electrical impulses of the heart; may be fatal

Comorbid – Two or more medical conditions that exist at the same time and may be unrelated

Complex regional pain syndrome (CRPS) – Overactivity of the sympathetic nervous system that incorporates signs and symptoms of both RSD and causalgia

Congenital aortic valve stenosis (AS) – Condition characterized by impaired left ventricular outflow with compensatory hypertrophy of the interventricular septum and left ventricular free wall, most commonly caused by bicuspid valve formation

Congestive heart failure (CHF) – Condition marked by impaired cardiac pumping due to cardiomyopathy, ischemia, or myocardial infarction

Conjunctivitis – Inflammation of the vascular tissue covering the anterior sclera and posterior surface of the eyelids; commonly caused by bacteria, allergies, or viral infection

Constitutional – Relating to the body as a whole

Contact dermatitis – Inflammation of the skin caused by direct contact with a specific allergen

Contraindication – Situation in which a drug or treatment should be avoided

Contrast venography – Radiographic examination of veins injected with a radiopaque dye

Crackles – Adventitious sounds that occur as a result of disruption of airflow in smaller airways, usually by fluid; also known as rales

CREST syndrome – When **C**alcinosis, **R**aynaud's phenomenon, **E**sophageal dysfunction, **S**clerodactyly, and **T**elangiectasis occur together; this is a progressive systemic condition

Cribiform plate – A perforated structure in the posterior portion of the ethmoid bone

Crohn's disease – Chronic inflammatory bowel disease that usually affects the small intestines

Croup – Acute viral infection of upper and lower respiratory tract

Cryptorchidism – Developmental defect in which one or both testes fail to descend into the scrotum and are retained in the abdomen or inguinal canal

Cushing's syndrome – Metabolic disorder characterized by excessive production of cortisol by the adrenal cortex or by administering large doses of glucocorticoids

Cyclothymia – Fluctuating depression typified by periods of elevated and depressed mood

Cystoscopy – Direct visualization of the urinary tract by means of a cystoscope inserted into the urethra

Decubitus ulcer – Pressure sore

Deep vein thrombosis (DVT) – A blood clot that becomes lodged in a large vein

Déjà vu – The illusion of having previously experienced something encountered for the first time

Dermatitis – General inflammation of the skin

Dermatographia – Wheals resulting from tracing on the skin with a blunt object or fingernail

Dermatographism – Hives induced by rubbing or stroking the skin or rubbing the skin with clothing

Dermatophyte – A fungus that causes a parasitic skin disease

Diabetes insipidus – A metabolic disorder marked by copious urine output and excessive thirst; is caused by deficient production or response to antidiuretic hormone (ADH)

Diabetes mellitus – Disease where the body is unable to produce or use insulin effectively; type I is characterized by the body's inability to produce insulin, whereas type II is characterized by the body's inability to use insulin effectively

Diabetic ketoacidosis (DKA) – Diabetic coma that is a life-threatening condition in uncontrolled diabetes mellitus

Diaphoresis – Sweating

Diethylstilbestrol (DES) – Synthetic hormone with estrogenic properties

Dilation – Stretching or dilating

Diplopia – Condition in which the patient sees two of a single object; also known as *double vision*

Dissolution – Separation of a complex chemical compound into simpler molecules

Distribution – The process of getting drugs delivered throughout the tissues and fluids of the body

Diverticulitis – Inflammation of the diverticula, especially in the colon, due to fecal material penetrating the wall lining of diverticula

Down syndrome – Most common cause of intellectual disability; an autosomal chromosomal disorder characterized by a sloping forehead, low-set ears, and short broad hands with a single palmar crease

Ductal carcinoma in situ – Cancer of the cells lining the milk ducts of the breast

Dysarthria – Impaired speech as a result of impairment of the tongue, injury to the peripheral or central motor nerve critical to speech, or because of emotional stress

Dysautonomic cephalgia – Headache that occurs with trauma to the anterior triangle of the neck injuring the sympathetic nerve fibers close to the carotid artery

Dysdiadochokinesis – Inability to perform rapidly alternating movements

Dyshidrosis – Any disorder of the sweat glands

Dysmenorrhea – Abnormally painful or irregular menstruation

Dysmetria – Impairment of muscle coordination and action

Dyspareunia – Painful intercourse

Dysphagia – Difficulty swallowing

Dyspnea – Difficulty in breathing, labored or shortness of breath; causes include certain heart conditions, strenuous exercise, or anxiety

Dysuria – Painful urination

Eczema – Dermatitis that may be pruritic or erythematous and that may later become crusted and scaly

Egophony – Altered voice sound in a patient with pleural effusion

Ehlers Danlos syndrome – Connective tissue disorder that is hereditary; characterized by increased mobility of joints and hyperplasticity of skin

Electrocardiogram (ECG, EKG) – Graphic record produced by a device that records the electrical activity of the heart

Electrocardiography – Study of electrical activity generated by the heart muscle

Electrophoresis – Movement of charged suspended particles through a liquid medium as a result of change in the surrounding electrical field

Elimination – Process of getting a drug out of the body

Emphysema – Abnormal condition of pulmonary system characterized by over inflation and destructive changes in the alveolar wall

Empiric therapy – Treatment of an infection not on the basis of culture results but on the basis of the knowledge of which organisms are the most common cause of the particular infection being treated

Encephalitis – Inflammation of the brain; often caused by an arbovirus infection transmitted by the bite of an infected mosquito

Endocarditis – Inflammation of the endocardium and the heart valves

Endoscopy – Procedure that uses an illuminating optic instrument to view the inside of a body cavity or organ

Enophthalmos – Recession of the eyeball deeper into the orbit

Enterovirus – A virus spread through direct contact with respiratory secretions

Epilepsy – Chronic condition consisting of unprovoked, randomly recurring seizures

Epiphysiolysis – Separation of the enlarged proximal or distal end of a long bone

Epistaxis – Bleeding from the nose, caused by inflammation or irritation of the mucous membranes; also known as nosebleed

Equilibrium – A state of balance resulting from the equal action of opposing forces

Erythea migrans – Red, circular rash that appears in early stages of Lyme disease

Erythema – Redness or inflammation of the skin or mucous membrane resulting from dilation of the superficial capillaries

Eustachian tube – A mucous membrane–lined tube that joins the nasopharynx and the middle ear cavity and that is opened during yawning, chewing, and swallowing to allow for equalization of air pressure

Exophthalmos – Bulging out of the eyes commonly seen in patients with hyperthyroidism

Exudates – Fluid or other substances that have slowly been released through small pores or breaks in the cell membranes

Exudative – Oozing of fluid from cells or tissues as a result of injury or inflammation

Factor V Leiden anticoagulant gene mutation – Genetic disorder characterized by blood clotting dysfunction resulting from an unstable procoagulant needed to convert prothrombin into thrombin

Faun's beard – Small patch of hair present on the lower back, which may be indicative of spina bifida occulta

Febrile – Having a fever

Felty's syndrome – Usually occurring with rheumatoid arthritis, a condition that results in a collection of pathological changes such as splenomegaly, infections, and anemia

Fibroadenoma – Benign tumor composed of dense epithelial and fibroblastic tissue

Fibromyalgia – Chronic, noninflammatory, diffuse pain syndrome characterized by multiple areas of musculoskeletal pain, sleep disturbances, fatigue, and depression

Flaccid – Loss of tone

Folliculitis – Bacterial skin infection that causes an inflammatory reaction in the hair follicle

Fornices – Most posterior portions of the upper and lower conjunctiva where the bulbar and palpebral conjunctiva join

Frenulum – A thin mucous membrane which connects the underside of the tongue to the floor of the mouth

Furuncle – Bacterial skin infection that is a walled-off abscess containing pus; also known as a boil

Gastritis – Diffuse inflammation of the lining of the stomach

Gastroesophageal reflux disease (GERD) – Condition in which stomach acid travels up through the lower esophageal sphincter into the esophagus or even into the back of the throat

Gastroenteritis – Inflammatory condition of the stomach and intestines that is usually caused by a bacteria or virus

Gaucher's disease – Disorder that alters fat metabolism as a result of enzyme deficiency; may result in splenomegaly, hepatomegaly, and bone marrow lesions

Generalized anxiety disorder (GAD) – Disorder marked by worry over or nervousness about many or most things in life

Gingivae – The gum tissue of the mouth that encircles the necks of the teeth

Gingivitis – An inflammation of the gingivae in which the margins close to the teeth are red, swollen, and bleeding

Glaucoma – Group of eye diseases characterized by increased intraocular pressure

Glomerulonephritis – Nephritis with inflammation in the renal glomeruli capillary loops; may follow group A streptococci infection

Gonorrhea – Sexually transmitted disease that affects the epithelium of the pharynx, eyes, urethra, cervix, and rectum; presents with yellow-green urethral discharge in males and vaginal discharge in females

Graves' disease – Hyperthyroidism caused by an autoimmune attack on the thyroid

Guillain-Barré syndrome (GBS) – Acute, diffuse demyelinating disorder of the spinal roots and peripheral nerves characterized by bilateral muscle weakness or even paralysis initiating in the legs

Gustatory hallucinations – False sense of taste of food or drink

Hairy leukoplakia – White plaque found on the lateral borders of the tongue that may be folded or smooth in appearance; associated with severe immunodeficiency

Hamilton Anxiety Scale (HAMA) – Scale developed to quantify the severity of the signs and symptoms of anxiety

Hashimoto's thyroiditis – Inflammatory condition of the thyroid gland that is the most frequent cause of goiter and is characterized by a lymphocytic infiltration of the thyroid gland

Heberden's nodes – Bony or cartilaginous nodes that form in the distal interphalangeal joint as a result of degenerative arthritis

Heliotrope rash – Rash that is exacerbated by exposure to the sun

Hematoma – Accumulation of blood in an organ, space, or tissue

Hematuria – Abnormal presence of blood in the urine

Hemoglobinuria – Abnormal presence in the urine of hemoglobin that is not attached to red blood cells

Hemolysis – Breakdown of red blood cells and the release of hemoglobin

Hemoptysis – Productive cough of sputum that may contain blood

Hepatomegaly – Enlarged liver

Herpes gladiatorum – Herpes simplex virus that occurs on the face and the trunk and is characterized by flu-like symptoms and vesicles on an erythematous base

Herpes keratoconjunctivitis – Herpes simplex virus that infects the cornea of the eye; may lead to corneal scarring or even blindness

Herpes zoster (i.e., shingles) – An acute infection primarily found in adults when the latent varicella zoster virus (VZV) is reactivated; virus presents with painful vesicular skin eruptions, which follow the underlying route of spinal nerves that are inflamed by the virus

Hidradenitis suppurativa – A chronic suppurative disease of the sweat glands; causes occlusion of the pores and bacterial infection in the apocrine sweat glands

Hirsutism – Presence of excessive body hair in a masculine distribution pattern as a result of hereditary, hormonal dysfunction or medication

Hodgkin's lymphoma – Malignant disorder of lymphoreticular origin, characterized histologically by the presence of Reed-Sternberg cells (multinucleated giant cells)

Holter monitor – A device used to record prolonged electrical activity of the heart on a tape recorder while the patient performs activities of daily living

Homocystinuria – Abnormal presence of homocystine in the blood and urine caused by enzyme deficiencies

Horner's syndrome – Neurological condition characterized by constricted pupils, drooping of the eyelid, and facial anhidrosis resulting from a spinal cord lesion

Human papillomavirus (HPV) – Virus that is the common cause of warts on the hands and feet, as well as lesions of the mucous membrane of the oral, anal, and genital cavities

Hydrocele – Fluid collection within the tunica vaginalis of the scrotum or along the spermatic cord

Hydrocephalus – Accumulation of cerebrospinal fluid within the ventricles of the brain

Hydronephrosis – Distention of the kidneys and calyces of kidney by urine that cannot flow past an obstruction in the ureter

Hydrophilicity – Water solubility

Hyperandrogenism – Excessive production of androgen in women

Hyperanhydrosis – Increased sweating

Hyperemia – An increase in blood flow to a body part characterized by reddening of the skin

Hyperhidrosis – Endocrine disorder characterized by elevated levels of insulin

Hyperlipidemia – Presence of excess lipids in the plasm

Hyperopia – Farsightedness, in which individuals can see objects in the distance clearly, whereas objects closer are out of focus

Hyperoxaluria – Excessive level of oxalic acid and oxalates in the urine, which may lead to the formation of renal calculi or renal failure

Hyperparathyroidism – Condition characterized by increased activity of the parathyroid glands, with excessive secretion of the parathyroid hormone; causes increased resorption of calcium from the skeletal system and increased absorption of calcium by the kidneys

Hyperpnea – Rapid breathing with very large breaths; >24 breaths/min

Hyperthyroidism – Hyperactivity of the thyroid gland due to excessive levels of thyroid hormone in the body

Hypertrophic cardiomyopathy – Condition characterized by abnormally hypertrophied left ventricle in the absence of physiological conditions; leading cause of sudden death in the United States of athletes under the age of 35

Hyperuricemia – Excessive amount of uric acid in the blood

Hyperuricosuria – Excess of uric acid or urates in the urine

Hyphema – Blood in the anterior chamber of the eye

Hypocitraturia – Abnormally low concentration of citrate in the urine

Hypogonadism – Absent or decreased gonadal function resulting from absence of gonadal stimulating pituitary hormones FSH and LH

Hypomagnesemia – Abnormally low concentration of magnesium in the urine

Hypopnea – Shallow, slow breaths

Hypotonia – Loss of muscle tone

Hysteroscopy – Direct visual inspection of the cervix and uterine cavity through a hysteroscope

Iatrogenic – An adverse physical or mental reaction as a result of receiving treatment

Immunosuppressed, immunocompromised – A weakened immune system

Impetigo – Highly contagious bacterial infection characterized by a yellow or honey-colored crusted lesion on an erythematous base

Incontinence – Inability to restrain from urinary or bowel evacuation

Indication – Condition for which the drug has been found to have a therapeutic effect

Indirect laryngoscopy – Inspection of the larynx with the use of a mirror

Infectious mononucleosis – Disease caused by the Epstein-Barr virus; associated with symptoms of fatigue, pharyngitis, fever, and lymphadenopathy; also known as the kissing disease

Infectious myringitis – A contagious bacterial condition characterized by the development of painful vesicles on the eardrum

Intellectual disability – Disability characterized by significant limitations both in intellectual functioning and in adaptive behavior

Intravenous pyelogram (IVP) – Radiographic picture of the kidneys and ureter taken after intravenous administration of radiopaque contrast medium

Irritable bowel syndrome (IBS) – Disorder of gastrointestinal motility with abnormal cycles of muscle contraction and relaxation

Jamais vu – The sensation of being a stranger when accompanied by someone known or of feeling like a stranger in a familiar place

Junctional rhythm – Cardiac rhythm originating at the junction of the A-V node and A-V bundle

Juxtaarticular – Beside a joint

Kaposi's sarcoma – Malignant neoplasm characterized by purple or brown papules that can metastasize to lymph nodes or other organs

Kawasaki's disease – Rare, inflammatory condition of unknown origin characterized by an acute febrile illness of young children with lymphadenopathy that may lead to complications such as coronary artery aneurysms with resulting stenosis of the coronary artery; also known as mucocutaneous lymph node syndrome (MLNS)

Keratinous cyst – An epithelial cyst containing the fibrous component of epidermis, nails, and hair

Kernig's sign – A test that is typically a component of Brudzinski's sign; it involves flexion of one knee and hip to 90 degrees while maintaining cervical flexion; may be indicative of meningitis

Kiesselbachs plexus – An area of small fragile arteries and veins located in the nasal septum; the root of most nose bleeds

KOH stain – Potassium hydroxide used to prepare specimens for microscopic examination for fungi

Korotkoff sounds – A series of sounds produced by distention of an artery by the blood pressure cuff; the level at which the sound disappears is the diastolic pressure, often referred to as the fifth or last Korotkoff sound

Kussmaul breathing – Deep, rapid sighing breaths characterized by diabetic ketoacidosis

Kyphosis – Increased posterior curvature of the thoracic spine

Labial commissure – Juncture of the mouth and lip

Lactic acidosis – Condition characterized by an accumulation of lactic acid in the blood, resulting in lowered pH in the muscle and serum

Lagophthalmos – Inability to close the eyelids completely, usually as a result of a severe subconjunctival hemorrhage

Lanugo – Fine, downy hair covering

Laparoscopy – Surgical use of an instrument that relies on an illuminating optical to examine the abdominal cavity through one or two small incisions in the abdominal wall

Laryngitis – Inflammation of the larynx

Lavage – Washout or irrigate

Legg-Calvè-Perthes disease – Avascular necrosis that occurs in children ages 3-12, causing osteochondritis of the femoral epiphysis

Legionnaire's disease – Acute bacterial pneumonia characterized by flu-like symptoms

Leptomeninges – Thin, delicate meninges of the pia and arachnoid mater

Lesion – A defined area of pathological, altered tissue; a wound; or single infected area in a skin disorder

Leucopenia – An abnormal decrease in white blood cells (WBCs) to fewer than 5000/cu

Leukemia – Group of malignant diseases characterized by diffuse replacement of bone marrow with proliferating leukocyte precursors

Leukocyte count – Number of white blood cells in relation to the total blood count

Leukocytosis – Increased circulation of white blood cells

Lhermitte's phenomenon – Sudden electric-like shock radiating down the body when the neck is flexed; commonly associated with multiple sclerosis or cervical pathology

Lichen simplex chronicus – A patch of pruritic papules

Lipophilicity – Fat solubility

Lobular carcinoma in situ – Benign growth change in some of the cells lining the very ends of milk ducts in the breast

Long QT syndrome – Cardiac disorder marked by a long QT interval, which is characterized by syncopal episodes during physical activity

Lyme disease – Tick-borne illness that is a multisystem disorder; if left untreated can lead to serious arthritic and neurological symptoms

Lymphadenopathy – A disorder characterized by enlarged lymph nodes

Lymphocytosis – Increased circulation of lymphocytes as a result of chronic disease

Lymphogranuloma venereum – Sexually transmitted disease caused by bacterium

Lymphoreticular – Tissues of the lymph and reticuloendothelial system, which primarily fights against infection and phagocytosis; all considered as one system

Lymphosarcoma – A tumor arising from the lymph system

Macules – A small discoloration or blemish that is level with the skin, such as freckles and some rashes

Maculopapular rash – Skin disruption characterized by distinctive macules or papules

Malaise – A general feeling of discomfort or uneasiness; often the first symptom of an illness or infection

Malleus – One of the three ossicles in the middle ear; connected to the tympanic membrane; transmits sound vibrations

Marfan syndrome – Autosomal dominant, hereditary disorder of the connective tissue that is associated with abnormalities of the cardiovascular, musculoskeletal, and ocular systems

Mastication – The process of chewing

Measles – An acute and very contagious viral infection of the respiratory tract characterized by a cutaneous rash

Melanoma – Skin disorder defined as any group of malignant neoplasms that originate in the skin

Meningitis – Inflammation or infection of the membranes and fluids surrounding the brain and spinal cord; usually caused by bacteria or a virus

Meningoencephalitis – Inflammation of both the brain and meninges; caused by a bacterial infection

Meningomyelocele – Most common type of spina bifida, also known as myelomeingocele

Metabolism – Complex process by which a drug is changed into one or more chemical entities that differ from the parent drug

Metastatic, metastasize – When cancerous cells from one tumor are found in another region or organ of the body

Mikulicz's syndrome – Bilateral enlargement of the salivary and lacrimal glands often seen in leukemia, tuberculosis, or sarcoidosis

Mitral regurgitation – Backflow of blood from the left ventricle into the left atrium during systole; occurs across a diseased mitral valve

Mitral valve prolapse (MVP) – Protrusion of one or both cusps of the mitral valve back into the left atrium during systole

Mittelschmerz – Abdominal pain in the region of the ovary during ovulation

Molluscum contagiosum – Disease of the skin and mucous membranes caused by the poxvirus; characterized by scattered, smooth, flesh-toned or white dome-shaped papules with a central point

Morbidity – Consequences of a given illness

Mortality – Death from a particular illness or disease

Mucolytic agent – Agent that destroys or dissolves

Mucolytics – Anything that destroys or dissolves the mucous membranes

Multiple sclerosis – Neurodegenerative, life-long chronic disease characterized by the gradual accumulation of focal plaques of demyelination in the brain

Mumps – Contagious viral infection that manifests with enlarged parotid glands and, sometimes, enlarged sublingual or submaxillary glands

Murphy's sign – Sudden stop of inspiration upon deep palpation over the liver when the patient takes a deep breath; may be a result of gallstones

Myasthenia gravis – Motor disorder characterized by muscular fatigue that develops with repetitive muscle use and improves with rest; caused by the presence of antibodies on the acetylcholine receptor in the neuromuscular junction, which results in a decreased number of receptor sites for acetylcholine

Mycoplasma – Ultramicroscopic organism that lacks a rigid cell wall

Mydriatics – Drops that cause the pupils to dilate

Myocardial bridging – A condition whereby the coronary artery is surrounded by the myocardium for part of its course

Myocardial ischemia – Insufficient blood flow to the heart muscle via the coronary arteries

Myocarditis – Inflammation of the myocardium

Myocyte – Muscle cell

Myopia – When individuals can see objects up close clearly, but objects in the distance are out of focus; also known as nearsightedness

Nares – The pair of openings in the front and back of the nasal cavity allowing the passage of air to the pharynx

Nasopharynx – The uppermost portion of the three regions of the throat (pharynx), extending from the posterior nares to the level of the soft palate

Nebulizer – Machines that use compressed air to cause aerosolization of a liquid drug, which is then inhaled through a mask or a mouthpiece

Necropsy – Postmortem examination to determine cause of death

Necrotic arachnidism – The condition that results when a brown recluse spider deposits venom within a host that leads to tissue necrosis

Necrotizing fascitis – Streptococcal gangrene, also known as flesh-eating bacteria

Neoplastic disease – A disease characterized by abnormal tissue growing more rapidly than normal cells; can be either benign or malignant

Neurocardiogenic syncope (vasovagal) – Sudden loss of consciousness resulting from cerebral ischemia secondary to decreased cardiac output, peripheral vasodilation, and bradycardia

Neuroendocrine axis – Pertaining to the effects of the endocrine glands that are linked with the nervous system

Neutropenia – Decrease of neutrophils, a white blood cell, in the blood

Nodes of Ranvier – Gaps between the Schwann cells that expose unmyelinated axons

Nongonococcal urethritis (NGU) – Also known as nonspecific urethritis (NSU), a catch-all term for sexually transmitted disease characterized by dysuria, frequent need to void, and discharge

Non-Hodgkin's lymphoma – Heterogenous group of malignancies of lymphoreticular system

Nonsuppurative – The absence of discharge or pus

Nonunion – Fracture site that fails to heal properly after a minimum of nine months

Nuchal rigidity – Resistance to cervical flexion; associated with meningitis

Nystagmus – Involuntary lateral fluttering of the eye that can be an indicator of brain injury

Obersteiner-Redlich zone – Junction between the CNS and PNS

Obsessive-compulsive disorder (OCD) – Anxiety disorder characterized by persistent behaviors that markedly impair the functioning of an individual

Oligomenorrhea – Abnormally light menstruation or reduction in menstruation

Oncologist – A medical doctor who specializes in cancer research and treatment

Onychia – Inflammation of the nail bed

Oophoritis – Inflammation of one or both of the ovaries

Open comedones – Lesions characterized by an accumulation of keratin and sebum within the opening of a hair follicle; also known as blackheads

Open globe – Eyeball that has been ruptured following blunt trauma, allowing leakage of intraocular fluid or extrusion of intraocular tissue

Optic neuritis – Inflammation of the optic nerve, in which loss of vision is the primary symptom

Orbital emphysema – Crunchy sensation under the skin associated with an orbital fracture; results from air from the sinuses that is trapped under the skin

Orchiectomy – Removal of one or both testes

Orchitis – Inflammation of one or both testes

Orthopnea – Shortness of breath while lying down

Orthostatic hypotension – Fall in systolic blood pressure of 20 mm Hg or more associated with changes in body position; accompanied by symptoms such as light-headedness or fainting

Orthostatic syncope – Low blood pressure that occurs when an individual rises to a standing position and that produces a sudden loss of consciousness

Ossicular chain – The body parts necessary for hearing, including an intact tympanic membrane and inner ear ossicles (malleus, incus, and stapes)

Osteochondrosis – Condition that affects the ossification centers in the bone

Otalgia – Pain in the ear

Otolaryngologist – A physician who specializes in the treatment and evaluation of the ears, nose, and throat

Otorrhea – Any discharge from the external ear

Oxygenation – Exchange of gases in the alveolar-capillary beds

Paget's disease – Nonmetabolic disorder of bone of unknown origin; characterized by excessive bone destruction and unorganized bone repair

Palliative therapy – Therapy designed to reduce intensity relieve symptoms and support the patient; does not produce a cure

Palpebral conjunctiva – Conjunctiva lining the eyelids

Palpitations – Heart rhythm irregularities

Panic disorder – Anxiety disorder marked by an acute period of intense fear or anxiety

Papillomatosis – A condition characterized by the presence of widespread nipple-like growths

Paraplegia – Lesion below T1 that affects the lower extremities; individual will have use of the upper extremities and may or may not have trunk control and sitting balance

Parenchyma – Functional tissue or cells of an organ

Paronychia – Infection of the fold of the skin at the margin of the nail

Parotitis – Inflammation of one or both parotid salivary glands

Paroxysmal nocturnal dyspnea – Disorder characterized by sudden attacks of respiratory distress that awaken an individual after a few hours of sleeping in a reclining position

Patency – A state of being open or exposed

Pectus carinatum – Pigeon chest

Pectus excavatum – Chest depression

Pediculosis – Infection of lice on the body, head, or pubic region; characterized by intense itching and presence of nits

Pelvic inflammatory disease (PID) – Inflammation of the female pelvic organs; caused by a bacterial infection

Peptic ulcer disease (PUD) – Ulcer found in the stomach or duodenum

Pericarditis – Inflammation of the lining enclosing the heart and the base of the great vessels

Periodontist – A dentist who specializes in the treatment and evaluation of the supporting structures of the teeth

Periodontitis – An inflammation or infection of the supporting structures of the teeth

Peripheral arterial disease (PAD) – Systemic form of atherosclerosis producing symptoms in the cardiac, cerebral, and renal vascular systems

Perirenal fat – Layer of fat surrounding the outer fibrous capsules that enclose each kidney

Pertussis – Highly contagious respiratory disease characterized by a cough that often ends in a whooping inspiration; usually caused by gram-negative coccobacillus; also known as whooping cough

Petechiae – Purple or red spots appearing on the skin as a result of hemorrhage within the dermal or submucosal layer

Phantom pain syndrome – Pain that seems to come from an amputated body part; more prevalent in adults than in children

Pharmacodynamics – Study of the actions of a drug on the body, including mechanism of action and medicinal effect

Pharmacokinetics – Study of how the body acts on a drug, including the absorption, distribution, metabolism, and elimination of the drug

Pheochromocytoma – Tumor derived from neural crest cells of the sympathetic nervous system

Photophobia – Pain when light is shined into the eye

Photopsia – Sensation of flashes of light

Pilonidal cyst – A cyst in the sacral region of the body

Pleural rubs – Sounds that occur outside the respiratory tree and result from friction between visceral and parietal pleura

Pleurisy – Inflammation of the lining of the lungs

Pneumothorax – Presence of air or gas in the pleural space causing the lung to collapse

Poliomyelitis – Form of paralysis caused by a viral infection that affects the motor cells of the spinal cord

Polycystic ovarian disease – Endocrine disturbance characterized by anovulation, amenorrhea, hirsutism, and infertility

Polycythemia – An increased number of erythrocytes in the blood; may be caused by primary or secondary pulmonary disease, heart disease, or long-term exposure to high altitude

Polydipsia – Increased thirst

Polymenorrhea – A condition in which the menstrual cycle is abnormally recurrent; more than one cycle per month

Polymyositis – Inflammation of multiple muscles; characterized by pain, edema, tension, and insomnia

Polyp – A small tumor-like growth on a mucous membrane surface

Polyphagia – Persistent hunger

Polyuria – Increased urination

Posterior vitreous detachment (PVD) – When vitreous liquefies and peels away from the retina, resulting in "floaters" in the field of vision

Postphlebitic syndrome – Condition occurring weeks or months after a DVT that is characterized by pain, redness, thickening, and a glossy appearance of the skin

Posttraumatic stress disorder (PTSD) – Psychiatric disorder in response to a traumatic event resulting in intense psychological distress

Potassium hydroxide (KOH) – Preparation used for microscopic examination to diagnose eczema

Poultice – A form of moist heat and other compounds, powders, herbs, or medications applied to an area to produce counter irritation

Preauricular lymphadenopathy – Small tender lymph node located just in the front of the tragus of the ear and commonly associated with conjunctivitis

Premature atrial complex (PAC) – Atrial depolarization that occurs earlier than expected as a result of atrial enlargement or ischemia; may lead to atrial fibrillation

Premature ventricular complex (PVC) – Ventricular depolarization that occurs earlier than expected as a possible result of stress, ischemia, or electrolyte imbalances

Presbycusis – Hearing loss due to aging

Presbyopia – Loss of flexibility of the crystalline lens inside the eye, resulting in inability to focus on near objects

Prodromal – Early symptoms that indicate the onset of a disease

Proptosis – Downward or forward displacement of the eyeball as a result of swelling; also referred to as exophthalmos

Prostatic calculi – Solid calcification formed in the prostate

Prostatic tuberculosis – Descending infection in which prostatic tuberculous cavities and abscesses may rupture into surrounding tissues, resulting in sinuses and fistulae to the perineum or rectum

Prostate-specific antigen (PSA) – Blood test used to detect prostate cancer and monitor patient's response to cancer

Prothrombin time (PT) – Test used to time clot formation; can detect defects in the ability of the plasma to coagulate, which are usually caused by a deficiency of Factor V, VII, or X (normal time: 11-12.5 seconds)

Pruritic, pruritus – Itching

Psoriasis – Chronic skin disorder marked by scaly red patches on the skin; due to excessive growth of epithelial cells

Psychotropic medications – Medications that alter the psychic function or behavior of an individual

Pulmonary embolus (PE) – An obstruction that occurs when a blood clot becomes lodged in one of the pulmonary vessels; may be fatal if the clot is not dissolved in time

Purulent – Containing or producing pus

Pyelonephritis – Pyogenic infection of the pelvis and parenchyma of kidney characterized by fever, chills, pain in the flank, and nausea

Pyuria – Increased number of white blood cells in the urine; may indicate a urinary tract infection

Radiofrequency ablation – Use of high-frequency, unmodulated alternating current to destroy damaged or ineffective tissue

Radiofrequency catheter ablation – Application of unmodulated high-frequency alternating current flow to the heart tissue to raise its temperature and injure cells to destroy accessory pathways

Raynaud's disease, Raynaud's phenomenon – Intermittent attacks of ischemia of the extremities of the body, especially the fingers, toes, ears, and nose; caused by exposure to cold or by emotional stimuli

Reed-Sternberg cells – Multinucleated giant cells

Reflex sympathetic dystrophy (RSD) – Injury to the afferent pathway resulting in diffuse, persistent pain and limited joint mobility

Reiter's disease – Arthritic disorder primarily found in males; associated with infection or enterocolitis

Renin-angiotensin system – System that regulates sodium balance, fluid volume, and blood pressure by renal secretions

Retinopathy – Inflammatory eye disorders resulting from diseases such as diabetes, hypertension, or vascular disorders

Retractions – Visible sinking in of the soft tissue of the chest

Reye's syndrome – Acute encephalopathy and fatty infiltration of internal organs after acute viral infections such as varicella, influenza B, or the Epstein-Barr virus

Rhabdomyolysis – Paroxysmal, potentially fatal disease of skeletal muscle characterized by the presence of myoglobin in the urine

Rhinitis – Inflammation of the mucous membranes of the nose, typically accompanied by swelling of the mucosa and nasal discharge

Rhinoplasty – A procedure in which the structure of the nose is altered by plastic surgery

Rhinorrhea – Thin watery discharge from the nose, or flowing of cerebrospinal fluid from the nose following injury to the head

Rhinovirus – Ribonucleic acid virus that causes acute respiratory illness

Rhonci – Low-pitched, sonorous wheezes

Rubella – Contagious virus acquired through the upper respiratory tract or through placental blood exchange; associated with a low-grade fever, rash, and lymphadenopathy; also known as German measles

Rubeola – One of the most highly communicable diseases; associated with a erythematous rash and fever; also known as *measles*

Saccadic eye movement – Rapid movement of the eye between points of fixation

Salpingitis – Infection or inflammation of the fallopian tube

Sarcoidosis – Chronic disorder characterized by tubercle formation of nonnecrotizing epitheloid tissue

Scabies – Parasitic infection caused by a mite; usually spread by direct or sexual contact or by sharing infested clothing or bedding; marked by intense itching on the body, especially the wrists, fingers, and ankles

Scarlet fever – An acutely contagious strain of group A hemolytic *Streptococcus*; characterized by sore throat, fever, enlarged lymph nodes in the neck, prostration, and a diffuse bright red rash

Schmorl's nodes – Bone necrosis detectible on a radiograph, associated with Scheumann's disease

Scleroderma – Chronic hardening or thickening of the skin as a result of collagen formation

Scotoma – Blindspot in a visual field

Seasonal affective disorder (SAD) – Mood disorder characterized by lethargy and depression due to shorter exposure to light and longer exposure to darkness during the fall and winter

Sebaceous gland – One of the small sacculated organs in the dermis; the glands are located throughout the body, primarily in close association with areas abundant in hair follicles, such as the scalp and nose, as well as the face, mouth, and anus

Seborrhea – Any skin condition characterized by an overproduction of sebum resulting in excessive oiliness or dry scales

Seminoma – Malignant tumor of the testes

Sequela, sequelae – A condition (conditions) occurring as a consequence of a given illness or disease

Sheehan's syndrome – Hypopituitarism resulting from death or disease of the pituitary

Sickle cell anemia – Chronic, hemolytic anemia caused by a genetic defect in the hemoglobin most commonly found in African-Americans; characterized by decreased red blood cell survival, microvascular occlusions due to RBC sickling, and increased susceptibility to certain infections

Sideroblastic anemia – Normocytic or slightly macrocytic anemia characterized by hypochromic and normochromic red blood cells and a decrease in erythropoiesis and hemoglobin synthesis

Sinusitis – Acute or chronic inflammation of the sinus with or without purulent drainage

Slit lamp – An instrument that uses a high-intensity light source that can be focused to shine as a slit to examine the structures that are at the front of the eye for any existing pathologies

Spasticity – Condition associated with lesions above L1 in which spasms are caused by excessive reflex activity below the lesion level and appear as a sudden, involuntary jerk of the body

Splenomegaly – Abnormally enlarged spleen

Spina bifida – Congenital spinal cord disability in which the neural tube fails to close completely during the first four to six weeks of fetal development, resulting in bladder and bowel dysfunction, spasms, and skin lesions

Status epilepticus – Continuous tonic-clonic seizures

Stensen's duct – A canal approximately 7 cm long, extending from the anterior portion of the parotid gland to the mouth

Stevens-Johnson syndrome – Severe form of erythema multiforme caused by a dermatologic reaction to antibiotics; characterized by malaise, headache, fever, and arthralgia

Stridor – High-pitched sound caused by obstruction in the larynx or trachea

Subconjunctival hemorrhage – Bright, red blood appearing in a sector of the eye under the clear conjunctiva and in front of the white sclera; caused by a broken blood vessel

Sudeck's atrophy – A visual defect in a defined area of the visual field of one or both eyes

Sulfonylureas – Oral antidiabetic agent that stimulates the pancreas to produce insulin

Supportive – Nonpharmacological management of an illness including rest and administration of fluids

Suppurative – Forming pus; purulent

Symmetrical tonic neck reflex (STNR) – Pathological reflex marked by bilateral arm and leg responses to up and down head movements; associated with cerebral palsy

Syncope – A brief loss of consciousness, typically caused by lack of oxygen to the brain; fainting

Syphilis – Sexually transmitted disease caused by a spirochete; characterized by small, painless red pustules that erode to form chancres

Systemic lupus erythematosus (SLE) – Chronic autoimmune disorder affecting the musculoskeletal, skin, renal, cardiac, and nervous system; characterized by joint pain and swelling, a butterfly rash over the malar eminence of the face, and nephritis

Tachycardia – A resting heart rate of 100 beats/min or greater

Tachypnea – Rapid breathing; >24 breaths/min

Tactile fremitus – Palpable vibration generated from the larynx and transmitted through the bronchi and lungs to the chest wall

Tension pneumothorax – Air in the pleural space caused by a rupture through the chest wall

Tetraplegia (formerly called quadriplegia) – Condition associated with a complete lesion above T1 in which all four limbs are affected, with corresponding lack of trunk control or sitting balance

Thalassemia – Hemolytic anemia characterized by microcytic, hypochromic, and short-lived red blood cells; caused by deficient synthesis of hemoglobin polypeptide chains

Thermograph, thermography – Infrared detector that reacts to blood flow and is used to detect hot and cold areas of the body

Thoracentesis – Surgical procedure that perforates the chest wall or pleural space to aspirate fluid for diagnosis or treatment purposes

Thrombocytopenia – A reduction of the number of platelets in the blood

Thrombophlebitis – Inflammation of a vein accompanied by the formation of a clot

Thrush – Yeast infection found in the tissues of the mouth

Tinea corporis – Common fungal infection characterized by scaly, erythematous lesions on the skin; also known as ringworm

Tinea versicolor – Common yeast infection that is not contagious; characterized by multiple, small, round, scaly macules that enlarge radially

Tinnitus – The sensation of ringing in the ears

Todd's paresis – Postepileptic hemiplegia that may last anywhere from a few seconds to days after a seizure

Tonic labyrinthine reflex prone (TLR-prone) – Pathological reflex marked by an increased flexor tone elicited by a change in position of the head; associated with cerebral palsy

Tonic-clonic contractions/seizures – An epileptic seizure marked by involuntary muscular contraction and apnea, followed by clonic and tonic (prolonged contraction) contractions and resumption of breathing

Torsade de pointes – Ventricular tachycardia with spiral-like appearance and complexes that look positive, then negative on electrocardiogram

Traumatic iritis – Inflammation of the iris secondary to blunt trauma

Traumatic mydriasis – Condition in which one pupil is dilated; usually associated with traumatic iritis

Trichomoniasis – Vaginal infection caused by *Trichomonas vaginalis;* characterized by itching, burning, and frothy, pale yellow to green, malodorous vaginal discharge

Trigeminal neuralgia – Neurological condition of the trigeminal nerve resulting in sharp pain radiating along the course of the nerve

Tuberculosis – Chronic granulomatous infection transmitted by inhalation or ingestion of infected droplets that usually affect the lungs

Turner's syndrome – Rare chromosomal disorder of females characterized by short stature and the lack of sexual development at puberty

Tympanogram – A test providing graphic representation of the acoustic impedance and air pressure in the middle ear, as well as the mobility of the tympanic membrane

Ulcerative colitis – Chronic inflammatory disease of the colon and large intestine characterized by watery diarrhea

Universal precautions – Guidelines for the treatment of all human waste as infectious materials with emphasize on the need to protect all health care workers and patients in every situation in which body fluid is exposed; mucous membranes in the eyes, mouth, or nose, genital secretions, or blood are examples of body fluids that may be infectious; any sharp object that may be contaminated with infectious waste, such as needles, scalpels, or broken glass, is also considered potentially hazardous material

Upper GI series – Radiographic or fluoroscopic evaluation of the upper gastrointestinal tract after ingestion of a barium sulfate solution

Uterine synechiae – Gradual decrease in menstrual flow, increased cramping and abdominal pain, eventual cessation of menstrual cycles (amenorrhea), and infertility due to inflammation of the uterus and formation of adhesions

Varicella (i.e., Chicken pox) – Highly contagious infection spread by respiratory droplets or direct contact; marked by a low grade fever, headache, malaise, and a vesicular rash that begins on the trunk and spreads

Varicocele – Dilatation of the pampiniform venous plexus and the internal spermatic vein within the scrotum

Ventilation – Process whereby air moves through the respiratory tract

Ventilation-perfusion scan – Radiographic examination of the lungs performed while the patient inhales a radioactive gas as a contrast medium; the lungs are scanned to detect nonfunctional or impaired areas

Vesicular breath sounds – Normal sound of rustling or swishing that represents air that moves into smaller airways

Vitiligo – A benign skin condition with irregular patches lacking pigment

Wernicke's aphasia – Aphasia impairing the ability to comprehend written and oral communication

Western blot – A blood test to detect presence of antibodies or antigens

Wheezes – Adventitious breath sounds that represents airway obstruction either from mucus, spasm, or even a foreign body

Whispered pectoriloquy – Whispered speech heard clearly through the stethoscope

Wolff-Parkinson-White syndrome – Condition manifested by ventricular preexcitation and tachycardia as the result of electrical conduction over accessory pathways

Wood's lamp – An ultraviolet lamp that emits electromagnetic radiation in the range of 4 to 400 nm

Zung Self-Rating Depression Scale – A 20-item instrument for use with patients being evaluated for depression

Note: Page numbers followed by *f* indicate figures; page numbers followed by *t* indicate tables; page numbers followed by *b* indicate boxes.